IMMUNOLOGY

THIRD EDITION

A slide atlas of Immunology, based on the contents of this book, is available. In the slide atlas format, the material is split into six volumes, each of which is presented in a binder together with numbered 35mm slides of each illustration. Each slide atlas volume also includes lists of abbreviated slide captions for easy reference when using the slides. Further information can be obtained from:

Mosby–Year Book Europe Ltd
Lynton House
7–12 Tavistock Square
London WC1H 9LB
England

IMMUNOLOGY

THIRD EDITION

Ivan M Roitt MA DSc(Oxon) Hon MRCP(Lond) FRCPath FRS
Emeritus Professor of Immunology
Director of the Institute of Biomedical Science
University College London Medical School
London, UK

Jonathan Brostoff MA DM(Oxon) DSc FRCP FRCPath
Reader in Clinical Immunology
Department of Immunology
University College London Medical School
London, UK

David K. Male MA PhD
Senior Lecturer in Neuroimmunology
Department of Neuropathology
Institute of Psychiatry
London, UK

Editorial Consultant
Linda Gamlin BSc(Hons) MSc

M Mosby

St. Louis Baltimore Boston Chicago London Philadelphia Sydney Toronto

The cover picture shows a diagrammatic representation of the pentameric polypeptide structure of human IgM (see page 4.5).

Publisher:	Fiona Foley
Project Manager:	Stephen McGrath
Design:	Pete Wilder Balvir Koura
Illustration:	Dereck Johnson
Production:	Susan Bishop
Index:	Nina Boyd

Text set in Garamond; captions set in Univers.
Originated in Hong Kong By Mandarin Offset (HK) Ltd.
Printed in Hong Kong.
Produced by Mandarin Offset (HK) Ltd.

Cataloguing in Publication data:
Catalogue records for this book are available from the US Library of Congress and the British Library.

ISBN 0-397-44765-5

Preface

There is no shortage of immunology textbooks on the booksellers' shelves, but this book stands out through its deliberate, free and unashamed use of lucid, colourful and visually appealing diagrams to focus and explain the main textual points and concepts. That this strategy has been so successful, explains the need for this third edition to bring the reader up to date with the compelling new discoveries being made in this exciting field. Aside from the changes in content driven by the great expansion in knowledge since the last edition, we have made some alterations to the chapters, such as a merger of chapters dealing with antibodies, T-cell receptors and major histocompatibility complex into one covering *Antigen Receptor Molecules*, and an amalgamation of the chapters on *Genetic Control of Immunity* and *Regulation of the Immune Response*. It was also clear that the striking importance of AIDS research warranted a separate chapter for *Immunodeficiency*, the same being true for *Cell Migration and Inflammation*.

With just a few changes, we have virtually the same powerful line-up of authors who produced such an impact in earlier editions, but to cope with the inevitable inconsistencies of style which are bound to creep in on a multi-author work, we have had the benefit of a professional scientific journalist, Linda Gamlin, who has tried to harmonize the contributions and generate a feeling of continuity without damaging the writing style of the individual authors. In so far as presentation is concerned, we have altered the format of the legends, to delineate their separation from the text itself more positively than hitherto. Furthermore, the artworks themselves have been redrawn. Immunology is a big and explosive subject with many ramifications, but it is our earnest hope that the style of presentation will bring pleasure and comprehension to our many readers at the undergraduate, graduate and clinical stages of their careers.

Ivan M Roitt
Jonathan Brostoff
David K Male

User Guide

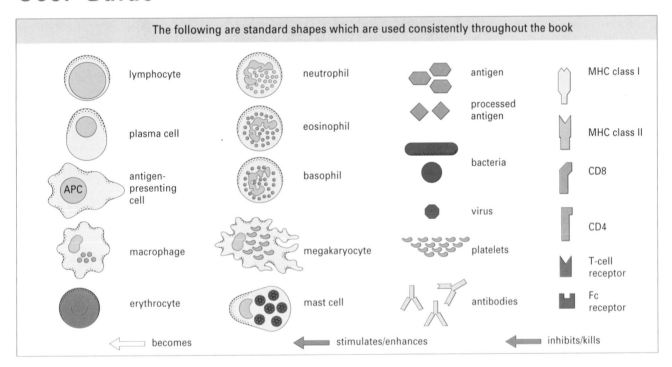

The following are standard shapes which are used consistently throughout the book

lymphocyte — neutrophil — antigen — MHC class I

plasma cell — eosinophil — processed antigen — MHC class II

antigen-presenting cell (APC) — basophil — bacteria — CD8

macrophage — megakaryocyte — virus — CD4

erythrocyte — mast cell — platelets — T-cell receptor

antibodies — Fc receptor

becomes — stimulates/enhances — inhibits/kills

Acknowledgements

The editors have a particular debt of gratitude to the Project Manager, Stephen McGrath, who guided the edition securely through its gestation. We also wish to extend our warmest thanks to Dereck Johnson, Pete Wilder, Balvir Koura, Susan Bishop and Nina Boyd for their invaluable contributions. It is a pleasure to acknowledge the vital support given by the publisher, Fiona Foley.

Contents

6. ANTIGEN RECOGNITION

Dr Michael Owen and Professor Michael Steward

7. CELL COOPERATION IN THE ANTIBODY RESPONSE

Professor Marc Feldmann

8. CELL-MEDIATED IMMUNE REACTIONS

Dr Graham Rook

9. REGULATION OF THE IMMUNE RESPONSE

Dr Anne Cooke

15. IMMUNITY TO VIRUSES, BACTERIA AND FUNGI

Dr Graham Rook

16. IMMUNITY TO PROTOZOA AND WORMS

Dr Janice Taverne

17. TUMOUR IMMUNOLOGY

Professor Peter Beverley

23. TRANSPLANTATION AND REJECTION

Professor Ian Hutchinson

24. AUTOIMMUNITY AND AUTOIMMUNE DISEASE

Professor Ivan Roitt

25. IMMUNOLOGICAL TECHNIQUES

Professor Michael Steward and Dr David Male

Appendices

Glossary
Index

Contributors

Professor Ross StC Barnetson
Department of Dermatology
University of Sydney
NSW 2006, Australia

Professor Peter C L Beverley
Department of Oncology
Courtauld Institute of Biochemistry
London, UK

Dr Jonathan Brostoff
Department of Immunology
University College London Medical School
London, UK

Dr Anne Cooke
Immunology Division
Department of Pathology
University of Cambridge
Cambridge, UK

Professor Marc Feldman
Charing Cross Sunley Research Centre
Charing Cross Hospital
London, UK

Dr David J Gawkrodger
University Department of Dermatology
Royal Hallamshire Hospital
Sheffield, UK

Professor Carlo Enrico Grossi
Department of Human Anatomy
University of Genoa
Genoa, Italy

Dr Tony Hall
Ciba-Geigy AG
CH-4002 Basel
Switzerland

Professor Frank C Hay
Division of Immunology
St George's Hospital Medical School
London, UK

Dr John Horton
Department of Biological Science
University of Durham
Durham, UK

Profesor Ian V Hutchinson
Department of Cell and Structural Biology
University of Manchester School of Biological Sciences
Manchester, UK

Dr Peter Lydyard
Department of Immunology
University College London Medical School
London, UK

Dr Jaques F A P Miller
Experimental Pathology Unit
Walter and Eliza Hall Institute of Medical Research
Melbourne
NSW 3050, Australia

Dr David K Male
Department of Neuropathology
Institute of Psychiatry
London, UK

Dr Michael J Owen
Lymphocyte Molecular Biology Laboratory
Imperial Cancer Research Fund
London, UK

Professor Norman Ratcliffe
School of Biological Science
University College of Swansea
Swansea, UK

Professor Ivan M Roitt
Institute of Biomedical Science
University College London Medical School
London, UK

Professor Fred S Rosen
The Center of Blood Research
Harvard University Medical School
Boston, USA

Dr Graham Rook
School of Pathology
University College London Medical School
London, UK

Professor Michael Steward
Department of Immunology
London School of Hygiene and Tropical Medicine
London, UK

Dr Janice Taverne
Department of Immunology
University College London Medical School
London, UK

Dr Malcom W Turner
Hugh Greenwood Department of Immunology
Institute of Child Health
University of London
London, UK

Dr Mark J Walport
Royal Postgraduate Medical School
Hammersmith Hospital
London, UK

chapter 1

Introduction to the Immune System

Our environment contains a great variety of infectious microbes – viruses, bacteria, fungi, protozoa and multi-cellular parasites. These can cause disease, and if they multiply unchecked they will eventually kill their host. Most infections in normal individuals are short-lived and leave little permanent damage. This is due to the immune system, which combats infectious agents.

Since microorganisms come in many different forms, a wide variety of immune responses are required to deal with each type of infection. In the first instance, the exterior defences of the body present an effective barrier to most organisms, and very few infectious agents can penetrate intact skin (Fig. 1.1). However, many gain access across the epithelia of the gastro-intestinal or urogenital tracts. Others can infect the nasopharynx and lung. A small number, such as malaria and hepatitis B, can only infect the body if they enter the blood directly.

The site of the infection, and the type of pathogen, largely determine which immune responses will be effective. The most important distinction is between those which invade the host's cells and those which do not. All viruses, some bacteria and some protozoan parasites replicate inside host cells, and to clear an infection, the immune system must recognize and destroy these infected cells. Many bacteria and larger parasites live in tissues, body fluids or other extracellular spaces, and the responses to these pathogens are quite different. During the course of an infection, however, viruses and other intracellular pathogens must reach their target cells by moving through the blood and tissue fluid. At this time they are susceptible to elements of the immune system which normally counter extracellular pathogens (see Fig. 1.2).

This chapter introduces the basic elements of the immune system and of immune responses, which are detailed in Chapters 2–16. There are various ways in which the immune system can fail, leading to immunopathological reactions, and these are outlined in the second half of the book. However, it is important to stress that the primary function of the immune system is to eliminate infectious agents and to minimize the damage they cause.

ADAPTIVE AND INNATE IMMUNITY

Any immune response involves, firstly, recognition of the pathogen or other foreign material, and secondly, mounting a reaction against it, to eliminate it. Broadly speaking, the different types of immune response fall into two categories: innate (or non-adaptive) responses, and adaptive immune responses. The important difference between these is that an adaptive immune response is highly specific for a particular pathogen. Moreover, the response improves with each successive encounter with the same pathogen: in effect the adaptive immune system 'remembers' the infectious agent and can prevent it from causing disease later. For example, diseases such as measles and diphtheria induce adaptive immune responses which generate a lifelong immunity following an infection. The two key features of the adaptive immune response are thus specificity and memory.

Immune responses are produced primarily by leuco-cytes, of which there are several different types. One important group of leucocytes are the phagocytic cells, such as the monocytes, macrophages and polymor-phonuclear neutrophils. They bind to microorganisms, internalize them and destroy them. Since they use prim-itive non-specific recognition systems, which allow them to bind to a variety of microbial products, they are mediating innate immune responses. In effect they act as a first line of defence against infection.

Exterior defences

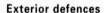

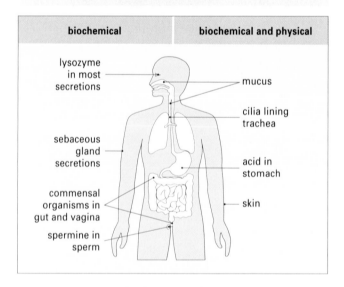

Fig. 1.1 Most of the infectious agents which an individual encounters do not penetrate the body surface, but are prevented from entering by a variety of biochemical and physical barriers. The body tolerates a number of commensal organisms which compete effectively with many potential pathogens.

Another important set of leucocytes are the lymphocytes. These cells are central to all adaptive immune responses, since they specifically recognize individual pathogens, whether they are inside host cells or outside in the tissue fluids or blood. In fact there are several different types of lymphocyte, but they fall into two basic categories – T lymphocytes (or T cells) and B lymphocytes (or B cells). B cells combat extracellular pathogens and their products by releasing antibody, a molecule which specifically recognizes and binds to a particular target molecule, called the antigen. The antigen may be a molecule on the surface of a pathogen, or a toxin which it produces. T lymphocytes have a wider range of activities. Some are involved in the control of B lymphocyte development and antibody production. Another group of T cells interacts with phagocytic cells to help them destroy pathogens they have taken up. A third set of T lymphocytes recognizes cells infected by virus and destroys them.

In practice there is a considerable amount of interaction between the lymphocytes and phagocytes. For example, some phagocytes can take up antigens and show them to T lymphocytes in a form they can recognize, a process which is called antigen presentation. In turn the T lymphocytes release soluble factors (cytokines), which activate the phagocytes and cause them to destroy the pathogens they have internalized. In another interaction phagocytes use antibodies released by B lymphocytes to allow them to recognize pathogens more effectively (Fig. 1.3). One consequence of these interactions, is that most immune responses to infectious organisms are made up of a variety of innate and adaptive components. In the earliest stages of infection, innate responses predominate, but later the lymphocytes start to generate adaptive immune responses. They then remember the pathogen, and mount more effective and rapid responses should the individual become reinfected with that agent.

Intracellular and extracellular pathogens

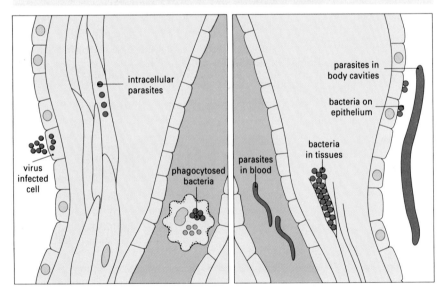

intracellular parasites

virus infected cell

phagocytosed bacteria

parasites in blood

parasites in body cavities

bacteria on epithelium

bacteria in tissues

Fig. 1.2 The immune system must recognize and react against pathogens in a number of different locations. For example, viruses must invade cells to reproduce, while protozoa such as *Plasmodium* species (malaria) and *Trypanosoma cruzi* (Chagas' disease), and bacteria such as *Salmonella typhi* all have intracellular phases (left). Some protozoan parasites (e.g. African trypanosomes) live in the blood, while many large multicellular parasites live in tissues or organs (e.g. tapeworms). Many bacteria colonize epithelial surfaces and may invade the host to multiply in tissues.

Interaction between lymphocytes and phagocytes

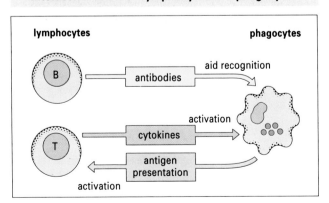

lymphocytes

phagocytes

B

antibodies

aid recognition

T

cytokines

activation

antigen presentation

activation

Fig. 1.3 B lymphocytes release antibodies which bind to pathogens and their products and so aid recognition by phagocytes. Cytokines released by T cells activate the phagocytes to destroy the material they have taken up. In turn, mononuclear phagocytes can present antigen to T cells to activate them.

CELLS OF THE IMMUNE SYSTEM

Immune responses are mediated by a variety of cells, and by the soluble molecules which they secrete. Although the leucocytes are central to all immune responses, other cells in the tissues also participate, by signalling to the lymphocytes and responding to the cytokines released by T lymphocytes and macrophages. Figure 1.4 lists the main cells and molecules involved in immune reactions.

Components of the immune system

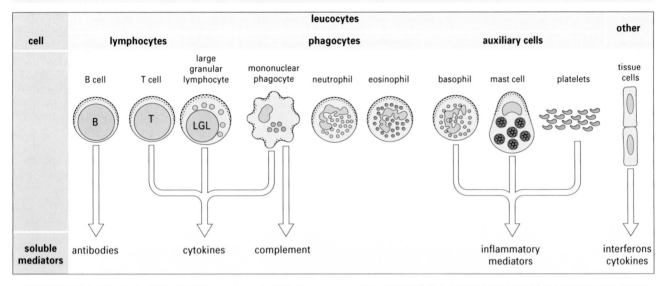

Fig. 1.4 The principle components of the immune system are listed, indicating which cells produce which soluble mediators. Complement is made primarily by the liver, with some synthesis by mononuclear phagocytes. Note that each cell only produces a particular set of cytokines, mediators etc.

Phagocytes of the monocyte/macrophage series

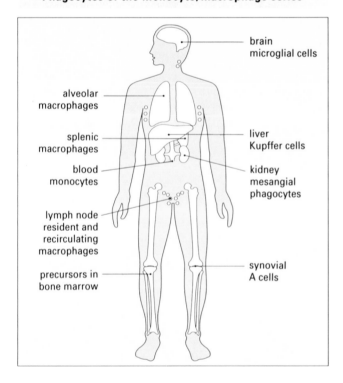

PHAGOCYTES

The most important group of long-lived phagocytic cells belong to the mononuclear phagocyte lineage. These cells are all derived from bone marrow stem cells, and their function is to engulf particles, including infectious agents, internalize them and destroy them. For this purpose they are strategically placed where they will encounter such particles. For example, the Kupffer cells of the liver line the sinusoids along which blood flows, while the synovial A cells line the synovial cavity (Fig. 1.5). In the blood, cells known as monocytes belongs to this lineage. In time, they migrate out into the tissues, where they develop into tissue macrophages. These cells are very effective at presenting antigens to T lymphocytes.

Fig. 1.5 Many organs contain phagocytic cells derived from blood monocytes which are manufactured in the bone marrow. Monocytes pass out of the blood vessel and become macrophages in the tissues. Resident phagocytic cells of different tissues (listed right) were previously referred to as the reticuloendothelial system, but they too appear to belong to the monocyte lineage.

A second important phagocytic cell is the polymorphonuclear neutrophil, often just called a neutrophil or PMN (Fig. 1.6). These constitute the majority of the blood leucocytes. Like monocytes, they too migrate into tissues, in response to certain stimuli, but neutrophils are short-lived cells, which engulf material, destroy it and then die.

LYMPHOCYTES

Lymphocytes are wholly responsible for the specific immune recognition of pathogens, so they initiate adaptive immune responses. All lymphocytes are derived from bone marrow stem cells, but T lymphocytes then develop in the thymus, while B lymphocytes develop in the bone marrow (in adult mammals).

Each B cell specifically recognizes a particular antigen, using a receptor molecule on its surface. Having recognized its specific antigen, the B cells divide and differentiate into plasma cells, which produce large amounts of the receptor molecule in a soluble form which can be secreted. This is known as antibody. These antibody molecules are large glycoproteins found in the blood and tissue fluids: they bind to the antigen which initially activated the B cells. The presence of the antibodies activates other parts of the immune system, which then eliminate the pathogen carrying that antigen.

T lymphocytes come in several different types and they have a variety of functions. One group interacts with B cells and helps them to divide, differentiate and make antibody. Another group interacts with mononuclear phagocytes and helps them destroy pathogens. These two groups of cells are called T-helper cells (TH). A third group of T cells is reponsible for the destruction of host cells which have become infected by viruses or other intracellular pathogens – this kind of action is called cytotoxicity and these T cells are hence called T-cytotoxic cells (Tc). In every case, the T cells recognize antigens, but only in association with familiar markers on host cells. They use a specific receptor to do this, termed the T cell antigen receptor (TCR). This is related, both in function and structure, to the surface antibody which B cells use as their antigen receptors. T cells generate their effects, either by releasing soluble proteins, called cytokines, which signal to other cells, or by direct cell–cell interactions. The principle functions of lymphocytes are summarized in Figure 1.7.

CYTOTOXIC CELLS

Several cell types have the capacity to kill other cells. The Tc cell mentioned above is probably the most important, but mononuclear phagocytes also have some cytotoxic capacity, provided they can recognize the infected target cell. There is also a group of lymphocytes (large granular lymphocytes – LGLs) which have the capacity to recognize the surface changes that occur on a variety of tumour cells and virally infected cells. They damage these target cells, but unlike Tc cells, they use recognition systems which are rather non-specific. This action is sometimes called natural killer (NK) cell activity. Both macrophages and LGLs may also recognize and destroy some target cells (or pathogens) which have become coated with specific antibody.

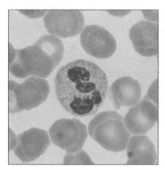
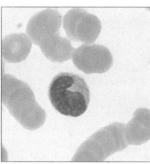

Fig. 1.6 Phagocytes. Apart from the fixed cells, there are polymorphonuclear neutrophils (left) and blood monocytes (right), both derived from bone marrow stem cells. (Courtesy of Dr P. M. Lydyard.)

Functions of lymphocytes

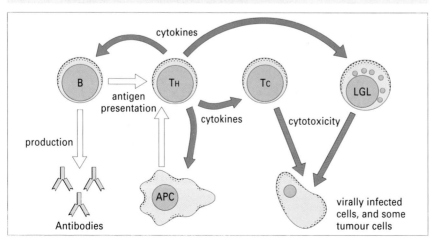

Fig. 1.7 B cells produce antibodies, while T helper cells (TH) are stimulated by antigen presenting cells (APCs) and B cells to produce cytokines which control immune responses. Cytotoxic T cells (Tc) and large granular lymphocytes (LGLs) can recognize and kill target host cells.

Eosinophil polymorphs (eosinophils) are a specialized group of leucocytes which have the ability to engage and damage large extracellular parasites, such as schistosomes. All of these cell types damage their different targets by releasing the contents of their intracellular granules close to them. Other molecules secreted by the cytotoxic cells, but not stored in granules, contribute to the damage.

AUXILIARY CELLS

A number of other cells are involved in the development of immune responses. For example, basophils and mast cells have granules containing a variety of mediators that produce inflammation in surrounding tissues. These mediators are released when the cells are triggered. They can also synthesize and secrete a number of mediators which control the development of immune reactions. Mast cells lie close to blood vessels in all tissues, and some of the mediators act on cells in the vessel walls. Basophils are functionally similar to mast cells but are circulating cells.

Platelets can also release inflammatory mediators when they are activated during thrombogenesis. The main purpose of inflammatory reactions, detailed below, is to attract leucocytes and the soluble mediators of immunity towards a site of infection.

 SOLUBLE MEDIATORS OF IMMUNITY

A wide variety of molecules are involved in the development of immune responses. These include antibodies and cytokines, produced by lymphocytes and a variety of other molecules which are normally present in serum. The serum concentration of a number of these proteins increases rapidly during infection and they are therefore called acute phase proteins. One example is C-reactive protein (CRP), so called because of its ability to bind to the C-protein of pneumococci. C-reactive protein, when bound to bacteria, promotes the binding of complement, which stimulates phagocytes to engulf the bacteria (Fig. 1.8). This process of protein-coating to enhance phagocytosis is known as opsonization. Both the CRP and the complement proteins are said to be acting as opsonins.

COMPLEMENT

The complement system is a group of about twenty serum proteins whose overall function is the control of inflammation. Several of the components are acute phase proteins. The components interact with each other, and with other elements of the immune system. For example, a number of microorganisms spontaneously activate the complement system, via the so-called 'alternative pathway', which is an innate, non-specific reaction. This results in a coat of complement molecules on the microorganism, leading to its uptake by phagocytes. The complement system can also be activated by antibodies bound to the pathogen surface, (the 'classical pathway'), when it constitutes a specific, adaptive response.

Complement activation is a cascade reaction, with each component sequentially acting on others, in a similar way to the blood-clotting system. Activation by either the classical or the alternative pathway generates peptides which have the following effects.
1. Opsonization (coating) of microorganisms for uptake by phagocytes.
2. Attraction of phagocytes to sites of infection (chemotaxis).
3. Increased blood flow to the site of activation and increased permeability of capillaries to plasma molecules.
4. Damage to plasma membranes on cells, gram-negative bacteria, enveloped viruses or other organisms which have induced the activation. This in turn can produce lysis of the cell.

These functions are outlined in Figure 1.9 overleaf and detailed in Chapter 12.

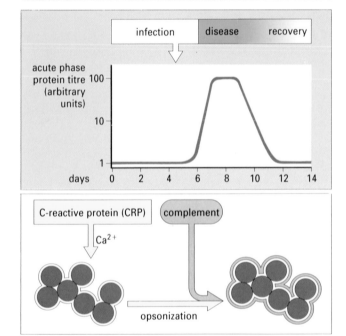

Fig. 1.8 Acute phase proteins (here exemplified by C-reactive protein) are serum proteins which increase rapidly in concentration (up to 100-fold) following infection (graph). They are important in the innate immunity to infection. C-reactive protein (CRP) recognizes and binds, in a Ca^{2+}-dependent fashion, to molecular groups found on a wide variety of bacteria and fungi. In particular it binds the phosphorylcholine moiety of pneumococci. CRP acts as an opsonin and also activates complement with all the associated sequelae.

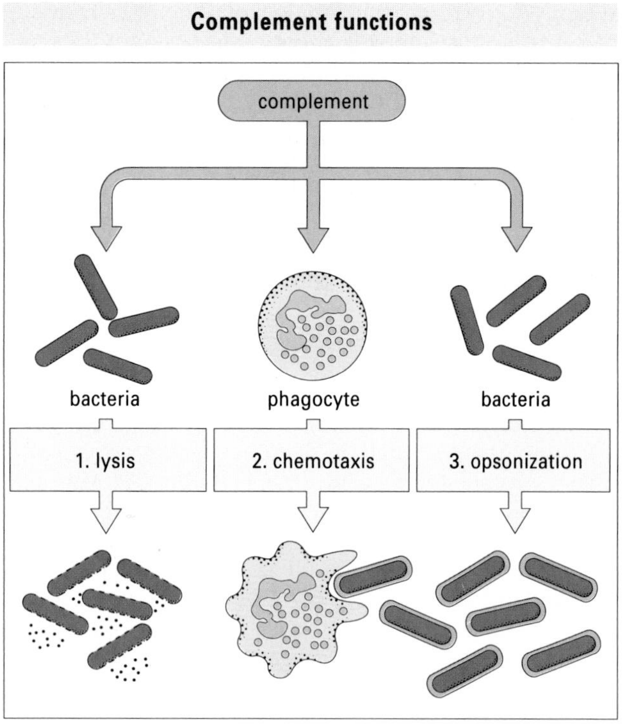

Complement functions

Fig. 1.9 The complement system has an intrinsic ability to lyse the cell membranes of many bacterial species (1). Complement products released in this reaction attract phagocytes to the site of the reaction – chemotaxis (2). Complement components coat the bacterial surface – opsonization – allowing the phagocytes to recognize the bacteria and engulf them (3). These are all functions of the innate immune system, although the reactions can also be triggered by the adaptive immune system, via antibodies coating the bacteria which activate the 'classical pathway'.

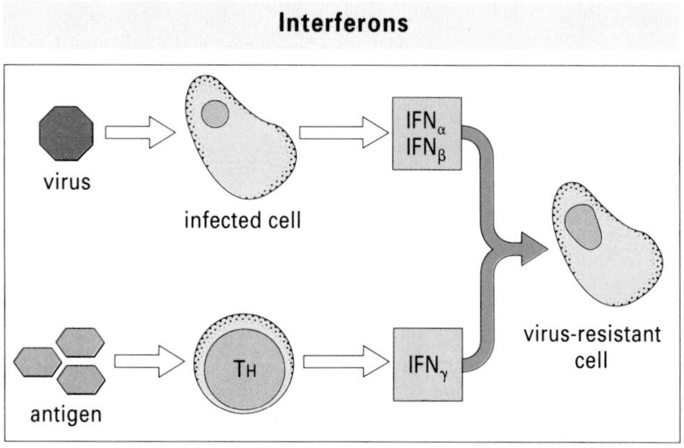

Interferons

Fig. 1.10 When host cells become infected by virus, they may produce interferon. Different cell types produce interferon-α (IFN_α) or interferon-β (IFN_β); interferon-γ (IFN_γ) is produced by some types of lymphocyte (TH) after activation by antigen. Interferons act on other host cells to induce a state of resistance to viral infection. IFN_γ has many other effects as well.

CYTOKINES

This is general term for a large group of molecules involved in signalling between cells during immune responses. All are proteins or peptides, some with sugar molecules attached (glycopeptides). The different cytokines fall into a number of categories.

Interferons (IFNs) are particularly important in limiting the spread of certain viral infections. One group (IFN_α and IFN_β) is produced by cells which have become virally infected; another type is released by certain activated T cells. Interferons induce a state of antiviral resistance in uninfected tissue cells (Fig. 1.10). They also determine how effectively the tissue cells can interact with lymphocytes and cytotoxic cells. IFNs are produced very early in infection and are the first line of resistance to many viruses.

Interleukins are a large group of cytokines (IL-1 to IL-10) produced mainly by T cells, although some are also produced by mononuclear phagocytes, or by tissue cells. Those produced by lymphocytes (T cells) are often called lymphokines. They have a variety of functions, but most of them are involved in directing other cells to divide and differentiate. Each interleukin acts on a specific, limited group of cells which express the correct receptors for that interleukin.

The colony-stimulating factors (CSFs) are involved in directing the division and differentiation of the bone marrow stem cells, and the precursors of the blood leucocytes. The balance of different CSFs partly determines the proportions of different cell types which will be produced. Some CSFs also promote further differentiation of cells outside the bone marrow.

Other cytokines include the tumour necrosis factors (TNF_α and TNF_β) and transforming growth factor-β (TGF_β), which have a variety of functions, but are particularly important in mediating inflammation and cytotoxic reactions.

ANTIBODIES

Antibodies (Ab), also called immunoglobulins (Ig), are a group of serum molecules produced by B lymphocytes. In fact they are the soluble form of the B cells' antigen receptor. All antibodies have the same basic structure, but they are diverse in the region that binds to the antigen. In general, each antibody can bind specifically to just one antigen.

While one part of an antibody molecule binds to antigen (the Fab portion), other parts interact with other elements of the immune system, such as phagocytes, or one of the complement molecules. In effect antibodies act as flexible adaptors, allowing elements of the immune system to recognize specific pathogens and their products (Fig. 1.11).

The part of the antibody molecule that interacts with cells of the immune system, is termed the Fc portion. Neutrophils, macrophages and other mononuclear phagocytes have Fc receptors on their surface. Consequently, if antibody is bound to a pathogen, it can then link to a phagocyte via the Fc portion. This allows the pathogen to be ingested and destroyed by the phagocyte (phagocytosed) – the antibody acts as an opsonin. Phagocytes can recognize material using either activated complement (C3b) or antibody as the opsonin, but phagocytosis is most effective when both are present (Fig. 1.12).

 ANTIGENS

Originally the term antigen was used for any molecule which induced B cells to produce a specific antibody (antibody generator). Now however the term is much more widely used to indicate any molecule which can be specifically recognized by the adaptive elements of the immune system, that is by B cells or T cells, or both.

Antibody molecules do not bind to the whole of an infectious agent. Each antibody molecule binds to one of the many molecules on the microorganism's surface. There may be several different antibodies for a given pathogen, each binding to a different antigen on that pathogen's surface.

The way in which a sufficient diversity of antibody molecules is generated, to bind to all the different antigens encountered in a lifetime, is explained in Chapter 5. Each antibody binds to a particular part of the antigen called an antigenic determinant, or epitope (these terms are synonymous). A particular antigen can have several different epitopes or repeated epitopes (see Fig. 1.13). Antibodies are specific for the epitopes rather than the whole antigen molecule.

T cells also recognize antigens, but they recognize antigens originating from within cells: small polypeptide fragments which are presented at the surface of other host cells. For example a host cell which has been infected with a virus, will express small fragments of viral proteins on its surface, thus making it instantly recognizable by cytotoxic T cells. The antigen fragments are presented on the surface of the cell by a specialized group of molecules. These are encoded in a set of genes known as the major histocompatibility complex (MHC), and are consequently called MHC molecules. The T cells use their antigen-specific receptors (TCRs) to recognize the antigenic peptides bound to these MHC molecules.

Antibody – a flexible adaptor

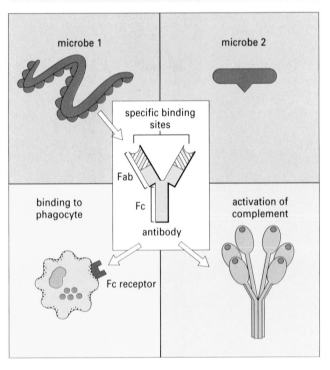

Fig. 1.11 When a microorganism lacks the inherent ability to activate complement or bind to phagocytes, the body provides antibodies as flexible adaptor molecules. The body can make several million different antibodies able to recognize a wide variety of infectious agents. Thus the antibody illustrated binds microbe 1, but not microbe 2, by its 'antigen-binding portion' (Fab). The 'Fc portion' may activate complement or bind to Fc receptors on host cells, particularly phagocytes.

Opsonization

	phagocyte	opsonin	binding
1		–	±
2		complement C3b	+ +
3		antibody	+ +
4		antibody and complement C3b	+ + + +

Fig. 1.12 Phagocytes have some intrinsic ability to bind directly to bacteria and other microorganisms (1), but this is much enhanced if the bacteria have activated complement. They will then have bound C3b so that the cells can bind the bacteria via C3b receptors (2). Organisms which do not activate complement well, if at all, are opsonized by antibody (Ab) which can bind to the Fc receptor on the phagocyte (3). Antibody can also activate complement and if both antibody *and* C3b opsonize the microbe, binding is greatly enhanced (4).

The essential point to remember about antigen, is that it is the initiator and driving force for all adaptive immune responses. The immune system has evolved to recognize antigens, destroy them and eliminate the source of their production – bacteria, virally infected cells etc. When antigen is eliminated immune responses switch off.

IMMUNE RESPONSES

You will recall that there are two major phases of any immune response:
1. recognition of the antigen
2. a reaction to eradicate it.

In adaptive immune responses, lymphocytes are responsible for immune recognition, and this is achieved by clonal selection.

CLONAL SELECTION

Each lymphocyte (whether a B cell or T cell) is capable of recognizing only one particular antigen. The immune system as a whole can specifically recognize many thousands of antigens, so the lymphocytes recognizing any particular antigen must represent only a minute proportion of the total. How then is an adequate immune response to an infectious agent generated? The answer is that when an antigen binds to the few cells that can recognize it, this induces them to proliferate rapidly. Within a few days there are enough of them to mount an adequate immune response. In other words, the antigen selects for the specific clones of its own antigen-binding cells (Fig. 1.14): a process called clonal selection. This operates for both B cells and T cells.

One might wonder how the immune system can 'know' which specific antibodies will be needed during an individual's lifetime. In fact, it does not. The immune system generates antibodies that can recognize an enormous range of antigens even before it encounters them. Many of these will never be called upon to protect the individual against infection. However, the tremendous number of infectious organisms, and their capacity to change their antigens through mutation, makes it necessary for all these different antibodies to be available.

Lymphocytes that have been stimulated, by binding to their specific antigen, take the first steps towards cell division. They express new receptors which allow them to respond to cytokines from other cells, which signal proliferation. The lymphocytes may also start to secrete cytokines themselves. They will usually go through a number of cycles of division, before differentiating into

Clonal selection

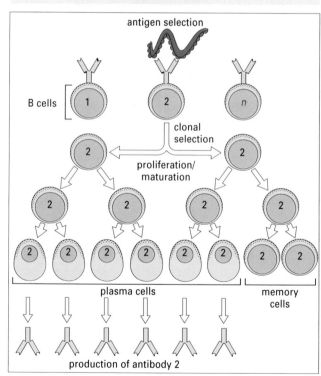

Fig. 1.14 Each antibody-producing cell (B cell) is programmed to make just one antibody, which is placed on its surface as an antigen receptor. Antigen binds to only those B cells with the appropriate surface receptor. These cells are stimulated to proliferate and mature into antibody-producing cells, and the longer-lived memory cells, all with the same antigen-binding specificity.

Antigens

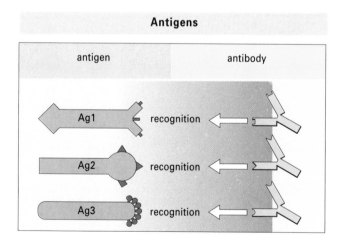

Fig. 1.13 Molecules which generate antibodies are called antigens. Antigen molecules each have a set of antigenic determinants, also called epitopes. The epitopes on one antigen (Ag1) are usually different from those on another (Ag2). Some antigens (Ag3) have repeated epitopes. Epitopes are molecular shapes recognized by the antibodies and T cell receptors of the adaptive immune system. Each antibody receptor recognizes one epitope rather than the whole antigen. Even simple microorganisms have many different antigens.

mature cells, again under the influence of cytokines. For example, proliferating B cells eventually mature into antibody-producing plasma cells. Even when the infection has been overcome some of the newly produced lymphocytes remain, available for restimulation if the antigen is encountered again. These cells are sometimes called memory cells, since they retain the immunological memory of particular antigen. It is memory cells that confer lasting immunity to a pathogen.

IMMUNE EFFECTOR MECHANISMS

There are numerous ways in which the immune system can destroy pathogens, each being suited to a particular type of infection at a particular stage of its life cycle. These defence mechanisms are often referred to as effector systems.

In one of the simplest effector systems, antibodies can combat certain pathogens just by binding to them. For example, antibody to the outer coat proteins of some rhinoviruses (which cause colds) can prevent the viral particles from binding to host cells.

More often antibody is important in activating complement, or acting as an opsonin to promote ingestion by phagocytes. Phagocytic cells, which have bound to an antigen-carrying microbe, proceed to engulf it by extending pseudopodia around it. These fuse and the microorganism is internalized (endocytosed) in a phagosome (Fig. 1.15). The phagocytes have several

ways of dealing with this material. For example macrophages can secrete reactive oxygen intermediates (ROIs), which are toxic to some bacteria, into the phagosome. Neutrophils can secret transferrin, which chelates iron and prevents some bacteria from obtaining that vital nutrient. Finally granules and lysosomes fuse with the phagosome, pouring enzymes into the phagolysosome, which digest the contents (Fig. 1.16). The mechanisms involved are described fully in Chapters 8 and 15.

Cytotoxic reactions are effector systems directed against whole cells, which are in general too large for phagocytosis. The target cell may be recognized either by specific antibody bound to the cell surface, or by T cells using their specific TCRs. In cytotoxic reactions the attacking cells direct their granules towards the target cell, in contrast to phagocytosis where the contents are directed into the phagosome. The granules of cytotoxic T cells contain molecules called perforins which

Phagocytosis

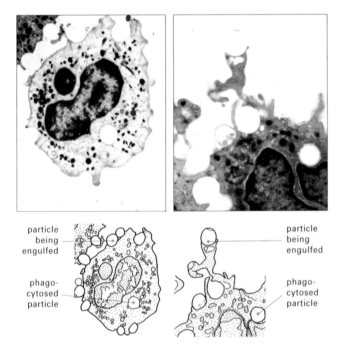

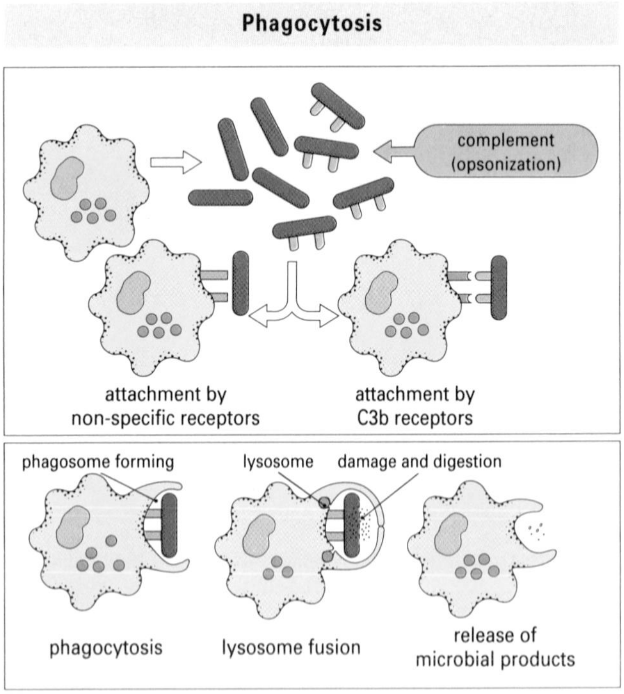

Fig. 1.16 Phagocytes arrive at a site of inflammation by chemotaxis. They may then attach to microorganisms via their non-specific cell surface receptors. Alternatively, if the organism is opsonized with a fragment of the third complement component (C3b), attachment will be through the phagocyte's receptors for C3b. If the phagocyte membrane now becomes activated by the infections agent, it is taken into a phagosome by pseudopodia extending around it. Once inside, lysosomes fuse with the phagosome to form a phagolysosome and the infectious agent is killed. Undigested microbial products may be released to the outside.

Fig. 1.15 Electronmicrographic study of phagocytosis. These two micrographs show human phagocytes engulfing latex particles. × 3000 (left); × 4500 (right). (Courtesy of Professor C. H. W. Horne.)

can punch holes in the outer membrane of the target. (In a similar way, antibody bound to the surface of a target cell can direct complement to make holes in its plasma membrane.) Some cytotoxic cells can also signal to the target cell to start a programme of self-destruction resulting in fragmentation of the DNA in a process called apoptosis.

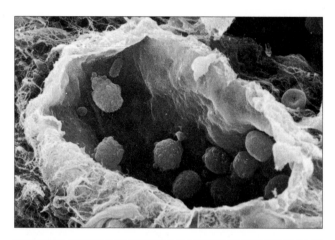

Fig. 1.17 Scanning electronmicrograph showing leucocytes adhering to the wall of a venule in inflamed tissues. × 16 000. (Courtesy of Professor M. J. Karnovsky.)

Chemotaxis

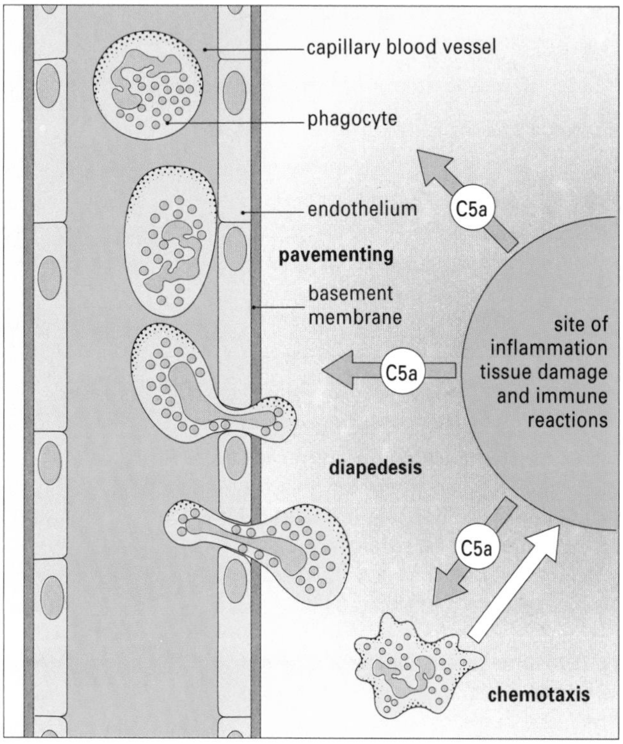

capillary blood vessel

phagocyte

endothelium   C5a

pavementing

basement membrane

C5a

site of inflammation tissue damage and immune reactions

diapedesis

C5a

chemotaxis

INFLAMMATION

The cells of the immune system are widely distributed throughout the body, but if an infection occurs it is necessary to concentrate them and their products at the site of infection. The process by which this occurs manifests itself as inflammation. Three major events occur during this response.

1. An increased blood supply to the infected area.

2. Increased capillary permeability caused by retraction of the endothelial cells. This permits larger molecules than usual to escape from the capillaries, and thus allows the soluble mediators of immunity to reach the site of infection.

3. Leucocytes migrate out of the capillaries into the surrounding tissues. In the earliest stages of inflammation, neutrophils are particularly prevalent, but later monocytes and lymphocytes also migrate towards the site of infection.

The process of cell migration is controlled by the adhesion of cells to the endothelium of inflamed tissues (pavementing). This occurs because molecules on the surface of the leucocytes interact with corresponding ones on the activated endothelium (Fig. 1.17). Once in the tissues, cells migrate towards the site of infection by a process of chemical attraction known as chemotaxis.

Phagocytes will actively migrate up concentration gradients of certain (chemotactic) molecules. Particularly active is C5a, a fragment of one of the complement components (Fig. 1.18), which attracts both neutrophils and monocytes. When purified C5a is applied to the base of an ulcer *in vivo*, neutrophils can be seen sticking to the endothelium of nearby capillaries shortly afterwards. The cells then squeeze between the endothelial cells and open the basement membrane of the microvessels (the whole process is called 'diapedesis') to reach the tissues. This process is described more fully in Chapter 13.

Fig. 1.18 At a site of inflammation, tissue damage and complement activation by the infectious agent cause the release of chemotactic peptides (e.g. C5a, a fragment of complement and one of the most important chemotactic peptides). These peptides diffuse to the adjoining capillaries, causing passing phagocytes to adhere to the endothelium (pavementing). The phagocytes insert pseudopodia between the endothelial cells and dissolve the basement membrane (diapedesis). They then pass out of the blood vessels and move up the concentration gradient of the chemotactic peptides towards the site of inflammation.

DEFENCES AGAINST EXTRACELLULAR AND INTRACELLULAR PATHOGENS

It will be clear that there is a fundamental difference between immune responses to extracellular and intracellular pathogens. In dealing with extracellular pathogens the immune system aims to destroy the pathogen itself and neutralize its products. In response to intracellular pathogens, there are two options. Either the T cells can destroy the infected cell – cytotoxicity – or they can activate the cell to deal with the pathogen for itself. This occurs, for example, when helper T cells release cytokines which activate macrophages to destroy organisms they have endocytosed.

Since many pathogens have both intracellular and extracellular phases of infection, different mechanisms are usually effective at different times. For example, the influenza virus travels through the blood stream to infect its target cells. Antibody is particularly effective at blocking this early phase of the infection. However, to clear an established infection, cytotoxic T cells must kill any cell that has become infected. Consequently, antibody is important in limiting the spread of infection, and preventing reinfection with the same virus, while cytotoxic T cells are essential to deal with infected cells (Fig. 1.19). These considerations play an important part in the development of effective vaccines.

Reaction to extracellular and intracellular pathogens

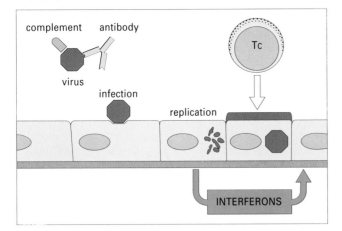

Fig. 1.19 Different immunological systems are effective against different types of infection, here illustrated as a virus infection. Antibodies and complement can block the extracellular phase of the life cycle, and promote phagocytosis of the virus. Interferons produced by infected cells can signal to uninfected cells, and induce a state of anti-viral resistance in them. Cytotoxic T cells are effective at recognizing and destroying the infected cells.

VACCINATION

One area in which immunological studies have had most immediate and successful application is in the field of vaccination. The principle of vaccination is based on two key elements of adaptive immunity, namely specificity and memory. Memory cells allow the immune system to mount a much stronger response on second encounter with antigen. This secondary response is both faster to appear and more effective than the primary response. The aim in vaccine development is to alter a pathogen or its toxins in such a way that they become innocuous without losing antigenicity. This is possible because antibodies and T cells recognize particular parts of antigens, the epitopes, and not the whole organism or toxin. Take, for example, vaccination against diphtheria. The diphtheria bacterium produces a toxin which destroys muscle cells. The toxin can be modified by formalin treatment so that it retains its epitopes but loses its toxicity; the resulting toxoid is used as a vaccine (Fig. 1.20). Whole infectious agents, such as the polio virus, can be attenuated so they retain their antigenicity but lose their pathogenicity.

Principle of vaccination

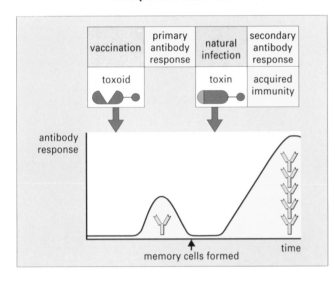

Fig. 1.20 The principle of vaccination is illustrated by immunization with diphtheria toxoid. Diphtheria toxoid retains some of the epitopes of the diphtheria bacillus toxin so that a primary antibody response to these epitopes is produced following vaccination with toxoid. In a natural infection the toxin restimulates B memory cells which produce the faster and more intense secondary antibody response to the epitope, so neutralizing the toxin.

IMMUNOPATHOLOGY

Up to this point, the immune system has been presented as an unimpeachable asset. It is certainly true that deficiencies in any part of the system leave the individual exposed to a greater risk of infection, although other parts of the system may partially compensate for such deficiencies. Clearly, strong evolutionary pressure from infectious microbes has lead to the development of the immune system in its present form. However, there are occasions when the immune system is itself a cause of disease or other undesirable consequences (Fig. 1.21).

In essence the system can fail in one of three ways.
1. Mistaken recognition of self antigens – autoimmunity. Normally the immune system recognizes all foreign antigens and reacts against them, while recognizing the body's own tissues as 'self' and making no reaction against them. If the system reacts against self components, autoimmune disease occurs. Examples of autoimmune disease are rheumatoid arthritis and pernicious anaemia.
2. An ineffective immune response – immunodeficiency. If any elements of the immune system are defective, the individual may not be able to fight infections adequately. These conditions are termed immunodeficiency. Some are hereditary deficiencies which start to manifest themselves shortly after birth, while others, such as acquired immunodeficiency syndrome (AIDS), develop later.
3. An overactive immune response – hypersensitivity. Sometimes immune reactions are out of all proportion to the damage that may be caused by a pathogen. The immune system may also mount a reaction to a harmless antigen, such as a food molecule. The immune reactions may cause more damage than the pathogen, or antigen, and in this case we speak of hypersensitivity. For example, molecules on the surface of pollen grain are recognized as antigens by some individuals, generating symptoms of hay fever or asthma.

Finally, there are occasions when the immune system acts normally, but the immune responses it produces are inconvenient in the context of modern medicine. The most important examples of this are in blood transfusion and graft rejection. In these cases it is necessary to match carefully the donor and recipient tissues so the immune system of the recipient does not attack the donated blood or graft tissue. These problems are, however, a small price to pay for an essential system of the body, which is absolutely vital to protect individuals against infection.

Failure of the immune system

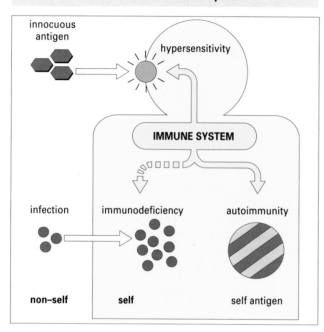

Fig. 1.21 There are three principle ways in which the immune system can fail – hypersensitivity, immuno-deficiency and autoimmunity. The first two are due to an inappropriately large or small immune response, respectively. Autoimmunity is caused by a failure of self/non-self discrimination in immune recognition.

chapter 2

Cells Involved in Immune Responses

The immune system of vertebrates consists of organs and tissues composed of many different types of cell plus a variety of actively trafficking cells. This complex system depends on multiple interactions between its component parts, and has evolved to specifically recognize microorganisms and eliminate them. By contrast, lower animals rely on more primitive defence mechanisms to protect themselves. These include lipid-binding and sugar-binding proteins (with low specificity) which can agglutinate and/or opsonize a wide variety of microorganisms, and the cells which are capable of engulfing and digesting the microbes – phagocytes. These are important cells for the defence of all animals, including vertebrates.

The key development which has occurred in vertebrates is the evolution of lymphoid cells and lymphoid organs. The lymphoid cells produce the high degree of specificity typical of vertebrate immune systems.

All the cells of the immune system arise from pluripotent stem cells through two main lines of differentiation (Fig. 2.1):
1. the lymphoid lineage – producing lymphocytes
2. the myeloid lineage – producing phagocytes (monocytes, macrophages and neutrophils) and other cells.

There are two main kinds of lymphocytes which carry out different functions, called T cells and B cells. Both are equipped with surface receptors for antigen. T cells develop from their precursors in the thymus, whereas mammalian B cells differentiate in the fetal liver and in the adult bone marrow. In birds, B cells differentiate in a uniquely avian organ, the bursa of Fabricius. These sites of lymphocyte differentiation are called the central or primary lymphoid organs. It is here that the lymphocyte precursors acquire the ability to recognize antigens through the development of specific surface receptors.

A third population of lymphocytes which do not express antigen receptors (see below) are called the natural killer (NK) cells. NK cells are derived from bone marrow and can be functionally distinguished from T and B cells by their ability, *in vitro*, to lyse certain tumour cell lines (but not fresh tumours) without prior sensitization. These cells are morphologically large granular lymphocytes (LGLs).

The phagocytes are also of two basic kinds – monocytes/macrophages and polymorphonuclear granulocytes. The latter have a distinctive lobed, irregularly shaped (polymorphic) nucleus. They are often referred to as polymorphs or granulocytes, and may be divided

Origin of cells involved in the immune response

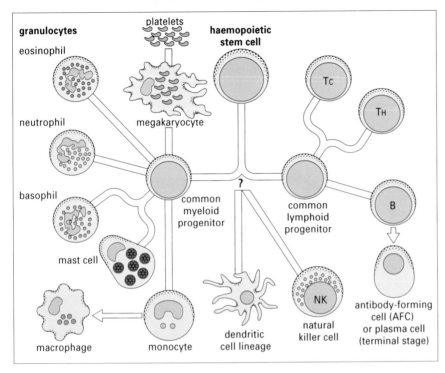

Fig. 2.1 All these cells are derived from pluripotent stem cells which give rise to two main lineages; one for lymphoid cells and the other for myeloid cells. The common lymphoid progenitor has the capacity to differentiate into either T cells or B cells depending on the microenvironment to which it homes. In mammals, T cells develop in the thymus while B cells develop in the fetal liver and bone marrow. The precise origin of some antigen-presenting cells (APCs) and the NK cells is not certain, although they do develop ultimately from the haemopoietic stem cells. The myeloid cells differentiate into the committed cells shown on the left. The collective name 'granulocyte' is sometimes used for eosinophils, neutrophils and basophils.

into neutrophils, basophils and eosinophils, on the basis of how the cytoplasmic granules respond to different types of staining agent when prepared for microscopy. The three types of cell also have distinct effector functions. The most numerous are the neutrophils, also called PMNs (polymorphonuclear neutrophils), which constitute the majority of leucocytes (white blood cells) in the bloodstream.

In addition to lymphocytes and phagocytes, there are a number of accessory cells which include:

1. a variety of cells specialized to present antigen to T cells, referred to as antigen-presenting cells (APCs)
2. platelets, which are involved in blood clotting and inflammation
3. mast cells, which have structural and functional similarities to basophil polymorphs
4. endothelial cells, which express molecules capable of recognizing certain lymphocytes but not others, thus controlling the traffic and distribution of lymphocytes.

The important features of these cell types will now be described in detail.

LYMPHOID CELLS

Lymphocytes are produced in the primary or central lymphoid organs (thymus and adult bone marrow) at a high rate (10^9 per day). Some of these cells migrate via the circulation into the secondary lymphoid tissues (the spleen, lymph nodes, tonsils, and mucosa-associated lymphoid tissue). The average human adult has about 10^{12} lymphoid cells and the lymphoid tissue as a whole represents about 2% of total body weight. Lymphoid cells represent about 20% of the total white blood cells (leucocytes) present in the adult circulation. Many mature lymphoid cells are long-lived, and may persist as memory cells for several years, or even for the lifetime of the individual.

MORPHOLOGICAL HETEROGENEITY OF LYMPHOCYTES

Lymphocytes in a conventional blood smear vary greatly in both size (6-10 μm in diameter) and morphology. Differences are seen in the nuclear to cytoplasmic ratio

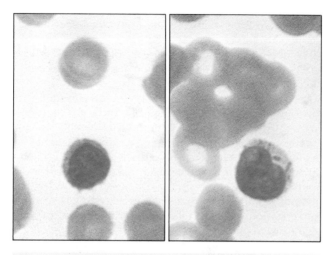

Fig. 2.2 Morphological heterogeneity of lymphocytes. Left: The small lymphocyte has no granules and a high N:C ratio. Right: The large granular lymphocyte has a lower N:C ratio and azurophilic granules in the cytoplasm. Condensed chromatin produces dark nuclear staining. Giemsa stain, × 1000.

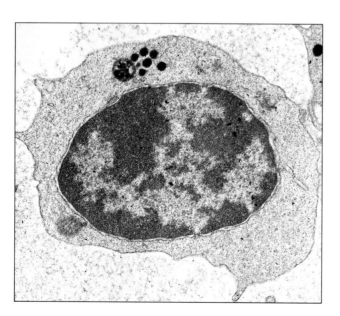

Fig. 2.3 Ultrastructure of a non-granular T cell. This electronmicrograph shows the Gall body which is characteristic of the majority of resting T cells. × 10 500.

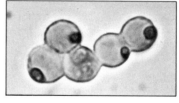

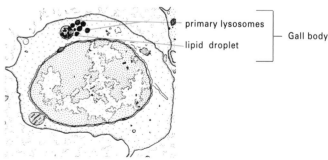

primary lysosomes
lipid droplet
Gall body

Insert: This structure is also seen as a single 'spot' following staining for non-specific esterase in light microscopy. × 400.

(N:C ratio), the degree of cytoplasmic staining with histological dyes, and the presence or absence of azurophilic granules.

Among resting lymphoid cells, two distinct morphological types can be distinguished in the circulation by light microscopy, using a haematological stain such as Giemsa. The smaller of the two is typically agranular and has a higher N:C ratio. The larger ones have a lower N:C ratio and contain intracytoplasmic azurophilic granules. These are currently referred to as large granular lymphocytes (LGLs), not to be confused with granulocytes (neutrophils, eosinophils and basophils) or with monocytes, which also have azurophilic granules (Fig. 2.2).

Resting blood T cells show two distinct morphological patterns. The majority of T helper (TH) cells and T cytotoxic (Tc) cells are of the smaller type, non-granular with a high N:C ratio. They also carry a cytoplasmic structure termed the 'Gall body', which consists of a cluster of primary lysosomes associated with a lipid droplet. The Gall body is easily identified by lysosomal enzyme cytochemistry and electron microscopy (Fig. 2.3). The other morphological pattern is shown by up to 10% of TH cells and 35% of Tc cells. These display LGL morphology, with primary lysosomes dispersed in the cytoplasm and a well-developed Golgi apparatus (Fig. 2.4).

Another subset of T cells with LGL characteristics is the gamma/delta ($\gamma\delta$) or TCR-1$^+$ lymphocyte population (see below). Within the lymphoid tissues, these cells display a dendritic morphology (Fig. 2.5) and when cultured *in vitro* they may adhere to the substrate,

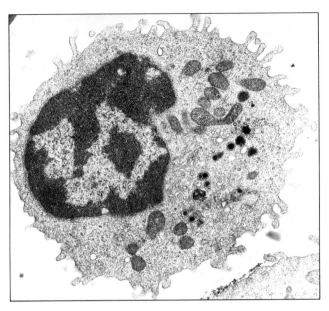

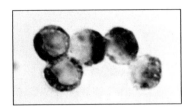

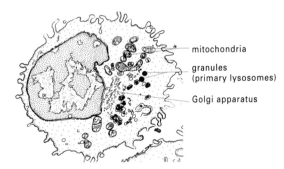

mitochondria

granules
(primary lysosomes)

Golgi apparatus

Fig. 2.4 Ultrastructure of T cells with granular morphology. These cells characteristically have electron-dense peroxidase-negative granules (primary lysosomes). These granules are dispersed in the cytoplasm with some

close to the well-developed Golgi apparatus. There are many mitochondria present. × 10 000. Insert: Cytochemical staining for acid phosphatase shows a granular pattern of staining under light microscopy. × 400.

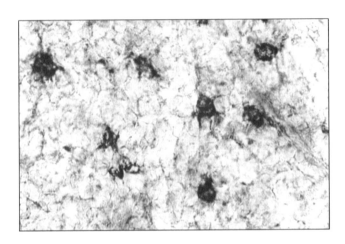

Fig. 2.5 Dendritic morphology of $\gamma\delta$ TCR-1$^+$ cells in the tonsil. This T cell population is predominantly localized in the interfollicular T-cell dependent zones in the lamina propria, and within the surface epithelium. Note the dendritic morphology of the cells. Anti-TCR-1 mAb and immunoperoxidase, × 900. (Courtesy of Dr. A. Favre, from *Eur J Immunol* 1991:**21**;173, with permission.)

showing a variety of morphological changes (Fig 2.6).

Resting blood B cells do not display Gall bodies or LGL morphology and their cytoplasm is predominantly occupied by scattered single ribosomes (Fig. 2.7). Occasionally, activated B cells are found with developing rough endoplasmic reticulum (Fig. 2.8).

NK cells, like γδ T cells and some Tc cells, are characterized by LGL morphology. They do, however, display a larger number of azurophilic granules than do granular T cells.

MARKERS

Lymphocytes (and other leucocytes) express a large number of different molecules, or 'markers' on their surfaces which can be used to distinguish cell populations. Many of these molecules can now be identified by specific monoclonal antibodies, and a systematic nomenclature has been developed, namely the CD system, in which the molecules are numbered CD1, CD2, etc. The term CD (cluster of differentiation), refers

to groups, or clusters, of monoclonal antibodies, each cluster binding specifically to a particular cell marker. The CD system depends on computer analysis of monoclonal antibodies (mAb), produced mainly in mice, against human leucocyte antigens. The work was carried out in a number of laboratories worldwide, and a series of International Workshops have determined the patterns of mAb binding on different leucocyte populations, and the molecular weights of the markers. Monoclonal antibodies with similar characteristics, defined by these criteria, were grouped together and given a CD number. This number is now also used to indicate the cell-marker molecule recognized by a group of monoclonal antibodies (see appendix for list of CD molecules).

Different molecules may be characteristic of different lineages (lineage markers), or of different stages of cell maturation (maturation markers). Some markers only appear following activation of the cell by a variety of stimuli (activation markers). An example of a lineage

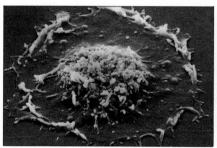 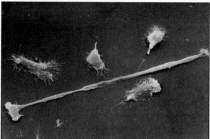 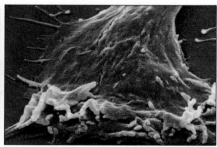

Fig. 2.6 Morphological changes in cloned γδ **T cells** *in vitro*. Left: Cells adhere to the substrate in a similar way to macrophages. × 6000. Centre: The cells become elongated with uropod formation, extending two polar filopodia. ×

6000. Right: Adhesion plaques are formed at the terminal ends of the filopodia. × 20 000. (Courtesy of Dr. G. Arancia and Dr A. Malorni, from *Eur J Immunol* 1991:**21**;173, with permission.)

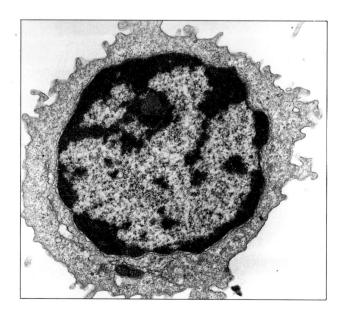

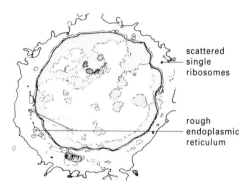

scattered single ribosomes

rough endoplasmic reticulum

Fig. 2.7 Ultrastructure of a resting B cell. These cells have no Gall body or granules. Scattered ribosomes and isolated profiles of rough endoplasmic reticulum (RER) are seen in the cytoplasm. Development of the Golgi lysosomal system in the B cell occurs only on activation. × 11 500.

marker is CD3, which is virtually exclusive to T cells and is involved in cell triggering. A maturation marker of T cells is CD1, which is only found on cells developing in the thymus and is not present on peripheral T cells. T-cell growth factor receptor (IL2 receptor, CD25) is an activation marker of T cells, only being expressed when the cell is stimulated by antigen.

Although it is sometimes useful to define markers in this way, it is not always possible to do so. Sometimes, a maturation marker for one lineage is an activation marker for another. For example, B cells express MHC class II antigens during most of their lifetime, but human T cells only express these molecules following activation. Furthermore, 'activation' markers may already be present on a cell in reduced numbers, which increase following activation. An example of this is CD11a (LFA-1) on monocytes.

Cell surface molecules exist as a number of different families which probably originate, in evolutionary terms, from a few ancestral genes. These families include the following major groups.

There are a number of integrin subfamilies – all members of a particular subfamily share a common β chain, but each has a unique α chain.

1. Molecules of the immunoglobulin supergene family have particular structural characteristics of the immunoglobulins and include CD2, CD3, CD4, CD8, murine Thy-1, and many more.

2. The integrin family consists of heterodimeric molecules containing α and β chains. One subfamily (β_2 integrins) uses CD18 as the β chain. This chain can be associated with CD11a, CD11b or CD11c – these combinations make up the lymphocyte function antigen LFA-1, Mac-1 (CR3) and p150,95 (CR4) surface molecules respectively – and are commonly found on leucocytes. The second subfamily (β_1 integrins) has various polypeptides associated with CD29 as the β chain. These include the VLA markers which are 'very late' activation markers (see below).

Surface molecules (markers) may be demonstrated using fluorescent antibodies as probes (Fig. 2.9). Flow cytometry, which can enumerate and separate cells on the basis of their size and fluorescence intensity (see Chapter 25), has revolutionized studies on lymphoid cell populations.

T CELLS

Historically, the first way in which human T cells were distinguished from B cells was by their fortuitous ability to bind to sheep erythrocytes – now known to bind through the CD2 molecule on T cells (Fig. 2.10). However the definitive T-cell lineage marker is the T-cell antigen receptor (TCR). There are presently two defined types of TCR; TCR-2 is a heterodimer of two disulphide-linked polypeptides (α and β); TCR-1 is structurally similar but consists of γ and δ polypeptides. Both receptors are associated with a set of five polypeptides, the CD3 complex, to give the T-cell receptor complex (TCR–CD3 complex; see chapter 4).

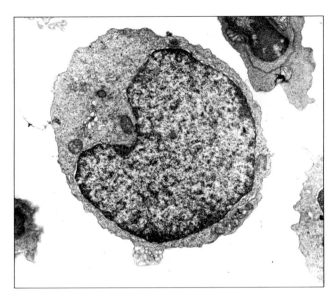

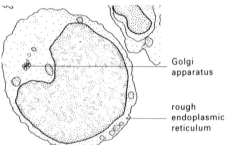

Fig. 2.8 The ultrastructure of a B cell blast. The main feature of activated B cells is the development of the machinery for immunoglobulin synthesis. This includes rough endoplasmic reticulum, free polyribosomes and the Golgi apparatus, which is involved in glycosylation of the immunoglobulins. × 7500.

Immunofluorescent demonstration of T cell markers

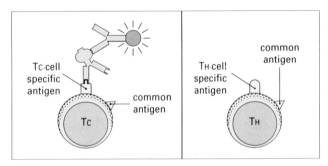

Fig. 2.9 Mouse antibodies directed towards a T cell subset-specific antigen on a T cytotoxic (Tc) cell will bind to such cells, but not to T helper (TH) cells. The bound antibody is detected using antibodies to mouse immunoglobulin coupled to a fluorescent molecule. This provides a method for enumerating T-cell subsets.

Thus a T cell is a cell that expresses either TCR-1 or TCR-2. Approximately 85–95% of blood T cells express TCR-2, and up to 15% of cells are TCR-1[+].

TCR-2[+] T cells

The TCR-2-bearing cells can be subdivided further into two distinct non-overlapping populations; a subset which carries the CD4 marker and mainly 'helps' or 'induces' immune responses (Tн), and a subset which carries the CD8 marker and is predominantly cytotoxic (Tc). Whereas CD4[+] T cells recognize their specific antigens in association with major histocompatibility complex (MHC) class II molecules, CD8[+] T cells recognize antigens in association with MHC class I molecules (See Chapter 4). This influences the type of cell they can interact with. Most circulating TCR-1[+] cells do not express either the CD4 or the CD8 marker, although a few of them may be CD8[+].

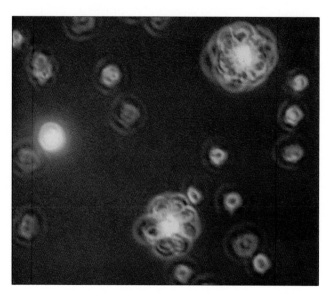

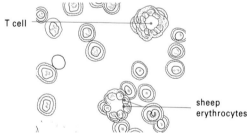

Fig. 2.10 Marker of human T cells. Human T cells from blood and tissues have the fortuitous property of binding to sheep erythrocytes (SEs). Following their centrifugation together, the cells form rosettes, with many SEs clustered around each human T cell. To facilitate enumeration, the nucleated T cells can be distinguished from the non-nucleated SEs by using a green fluorescent stain which is specific for nuclei. This rosette formation with SEs provides a means of physically separating T from non-T cells (see Chapter 25).

CD4[+] cells

The CD4[+] set have been functionally divided into two further subsets.
1. cells which positively influence the response of T cells and B cells - the helper cell function – are CD29[+]. This same population practically overlaps, with a population which expresses a low molecular weight isoform of the CD45 common leucocyte antigen This isoform is designed CD45R0[+].
2. Cells which induce the suppressor/cytotoxic functions of CD8[+] cells - the suppressor/inducer function express a different isoform of the CD45 molecule, and are CD45RA[+].

Over the last 5 years, the CD45RA[+] and CD45R0[+], TH cells have been designated 'naïve' and 'memory' cells respectively. However, current opinion is that expression of CD45R0/CD29 by CD4[+] TH cells is more relevant to the state of activation of the cell (see activation markers).

Functional diversity of T cells has also been demonstrated by analysis of Tн clones for cytokine secretion patterns. In both mice and now more convincingly in man, two groups CD4[+] T cell clones have been found. One secretes IL-2 and IFN$_\gamma$, the other produces IL-4, IL-5, IL-6 and IL-10. These are known as the Tн1 and Tн2 cell subsets (see Chapter 8). Tн1 cells mediate several functions associated with cytotoxicity and local inflammatory reactions. Consequently these cells are important for combating intracellular pathogens including viruses, bacteria and parasites. Tн2 cells are more effective at stimulating B cells to proliferate and produce antibodies, and therefore function primarily to protect against free-living microorganisms (humoral immunity).

Other criteria have been used to subdivide the CD4[+] set. For example, there is a rare subset of CD4[+] cells expressing NK cell markers, which do not produce the lymphokine IL-2 and do not proliferate in response to antigens and mitogens.

CD8[+] cells

CD8[+] T cells can also be subdivided, according to a number of criteria and using a variety of monoclonal antibodies, into specific functional subsets.

One subset expresses CD28 molecules, and produces IL-2 in response to activation signals, while another subset responds to (but does not produce) IL-2 and expresses the heterodimeric CD11b/CD18 molecule. Interestingly, cells of the former subset have a distinct Gall body (see above) whereas cells of the latter subset show LGL morphology. Granule contents are known to be involved in the cytotoxic function of T cells and NK cells, but the function of the Gall body is not known.

TCR-1[+] T cells

CD3[+]TCR-1[+] cells are a minor subpopulation of circulating T cells and tend to home into mucosal epithelia. The majority of intra-epithelial lymphocytes (IEL) are TCR-1[+] and express the CD8 marker, but this is not found on most circulating TCR-1[+] cells. It has recently been shown that these cells have a specific repertoire of T-cell receptors biased towards bacterial antigens, and current opinion is that these cells may play an important role in protecting the mucosal surfaces of the body. Recently, a small subset of double negative (CD4⁻ CD8⁻) cells expressing TCR-2 has also been described.

Major T cell subsets

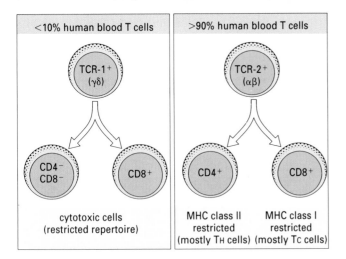

Fig. 2.11 T cells can be subdivided into different subsets based on the expression of one or other T cell receptor (TCR-1 or TCR-2). TCR-1⁺ cells are thought to have a restricted repertoire and to be mainly non-MHC restricted. On the other hand, TCR-2⁺ cells express either CD4 or CD8 which determines whether they see antigen in association with MHC class II or MHC class I molecules.

Functional subsets of CD4⁺ T cells

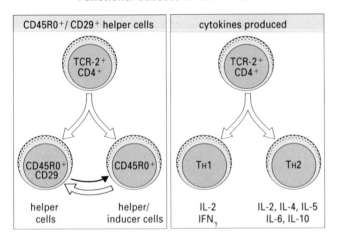

Fig. 2.12 These MHC class II restricted T cells have been divided into subsets on the basis of expression of isoforms of the CD45 and CD29 molecules (left). In addition, they can be subdivided into TH1 and TH2 populations based on their profiles of cytokine production (right).

Division of the TCR-, CD4- and CD8-bearing cells into different functional subsets is illustrated in Figs 2.11 and 2.12.

Thus far we have described the cell markers and antigen-specific receptors which define T-cell subsets. There are also a number of other surface molecules, expressed on all T cells (pan T-cell markers), which are also found on cells of other lineages. The receptors for sheep erythrocytes (CD2) are a good example. Under normal circumstances, *in vivo*, the CD2 molecule, together with the TCR–CD3 complex and other membrane-bound glycoproteins, is involved in activating cells when it binds to the appropriate ligand. CD2 is also found on about 75% of CD3⁻ NK cells. Another molecule, CD5, also involved in T-cell activation, is expressed on all T-cells and on a subpopulation of B cells. The ligand for this molecule has recently been shown to be CD72 on B cells. CD7 is present on the majority of NK cells. A complete list of CD molecules on T cells, some of which are shared by other haemopoietic cells, is given in the Appendix.

Murine T cells express markers similar to those detected on human T cells. All murine T cells carry a molecule, Thy-1 or θ, with a molecular weight of 19–35 kDa; a human equivalent has been described but little studied.

It is currently unclear whether T suppressor (Ts) cells really exist as a subpopulation functionally separate from other subsets, but it has been documented that murine T cells having suppressor activity carry I–J molecules, the expression of which is controlled by genes in the MHC (see chapter 10). Furthermore, the binding of a Vicia villosa lectin might also mark a functional population in man and mouse which is involved in 'contrasuppression'. (A lectin is a protein which binds to specific carbohydrate residues.) A summary of major TCR-2⁺ cell markers in man and mouse is shown in Fig. 2.13.

Surface markers of human and murine T cells

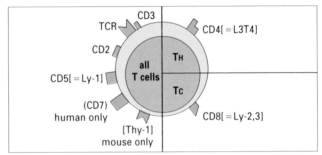

Fig. 2.13 The molecule CD7 has thus far only been detected in man, while Thy-1 is specific for the mouse. Other markers in square brackets are mouse equivalents of human markers. Most of these molecules belong to the immunoglobulin superfamily of adhesion molecules.

B CELLS

B lymphocytes represent about 5–15% of the circulating lymphoid pool, and are classically defined by the presence of surface immunoglobulins. (These immunoglobulin markers are made by the cells themselves, in contrast to the immunoglobulin molecules on a mast cell, for example, which originate elsewhere.) The immunoglobulin molecules are inserted into the surface membrane of the B cell where they act as specific antigen receptors. They are detected on the surface of mature cells with fluorochrome-labelled antibodies specific for immunoglobulin of the species under investigation. Staining of cells in the cold results in the detection of the fluorescence with a 'ring-like' (or patchy) appearance over the B cell (Fig. 2.14). Divalent antibodies to the surface immunoglobulin attach to and cross-link the surface receptors, producing 'patches' of cross-linked immunoglobulin on the cell surface. On warming up, most of these complexes are actively swept along the cell surface and are seen as a 'cap' over one pole of the cell (see Fig. 2.14). This phenomenon, although first shown for immunoglobulin on B cells, may also be seen with other surface glycoproteins, both on B cells and other cell types.

The majority of human B cells in peripheral blood express two immunoglobulin isotypes on their surface, IgM and IgD (see Chapter 4). On the same cell, their antigen-binding sites are identical. Very few cells in the circulation express IgG, IgA or IgE, although these are present in larger numbers in specific locations in the body, for example, IgA-bearing cells in the intestinal mucosa. It has recently been shown that surface IgM is associated with other molecules forming the 'B-cell antigen receptor complex'. IgMα, a 34 kDa molecule and product of the *mb-1* gene is required for the transport and assembly of IgM monomers in the cell membrane. Igβ, and a probable isoform Igγ, are other accessory molecules, of approximately 39 kDa, which interact with the transmembrane segments of IgM. These molecules are also involved in activation of the B cell.

A number of other markers are expressed by both mouse and human B cells (Fig. 2.15). The majority of B cells carry MHC class II antigens which are important for cooperative interactions with T cells. These class II molecules consist of I–A or I–E in the mouse and HLA-DP, DQ and DR antigens in man. Complement receptors for C3b (CR1, CD35) and C3d (CR2, CD21) are commonly found on B cells and are associated with activation and possibly 'homing' of the cells. Fc receptors for exogenous IgG (FcγRII, CD32) are also present and play a role in negative signalling to the B cell. CD19, CD20 and CD22 are the main markers currently used to identify human B cells. Other molecules which identify human B cells are CD72 through 78. The CD72 molecule has also been described for murine B cells (Lyb-2) together with B220, a high molecular weight (220 kDa) isoform of CD45 (Lyb-5).

A marker originally found only on T cells (Ly1, CD5) has now been shown to be present on some B cells; it identifies a subset which is predisposed to autoantibody production. These cells (recently termed B1 cells) are found predominantly in the peritoneal cavity in mice and there is some evidence for a separate differentiation pathway from 'conventional' B cells (B2 cells). Some human B cells bind to (and form rosettes with) mouse erythrocytes (ME-R). This property, together with expression of the CD5 molecule, identifies a subset whose immunoglobulin repertoire is biased towards autoantigens including DNA, Fc of IgG, phospholipids and cytoskeletal components.

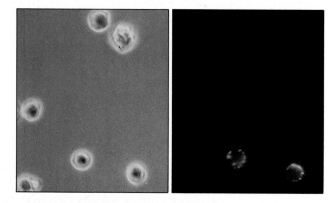

Fig. 2.14 B cells stained for surface immunoglobulin. Human blood B cells stained in the cold with fluoresceinated anti-human immunoglobulin show a patchy surface fluorescence viewed under ultraviolet light (right). Under phase contrast light microscopy (left) it can be seen that only 2 out of 6 in this field are B cells. The lower cell shows 'capping' of the fluorescent antibody.

Surface markers of human and murine peripheral B cells

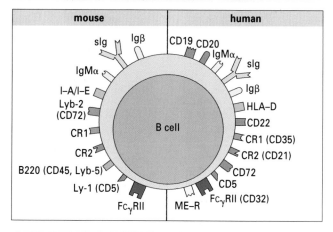

Fig. 2.15 Many of these molecules are homologous; they are shown in the same colour.

NATURAL KILLER CELLS

Natural killer (NK) cells account for up to 15% of blood lymphocytes and can be negatively defined as lymphocytes having no conventional surface antigen receptors (TCR or immunoglobulin). Most surface antigens detectable on NK cells by monoclonal antibodies are shared with T cells or cells of the myelomonocytic series. The major markers of human NK cells and their shared specificities are shown in Fig. 2.16. A reagent commonly used to identify NK cells in purified lymphocyte populations is the monoclonal antibody to CD16 (Fc$_\gamma$RIII); CD16 is involved in one of the activation pathways of NK cells. It is also expressed by neutrophils, some macrophages and probably some T cells.

On granulocytes, CD16 is linked to the surface membrane by a phosphatidylinositol glycan (PIG) linkage, whereas NK cells express the transmembrane form of the molecule. Another important marker of NK cells is the CD56 molecule. The absence of CD3, but the presence of CD56 and/or CD16 is currently in use as a definitive marker for NK cells in man. Resting NK cells also express the α chain of the IL-2 receptor, an intermediate affinity receptor of 70 kDa. Therefore, direct stimulation with IL-2 results in activation of NK cells. Interestingly, this 70 kDa receptor is also expressed on all of the T cells which display LGL morphology, namely TCR-1$^+$ cells and a proportion of TCR-2$^+$CD8$^+$ cells. All of these respond to IL-2 by acquiring non-specific cytotoxic functions. Collectively, these cells are termed lymphocyte activated killer (LAK) cells, which kill fresh tumour cells and a broader spectrum of neoplastic targets in comparison to those lysed by resting NK cells.

Murine NK cells have been defined primarily by using allo- or hetero-antisera. A distinctive difference between human and murine NK cells is the presence in mouse cells of fewer, but much larger, azurophilic granules. A summary of phenotypic markers of murine NK cells is shown in Fig. 2.17.

NK cells, in addition to being able to kill certain tumour cells (Fig 2.18) are also cytotoxic for virus-infected cells, and to targets coated with IgG antibodies.

Surface markers of human NK cells

marker	shared specificities
CD16 (Fc$_\gamma$RIII)	minority of T cells, granulocytes, some macrophages
CD11b	granulocytes, monocytes, some T cells
CD38*	activated T cells, plasma cells, haemopoietic precursors
CD2*	all T cells
CD7	all T cells
CD8*	some T cells
CD56	minority of T cells
CD57	some T cells
IL-2R (β chain, p70)	activated T cells
*expressed on 10–80% of NK cells.	

Fig. 2.16 None of these markers are lineage-specific.

Surface markers of murine NK cells

marker	shared specificities
Thy-1*	T cells
Lyb-5 (B220)	B cells
NK1	–
NK2	–
Fc$_\gamma$RIII*	some T cells, granulocytes, some monocytes/macrophages
Asialo-GM1	–
CR3 (CD11b, MAC-1)	granulocytes, monocytes
*expressed on some but not all murine NK cells	

Fig. 2.17 Although some molecules are shared by other cell types, some lineage-specific markers have been defined.

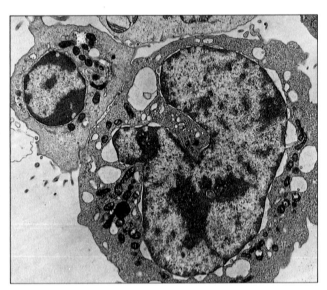

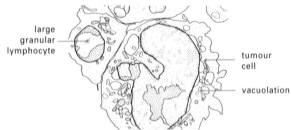

Fig. 2.18 A large granular lymphocyte (LGL) killing a tumour cell. LGLs bind to and kill IgG antibody-coated, and even non-coated, tumour cells. It is essential for the membranes of the two cells to be closely apposed in order for the LGL to deliver its cytotoxic factors. × 4500.

The latter property is referred to as antibody-dependent cellular cytotoxicity (ADCC) and is mediated through the receptor for IgG (Fc$_\gamma$RIII). NK cells may also release interferon-γ (IFN$_\gamma$) and other cytokines (e.g. IL-1 and GM–CSF) which may be important in the regulation of haemopoiesis and immune responses.

B cells, T cells and NK cells have other important surface molecules which are common to all leucocytes. For example, the leucocyte function antigen (LFA-1), also found on granulocytes and macrophages, is important for cell adhesion and intercellular communication.

LYMPHOCYTE ACTIVATION

Both T and B cells are activated on binding their specific antigens. T cells need to 'see' antigen in the context of MHC molecules on accessory cells, whereas B cells can bind to free antigens, but generally need T-cell help to become activated.

Following interaction of resting lymphocytes with their antigens, there are a number of early biochemical events which result in the generation of 'second messengers' within the B cell or T cell. These are responsible for changes at the level of the cell's DNA.

Both T and B cells utilize a GTP-dependent component (or G-protein) to induce these signalling reactions.

These G-proteins stimulate phosphatidylinositol metabolism. This reaction generates two secondary messengers, inositol 1,4,5-trisphosphate (IP$_3$) and diacylglycerol. The former triggers the release of Ca^{2+} ions from internal stores, while the latter activates protein kinase C. Together with other kinases, protein kinase C phosphorylates a number of surface molecules.

At the same time, a number of surface receptors for cytokines such as IL-2 are produced. Interaction with these cytokines results in proliferation and maturation of the lymphocytes.

Clonal selection through antigen recognition results in expansion of specific clones, which either terminally differentiate into effector cells or gives rise to memory cells (Fig. 2.19). Memory cells recirculate and home to T- or B-dependent areas of lymphoid tissues where they stay, ready to respond it the same antigen is encountered again. Antigen-induced lymphocyte proliferation normally occurs in the lymphoid tissues and can be visualized *in vitro* by cultivating lymphoid cells with specific antigens. Even in the absence of antigens, mitogenic lectins (carbohydrate-binding proteins which stimulate cell division) will polyclonally stimulate lymphoid cells. These mitogenic lectins (mitogens) are derived from various plants and bacteria. Monoclonal antibody to the surface molecules CD3–TCR, or to one epitope of CD2, are also mitogenic for all T cells. Their use *in vitro* has shown that activation of T and B cells results in the production of cytokines, and their receptors, which together drive the cells through their cell cycle (proliferation) and ultimately to effector function (maturation). Lymphocyte activation, by either antigens or mitogens, results in intracellular changes and subsequent development into lymphoblasts. Mitogen stimulation of lymphocytes *in vitro* is believed to mimic stimulation by specific antigens fairly closely.

T and B cells are activated by different mitogens. Phytohaemagglutinin (PHA) and Concanavalin-A (Con-A) stimulate human and mouse T cells. Lipopolysaccharide (LPS) stimulates mouse B cells, while pokeweed mitogen (PWM) stimulates both human T cells and B cells (Fig. 2.20).

Following T and B cell activation by mitogen or antigen, distinctive differentiation features are observed at the ultrastructural level (see Figs 2.8 and 2.21). Ultimately, many B cell blasts mature into antibody forming cells (AFCs), which progress *in vivo* to terminally differentiated plasma cells. Some B blasts do not develop rough endoplasmic reticulum cisternae. These cells are found in germinal centres and are named follicle centre cells or centroblasts and centrocytes. It seems likely that these are the B memory cells whose existence is inferred from the ability of the immune system to develop lasting immunity (Fig. 2.22).

Under light microscopy, the cytoplasm of the plasma cells is basophilic; this is due to the large amount of RNA being utilized for antibody synthesis in the rough endoplasmic reticulum (Fig. 2.23). At the ultrastructural level, the rough endoplasmic reticulum can often be

Clonal expansion of lymphocytes

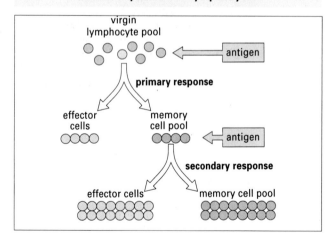

Fig. 2.19 T and B cells carrying antigen receptors are produced in the primary lymphoid organs and form the 'virgin' lymphoid pool. Following stimulation by antigen, those cells whose receptors are specific for that antigen proliferate and form clones. These may either become effector cells (e.g. T cells with cytotoxic or other functions, or antibody-secreting plasma cells from mature B cells), or memory cells. This cellular proliferation is the primary response. When the memory cells are again stimulated by antigen they also proliferate (the secondary response). Some cells of the clone mature into effector cells, while others again become memory cells, thus increasing the size of both effector and memory cell pools.

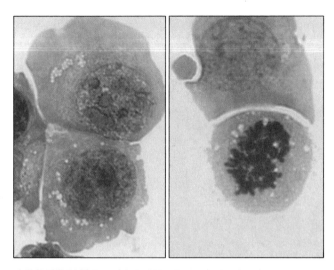

Fig. 2.20 Mitogen/antigen-induced lymphocyte blastogenesis. The human T cells and B cells shown here have been stimulated by pokeweed mitogen. Left: There is increased basophilia in the cytoplasm and an increase in the cell volume. Right: The chromosomes condense during cell division, and can be clearly seen during metaphase. Giemsa stain, × 2000.

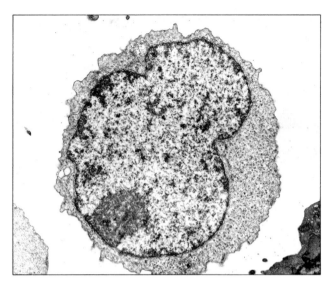

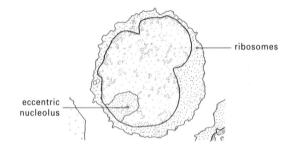

Fig. 2.22 A small follicle centre cell. This shows extended cytoplasm largely occupied by polyribosomes and a few strands of rough endoplasmic reticulum (ER) but no cisternae (parallel arrays of ER). The large eccentric nucleolus adjacent to the nuclear envelope is of note. This cell, which may correspond to the memory B cell, is also frequently seen as a tumour cell in lymphomas. × 8500.

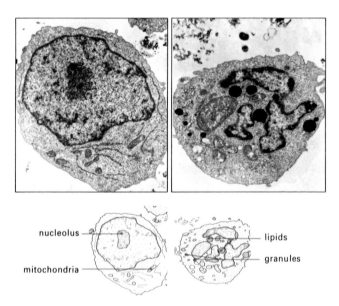

Fig. 2.21 The ultrastructure of T cell blasts. T cell blasts, developing after antigen or mitogen stimulation, are large cells with extended cytoplasm containing a variety of organelles, including mitochondria and free polyribosomes. The blasts may be 'agranular' (left) or granular (right) depending on the presence or absence of electron-dense granules. Note also the lipid droplets in the granular blast. Studies on T cell clones (i.e. population derived from a single cells) have shown that in humans all cytotoxic clones are granular. Studies in the mouse have shown that both cytotoxic and suppressor clones are granular, whereas those clones without these functions are agranular. × 3200.

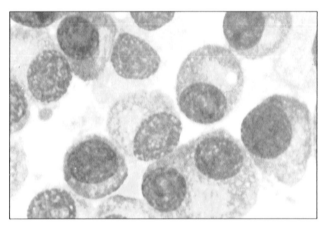

Fig. 2.23 Morphology of the plasma cell. The mature plasma cell has an eccentric nucleus and a large amount of basophilic cytoplasm, which is due to the abundant RNA required for protein synthesis. May–Grünwald–Giemsa stain, × 1500.

seen in parallel arrays (Fig. 2.24). Plasma cells are seldom seen in the circulation (less than 0.1% of lymphocytes) and are normally restricted to the secondary lymphoid organs and tissues. Antibodies produced by a single plasma cell are of one specificity and immunoglobulin class. Immunoglobulins can be visualized in the plasma cell cytoplasm by staining with fluorochrome-labelled specific antibodies (Fig. 2.25).

ACTIVATION MARKERS

Activation of T and B cells results in increased expression of some existing surface molecules, and the *de novo* appearance of others (activation markers). These molecules include adhesion molecules, which allow a more efficient interaction with other cells, and receptors for growth and differentiation 'factors,' required for continued cell proliferation and differentiation. As indicated above, the IL-2 receptor (IL-2R) is expressed following T cell activation. This is composed of a low-affinity receptor of 55 kDa (CD25) and a larger intermediate-affinity molecule of 70 kDa. Together they make up a heterodimer – the high affinity IL-2R. Receptors for CD71 (transferrin, important for proliferation) and CD38 are also generated on activated T cells. These two markers are also expressed in the early phase of T cell ontogeny, but disappear during intrathymic development (see Chapter 11). Class II MHC molecules are expressed by human T cells as late activation markers, but not by murine T cells. CD29, is expressed as a very late activation marker on T cells and by the cells designated as 'memory cells'. The 'memory' function of the CD4+CD29+ cell population might therefore be explained as an activation-induced increase in various adhesion molecules, which facilitates interaction with other cells should the animal encounter the antigen again.

Activation markers on B cells include the high affinity IL-2R, and other receptors for growth and differentiation factors such as IL-3, IL-4, IL-5 and IL-6 (see Chapter 8). These receptors have recently all been cloned and sequenced. Transferrin receptors (CD71) and elevated levels of membrane class II MHC molecules are also detected. CD23 (Fc$_\epsilon$RII, a low-affinity IgE receptor) is present on murine and human activated B cells and is involved in driving B cells into proliferation. CD38, although not present on mature human B cells, is found on terminally differentiated plasma cells (as well as in the very early stages of B cell development). PCA-1 molecules are only found on the plasma cell stage of human B cell differentiation. Memory cells within the germinal centres of secondary follicles (see chapter 11) do not express surface IgD or CD22.

Activation markers of NK cells include the class II MHC molecules.

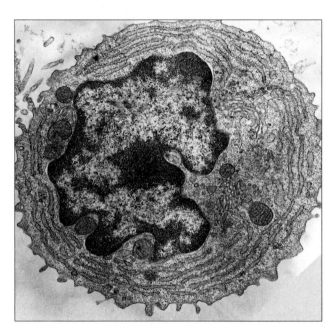

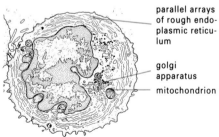

parallel arrays of rough endo-plasmic reticulum

golgi apparatus

mitochondrion

Fig. 2.24 The ultrastructure of the plasma cell. The plasma cell is characterized by parallel arrays of rough endoplasmic reticulum. In mature cells, these cisternae become dilated with immunoglobulins. Mitochondria and a well-developed Golgi apparatus are also seen. × 9500.

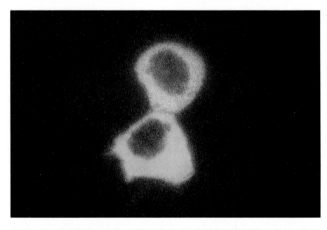

Fig. 2.25 The immunofluorescent staining of intracytoplasmic immunoglobulin in plasma cells. Fixed human plasma cells, treated with fluoresceinated anti-human–IgM (green) and rhodaminated anti-human-IgG (red) show extensive intracytoplasmic staining. As the distinct staining of the two cells shows, plasma cells normally only manufacture one class (isotype) of antibody. × 3000.

MONONUCLEAR PHAGOCYTES

Bone-marrow derived stem cells give rise to mono-nuclear phagocyte system. This system has two main functions, performed by two different types of cells:
1. the 'professional' phagocytic macrophages whose predominant role is to remove particulate antigens
2. antigen-presenting cells (APCs) whose role is to present antigen to lymphocytes.

THE MONONUCLEAR PHAGOCYTE SYSTEM

The phagocytic tissue macrophages form a network, known as the mononuclear phagocyte system, (previously included with endothelial cells and polymorphs under the term 'the reticuloendothelial system' or RES), which is found in many organs (Fig. 2.26). Intravenously injected carbon particles become localized in these tissues (Fig. 2.27).

The mononuclear phagocyte system

circulating blood monocytes
capillary endothelial cell

Kupffer cells in the liver
sinusoidal space
endothelial cell
hepatocyte
Kupffer cell

intraglomerular mesangium of the kidney
basement membrane
mesangial macrophage
endothelium
podocyte

alveolar macrophages in the lung
pneumocyte type II
macrophage
air space
pneumocyte type I
basement membrane
capillary

serosal macrophages
mesothelium
basement membrane
reticular fibres
macrophage
capillary

brain microglia
ependyma
microglial cell
capillary
nerve cell

spleen sinus macrophages
macrophage
reticular fibres
erythrocyte
sinus endothelium

lymph node sinus macrophages
macrophages
endothelial cell

Fig. 2.26 This system includes blood monocytes, and phago-cytes resident in tissues or fixed to the endothelial layer of blood capillaries. In the liver the latter are known as Kupffer cells, while in the kidney they are called the intraglomerular mesangial cells. Alveolar and serosal (eg. peritoneal) macrophages are examples of 'wandering' macrophages, while brain microglia are cells which enter the brain around the time of birth and differentiate into fixed cells.

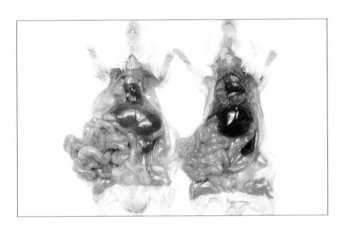

liver
gut
lung
spleen

Fig. 2.27 Localization of intravenously injected particles in the reticuloendothelial system. A mouse was injected intravenously with fine carbon particles and killed 5 minutes later. Carbon accumulates in organs rich in mononuclear phagocytes – lungs, liver, spleen and areas of the gut wall. Normal organ colour is shown in the control mouse (left).

The progenitors of the myeloid cells give rise to promonocytes in the bone marrow (see Chapter 11). These differentiate into blood monocytes, which represent a circulating pool. They migrate (through the blood-vessel walls) into the various organs and tissue systems to become macrophages. Since blood mono-

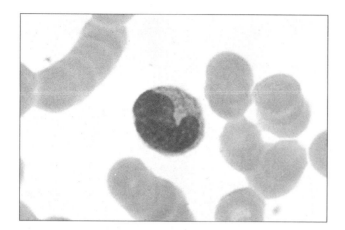

Fig. 2.28 Morphology of the monocyte. Blood monocytes have a characteristic horseshoe-shaped nucleus and are larger than most circulating lymphocytes. Giemsa stain, × 1200.

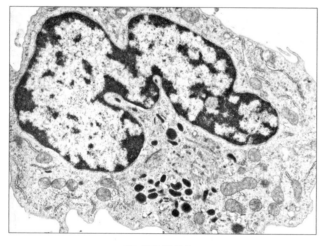

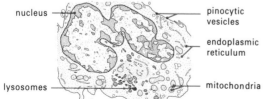

Fig. 2.29 The ultrastructure of the monocyte. This shows the horseshoe-shaped nucleus, the pinocytic vesicles, lysosomal granules, mitochondria and isolated rough endoplasmic reticulum cisternae. × 8000. (Courtesy of Dr B. Nichols, from *J Cell Biol* 1971:**50**;498, with permission.)

cytes are more easily obtained than macrophages they have been studied in greatest detail. The human blood monocyte is large (10–18 μm diameter) relative to the lymphocyte. It usually has a horseshoe-shaped nucleus and often contains faint azurophilic granules (Fig. 2.28). Ultrastructurally, the monocyte possesses ruffled membranes, a well-developed Golgi complex and many intracytoplasmic lysosomes (Fig. 2.29). These lysosomes contain peroxidase and several acid hydrolases which are important in intracellular killing of microorganisms.

Monocytes/macrophages adhere strongly to glass and plastic surfaces, and actively phagocytose organisms or even tumour cells *in vitro*. Adherence and ingestion by monocytes occurs when the cells bind the microorganisms through specialized receptors. The receptors may bind to certain carbohydrates of the microbial cell wall, or to IgG and complement, with which the microorganism has become coated.

Human and murine monocyte/macrophages have mannosyl–fucosyl receptors (MFR) which bind to these sugars on the surface of microorganisms. Monocytes/macrophages also have CD14, a receptor for lipopolysaccharide binding protein (LBP) which is normally present in serum and coats Gram-negative bacteria. There are also three distinct Fc receptors for IgG on human and murine macrophages. Fc$_\gamma$RI (CD64) on human cells has a high affinity for IgG. This is homologous to the Fc$_\gamma$RIIa receptor in the mouse. Fc$_\gamma$RII (CD32) is of medium affinity and is equivalent to the Fc$_\gamma$RIIb/1 receptor in the mouse. Finally, Fc$_\gamma$RIII (CD16) or Fc$_\gamma$RIIIlo (mouse equivalent) is of low affinity. These receptors probably have different functions which include triggering extracellular killing, or opsonization and phagocytosis. Other receptors are important in

Summary of the main surface markers on murine and human monocytes/macrophages

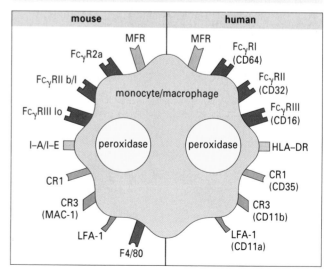

Fig. 2.30 Equivalent molecules are shown in the same colour.

uptake of microorganisms including the complement receptor, CR1 (C3b receptor, CD35). Additional molecules, probably involved mainly in adhesion, include the complement receptor CR3 (C3bi receptors, CD11b, MAC-1), present especially on activated macrophages, together with the 'leucocyte function antigen' LFA-1 (CD11a) and p150,95 (CD11c). Both CD11b and CD11c are found in intracytoplasmic vesicles (of macrophages) and are rapidly expressed following activation. Class II MHC antigens are present on some of the monocytes/macrophages and are important in presentation of antigens to T cells. A low affinity receptor for the Fc of IgE (Fc$_\epsilon$RII; CD23) is also present on some macrophages. Other molecules found on human macrophages include CD13, CD15, CD68 and VLA-4 (CD29/CD49d). It should be stressed that none of these markers so far discussed are lineage specific, although Fc$_\gamma$RI is a particularly useful marker. Lineage specific markers in the mouse include F480 (160 kDa), sheep erythrocyte receptor (SER, not to be confused with CD2) and erythroblast receptor (EbR). The main markers on human and mouse monocytes are summarized in Fig. 2.30.

In addition to all of these molecules, monocytes and macrophages also have receptors for cytokines such as IL4, IFNγ and migration inhibition factor. The functions of monocytes and macrophages can therefore be enhanced by T-cell derived cytokines through these receptors. Such 'activated' monocytes/macrophages also generate cytokines including IFNs, IL-1 and TNF (see Chapter 8). Complement components and prostaglandins are also produced. Like neutrophils, monocytes and macrophages contain peroxidase, which inactivates the peroxide ions that they generate while killing ingested microorganisms.

ANTIGEN-PRESENTING CELLS

APCs are a heterogeneous population of leucocytes with exquisite immunostimulatory capacity. Some have a pivotal role in the induction of functional activity of TH cells; some communicate with other leucocytes. Cells other than leucocytes, such as endothelial or epithelial cells, can acquire the ability to 'present' antigens when stimulated by cytokines. Such cells do not usually express class II MHC molecules, but are induced to express them when they act as APCs.

APCs are found primarily in the skin, lymph nodes, spleen and thymus (Fig. 2.31). The archetypal APCs are the Langerhans' cells in the skin. They migrate, as 'veiled cells', via the afferent lymphatics into the lymph node paracortex of the draining lymph nodes. Within the paracortex the cells 'interdigitate' with many T cells (Fig. 2.32). This migration provides an efficient mechanism for carrying antigen from the skin to the TH cells located in the lymph nodes. These APCs are rich in class II MHC molecules, which are important for presenting antigen to TH cells.

Other specialized APCs, the follicular dendritic cells, are found in the secondary follicles of the B cell areas of the lymph nodes and spleen. They present antigen

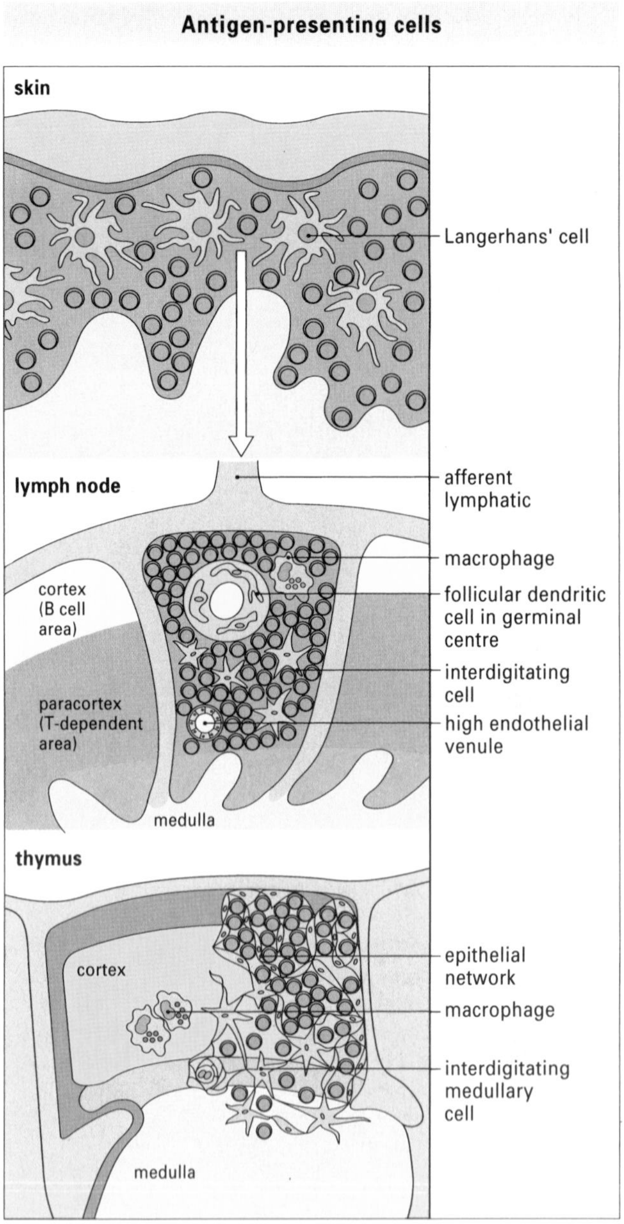

Antigen-presenting cells

skin — Langerhans' cell

— afferent lymphatic

lymph node — macrophage
cortex (B cell area) — follicular dendritic cell in germinal centre
— interdigitating cell
paracortex (T-dependent area) — high endothelial venule
medulla

thymus
cortex — epithelial network
— macrophage
— interdigitating medullary cell
medulla

Fig. 2.31 Bone-marrow derived antigen-presenting cells (APCs) are found especially in lymphoid tissues and in the skin. APCs are represented in the skin by Langerhans' cells, found in the epidermis and characterized by special granules (the tennis-racket-shaped Birbeck granules). These cells, rich in Ia (mouse) or HLA-DR (human) determinants, are believed to carry antigens and migrate via the afferent lymphatics (where they appear as 'veiled' cells) into the paracortex of the draining lymph nodes. Here they interdigitate with T cells. These 'interdigitating cells', localized in the T cell-dependent cells areas of the lymph node, present antigen to lymphocytes. Presentation to B cells is by follicular dendritic cells, which are found in the B cell areas of the lymph nodes, and in particular in the germinal centres. Some macrophages located in the outer cortex and marginal sinus may also act as APCs. In the thymus, APCs occur as interdigitating medullary cells.

to B cells and lack class II MHC molecules, but have the complement receptor CRI (CD35) for interaction with immune complexes. Some markers on the different kinds of APCs are shown in Fig. 2.33.

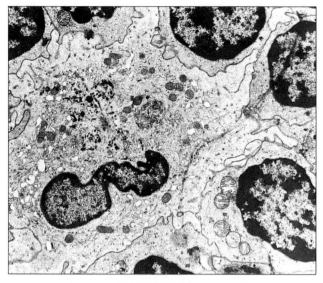

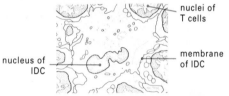

nuclei of
T cells

nucleus of
IDC

membrane
of IDC

Fig. 2.32 The ultrastructure of an interdigitating cell (IDC) in the T cell area of the rat lymph node. Intimate contacts are made with the membranes of the surrounding T cells. The cytoplasm contains relatively few organelles and does not show the Birbeck granules characteristic of the skin Langerhans' cells, which appear after antigenic stimulation. × 2000. (Courtesy of Dr B. H. Balfour.)

APCs have recently been found in the thymus, and are especially abundant in the thymic medulla. They are rich in self antigens, including class II MHC molecules. The thymus is of crucial importance in the development and maturation of T cells, and it appears that the interdigitating cells play a role in deleting T cells that react against self antigen. This process is referred to as 'negative selection' (see chapter 10).

B cells, which are rich in class II MHC molecules (especially after 'activation'), can also process and present antigen, particularly when the B cell is specific for the antigen being presented (see Chapter 7).

Somatic cells other than immune cells do not normally express class II MHC molecules, but cytokines such as IFN_γ and TNF can induce these molecules on some cell types and thus allow them to present antigen. Such induction of 'inappropriate' class II expression might contribute to the pathogenesis of autoimmune diseases.

POLYMORPHONUCLEAR GRANULOCYTES AND PLATELETS

Polymorphonuclear granulocytes (polymorphs) are produced in the bone marrow at a rate of 80 million per minute and are short-lived (2-3 days) relative to monocytes/macrophages which may live for months or years. Granulocytes make up about 60–70% of the total normal blood leucocytes but are also found in extravascular sites. Like monocytes polymorphs can adhere to endothelial cells lining the blood vessels, and extravasate (squeeze between them to escape from the blood vessel). This process is known as diapedesis. The adhesion is mediated by polymorph receptors, and their ligands on the endothelial cell (see chapter 13). As the name suggests, mature polymorphs usually contain a multilobed nucleus and many granules. They are classified into neutrophils, eosinophils and basophils, on

Markers on different antigen-presenting cells

cell markers	cell type				
	Langerhans' cells	interdigitating cells	follicular dendritic cells	B cells	macrophages
MHC class II	+	+	–	+	(+)
FcγR	+	–	+	+	+
CR1 (CD35)	+	–	+	+	+
phagocyte function	–	–	–	–	+

Fig. 2.33 The Langerhans' cells (LCs), and the interdigitating cells derived from them, are rich in class II MHC for communicating with CD4+ T cells. LCs also possess receptors for IgG (FcγR) and for the complement protein C3b (CR1). Follicular dendritic cells located within the secondary follicles do not express class II MHC but have high levels of FcγR and CR1 to enable them to trap immune complexes and interact with B cells. B cells and macrophages are also efficient as antigen-presenting cells and have been included for completeness.

the basis of the staining reaction of their granules with histological dyes.

Polymorphs do not show any inherent specificity for antigens, but they play an important role in acute inflammation (with antibodies and complement) in pro-tection against microorganisms. Their predominant role is phagocytosis. The importance of polymorphs is shown in individuals with low numbers of circulating polymorphs, or in rare genetic defects which prevent polymorph extravasation in response to chemotactic stimuli. Both defects markedly increase susceptibility to infection.

NEUTROPHILS

Neutrophils constitute over 90% of the circulating poly-morphs and are 10–20 μm in diameter (Fig. 2.34).

Chemotactic agents for neutrophils include protein fragments released when complement is activated (e.g. C5a), factors derived from the fibrinolytic and kinin sys-tems, the products of other leucocytes, and platelets, and the products of certain bacteria. Chemotactic stim-uli result in neutrophil margination (adhesion to endothelial cells) and diapedesis (movement through the capillary wall). Neutrophils possess two main types of granules. The primary (azurophilic) granules are lysosomes containing acid hydrolases, myeloperoxidase and muramidase (lysozyme). The secondary or specific granules contain lactoferrin in addition to lysozyme. These granules are shown in Fig. 2.35. Ingested organ-isms are contained within vacuoles termed phago-somes, which fuse with the lysosomes to form phagolysosomes (Fig. 2.36).

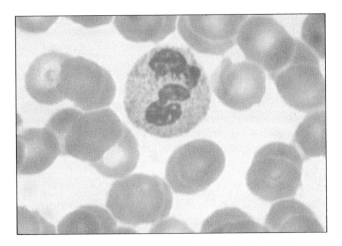

Fig. 2.34 Morphology of the neutrophil. This shows a neutrophil with its characteristic multilobed nucleus and neutrophilic granules in the cytoplasm. Giemsa stain, × 1500.

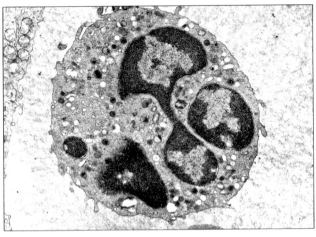

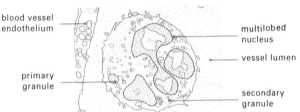

Fig. 2.35 The ultrastructure of the neutrophil. This mouse neutrophil lies within a skin blood vessel. The neutrophil cytoplasm contains primary and secondary granules of different electron opacity. × 6000. (Courtesy of Dr D. McLaren.)

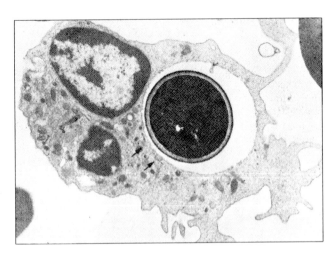

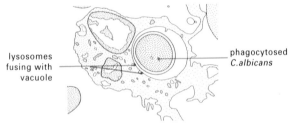

Fig. 2.36 A neutrophil that has phagocytosed a *Candida albicans* **cell.** Two lysosomal granules can be seen fusing with the vacuole containing the yeast cell. × 7000. (Courtesy of Dr H. Validimarsson.)

Extracellular release of granules and cytotoxic substances by neutrophils can also occur, when they are activated through their Fcγ receptors by immune complexes. This may be an important pathogenic mechanism in immune-complex diseases (Type III hypersensitivity, see Chapter 21).

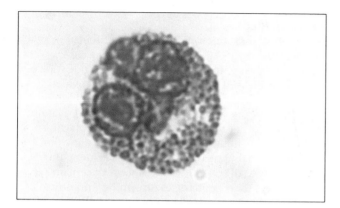

Fig. 2.37 Morphology of the eosinophil. The multilobed nucleus is stained blue and the cytoplasmic granules are stained red. Leishman stain, × 1800.

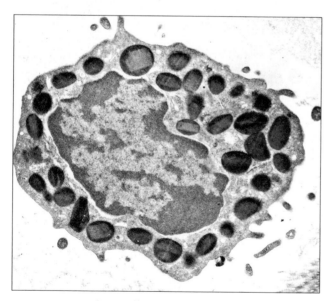

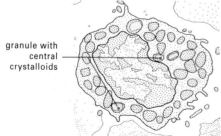

granule with central crystalloids

Fig. 2.38 The ultrastructure of a guinea-pig eosinophil. The mature eosinophil contains granules with central crystalloids. × 8000. (Courtesy of Dr D. McLaren.)

EOSINOPHILS

Eosinophils (Fig. 2.37) comprise 2–5% of blood leucocytes in healthy, non-allergic individuals. They appear to be capable of phagocytosing and killing ingested microorganisms, although it is not their primary function. The granules in mature eosinophils are membrane-bound organelles with a 'crystalloid' core, differing in electron opacity from the surrounding matrix (Fig. 2.38). Human blood eosinophils usually have only a bilobed nucleus and many cytoplasmic granules.

Eosinophils (as well as basophils and mast cells both described below) can be triggered to 'degranulate' by appropriate stimuli. Degranulation involves fusion of the intracellular granules with the plasma membrane. The contents are released to the outside of the cell. This type of reaction is the only way that these cells can use their 'granule armament' against large targets which cannot be phagocytosed. Eosinophils are thought to play a specialized role in immunity to parasitic worms using this mechanism (see Chapter 16).

Eosinophils are attracted by products released from T cells, mast cells and basophils (eosinophil chemotactic factor of anaphylaxis, or ECF-A). They bind schistosomules (worm larvae) coated with IgG or IgE, degranulate, and release a toxic protein ('major basic protein'). Eosinophils also release histaminase and aryl sulphatase, which inactivate two mast cell products, histamine and the slow reactive substance of anaphylaxis (SRS-A), respectively. The effect of these two factors is to dampen down the inflammatory response and reduce granulocyte migration into the site of invasion.

BASOPHILS AND MAST CELLS

Basophils are found in very small numbers in the circulation (less than 0.2% of leucocytes) and are characterized by deep violet blue granules (Fig. 2.39). The mast cell, which is not found at all in the circulation, only resident in body tissues, is often indistinguishable from

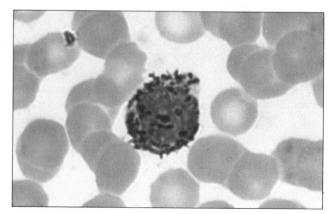

Fig. 2.39 Morphology of the basophil. This blood smear shows a typical basophil with its deep violet-blue granules. Wright's stain, × 1500.

the basophil in a number of its properties. Its relationship to the basophil is not completely clear.

There are two different kinds of mast cell; the mucosal mast cell (MMC) associated with mucosal epithelia, and the connective tissue mast cell (CTMC). MMCs appear to be dependent on T cells for their proliferation, while the CTMCs are not. Under light microscopy, both types can be visualized with Alcian blue staining (Fig. 2.40).

Mature blood basophils have randomly distributed granules surrounded by membranes (Fig. 2.41). The granules in both basophils and mast cells contain heparin, SRS-A and ECF-A, and these substances are released on degranulation (Fig. 2.42). The stimulus for degranulation is usually an allergen (an antigen causing allergic reaction). To be effective, an allergen must cross-link IgE molecules bound to the surface of the mast cell or basophil via its high-affinity Fc receptors for IgE ($Fc_\epsilon RI$). Characteristically, the degranulation of basophil or mast cell is substantial, with all the contents of the granules being released simultaneously. This is due to intracytoplasmic fusion of the granules prior to rapid expulsion of their contents to the exterior. Mediators such as histamine, released by degranulation, cause the adverse symptoms of allergy but, on the positive side, they may also play a role in immunity against parasites. Granulocyte and mast cell functional markers are summarized in Fig. 2.43.

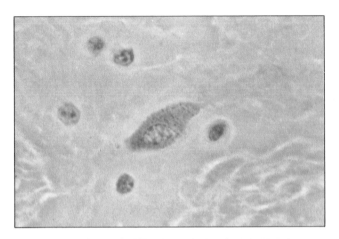

Fig. 2.40 Histological appearance of human connective tissue mast cells. This micrograph shows the dark blue cytoplasm with purple granules. Alcian blue and safranin stain, × 600. (Courtesy of Dr T. S. Orr.)

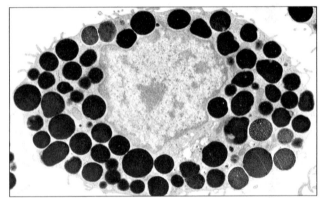

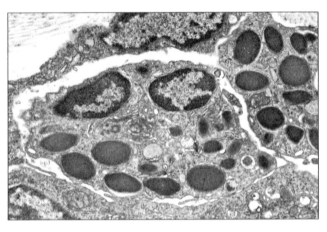

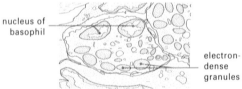

nucleus of basophil

electron-dense granules

Fig. 2.41 The ultrastructure of the basophil. Basophils in guinea-pig skin showing the characteristic randomly distributed granules. ×6000. (Courtesy of Dr D. McLaren.)

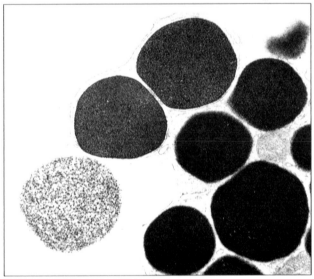

Fig. 2.42 Rat peritoneal mast cells. Upper: A non-degranulated cell with its electron-dense granules. × 6000. Lower: A granule leaving the cell. × 30 000. (Courtesy of Dr T. S. C. Orr.)

Human granulocyte and mast cell functional markers

cell type	cell surface markers									granules		
	C5aR	CR1 (CD35)	CR3 (CD11b)	LFA-1 (CD11a)	VLA-4 (CD49d)	FcγRII (CD32)	FcγRIII (CD16)	Fc$_\epsilon$RI	Fc$_\epsilon$RII (CD23)	peroxidase	acid phosphatase	alkaline phosphatase
neutrophils	+	+	+	+	+	+	+	–	–	+	+	+
eosinophils	+	+	+	+	+	+	±	–	+	+	+	
basophils	+	+	+	+	+		+	+	–	+		
mast cells	+	+	+	+			+	+	–		+	+

Fig. 2.43 Neutrophils, eosinophils, basophils and mast cells all respond to C5a by chemotaxis and therefore must have a receptor for it. They all have receptors for C3 and express the adhesion molecules LFA-1 (CD11a) and VLA-4 (CD49d). They express FcγRII (CD32) and FcγRIII (CD16). Only basophils and mast cells have the high affinity receptor for IgE (Fc$_\epsilon$RI). Several other glycoproteins, including CD13 and CD14 (weakly expressed), are found on some granulocytes. In addition, glycolipid molecules such as the Le x hapten (CD15) and lactosyl ceramide (CD17) are expressed by these cells. The granules in different cell types vary qualitatively in their enzyme content.

PLATELETS

The final myeloid cell to be considered here is the blood platelet. Platelets are derived from megakaryocytes in the bone marrow and contain granules (Fig. 2.44). In addition to their role in blood clotting, platelets are also involved in the immune response, especially in inflammation. They express class I MHC products and receptors for IgG (FcγRII), and low-affinity receptors for IgE (FcγRII; CD23). In addition, megakaryocytes and platelets carry receptors for factor VIII and other molecules important for their function, such as the GpIIb/IIIa complex (CD41) and GpIb/GpIx complex (CD42). The GpIIb/IIIa complex, also termed a cytoadhesin, is responsible for binding to fibrinogen, fibronectin, and vitronectin. In addition, both this complex and the GpIb/GpIx complex are receptors for von Willebrand factor. There is an additional vitronectin receptor, CD51. Both receptors and adhesion molecules are important in activation of platelets. Following injury to endothelial cells, platelets adhere to, and aggregate at, the endothelial surface of damaged vascular tissue. They release substance that increase permeability and factors that activate complement and hence attract leucocytes.

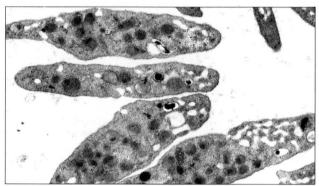

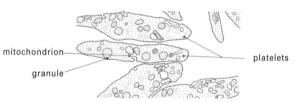

Fig. 2.44 The ultrastructure of a platelet. The cytoplasmic organelles, including granules and mitochondria, are randomly dispersed. × 20 000. (Courtesy of Dr J. G. White.)

FURTHER READING

Gordon JR, Burd PR, Galli SJ. Mast cells as a source of multifunctional cytokines. *Immunol Today* 1990;**11**:458.

Lloyd AR, Oppenheim JJ. Poly's lament: the neglected role of the polymorphonuclear neutrophil in the afferent limb of the immune response. *Immunol Today* 1992;**13**:169.

Playfair JHL. *Immunology at a Glance.* 5th ed. Oxford: Blackwell Scientific Publications, 1992.

Reth M, *et al.* The B-cell antigen receptor complex. *Immunol Today* 1991;**12**:201.

Roitt IM. *Essential Immunology.* 7th ed. Oxford: Blackwell Scientific Publications, 1991.

Romagnini S. Human T$_H$1 and T$_H$2 subsets: doubt no more. *Immunol Today* 1991;**11**:256.

Silverstein S, Unkeliss J, eds. Innate Immunity. *Curr Opin Immunol* 1991;**3**:47–97.

Steinman RM. The dendritic cell system and its role in immunogenicity. *Annu Rev Immunol* 1991;**9**:271.

chapter 3

The Lymphoid System

The cells involved in the immune response are organized into tissues and organs in order to perform their functions most effectively. These structures are collectively referred to as the lymphoid system.

PRIMARY AND SECONDARY LYMPHOID TISSUES

The lymphoid system comprises lymphocytes, accessory cells (macrophages and antigen-presenting cells) and, in some tissues, epithelial cells. It is arranged into either discretely capsulated organs or accumulations of diffuse lymphoid tissue. The major lymphoid organs and tissues are classified into either primary (central) or secondary (peripheral) lymphoid organs (Fig. 3.1).

Major lymphoid organs and tissues

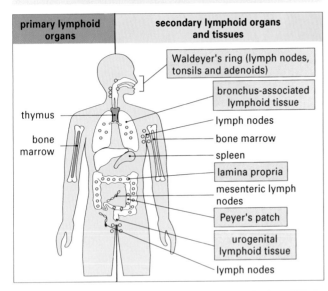

primary lymphoid organs	secondary lymphoid organs and tissues

Waldeyer's ring (lymph nodes, tonsils and adenoids)

bronchus-associated lymphoid tissue

lymph nodes

bone marrow

spleen

lamina propria

mesenteric lymph nodes

Peyer's patch

urogenital lymphoid tissue

lymph nodes

thymus

bone marrow

Fig 3.1 Thymus and bone marrow are primary lymphoid organs. They are the sites of maturation for T and B cells respectively. Cellular and humoral immune responses occur in the secondary (peripheral) lymphoid organs and tissues; effector and memory cells are generated here. Secondary lymphoid organs can be classified according to the body regions which they defend. The spleen responds predominantly to blood-borne antigens. Lymph nodes mount immune responses to antigens circulating in the lymph, absorbed either through the skin (superficial nodes) or from internal viscera (deep lymph nodes). Tonsils, Peyer's patches and other mucosa-associated lymphoid tissues (blue boxes) respond to antigens which have penetrated the mucosal barriers. Note that bone marrow is both a primary and a secondary lymphoid organ.

Primary lymphoid organs are the major sites of lymphopoiesis. Here, lymphocytes differentiate from lymphoid stem cells, proliferate and mature into functional cells. In mammals, T cells mature in the thymus, B cells in the fetal liver and bone marrow (see Chapter 11). Birds have a specialized site of B-cell maturation, the bursa of Fabricius. In primary lymphoid organs the lymphocytes acquire their repertoire of specific antigen receptors, in order to cope with antigenic challenges the individual receives during its life. The cells are selected for tolerance to self-antigens, and are capable of recognizing only non-self antigens; this recognition is needed in order to make an immune response.

Secondary lymphoid organs include the spleen, lymph nodes and mucosa-associated tissues, including the tonsils and the Peyer's patches of the gut. Secondary lymphoid tissue provides an environment in which lymphocytes can interact with each other and with antigens. It also disseminates the immune response. These functions are performed by phagocytic macrophages, antigen-presenting cells (APCs), and mature T and B cells in the secondary lymphoid organs.

PRIMARY LYMPHOID ORGANS

THE THYMUS

The thymus in mammals is bilobed and located in the thorax, overlying the heart and major blood vessels. Each lobe is organized into lobules separated by connective tissue trabeculae (Fig. 3.2). Within each lobule the lymphoid cells (thymocytes) are arranged into an outer cortex and an inner medulla (Fig. 3.3). The tightly packed cortex contains the majority of relatively immature proliferating thymocytes whereas the medulla contains more mature cells, implying a differentiation gradient from cortex to medulla. Mature thymocytes in the medulla express CD44, which is not detected on cortical thymocytes. This receptor, which binds to hyaluronate and other connective tissue components, is found on all trafficking T cells and is not expressed on sessile lymphocytes. There is a network of epithelial cells throughout the lobules which plays a role in the differentiation process from bone marrow-derived stem cells to T cells. At least three types of epithelial cells can be distinguished in the thymic lobules according to structure, function and phenotype. These are the epithelial nurse cells of the outer cortex, the cortical epithelial cells forming a network, and the medullary epithelial cells, mostly organized into clusters (see Chapter 11). In addition, interdigitating (ID) cells and macrophages, both derived from bone marrow, are found in thymic lobules, particularly at the corti-comedullary junction. Traffic of cells into and out of the thymus occurs via high endothelial venules (HEVs) in this region. Epithelial cells, ID cells and macrophages express MHC molecules, which are vital for T cell development.

Hassall's corpuscles are found in the thymic medulla. Their function is unknown but they appear to contain degenerating epithelial cells, rich in high molecular weight cytokeratins.

The mammalian thymus involutes with age – in man, atrophy begins at puberty and continues throughout life. Thymic involution begins within the cortex and this region may disappear completely; medullary remnants persist. Cortical atrophy is related to corticosteroid sensitivity of the cortical thymocytes. Thus, all conditions associated with acute increase in steroids (e.g. pregnancy, stress) promote thymic atrophy. However, it is conceivable that T-cell generation within the thymus continues into adult life, albeit at a low rate.

THE BURSA OF FABRICIUS AND ITS MAMMALIAN EQUIVALENT

In birds, B cells differentiate in the bursa of Fabricius, hence the term 'B' cells. The bursa is a modified section of the dorsal wall of the cloaca – the common exit of the intestinal and genitourinary tracts in birds. It is composed of folds or plicae (like villi in the intestine) which are directed towards a central lumen (Fig. 3.4). Bursal follicles are organized into a cortex and a medulla and lie along the outer margins of the plicae, arranged along this surface in close contact with the surface epithelium.

Mammals have no bursa; instead, islands of haemopoietic cells in the fetal liver, and in the fetal and adult bone marrow, give rise directly to B lymphocytes. As well as being a site of B-cell generation, the adult bone marrow contains mature T cells and numerous plasma cells. Thus, in man, the bone marrow is also an important secondary lymphoid organ.

SECONDARY LYMPHOID ORGANS AND TISSUES

The generation of lymphocytes in primary lymphoid organs (lymphopoiesis) is followed by their migration into the secondary peripheral tissues. The secondary lymphoid tissues comprise well-organized encapsulated organs – the spleen and lymph nodes – and non-encapsulated accumulations throughout the body. The bulk of this non-encapsulated lymphoid tissue is found in association with mucosal surfaces and is called the mucosa-associated lymphoid tissue (MALT).

The secondary lymphoid tissues, in which T-cell-mediated and humoral effector mechanisms are generated, can be functionally divided into systemic organs and a mucosal system. Among the systemic organs, the spleen is responsive to blood-borne antigens whereas the lymph nodes protect the organism from antigens which come from tissues via the lymphatic system. Responses to antigens encountered via these routes result in secretion of antibodies into the circulation, and in local cell-mediated responses. In contrast, the mucosal system protects the organism from antigens

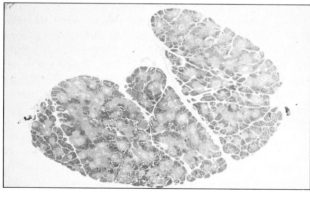

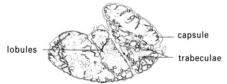

lobules — capsule
trabeculae

Fig. 3.2 Thymus section showing the lobular structure.
This low power cross-section shows a fibrous capsule with the thymocytes (developing T cells) organized into lobules separated from each other by connective tissue trabeculae. H&E stain, × 3.5.

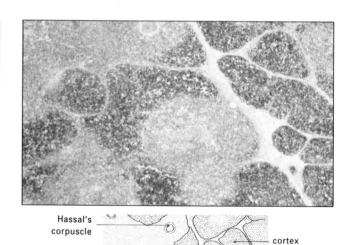

Hassal's corpuscle

medulla

cortex

trabecula

Fig. 3.3 Thymus section showing the lobular organization.
This section shows the two main areas of the thymus lobule – an outer cortex of rapidly dividing immature cells and an inner medulla of more mature cells. Hassall's corpuscles are found in the medulla. H&E stain, × 25.

entering the body directly through mucosal epithelial surfaces. Lymphoid tissues are found associated with surfaces lining the intestinal tract (gut-associated lymphoid tissues, or GALT), the respiratory tract (bronchial-associated lymphoid tissue, or BALT) and the genitourinary tract. The major effector mechanism at these sites is sIgA, secreted directly onto the mucosal epithelial surfaces of the tract. It is perhaps not surprising that the bulk of the body's lymphoid tissues are found associated with the mucosal system, especially the GALT, since this is a major pathway of entry for external antigens.

THE SYSTEMIC LYMPHOID ORGANS
The Spleen

The spleen lies at the upper left of the abdomen, behind the stomach and close to the diaphragm. Its outer layer consists of a capsule of collagenous bundles of fibres which penetrate into the parenchyma of the organ as trabeculae. These, together with a reticular framework, support the variety of cells found within the organ (Fig. 3.5). There are two main types of tissue, the red pulp and the white pulp (Fig. 3.6). The red pulp is mainly concerned with the destruction of aged erythrocytes and is the emergency source of erythrocytes,

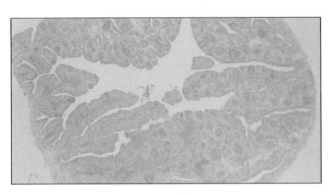

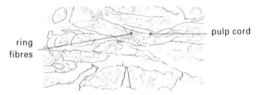

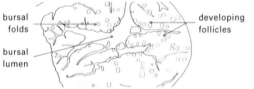

Fig. 3.4 Section of embryonic bursa of Fabricius, showing the follicular structure. The avian bursa of Fabricius is a lympho-epithelial organ (like the thymus) and is found dorsal to the hindgut. The lumen of the bursa opens into the cloaca. Like the thymic lobules, bursal follicles are arranged into an outer cortex and inner medulla. The bursa, like the thymus, atrophies with age. H&E stain, × 10.

Fig. 3.5 Spleen section showing the connective tissue framework. This section is stained for reticulin and shows the architecture of the red pulp cords and the ring fibres which support the endothelial cells of the venous sinuses. The latter blood vessels have a discontinuous wall which allows free flow of plasma into their lumen, and selective passage of cells from the red pulp cords. × 125.

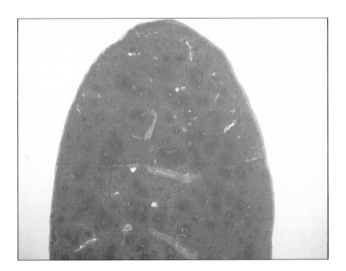

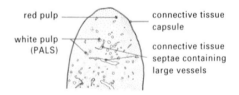

Fig. 3.6 Spleen section showing the tissue organization. This cross-section of the spleen shows the lymphoid tissue localized in the white pulp around the arterioles. The lymphoid tissue in the periarteriolar lymphoid sheaths (PALS) is easy to distinguish from the red pulp of the spleen. The red pulp is mainly involved in the destruction of aged erythrocytes and platelets, but also contains some lymphocytes, the majority of the plasma cells and a population of resident macrophages. H&E stain, × 7.

granulocytes and platelets which can be instantly delivered into the circulation whenever needed (see below). The white pulp consists of lymphoid tissue – the bulk of which is arranged around a central arteriole – the periarteriolar lymphoid sheath (PALS). The PALS is composed of T and B cell areas, the T cells being found around the central arteriole. B cells may be organ-ized into either primary unstimulated follicles (aggregates of B cells), or secondary stimulated follicles which possess a germinal centre (Figs 3.7 and 3.8).

Follicular dendritic cells and phagocytic macrophages are also found in germinal centres. Specialized macrophages are found in the marginal zone – the area surrounding the PALS. These, together with the follicular dendritic cells of the primary follicles, are the cells which present antigen to B cells in the spleen. Lymphocytes are free to leave and enter the PALS via capillary branches of the central arterioles in the marginal zone, and both T and B cells are found in this area. Some lymphocytes, especially maturing plasmablasts, can pass across the marginal zone via bridges into the red pulp. The red pulp consists of sinuses and cellular cords containing phagocytic macrophages (Fig. 3.9), erythrocytes, platelets, granulocytes, lymphocytes and numerous plasma cells. In addition to immunological functions, the spleen serves as a reservoir for platelets, erythrocytes and granulocytes and is the site where aged platelets and erythrocytes are destroyed.

These functions are made possible by the vascular organization of the spleen. Central arteries surrounded by PALS end with arterial capillaries which open freely within the red pulp cords. Thus, circulating cells reach these cellular cords, where they are trapped. Aged platelets and erythrocytes are recognized and phagocytosed by macrophages; blood cells that are not ingested and destroyed can re-enter the blood circulation by crossing the highly discontinuous walls of the venous sinuses, since plasma flows freely through these sinuses.

LYMPH NODES AND THE LYMPHATIC SYSTEM

The lymph nodes form part of a network which filters antigens from the interstitial tissue fluid and lymph during its passage from the periphery to the thoracic

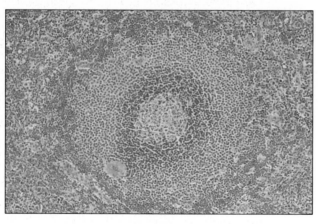

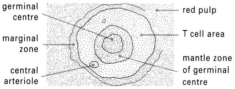

Fig. 3.7 Spleen section showing a periarteriolar lymphoid sheath (PALS). This view shows the lymphoid tissue arranged around an arteriole. The T cells are found close to the central arteriole and the B cell area has a germinal centre. In the unstimulated state the B cell area consists of a primary follicle. The lymphoid tissue is separated from the red pulp by the marginal zone. This contains blood vessels and is the site of entry of blood-borne lymphocytes into the splenic lymphoid areas. H&E stain, × 125.

Schematic organization of lymphoid tissue in the spleen

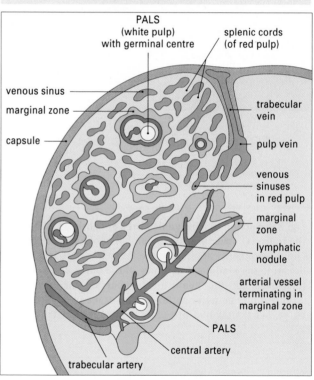

Fig. 3.8 The white pulp is composed of periarteriolar lymphoid sheaths (PALS), frequently containing germinal centres with mantle zones. The white pulp is surrounded by the marginal zone, which contains numerous macrophages, APCs, slowly recirculating B cells and NK cells. The red pulp contains venous sinuses separated by splenic cords. Blood enters the tissues via the trabecular arteries which give rise to the central arteries producing many branches; some end in the white pulp, supplying the germinal centres and mantle zones, but most empty into or near the marginal zones. Some arterial branches run directly into the red pulp, mainly terminating in the cords. The venous sinuses drain blood into the pulp veins and then into the trabecular veins.

duct (Fig. 3.10). Lymph nodes frequently occur at branches of the lymphatic vessels. Clusters of lymph nodes are strategically placed in areas such as the neck, axillae, groin, mediastinum and the abdominal cavity, which drain different superficial and deep regions of the body. Human lymph nodes are 1–15 mm in diameter, are round or kidney-shaped, and have an indentation, the hilus, where blood vessels enter and leave the node. Lymph arrives at the lymph node via several afferent lymphatic vessels, and leaves the node through one efferent lymphatic vessel at the hilus. A typical lymph node, like the spleen, is surrounded by a col-

lagenous capsule (Fig. 3.11). Radial trabeculae, together with reticulin fibres, support the various cellular components within the lymph nodes. The lymph node consists of a B cell area (cortex), a T cell area (paracortex) and a central medulla with cellular cords containing T cells, B cells, plasma cells and abundant macrophages (Fig. 3.12). The paracortex contains many APCs (interdigitating cells) which express high levels of MHC class II

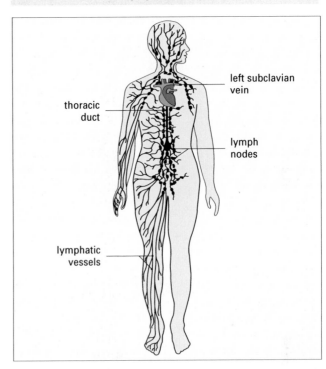

The lymph node system

Fig. 3.10 Lymph nodes are found at junctions of lymphatic vessels and form a complete network, draining and filtering lymph derived from the tissue spaces. They are either superficial or visceral, draining the skin or deep tissues and internal organs of the body. The lymph eventually reaches the thoracic duct which drains into the left subclavian vein and thus back into the circulation.

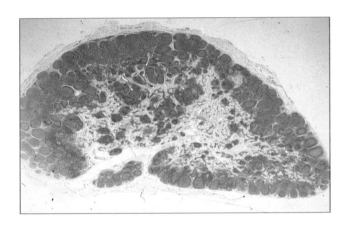

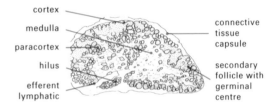

Fig. 3.9 Spleen section showing the red pulp macrophages. Microorganisms in the blood become trapped in the red pulp macrophages of the spleen, which are part of the reticuloendothelial system. This section shows intravenously injected mycobacteria phagocytosed by the red pulp macrophages. Modified Ziehl–Neelsen stain, × 125. (Courtesy of Dr I. Brown.)

Fig. 3.11 Lymph node section. The lymph node is surrounded by a connective tissue capsule and is organized into three main areas – the cortex (B cell area), the paracortex (T cell area) and the medulla, which contains cords of lymphoid tissue (T and B cell area, rich in plasma cells). H&E stain, × 5. (Courtesy of Mr C. Symes.)

surface antigens. The bulk of the lymphoid tissue is found in the cortex and paracortex. Some lymphoid tissue extends into the medulla. It is organized into cords separated by lymph (medullary) sinuses, which drain into the terminal sinus, the origin of the efferent lymphatic vessel (Fig. 3.12). Scavenger phagocytic cells are arranged along the lymph sinuses, especially in the medulla (Figs 3.13 and 3.14). During passage of the lymph across the nodes, from the afferent to the efferent lymphatic, particulate antigens are removed by the phagocytic cells and transported into the lymphoid tissue of the lymph node (Fig. 3.14).

The cortex contains aggregates of B cells (primary or secondary follicles), while T cells are localized primarily in the paracortex. If an area of skin is challenged by a T-dependent antigen, the lymph nodes draining that

Schematic structure of the lymph node

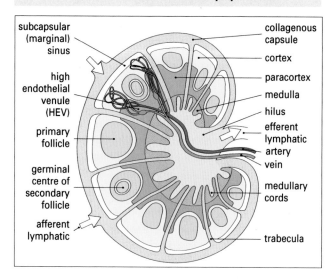

Fig. 3.12 Beneath the collagenous capsule is the subcapsular sinus which is lined by phagocytic cells. Lymphocytes and antigens (if present) pass into the sinus via the afferent lymphatics from surrounding tissue spaces or adjacent nodes. The cortex contains aggregates of B cells (primary follicles) most of which (secondary follicles) have a site of active proliferation (germinal centre). The paracortex contains mainly T cells, many of which are associated with the interdigitating cells (antigen-presenting cells). Each lymph node has its own arterial and venous supply. Lymphocytes enter the node from the circulation through the highly specialized high endothelial venules (HEVs) in the paracortex. The medulla contains both T and B cells and most of the lymph node plasma cells organized into cords of lymphoid tissue. Lymphocytes can only leave the node through the efferent lymphatic vessel.

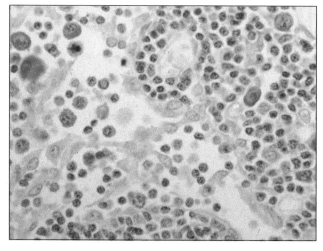

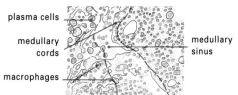

Fig. 3.13 Section of lymph node medulla. This section shows typical plasma cells in the medullary cords and sinuses. The plasma cell cytoplasm stains red with pyronin which binds to RNA. Macrophages are also abundant in this region. Methyl green pyronin stain, × 200.

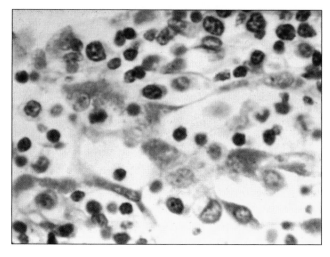

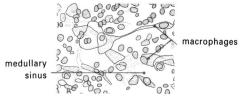

Fig. 3.14 Section of lymph node medulla showing phagocytic macrophages. The macrophages which line the medullary sinuses can be seen following the uptake of red dye. Lithium carmine stain with haematoxylin counterstain, × 330.

particular skin area show active T-cell proliferation in the paracortex (Fig. 3.15). On the other hand, patients with congenital thymic aplasia (DiGeorge syndrome) have fewer cells in the paracortex than normal, as do neonatally thymectomized, or congenitally athymic (nude) mice or rats (Fig. 3.16).

Germinal centres within secondary follicles are seen in antigen-stimulated lymph nodes. These are similar to the germinal centres seen in the B-cell areas of the splenic PALS, and in the B-cell areas of other peripheral lymphoid tissues. Centroblasts and centrocytes are the large and small follicular centre cells, respectively. Proliferating B cells within the germinal centres have a clearly defined nuclear shape (cleaved versus non-cleaved) which is useful in defining certain malignant lymphoproliferative disorders such as lymphomas.

Germinal centres are surrounded by a mantle of lymphocytes (Fig. 3.17). B cells in these areas are rich in surface IgM and IgD, as detected by immunohistochemical

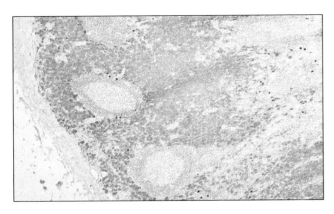

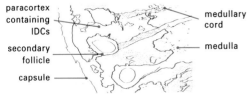

paracortex containing IDCs

secondary follicle

capsule

medullary cord

medulla

Fig. 3.15 Lymph node section showing paracortical proliferation. This shows a lymph node draining the skin area of a patient with chronic eczema. Antigens penetrating the skin are carried to draining lymph nodes by antigen-presenting cells which are normally present in the epidermis, namely Langerhans' cells. These cells are seen as veiled cells in the afferent lymphatics and they settle in the paracortex as interdigitating cells (IDCs), here stained brown with peroxidase-labelled monoclonal antibody. T cell proliferation, in response to specific antigen presented by IDCs, results in paracortical expansion. Haematoxylin counterstain, × 40.

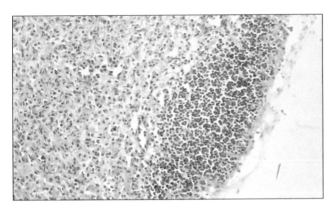

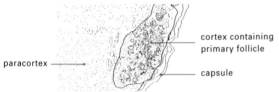

paracortex

cortex containing primary follicle

capsule

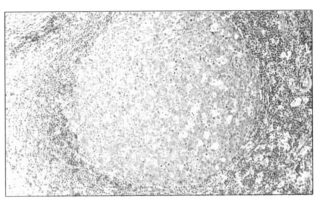

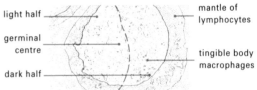

light half

germinal centre

dark half

mantle of lymphocytes

tingible body macrophages

Fig. 3.16 Lymph node section from a congenitally athymic (nude) mouse showing paracortical depletion. A genetic defect in the nude mouse causes thymic aplasia and failure of T cell development. This lymph node section from a 'T-less' mouse shows few cells in the T-dependent paracortex. There are, however, large numbers of interdigitating cells in the paracortex of this node. The cortex is also poorly developed since T cells are required for the organization of the follicles. H&E stain, × 125. (Courtesy of Dr H. Dockrell.)

Fig. 3.17 Secondary lymphoid follicle section showing a germinal centre. This human lymph node germinal centre contains actively proliferating B cells. Zoning of this centre may be seen as a light part and a more actively proliferating dark part, which contains tingible body macrophages. There is a well-developed mantle or corona of small resting lymphocytes, which have much less cytoplasm than the lymphoblasts and appear more densely packed. Giemsa stain, × 40. (Courtesy of Dr K. McLennan.)

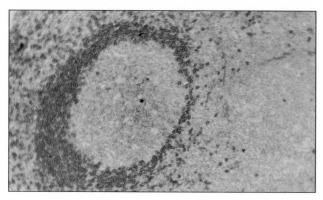

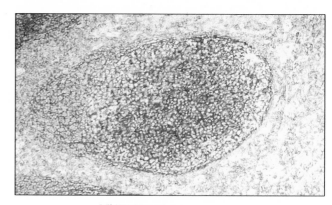

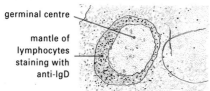

germinal centre
mantle of lymphocytes staining with anti-IgD

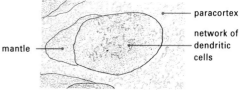

paracortex
network of dendritic cells
mantle

Fig. 3.18 Secondary lymphoid follicle showing the mantle of lymphocytes around the germinal centre. Human lymph node germinal centre stained with anti-human IgD antibody labelled with horseradish peroxidase. Note that there are few IgD-positive cells in the centre itself; both areas contain IgM-positive cells. × 40. (Courtesy of Dr K. McLennan.)

Fig. 3.19 Secondary lymphoid follicle section showing the reticular cell network. This lymph node follicle is stained with peroxidase-labelled monoclonal antibody to dendritic cells and macrophages. Note the extension of the network into the mantle. Haematoxylin counterstain, × 40. (Courtesy of Dr K. McLennan.)

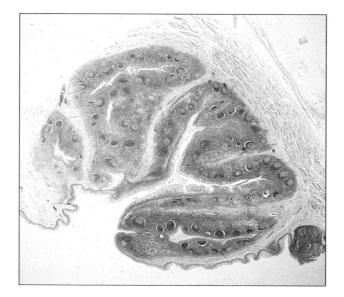

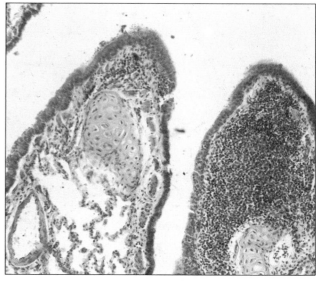

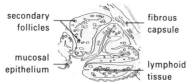

secondary follicles
mucosal epithelium
fibrous capsule
lymphoid tissue

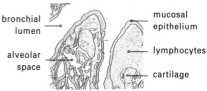

bronchial lumen
alveolar space
mucosal epithelium
lymphocytes
cartilage

Fig. 3.20 Section of human tonsil showing MALT. This view shows the large number of germinal centres frequently found in tonsillar lymphoid tissue. H&E stain, × 4. (Courtesy of Mr C. Symes.)

Fig. 3.21 Section of lung showing MALT. This section shows diffuse accumulation of lymphocytes in the bronchial wall. H&E stain, × 40.

staining (Fig. 3.18). In some secondary follicles, this thickened mantle or corona is more cellular towards the capsule of the node. Secondary follicles contain dendritic APCs and some macrophages in addition to a few CD4[+] T cells (Fig. 3.19). All these cells, together with specialized marginal sinus macrophages, appear to play a role in the development of B-cell responses and, in particular, the development of B-cell memory, which is probably the primary function of the germinal centres. (See Chapter 11 for a detailed description of the cellular organization of the germinal centre.)

THE MUCOSAL LYMPHOID SYSTEM
Mucosa-associated lymphoid tissue (MALT)

Aggregates of non-encapsulated lymphoid tissue are found especially in the lamina propria and submucosal areas of the gastrointestinal, respiratory and genitourinary tracts (see Fig. 3.1). The lymphoid cells are either present as diffuse aggregates, or are organized into solitary or aggregated nodules containing germinal centres (secondary follicles). In man, the tonsils contain a considerable amount of lymphoid tissue, often with many large germinal centres (Fig. 3.20). Similar accumulations of lymphoid tissue are seen lining the bronchi (Fig. 3.21) and along the genitourinary tract.

Diffuse accumulations of lymphoid tissue are seen in the lamina propria of the intestinal wall (Fig. 13.22). The Peyer's patches of the lower ileum are particularly prominent in young animals and contain secondary follicles (Fig. 3.23). The intestinal epithelium overlying the Peyer's patches is specialized to allow the transport of antigens into the lymphoid tissue. This particular function is carried out by epithelial cells termed 'M' (microfold) cells, due to the numerous microfolds on their luminal surface. M cells are able to absorb and transport antigens and, possibly, process and present them to subepithelial lymphoid cells. Humoral immune responses at the mucosal level are mostly of the IgA isotype. Secretory IgA is an antibody which can traverse mucosal membranes and helps prevent entry of infectious microorganisms (Fig. 3.24).

Mucosal lymphocytes

In addition to organized lymphoid tissue forming the MALT system, a large number of lymphocytes are found in the mucosa of the stomach, the small and large intestine, the bronchial airways and in the mucosa of several other organs. The lymphocytes are found in the connective tissue of the lamina propria and within the epithelial layer. The lamina propria lymphocytes (LPLs) are predominantly activated T cells, although numerous activated B cells and plasma cells are also detected. These particular plasma cells secrete mainly IgA, which is transported across the epithelial cells and released into the lumen (see above). The intra-epithelial lymphocytes (IELs) are mostly T cells which display phenotypic

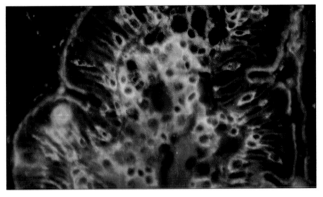

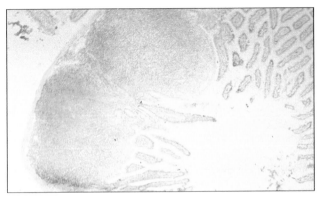

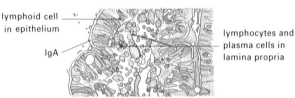

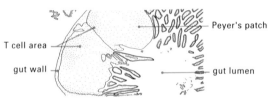

Fig. 3.22 Section of human jejunum showing MALT. Lymphoid cells in the epithelium and lamina propria fluoresce green (using anti-leucocyte monoclonal antibody, 2D1). Red cytoplasmic staining is obtained with anti-IgA antibody, which detects plasma cells in the lamina propria and IgA in the mucus. (Courtesy of Professor G. Janossy.)

Fig. 3.23 Section of mouse ileum showing Peyer's patches in the MALT. This shows the lymphoid tissue in the intestinal wall organized into Peyer's patches. The T cell areas are stained with peroxidase-labelled antibody to Thy-1 antigen on the T cells. Haematoxylin counterstain, × 40. (Courtesy of Dr E. Andrew.)

Transport of IgA across the mucosal epithelium

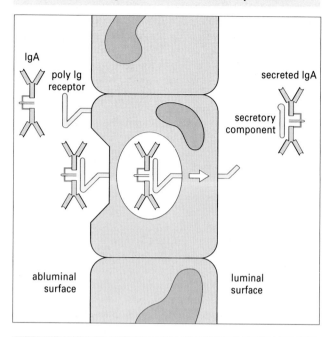

Fig. 3.24 Secretory IgA dimers secreted into the interstitial space by plasma cells bind to membrane receptors on the internal (abluminal) surface of the epithelial cells. The sIgA–receptor complex is then endocytosed and transported across the cell, bound to the membrane of transport vesicles. These vesicles fuse with the plasma membrane at the luminal surface, releasing IgA dimers and secretory component derived from cleavage of the receptor. The dimeric IgA is probably protected from proteolytic enzymes outside the cell by the presence of this secretory component.

features distinct from those of LPL (Fig. 3.25). Although the phenotype of LPLs is similar to that of cells circulating in the peripheral blood, a higher percentage of IELs are TCR γδ cells, most of which express CD8. This marker is not detected on the majority of γδ T cells in the circulation. Expression of CD8 on γδ IELs has been related to their state of activation.

Most LPL and IEL T cells belong to the CD45R0 subset of memory cells. They respond poorly to stimulation with antibodies to CD3, but may be triggered via other activation pathways (e.g. via CD2 or CD28).

HML-1, a monoclonal antibody raised against IELs, recognizes a molecule not found on resting circulating T cells but expressed following phytohaemagglutinin (PHA) stimulation. This antibody is mitogenic and induces IL-2 receptor (CD25) expression on peripheral blood T cells. Recently, it has been shown that HML-1

Phenotypic differences between human LPLs and IELs

cell type	TCR αβ	TCR γδ	CD4	CD8
lamina propria lymphocytes	>95%	<5%	70%	30%
intra-epithelial lymphocytes	60–90%	10–40%	<10%	70%

Fig 3.25 In general, the phenotype of lamina propria lymphocytes (LPLs) is similar to that of cells circulating in the peripheral blood. A higher percentage of intraepithelial lymphocytes (IELs) are TCR γδ cells, and more of this subset express CD8.

Lymphocyte traffic through the systemic lymphoid organs and tissues

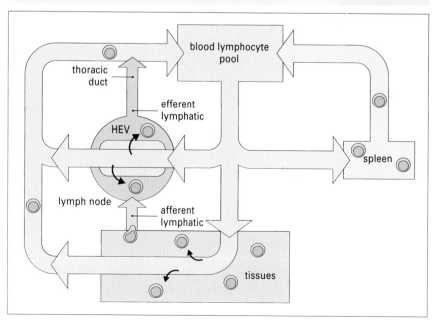

Fig. 3.26 The lymphocytes in a mature animal move through the circulation and enter the tissues and lymph nodes via the specialized endothelial cells of the post-capillary venules (HEV). They leave through the efferent lymphatic vessels and pass through other nodes, finally entering the thoracic duct which empties into the circulation at the left subclavian vein (in the human). Lymphocytes enter the white pulp areas of the spleen in the marginal zone; they pass into the sinusoids of the red pulp and leave via the splenic vein.

is a novel α chain of the integrin family, which is coupled with a β₇ chain to form an αHML-1/β₇ heterodimer, an integrin expressed by IELs and other activated leucocytes.

IELs are known to release cytokines including IFN$_\gamma$ and IL-5. One function suggested for IELs is immune surveillance against mutated or virus-infected host cells.

LYMPHOCYTE TRAFFIC

The migration of lymphocytes from primary to secondary lymphoid tissues has already been described. Once in the secondary tissues the lymphocytes do not simply remain there; many move from one lymphoid organ to another, via the blood and lymph (Fig. 3.26).

Although some lymphocytes leave the blood through non-specialized venules, the main exit route in most mammals is through a specialized section of the postcapillary venules known as the high endothelial venule (Fig. 3.27). In the lymph nodes these are mainly in the paracortex with some in the cortex; the medulla lacks high endothelial venules (HEVs). Some lymphocytes, primarily T cells, arrive from the drainage area of the node through the afferent lymphatics; this is the main route by which antigen enters the nodes.

Cuboidal epithelial cells, lining the HEVs, are activated cells which express a variety of adhesion molecules not found on the flat resting endothelial cells of ordinary venules. One mechanism by which endothelial cells are activated is through locally produced cytokines. These include IFN$_\gamma$, IL-1 and TNF, all of which can induce activation of endothelial cells. At sites of chronic inflammatory reactions the activated endothelial cells may develop into HEVs, for example in the skin and in the synovium, where HEVs are normally absent. This, in turn, may direct specific lymphocyte subsets to the area where HEVs are formed. Molecules expressed by activated endothelial cells belong to the immunoglobulin superfamily, such as ICAM-1 (CD54), ICAM-2 and VCAM, and to the selectin family, such as E-selectin (ELAM-1) and P-selectin (CD62, GMP-140). P-selectin is stored in the Weibel–Palade bodies of endothelial cells, and is rapidly moved to the cell surface following activation (see Chapter 13). The molecule CD44, a 90 kDa protein expressed by all leucocytes, plays a major role in lymphocyte adhesion to HEV. The pattern that is emerging is that several receptor–ligand interactions occur between lymphocytes and endothelial cells. These interactions not only direct lymphocytes to specific target organs, but also subserve specific functions in the different phases of lymphocyte migration out of blood vessels (extravasation). These phases include cell margination, rolling over the endothelial surface, and attachment and diapedesis between endothelial cells (Fig. 3.28). More seldom, cells migrate by emperipolesis, in which the lymphocyte moves through the endothelial cell. This is the the normal route into the CNS, where the endothelium has continuous tight junctions.

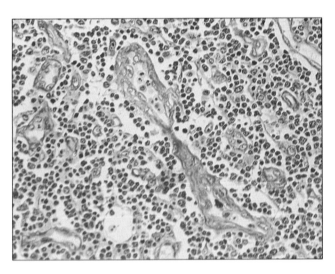

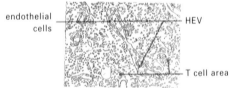

Fig. 3.27 Section of lymph nodes showing the high endothelial venule. This section of lymph node paracortex shows the specialized high endothelial cells lining the HEV through which lymphocytes leave the circulation and enter the node. Giemsa stain (resin section), × 180. (Courtesy of Dr K. McLennan.)

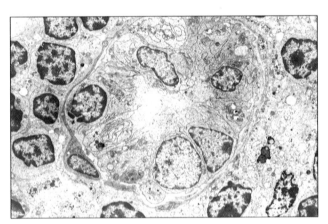

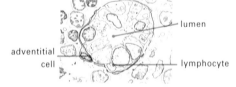

Fig. 3.28 Electron micrograph showing a high endothelial venule in the thymus-dependent area of a lymph node. A lymphocyte in transit from the lumen of the HEV can be seen close to the basal lamina. The HEV is partly surrounded by an adventitial cell. × 1600.

Lymphoid cells within lymph nodes return to the circulation by way of the efferent lymphatics, which pass via the thoracic duct into the left subclavian vein.

About 1–2% of the lymphocyte pool recirculates each hour. Overall, this process allows a large number of antigen-specific lymphocytes to come into contact with the appropriate antigen in the microenvironment of the peripheral lymphoid organs. This is particularly important since lymphoid cells are monospecific and there is only a finite number of lymphocytes capable of recognizing any particular antigenic conformation. Under normal conditions there is continuous active flow of lymphocyte traffic through the nodes, but when antigen enters the lymph nodes of an animal already sensitized to that antigen there is a temporary shutdown in the traffic which lasts for approximately 24 hours. Thus, antigen-specific lymphocytes are preferentially retained in the lymph nodes draining the source of antigen. In particular, blast cells do not recirculate but appear to remain in one site.

The main route of lymphocyte traffic into the spleen from the circulation is via the marginal sinus (the venous sinus surrounding the marginal zone of the PALS). Lymphocytes leave through the marginal zone bridging channels, into the red pulp sinuses and subsequently into the splenic vein.

One reason for considering the MALT as a distinct system – separate from the systemic lymphoid organs – is that mucosa-associated lymphoid cells mainly recirculate within the mucosal lymphoid system. Thus, lymphoid cells stimulated in Peyer's patches pass via regional lymph nodes to the blood stream and then 'home' back into mucosal sites (Fig. 3.29). Specific recirculation is brought about by the lymphoid cells being able to recognize adhesion molecules specifically expressed on endothelial cells of the mucosal post-capillary venules, but which are absent from lymph node HEVs. Based on this mechanism, antigen stimulation in one mucosal area elicits an antibody response in other mucosal areas.

Lymphocyte circulation within the mucosal lymphoid system

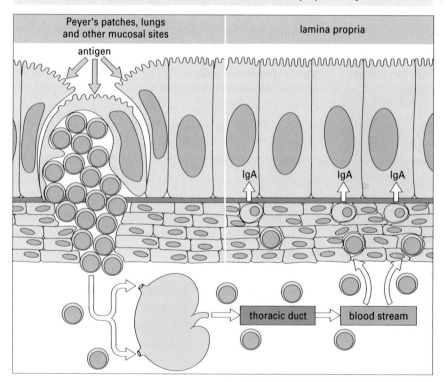

Fig. 3.29 Lymphoid cells which are stimulated with antigen in Peyer's patches (probably also lungs and other mucosal sites) migrate via the regional lymph nodes and thoracic duct into the blood stream, and hence to the lamina propria of the gut and probably to other mucosal surfaces. Thus lymphocytes stimulated at the mucosal level re-enter the mucosa.

FURTHER READING

Bros JD, Kapsenberg ML. The skin immune system. *Immunol Today* 1986;**7**:235.

Kuby J. *Cells and Organs of the Immune System*. New York: WH Freeman and Co, 1992:39–71.

Pardi R, Inverardi L, Bender JR. Regulatory mechanisms in leukocyte adhesion: flexible receptors for sophisticated travellers. *Immunol Today* 1992:**13**;224.

Playfair JHL. *Immunology at a Glance*. 7th ed. Oxford: Blackwell Scientific Publications, 1992.

Roitt IM. *Essential Immunology*. 7th ed. Oxford: Blackwell Scientific Publications, 1991:85–100.

chapter 4

Antigen Receptor Molecules

The recognition of foreign antigen is the hallmark of the specific adaptive immune response. Two distinct types of molecules are involved in this process – the immunoglobulins and the T-cell antigen receptors (TCRs) (Fig 4.1). Diversity and heterogeneity are characteristic features of these molecules. In both cases there is evidence of extensive gene rearrangements which generate different immunoglobulins or TCRs, able to recognize many different antigens.

The immunoglobulins are a group of glycoproteins present in the serum and tissue fluids of all mammals. Some are carried on cell surfaces where they act as receptors. Others (antibodies) are free in the blood or lymph. They are produced in large quantities by plasma cells, which develop from precursor B cells. Plasma cell is the original histological term used to describe antibody-forming cells (AFCs) seen in blood and tissues. Precursor B cells carry membrane-bound immunoglobulin of the same binding specificity as that produced by the AFC. Contact between these B cells and foreign antigen is needed for induction of antibody formation.

T-cell receptors are expressed exclusively on the membrane surface of T lymphocytes; there is no production of soluble molecules, analogous to the circulating antibodies. T-cell recognition of antigen through the T-cell receptor is the basis of a range of immunological phenomena including T-cell helper and suppressor activity, cytotoxicity and, possibly, NK (natural killer) activity.

IMMUNOGLOBULINS

Five distinct classes of immunoglobulin molecule are recognized in most higher mammals, namely IgG, IgA, IgM, IgD, and IgE. These differ in size, charge, amino acid composition and carbohydrate content.

In addition to the difference between classes, the immunoglobulins within each class are also very heterogeneous. Electrophoretically the immunoglobulins show a unique range of heterogeneity which extends from the γ to the α fractions of normal serum (Fig. 4.2). These fractions suffer marked depletion following

Antigen recognition molecules

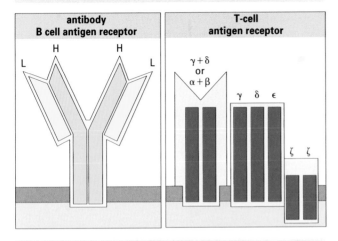

Distribution of the major human immunoglobulins

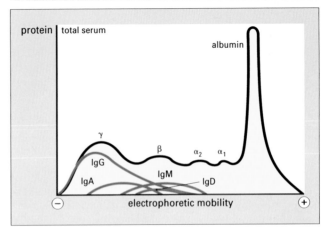

Fig. 4.1 The antigen receptors of T and B cells are probably derived from a common ancestor and both belong to the immunoglobulin supergene family. Immunoglobulin consists of two identical heavy (H) chains and two identical light (L) chains. The T-cell receptor has an antigen-binding portion consisting of an α and β chain (or a γ and δ chain) which are associated with four other transmembrane peptides (γ, δ, ϵ and ζ), structurally distinct from the chains of the receptor. Circulating antibodies are structurally identical to B cell antigen receptors except that they lack the transmembrane and intracytoplasmic sections.

Fig. 4.2 Electrophoresis of human serum showing the distribution of the four major immunoglobulin classes. Serum proteins are separated according to their charges in an electric field, and classified as α_1, α_2, β, and γ, depending on their mobility. (The IgE class has a similar mobility to IgD but cannot be represented quantitatively because of its low level in serum.) IgG exhibits most charge heterogeneity, the other classes having a more restricted mobility in the β and fast γ regions.

absorption with antigen. The basic four-chain polypeptide structure of the immunoglobulin molecule is shown in Fig. 4.3.

ANTIBODY FUNCTION

Each immunoglobulin molecule is bifunctional. One region of the molecule is concerned with binding to antigen while a different region mediates so-called effector functions. These include binding of the immunoglobulin to host tissues, including various cells of the immune system, some phagocytic cells, and the first component (C1q) of the classical complement system.

The basic chain structure of immunoglobulins

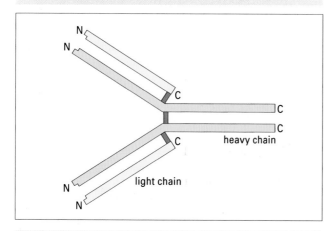

Fig. 4.3 The immunoglobin unit consists of two identical light polypeptide chains and two identical heavy polypeptide chains linked together by disulphide bonds (red). Note the position of the amino- (N) and carboxy- (C) terminal ends of the peptide chains.

IMMUNOGLOBULIN CLASSES AND SUBCLASSES

The basic structure of all immunoglobulin molecules is a unit consisting of two identical light polypeptide chains and two identical heavy polypeptide chains. These are linked together by disulphide bonds. The class and subclass of an immunoglobulin molecule (i.e. its isotype) are determined by its heavy chain type. Thus the four human IgG subclasses (IgG1, IgG2, IgG3 and IgG4) have heavy chains called γ_1, γ_2, γ_3 and γ_4 which differ slightly, although all are recognizably γ heavy chains.

The four subclasses of human IgG (IgG1, IgG2, IgG3 and IgG4) occur in the approximate proportions of 66%, 23%, 7% and 4%, respectively. There are also known to be subclasses of human IgA (IgA1 and IgA2), but none have been described for IgM, IgD, and IgE.

Immunoglobulin subclasses appear to have arisen late in evolution and the human subclasses cannot be compared with, for example, the four known subclasses of IgG which have been identified in the mouse.

GENERAL PROPERTIES OF IMMUNOGLOBULINS

All immunoglobulins are glycoproteins, but the carbohydrate content ranges from 2–3% for IgG to 12–14% for IgM, IgD, and IgE. The physicochemical properties of the immunoglobulins are summarized in Fig. 4.4.

IgG is the major immunoglobulin in normal human serum, accounting for 70–75% of the total immunoglobulin pool. IgG consists of a single immunoglobulin molecule with a sedimentation coefficient of 7S and a molecular weight of 146 000. However, IgG3 proteins are slightly larger than the other subclasses; this is due to the slightly heavier γ_3 chain. The IgG class, which is distributed evenly between the intravascular and extravascular pools, is the major antibody of secondary immune responses and the exclusive antitoxin class.

Physicochemical properties of human immunoglobulin classes

property	immunoglobulin type									
	IgG1	IgG2	IgG3	IgG4	IgM	IgA1	IgA2	sIgA	IgD	IgE
heavy chain	γ_1	γ_2	γ_3	γ_4	μ	α_1	α_2	α_1/α_2	δ	ϵ
mean serum conc. (mg/ml)	9	3	1	0.5	1.5	3.0	0.5	0.05	0.03	0.000 05
sedimentation constant	7s	7s	7s	7s	19s	7s	7s	11s	7s	8s
mol. wt ($\times 10^3$)	146	146	170	146	970	160	160	385	184	188
half-life (days)	21	20	7	21	10	6	6	?	3	2
intravascular distribution(%)	45	45	45	45	80	42	42	trace	75	50
carbohydrate(%)	2–3	2–3	2–3	2–3	12	7–11	7–11	7–11	9–14	12

Fig. 4.4 Each immunoglobulin class has a characteristic type of heavy chain. Thus IgG possesses γ chains; IgM, μ chains; IgA, α chains; IgD, δ chains and IgE, ϵ chains. Variation in heavy chain structure within a class gives rise to immunoglobulin subclasses. For example, the human IgG pool consists of four subclasses reflecting four distinct types of heavy chain. The properties of the immunoglobulins vary between the different classes. Note that in secretions, IgA occurs in a dimeric form (sIgA) in association with a protein chain termed the secretory piece. Serum concentration of sIgA is very low, whereas the level in intestinal secretions can be very high.

IgM accounts for approximately 10% of the immunoglobulin pool. The molecule has a pentameric structure in which individual heavy chains have a molecular weight of approximately 65 000 and the whole molecule has a molecular weight of 970 000. IgM is largely confined to the intravascular pool and is the predominant 'early' antibody, frequently seen in the immune response to antigenically complex infectious organisms.

IgA represents 15–20% of the human serum immunoglobulin pool. In man more than 80% of IgA occurs as a monomer of the four-polypeptide chain unit, but in most mammals the IgA in serum is mainly polymeric, occurring mostly as a dimer. IgA is the predominant immunoglobulin in seromucous secretions such as saliva, colostrum, milk, and tracheobronchial and genitourinary secretions.

Secretory IgA (sIgA), which may be either subclass IgA1 or IgA2, exists mainly in the 11S, dimeric form and has a molecular weight of 385 000. Secretory IgA is abundant in seromucous secretions where it is associated with another protein – the secretory component.

IgD accounts for less than 1% of the total plasma immunoglobulin but is present in large quantities on the membrane of many B cells. The precise biological function of this class is unknown but it may play a role in antigen-triggered lymphocyte differentiation.

IgE, though scarce in serum, is found on the surface membrane of basophils and mast-cells in all individuals, and also sensitizes cells on mucosal surfaces such as the conjunctival, nasal and bronchial mucosa. This class of immunoglobulin may play a role in immunity to helminthic parasites, but in developed countries is more commonly associated with allergic diseases such as asthma and hay fever.

ANTIBODY STRUCTURE

In 1962 Rodney Porter proposed a basic four-chain model for immunoglobulin molecules (Fig. 4.5), based on two distinct types of polypeptide chain. The smaller (light) chain has a molecular weight of 25 000 and is common to all classes, whereas the larger (heavy) chain has a molecular weight of 50 000–77 000 and is structurally distinct for each class or subclass. The polypeptide chains are linked together by covalent and non-covalent forces.

In the most abundant immunoglobulin, IgG, the hinge region can undergo proteolytic cleavage by papain to produce two identical fragments that can bind antigen – Fab (fragment antigen binding) and a third fragment which cannot bind antigen – Fc (fragment crystallizable).

Pepsin leaves at a different point and produces an F(ab')$_2$ and an Fc portion. The F(ab')$_2$ is divalent and can bind to antigen similarly to the original antibody (see Fig 4.19).

The light chains of most vertebrates have been shown to exist in two distinct forms called kappa (κ-type) and lambda (λ-type). They may be distinguished by their behaviour as antigens – antisera may be raised to one type which do not react with the other. Either of the light chain types may combine with any of the heavy chain types, but in any one molecule both light chains are of the same type – hybrid molecules do not occur naturally.

Hilschmann, Craig and others in 1965 established that light chains consist of two distinct regions. The C-terminal half of the chain (approximately 107 amino acid residues) is constant except for certain allotypic and isotypic variations (see below) and is called the C$_L$ (Constant:Light chain) region, whereas the N-terminal half of the chain shows much sequence variability and is known as the V$_L$ (Variable:Light chain) region.

The IgG molecule may be considered as a typical example of the basic antibody structure. IgG has two intrachain disulphide bonds in the light chain – one in the variable region and one in the constant region (Figs 4.6 and 4.7). There are four such bonds in the heavy

The basic structure of IgG1

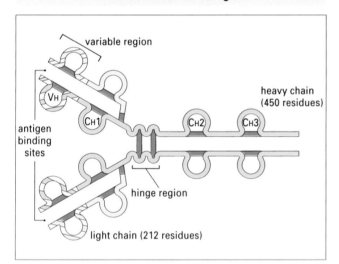

Fig. 4.5 The N-terminal end of IgG1 is characterized by sequence variability (V) in both the heavy and light chains, referred to as the V$_H$ and V$_L$ regions respectively. The rest of the molecule has a relatively constant (C) structure. The constant portion of the light chain is termed the C$_L$ region. The constant portion of the heavy chain is further divided into three structurally discrete regions: C$_H$1, C$_H$2 and C$_H$3. These globular regions, which are stabilized by intrachain disulphide bonds, are referred to as 'domains'. The sites at which the antibody binds antigen are located in the variable domains. The hinge region is a segment of heavy chain between the C$_H$1 and C$_H$2 domains. Flexibility in this area permits the two antigen-binding sites to operate independently. There is close pairing of the domains except in the C$_H$2 region (see Fig. 4.8). Carbohydrate moieties are attached to the C$_H$2 domains.

(γ) chain, which is twice the length of the light chain. Each disulphide bond encloses a peptide loop of 60–70 amino acid residues, and if the amino acid sequences of these loops are compared a striking degree of homology is revealed. Essentially this means that each immunoglobulin peptide chain is composed of a series of globular regions with very similar secondary and tertiary structure (folding). This is shown for the light chain in Fig. 4.6. The peptide loops enclosed by the disulphide bonds represent the central portion of a 'domain' of about 110 amino acid residues. In both the heavy and the light chains the first of these domains corresponds to the variable region, VH and VL respectively (Fig. 4.7). In the heavy chain of IgG, IgA and IgD there are three further domains, which make up the constant part of the chain, CH1, CH2 and CH3. In both μ and ε chains there is an additional domain after CH1. Thus, the C-terminal domains of IgM and IgE heavy chains (referred to as Cμ4 and Cε4) are homologous to the CH3 domain of IgG (Cγ3).

Fig. 4.7 shows the structure of the IgG1 molecule in a form which corresponds more closely to the actual molecule than Fig. 4.5. Although Fig. 4.7 is a useful model for all immunoglobulins, there are differences of detail between every class, and between subclasses.

IgG With human IgG, no two subclasses are identical in the number and distribution of interchain disulphide bonds. Indeed, the light–heavy chain bonds in IgG2, IgG3 and IgG4 are located at the junction between the variable and constant regions of the heavy chains and this pattern is the one most frequently observed in other classes. Similarly, the number of inter-heavy chain bonds may be two (IgG1 and Ig4), four (IgG2) or fifteen (IgG3) (Fig. 4.8).

IgM Although usually a pentamer (Fig 4.9), there is evidence that in both mouse and man some IgM is hexameric. The μ chains differ from the γ chains in amino acid sequence and have an extra constant region domain. The subunits are linked by disulphide bonds between the Cμ3 domains and possibly by disulphide bonds between the C-terminal 18-residue peptide tailpieces. The complete molecule consists of a densely packed central region with radiating arms, as seen in electron micrographs. Photographs of IgM antibodies

---

Basic folding in the light chain

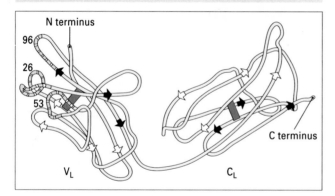

Fig. 4.6 The basic folding pattern of the variable and constant domains of the light chain. Within the past decade the tertiary structure of immunoglobulins has been investigated by X-ray diffraction techniques. Such studies have shown that the immunoglobulin domains share a basic folding pattern with several straight segments of polypeptide chain lying parallel to the long axis of the domain. Shown here is a light chain which has two domains – one constant and one variable. Within each domain, the polypeptide chain is arranged in two layers, running in opposite directions, with many hydrophobic amino acid side-chains between the layers. One of the layers has four segments (arrowed white), the other has three (arrowed black); both are linked by a single disulphide bridge (red). Folding of the VL domains causes the hypervariable regions to become exposed in three separate but closely disposed loops. One numbered residue from each hypervariable region is identified.

Structure of IgG1

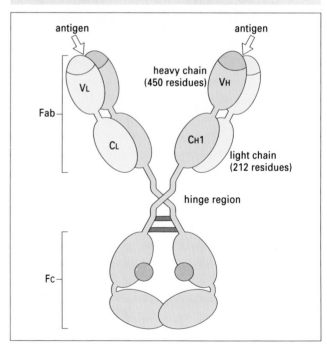

Fig. 4.7 A model of IgG1 indicating the globular domains of heavy (H) and light (L) chains. Note the apposition of the CH3 domains and the separation of the CH2 domains. The carbohydrate units (purple) lie between the CH2 domains. In this figure (and in Fig. 4.9 onwards) the interchain disulphide bonds between H and L chains are not shown.

binding to bacterial flagella show molecules adopting a 'staple' configuration (Fig. 4.10). The latter suggests that flexion readily occurs between the Cμ2 and Cμ3 domains although this region is not structurally homologous to the IgG hinge. The dislocation resulting in the 'staple' configuration appears to be related to the activation of complement by IgM.

Two other features characterize the IgM molecule: an abundance of oligosaccharide units associated with the μ chain, and an additional peptide chain, the J (joining) chain, thought to assist the process of polymerization prior to secretion by the AFC. The J chain is a cysteine-rich peptide of 137 amino acid residues. One J chain is incorporated into the IgM structure by disulphide bonding to the 18-residue peptide tailpiece of the separate monomers. Binding is to the penultimate cysteine residues of the tailpieces. If J chains are not freely available, hexameric IgM appears to become the preferred form, rather than pentameric IgM.

Structures of human IgG subclasses

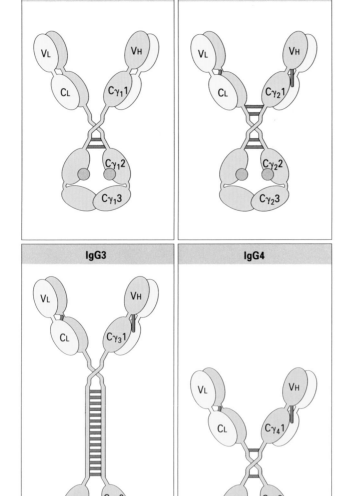

Fig. 4.8 Polypeptide chain structure of the four human IgG subclasses. The subclasses differ in the number and arrangement of the interchain disulphide bonds.

Structure of human IgM

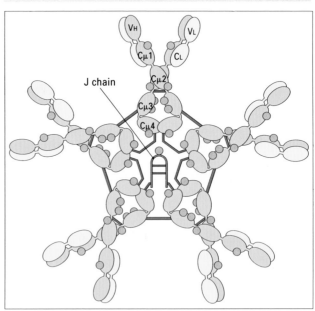

Fig. 4.9 IgM heavy chains have five domains with disulphide bonds cross-linking adjacent Cμ3 and Cμ4 domains. Also shown are the carbohydrate side-chains (purple) and possible location of the J chain. IgM does not have extended hinge regions, but flexion can occur about the Cμ2 domains.

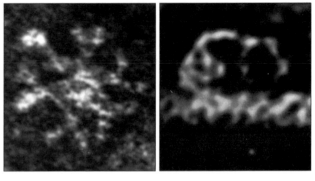

Fig. 4.10 Electron micrographs of IgM molecules. Left: In free solution, IgM adopts the characteristic star-shaped configuration. × 5 200 000. (Courtesy of Dr R. Dourmashkin.) Right: IgM bound to a single flagellum has adopted the crab-like, 'staple' configuration. × 5 200 000. (Courtesy of Dr A. Feinstein.)

IgA Polymeric serum IgA and all secretory IgA molecules also contain the J chain found in IgM. The 472 amino-acid residues of the α chain are arranged in four domains, VH, Cα1, Cα2 and Cα3 (Fig. 4.11). A feature shared with IgM is an additional C-terminal 18-residue peptide with a penultimate cysteine residue, which is able to bind covalently to the J chain to form dimers. Electron micrographs of IgA dimers show double Y-shaped structures which suggest that the monomeric subunits are linked end-to-end through the C-terminal Cα3 regions (Fig. 4.12). The Cα1 and Cα2 domains possess an additional intrachain disulphide bond, and in each Cα2 domain there are two cysteine residues of unknown function.

Secretory IgA (sIgA) exists mainly in the form of a molecule sedimenting at 11S (mol. wt. 380 000). The complete molecule is made up of two units of IgA, one secretory component (mol. wt 70 000) and one J chain (mol. wt 15 000) (Fig. 4.13). It is not clear how the various peptide chains are linked together. In contrast to the J chain, secretory component is not synthesized by plasma cells but by epithelial cells. IgA held in dimer configuration by a J chain, and secreted by submucosal plasma cells, actively binds secretory component as it traverses epithelial cell layers. Bound secretory component facilitates the transport of sIgA into secretions, as well as protecting it from proteolytic attack. IgA1 is the predominant subclass in serum, whereas IgA2 predominates in secretions. This may be because many microorganisms in the respiratory and gastrointestinal tracts release proteases that cleave IgA1.

Structure of human IgA1

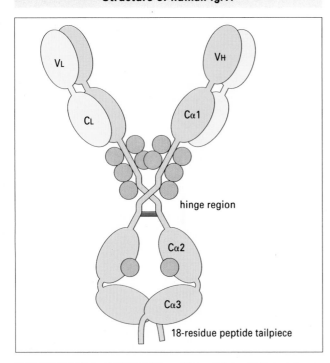

Fig. 4.11 This diagram shows the domain structure of IgA1 and the possible location of carbohydrate units (purple). Note the presence of the C-terminal 18-residue tailpiece (a feature shared with IgM) and a hinge region.

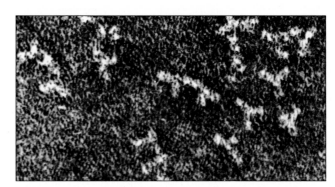

Fig. 4.12 Electron micrograph of a human dimeric IgA myeloma protein. The double Y-shaped appearance suggests that the monomeric subunits are linked end to end through the C-terminal Cα3 domain. × 1 600 000. (Courtesy of Dr R. Dourmashkin.)

Structure of human secretory IgA (sIgA)

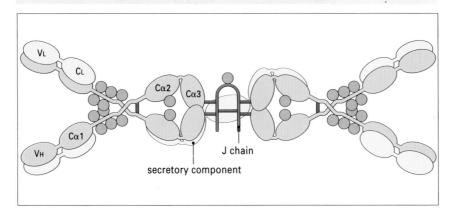

Fig. 4.13 The secretory component of sIgA is probably wound around the dimer and attached by disulphide bonds to the Cα2 domain of each IgA monomer. The J chain is required to join the two subunits.

IgD is a trace immunoglobulin in serum (less than 1% of the total). This protein is more susceptible to proteolysis than IgG1, IgG2, IgA or IgM and has a tendency to undergo spontaneous proteolysis. IgD structure is shown diagrammatically in Fig. 4.14. There appears to be a single disulphide bond between the δ chains and a large amount of carbohydrate distributed in multiple oligosaccharide units. One of these units is rich in *N*-acetylgalactosamine, a sugar which also occurs in IgA1, but in no other known immunoglobulin.

IgE The structure of IgE is shown in Fig. 4.15. The higher molecular weight of the ε chain (72 500) is explained by the larger number of amino acid residues (approximately 550) distributed over five domains (VH, Cε1, Cε2, Cε3 and Cε4).

THE GENETIC BASIS OF ANTIBODY HETEROGENEITY

The mRNA for an immunoglobulin polypeptide is made by a B cell by splicing together sections of mRNA coding for different parts of the polypeptide. For example, the production of light-chain mRNA involves the splicing together of two mRNA segments – one for the V domain and one for the C domain. The segment of DNA coding for the V genes is, in turn, produced by recombination of two germ-line genes (see Chapter 5).

Thus a single polypeptide is produced from several genes, which creates problems in analysing its genetic variability. Nevertheless the variability of antibodies can be divided into three types: isotypic, allotypic and idiotypic (Fig. 4.16).

Structure of human IgE

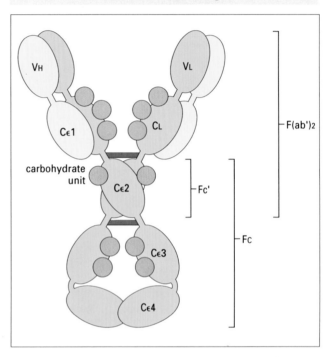

Fig. 4.15 IgE can be cleaved by enzymes to give the fragments F(ab')₂, Fc and Fc'. Note the absence of a hinge region.

Structure of human IgD

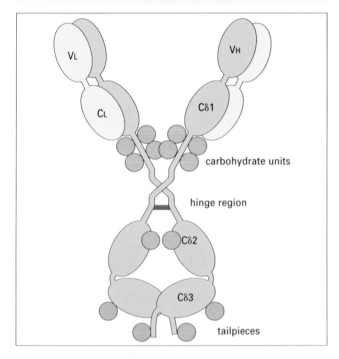

Fig. 4.14 This diagram of IgD shows the domain structure and a characteristically large number of oligosaccharide units. Note also the presence of a hinge region and short octapeptide tailpieces.

Antibody variants

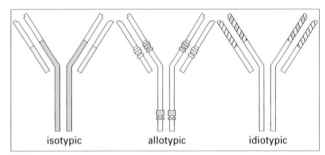

Fig. 4.16 Isotypic variation refers to the different heavy and light chain classes and subclasses: the variants produced are present in all healthy members of a species. Allotypic variation occurs mostly in the constant region: not all variants are present in all healthy individuals. Idiotypic variation occurs in the variable region only and idiotypes are specific to each antibody molecule.

Isotypic Variation The genes for isotypic variants are present in all healthy members of a species. For example, the genes for γ_1, γ_2, γ_3, γ_4, μ, α_1, α_2, δ, ϵ, κ, and λ chains are all present in the human genome and these are therefore isotypes.

Allotypic Variation This refers to genetic variation between individuals within a species, involving different alleles at a given locus. For example, the variant of IgG3 called G3m(b°) is characterized by a phenylalanine at position 436 of the γ_3 heavy chain. It is not found in all people and is therefore an allotype. Allotypes occur mostly as variants of heavy chain constant regions.

Idiotypic Variation Variation in the variable domain, particularly in the highly variable segments known as hypervariable regions, produces idiotypes. These determine the binding specificity of the antigen binding site. Idiotypes are usually specific for individual B-cell clones (private idiotypes), but are sometimes shared between different B-cell clones (public, cross-reacting or recurrent idiotypes). The precise genetic basis of idiotypic variability is only partially understood.

ANTIBODY EFFECTOR FUNCTIONS

The primary function of an antibody is to bind the antigen. In a few cases this has a direct effect, for example by neutralizing bacterial toxin, or by preventing viral penetration of cells. In general, however, the interaction of antibody and antigen is without significance unless secondary 'effector' functions come into play (Fig. 4.17).

The activation of the complement system is one of the most important effector mechanisms of IgG1 and IgG3 molecules. The complement system is a complex group of serum proteins which mediate inflammatory reactions. Having bound to antigen, IgM, IgG1 and IgG3 may activate the complement enzyme cascade. IgG2 appears to be less effective in activating complement, while IgG4, IgA, IgD and IgE are ineffective.

In man, IgG molecules of all subclasses cross the placenta and confer a high degree of passive immunity to the newborn. In species in which maternal immunoglobulin only reaches the offspring postnatally, for example the pig, IgG derived from the maternal milk selectively crosses the gastrointestinal tract.

The immunoglobulins display a complex pattern of interactions with various cell types (Fig. 4.18).

Three groups of human Fcγ receptor are now recognized on cell surfaces, namely FcγRI (CD64), FcγRII (CD32) and FcγRIII (CD16). They are all characterized by extracellular domains showing significant homology with immunoglobulin V regions, i.e. they belong to the Ig superfamily, as does FcαR, a fourth type of receptor. In contrast FcϵRII belongs to a family of serum lectins (molecules that bind carbohydrates).

Major functions of human antibody classes and subclasses

effector function	immunoglobulin							
	IgG1	IgG2	IgG3	IgG4	IgM	IgA	IgD	IgE
complement fixation (classical pathway)	++	+	+++	–	+++	–	–	–
placental transfer	+	+	+	+	–	–	–	–
binding to staphylococcal protein A	+++	+++	–*	+++	–	–	–	–
binding to streptococcal protein G	+++	+++	+++	+++	–	–	–	–

Fig. 4.17 Immunoglobulin classes and subclasses differ in their ability to fix complement, cross the placenta and react with various microbial proteins. These functions are mediated by different parts of the Fc region. For example, staphylococcal protein A (a cell-wall protein of staphylococci) binds to the Fc portion of certain immunoglobulins and therefore is a natural receptor for antibody. (*IgG3 of the G3m(g) and G3m(b) allotypes found in the sera of most Caucasians does not bind. In contrast, IgG3 G3m(st), characteristically found in Oriental populations, does bind.)

Selected cell binding functions of human immunoglobulins

receptor		immunoglobulin									
		IgG1	IgG2	IgG3	IgG4	IgM	IgA1	IgA2	sIgA	IgD	IgE
mononuclear cells	FcγRI	+++	–	+++	++	–	–	–	–	–	–
	FcγRIIa	+	–	+	–	–	–	–	–	–	–
	FcγRIII	+	–	+	–	–	–	–	–	–	–
	FcμR	–	–	–	–	+	–	–	–	–	–
	FcϵRII	–	–	–	–	–	–	–	–	–	++
neutrophils	FcγRIIa	+	–	+	–	–	–	–	–	–	–
	FcγRIII-1	+	–	+	–	–	–	–	–	–	–
	FcαR	–	–	–	–	–	++	++	++	–	–
mast cells/ basophils	FcϵRI	–	–	–	–	–	–	–	–	–	+++

Fig. 4.18 A complex family of receptor molecules able to bind immunoglobulin continues to be delineated (selected examples are listed here). FcμR is expressed by activated B cells but not by T cells or monocytes. FcϵRII is also expressed on eosinophils, platelets, T cells and B cells. A receptor designated FcγRIII-2 has been identified on NK cells.

IMMUNOGLOBULIN STRUCTURE AND FUNCTION

The plant protease papain cleaves the IgG molecule in the hinge region between the Cγ1 and Cγ2 domains, to give two identical Fab fragments and one Fc fragment. These papain-generated fragments have been of enormous value in structure/function studies on the antibody molecule. The Fab region binds to antigen, while the Fc region mediates effector functions such as complement fixation and monocyte binding. The Fc region is also important in placental transmission.

Papain also generates, after prolonged digestion, a degraded fragment of the Cγ3 region which is called the Fc' fragment. Some of these major points of enzymic cleavage are shown in Fig. 4.19.

Pepsin is another useful enzyme for structure/function studies, and generates two major fragments: the F(ab')₂ fragment, which broadly encompasses the two Fab regions linked by the hinge region, and the pFc' fragment, which corresponds to the Cγ3 domain of the molecule.

Many other enzymes are known to cleave the immunoglobulin molecule. Brief trypsin digestion of acid-treated Fc fragments yields the Cγ2 domain; isola-tion of this fragment has permitted structural and functional comparison with other subfragments such as pFc'.

Within the variable regions of both heavy and light chains, some short polypeptide segments show exceptional variability. Termed hypervariable regions these segments are located near amino acid positions 30, 50 and 95 (Fig. 4.20). Because they create the antigen-binding site, hypervariable regions are sometimes referred to as complementarity determining regions (CDRs). The intervening peptide segments are called framework regions (FRs). In both light and heavy chain V regions there are three CDRs (CDR1–CDR3) and four FRs (FR1–FR4).

The variable regions of the light and heavy chains are folded in such a way that the regions of hypervariability are brought together to create the surface structure which binds antigen. These regions are, in the main, associated with bends in the peptide chain (Fig. 4.6).

X-ray crystallography is now yielding structural data on complete IgG molecules and it is possible to construct both an α-carbon backbone and a computer-generated atomic model for this class of immunoglobulin

---

Enzymic cleavage of human IgG1

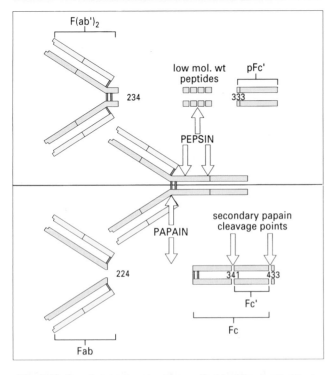

Fig. 4.19 Pepsin cleaves the heavy chain of human IgG1 at positions 234 and 333, to yield the F(ab')₂ and pFc' fragments. Further action reduces the central fragment to low molecular weight peptides. Papain splits the molecule in the hinge region (at residue 224) yielding two Fab fragments and the Fc fragment. Secondary action on the Fc fragment at residues 341 and 433 gives rise to Fc'.

Amino acid variability in the variable region of immunoglobulin light chains

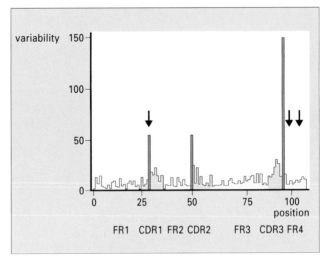

Fig. 4.20 Variability is calculated by comparing the sequences of many individual chains and, for any position, is equal to the ratio of the number of different amino acids found at that position, to the frequency of the most common amino acid. The areas of greatest variability, of which there are three in the VL domain, are the hypervariable regions. In some sequences studied, extra amino acids have been found, but these are excluded here to enhance comparison; their positions are indicated by arrows. The areas shaded orange denote regions of hypervariability (CDR), and the most hypervariable positions are shaded red. The four framework regions (FR) are shown in yellow. (Courtesy of Professor E. A. Kabat.)

(Figs 4.21 and 4.22). These show the general Y-shaped structure with three limbs which has also been visualized by electron microscopy.

Homologous domains of the light and heavy chains are paired in the Fab regions. Likewise the Cγ3 domains of the γ heavy chains are paired but the Cγ2 domains are separated by the carbohydrate moieties. Despite the structural similarities between domains there are striking differences at the level of domain interaction. For example, the variable domains associate with each other through their three segment layers, whereas the constant domains associate through the four segment layers.

In contrast to the rapid progress made in localizing the antigen binding sites of antibodies, the precise structural locations of most effector functions have proved to be elusive. Enzymic subfragments and peptide inhibition studies provided provisional data, but further progress was slow until the technique of site-directed mutagenesis began to be applied. By selectively altering amino acids at different positions in the known peptide sequence it is possible to assess the importance of specific residues for particular functions.

An investigation of complement activation by IgG was one of the first such applications. Earlier studies had already suggested that the C1q subcomponent of C1 interacted with the Cγ2 domain of IgG. Site-directed mutagenesis was used to localize the binding site for C1q to three side chains in the Cγ2 domain, Glu 318, Lys 320 and Lys 322. This IgG sequence motif appears to constitute a common core in the interactions between C1q and IgG molecules. In the case of IgM, however, complement activation seems to involve a different mechanism. Free circulating IgM in the star-shaped configuration is clearly incapable of activating complement, whereas a single molecule of IgM bound to antigen is a potent activator. Feinstein and colleagues have suggested that the process of IgM binding to a polymeric or latticed antigen dislocates the F(ab')₂ units out of their original plane and leads to the so-called 'staple' configuration visualized by electron microscopy (see Fig. 4.10). It is suggested that these conformational changes unveil a ring of C1q binding sites which are hidden in the star-shaped configuration of IgM by the close juxtaposition of the subunits.

IgG molecules interact with a wide range of cellular Fc receptors to promote phagocytosis (neutrophils, macrophages, monocytes), antibody-dependent cellular cytotoxicity (NK cells, monocytes), and maternal–fetal transport of IgG (placental syncitiotrophoblast). Site-

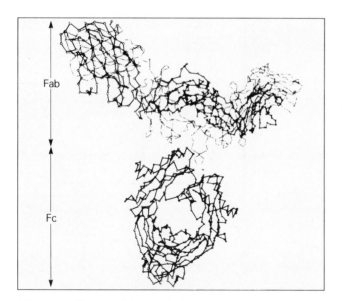

Fig. 4.21 Model of the α-carbon backbone of human IgG1. This model is based on X-ray crystallography studies which reveal that the polypeptide is folded into globular domains forming a Y-shaped structure. The antigen-binding surfaces formed between the variable regions of the light and heavy chains are located at the tips of the arms. The model clearly shows the hinge region between the Fab and Fc regions, as well as suggesting weak interaction between the Cγ2 domains and strong interaction between the Cγ3 domains. (Courtesy of Professor R. Huber.)

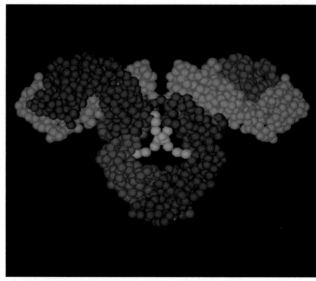

Fig. 4.22 Computer-generated model of the hinge-deleted human IgG1 protein Dob. One heavy chain is showed in blue and one in red, with two light chains being depicted in green. Carbohydrate bound to the Fc portion of the molecule is shown in turquoise. The structure of this immunoglobulin, which lacks a hinge region, was determined by David R. Davies *et al.* (*Proc. Nat. Acad. Sci. USA*, 1977; **74**). The computer graphics were generated using the system developed by Richard J. Feldmann at the National Institutes of Health.

Selected phagocyte receptors interacting with immunoglobulins

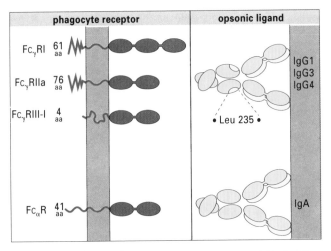

Fig 4.23 The receptor structures shown are those for Fc$_\gamma$RI (expressed by monocytes), Fc$_\gamma$RIIa (expressed by neutrophils) and Fc$_\gamma$RIII-I (expressed by neutrophils). The latter is attached by a phosphatidyl inositol glycan (PIG) membrane anchor, whereas the same receptor on NK cells is expressed as a normal transmembrane protein. The number of intracytoplasmic amino acids associated with each receptor is shown(left). Each receptor belongs to the immunoglobulin superfamily and expresses two or three extracellular immunoglobulin -like domains. In Fc$_\gamma$RI interactions, the structural motif of IgG that is probably involved is centred around Leu 235 in the C$_H$2 domain (red).

directed mutagenesis studies suggest that the high affinity Fc$_\gamma$RI receptor of monocytes interacts with a motif centred around a leucine residue at position 235 of the IgG heavy chain, between the Cγ2 domain and the hinge region (Fig. 4.23). The localization of sites interacting with other Fc receptors will probably require similar experimental approaches.

Another genetic engineering approach has been used to study the sites on the IgE molecule which interact with mast-cells through the Fc$_\epsilon$RI receptor, or with B cells through the Fc$_\epsilon$RII receptor. Recombinant peptides containing ε-chain sequences were synthesized by *Escherichia coli* expression and then used to inhibit IgE-receptor interactions. In the case of Fc$_\epsilon$RI interactions, a 76-residue peptide spanning the Cε2–Cε3 junction (Gln 301–Arg 376) appears to be critical (Fig. 4.24). In contrast, the Fc$_\epsilon$RII site appears to recognize a motif involving residues Lys 367–Val 370 of the Cε3 domains of both chains (Fig. 4.25).

One other effector function site has been mapped in some detail. The interaction between protein A of *Staphylococcus aureus* and the Fc region of IgG has been studied by both X-ray crystallography and circular dichroism. The data suggests that three contact areas exist spanning the Cγ2–Cγ3 junction in the Fc structure: these are residues 252–254 and 308–312 of the Cγ2 domain, and residues 433–436 of the Cγ3 domain. There appears to be a critical requirement for histidine at position 435. It is the replacement of histidine by arginine at position 435 of the γ$_3$ chain sequence which accounts for the inability of Caucasian IgG3 to bind to protein A.

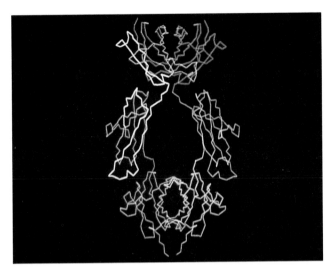

Fig. 4.24 Suggested location of the mast-cell receptor (Fc$_\epsilon$RI) binding site on human IgE. The Fc domains shown are (from top to bottom) Cε2, Cε3, and Cε4. The putative location of the peptide involved in binding is shown as a white segment extending from residue Gln 301 to residue Arg 376. (Reproduced from Helm *et al* [1988] with permission.)

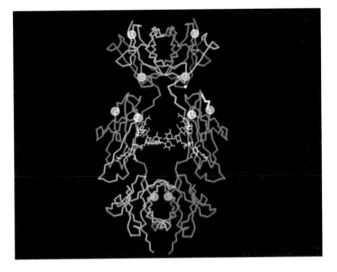

Fig. 4.25 Suggested location of the B-cell binding site (Fc$_\epsilon$RII) on human IgE. Model of IgE Fc showing the Cε2 on top, the Cε3 in the middle and the Cε4 at the bottom. The residues Lys 367–Val 370 of both ε chains (shown in white) are believed to contribute to the critical structure of the binding site. (Reproduced from Vercelli *et al* [1989], with permission.)

T-CELL ANTIGEN RECEPTORS

Antigen recognition by T lymphocytes is central to the generation and regulation of an effective immune response. Many important questions in immunology have centred on the nature of the receptor on T-cells that mediates specific antigen recognition. A T-cell receptor (TCR) was first defined and purified using specific antibodies directed against clone-specific (the equivalent of idiotypic) determinants on T-cells. It was called the αβ TCR because it was a heterodimeric molecule comprising an α chain and a β chain, linked by a disulphide bond. Independently, putative TCR α and β cDNA clones were isolated by either subtractive or differential hybridization of cDNA libraries. The amino acid sequence deduced from the nucleotide sequence of cDNA clones matched the partial sequence obtained from α and β TCR proteins purified using monoclonal antibodies. Thus, the two different approaches had identified the same entity. In further experiments, a second TCR, called γδ, was isolated.

THE CD3 COMPLEX
Structure of the CD3 polypeptides
The αβ and γδ forms of the TCR are both associated physically with a series of polypeptides, collectively called CD3. This association is required for surface expression of the TCR complex at the T-cell surface. The CD3 components show no amino acid variability on different T-cells and thus cannot generate the diver-

sity associated with TCRs. Rather, the CD3 component of the TCR is most probably required for signal transduction, following antigen recognition by the TCR heterodimer. CD3 comprises at least 5 invariant polypeptides, called γ, δ, ε, ζ and η (Fig. 4.26).

The CD3 γ, δ and ε chains are the products of three closely linked genes and are clearly related in their primary sequences. The polypeptides are members of the immunoglobulin superfamily, each containing an external domain followed by a transmembrane region and a highly conserved cytoplasmic tail of 40 or more amino acids. An unusual feature of the transmembrane regions is that they each contain a negatively-charged amino acid, rather than being completely apolar.

The CD3 ζ and η polypeptides are products of a single gene and differ at their C-terminal ends due to alternate splicing of the corresponding RNA. The CD3 ζη gene is on a different chromosome to the CD3 γδε gene complex and the ζη and γδε polypeptides are structurally unrelated. The ζ and η chains comprise a small extracellular domain of only nine amino acids, a transmembrane segment including a negatively-charged residue, and a large cytoplasmic tail. The cytoplasmic domains of the ζ and η chains diverge towards the C-terminal end with the cytoplasmic domain of CD3 η being 42 amino acids larger than that of CD3 ζ. The CD3 ζ and η chains exist as disulphide-linked dimers. Three dimeric forms exist (ζ–ζ, η–η and ζ–η) and have been postulated to perform different functions, perhaps varying the consequences of antigen recognition by the TCR at different stages of thymocyte development.

The stoichiometry of the TCR complex, and the way in which the CD3 chains are thought to interact with the αβ or γδ heterodimers, are discussed below.

CD3 phosphorylation
During T-cell activation, various components of the CD3 complex become phosphorylated on their intracytoplasmic portions. The murine and human CD3 γ chains are rapidly phosphorylated upon mitogen or antigen stimulation; this phosphorylation is mediated by the enzyme, protein kinase C. Minor phosphorylation of the murine δ chain also occurs. Protein kinase C-mediated phosphorylation of CD3 is thought to play a role in the downregulation of the TCR complex from the cell surface that occurs rapidly after occupancy of the TCR by antigen/MHC. This decrease in surface TCR levels may be involved in the desensitization of the T-cells that occurs after initial antigen stimulation.

Immune activation of T-cells also results in rapid and transient tyrosine phosphorylation of CD3 ζ. Two tyrosine kinases, p56[lck] and c-fyn, have been implicated as being important in T-cell activation. The product of the c-fyn oncogene is associated with the TCR complex and is, therefore, a good candidate for the kinase that phosphorylates CD3 ζ. Tyrosine phosphorylation on CD3 ζ is likely to form part of the signal transduction pathway that communicates signals from the T-cell surface to the nucleus, as both CD3 ζ and c-fyn are essential for T-cell activation.

Structure of CD3 polypeptides

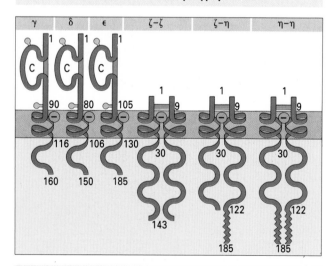

Fig. 4.26 The CD3 γ, δ and ε chains comprise an external immunoglobulin-like domain (C), a transmembrane segment containing a negatively charged amino acid (–) and a cytoplasmic tail. The numbers refer to the positions of the amino acid residues at the boundaries of the various domains. The external domains are glycosylated (purple). The ζ and η chains form disulphide-linked dimer combinations. These two chains are identical until position 122.

STRUCTURE OF THE αβ TCR HETERODIMER.

The αβ TCR comprises a disulphide-linked heterodimer of α (40–50 kDa) and β (35–47 kDa) subunits. The structural features of the αβ heterodimer are presented in Fig. 4.27. Each polypeptide chain comprises two immunoglobulin-like domains of approximately 110 amino acids, anchored into the plasma membrane by a transmembrane peptide and a short cytoplasmic tail. The difference in molecular weights of the α and β chains is accounted for by the presence of extra N-linked carbohydrate on the former.

The amino acid sequence variability resides in the N-terminal domains of the α and β polypeptides which are homologous with the variable domains of immunoglobulins. This domain is encoded by rearranging V, D and J gene segments for β, and the V and J gene segments for α (see Chapter 5). Analysis of different TCR V domain sequences has revealed areas of relatively greater variability which correspond to immunoglobulin hypervariable regions (CDRs).

The disulphide bond that links the α and β chains is in a peptide sequence between the constant domain and the transbilayer peptide. An unusual feature of both α- and β-chain transmembrane regions is the inclusion of positively-charged residues (see Fig. 4.27). These charged residues have been implicated in the assembly and intracellular transport of the TCR complex.

STRUCTURE OF THE TCR COMPLEX

The stoichiometry and subunit interactions of the components of the TCR complex are the subject of extensive study. *In vitro* mutagenesis studies have shown that the charged residues within the transmembrane regions are essential for the assembly and surface expression of the TCR complex. This presumably involves the generation of ion pairs within the lipid bilayer, between the basic amino acids in the TCR αβ peptides and the complementary acidic residues in the CD3 chains.

The immunoglobulin-like extracellular domains of the TCR (αβ or γδ) and CD3 (γ, δ and ε) polypeptides probably also form associations. In particular, the V domains of the αβ and γδ TCRs are thought to associate in much the same way as the VH/VL domains of Ig molecules, bringing the six TCR hypervariable regions together to form the antigen binding site. In the case of T-cells, this binding site must also bind sites on an MHC molecule that is alongside the antigen epitope. There are, however, no structural data to support this contention, although the key residues involved in VH/VL interactions are conserved in TCR V domains.

The subunit stoichiometry of the TCR–CD3 complex has not been clearly established, although various models have been proposed. Studies using transgenic mice have suggested that each complex contains two CD3 ε chains (Fig. 4.28).

Structure of human TCR heterodimers

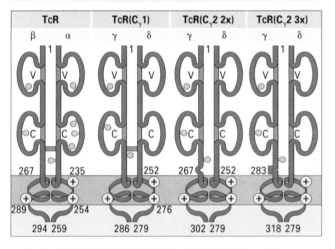

Fig. 4.27 The TCR α and β chains each comprise two external immunoglobulin-like domains (V and C), a transmembrane segment containing one (β) or two (α) positively-charged residues (+) and a short cytoplasmic tail. The positions of the domain boundaries are indicated. The α and β chains are disulphide linked. The human TCR γδ receptor can take several forms. The form containing a Cγ1 constant region contains an interchain disulphide bond, whereas Cγ2 forms are not disulphide linked. Duplication (2×) or triplication (3×) of a section of the γ chain generates different forms of the γ protein.

Suggested subunit interactions within the αβ TCR–CD3 complex

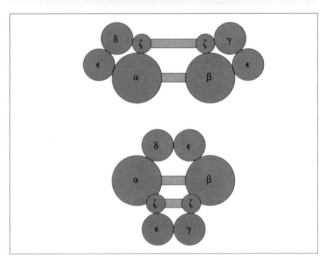

Fig. 4.28 The precise way in which the various subunits of the TCR–CD3 complex associate is unknown. However, various models have been proposed, based on biosynthetic experiments. Two alternatives are shown here. The α, β and CD3 ζ components form disulphide pairs. Other interactions (abutting circles) are based on non-covalent bonds. The TCR complexes may form higher order structures in the plasma membrane. (Taken from Manolios *et al*, 1991.)

STRUCTURE OF THE γδ TCR HETERODIMER

The overall structure of the γδ TCR is similar to that of its αβ counterpart, each chain being organized into external V and C domains, a transmembrane segment containing positively-charged residues and a short cytoplasmic tail (see Fig. 4.27). The human γδ TCR structure is more variable structurally than the mouse receptor. The human γ and δ chains are either disulphide linked or non-disulphide linked, these two forms correlating with the use of the Cγ1 or Cγ2 constant regions respectively, because Cγ2 possesses a cysteine in its second constant region exon. (See chapter 5 for TCR gene organization.) TCR γ chains containing a Cγ2 constant region vary in molecular weight due to duplication or triplication of the second exon. The biological significance of these structural differences remains unclear. In the mouse, non-disulphide linked forms for the γδ TCR have not been reported.

DISTRIBUTION OF αβ AND γδ FORMS OF TCR

The two forms of TCR show quite distinct anatomical locations. The αβ TCR is present on more than 95% of peripheral T cells and the vast majority of TCR-expressing thymocytes. In contrast, T cells expressing the γδ receptor often have defined anatomical locations. Although γδ T cells form only minor proportions of the T cells in the thymus and secondary lymphoid organs, they are abundant in various epithelia such as the epidermis (in mice but not humans), intestinal epithelium, uterus and tongue.

The various anatomically distinct γδ T-cell subsets differ structurally in terms of which V regions are expressed. The expression of different V gene segments by distinct γδ subsets may reflect their ontogeny. For example, γδ T cells residing in mouse skin (dendritic epidermal cells or DECs) express exclusively the Vγ3 and Vδ1 regions (see Chapter 5). Conversely, intraepithelial lymphocytes (IELs), from the gut epithelium,

express Vγ5 almost exclusively (in combination with predominantly Vδ4, Vδ5, Vδ6 or Vδ7). It is thought that these populations may arise at distinct stages during intrathymic T-cell development.

MAJOR HISTOCOMPATIBILITY COMPLEX ANTIGENS

The genetic loci involved in rejection of foreign or non-self tissues form a region known as the major histocompatibility complex (MHC). The highly polymorphic cell surface structures involved in rejection, called MHC antigens, were initially characterized using alloantibodies produced in one inbred strain of mice immunized with cells of other strains differing only at the MHC. Subsequently, specific antibodies to molecules encoded in subregions of the MHC, defined from crossovers in inbred strains, were used to map the MHC in detail. Similar techniques were used to define the human MHC, known as the human leucocyte antigen (HLA) system. The overall organisation of the human and murine MHCs is presented in Fig. 4.29. Three classes (I, II and III) have been identified as encoded within the murine and human MHCs. Class I and class II molecules represent distinct structural entities; that is, although multiple class I and class II genes exist within the MHC, all class I and class II gene products have similar overall structure. In contrast, the class III region contains a rather diverse collection of over 20 genes, including those encoding the components of the alternative complement activation pathway. There are no established functional or structural similarities between class III gene products and the class I or class II molecules. Therefore, only those loci involved in triggering T lymphocytes – the class I and II genes and their gene products – are described in this chapter.

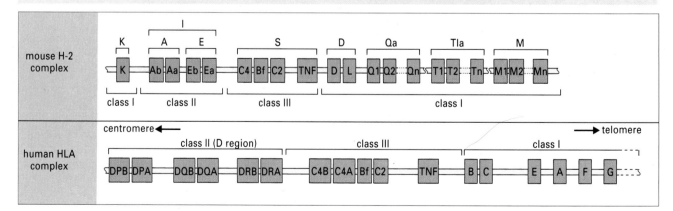

Organization of murine and human MHCs

Fig. 4.29 The locations of the subregions of the murine and human MHCs and the positions of the major genes within these subregions are shown. The human organization pattern, in which the Class II loci are positioned between the centromeric and the Class I loci, occurs in every other mammalian species so far examined.

THE STRUCTURE OF CLASS I MOLECULES

A scheme for the structure of MHC class I molecules is presented in Fig. 4.30. It comprises a glycosylated heavy chain (45 kDa) non-covalently associated with β_2-microglobulin (12 kDa) a polypeptide which is also found free in serum. The class I heavy chain consists of three extracellular domains, designated α_1 (N-terminal), α_2 and α_3, a transmembrane region and a cytoplasmic tail. The three extracellular domains each comprise about 90 amino acids and can be cleaved from the surface with the proteolytic enzyme papain. The α_2 and α_3 domains both have intrachain disulphide bonds enclosing loops of 63 and 86 amino acids respectively. The α_3 domain is homologous with immunoglobulin C domains. The extracellular portion of the class I heavy chain is glycosylated, the degree of glycosylation depending on the species and haplotype. The 25 amino acid, predominantly hydrophobic, transmembrane region traverses the lipid bilayer most probably in an α-helical conformation. The hydrophilic cytoplasmic domain of about 30–40 residues long may be phosphorylated *in vivo*.

β_2-microglobulin (β_2m) is a non-polymorphic protein in man, but is dimorphic in mice (a single amino acid change at position 85). It has the structure of an immunoglobulin C domain. This molecule also associates with a number of other class I-related structures, for example the products of the CD1 genes on chromosome 1 in man, and the Fc receptor that mediates the uptake of IgG from milk in intestinal cells of neonatal rats. Mouse mutants that lack the β_2m gene show that β_2m is required for expression of all class I antigens as well as for the gut Fc receptor at the cell surface.

The three-dimensional structures of the extracellular portion (α_1, α_2, α_3 domains and β_2m) of several human class I molecules have been elucidated by X-ray diffraction (Fig. 4.31). As predicted, the α_3 and β_2m domains

An intact human MHC class I antigen

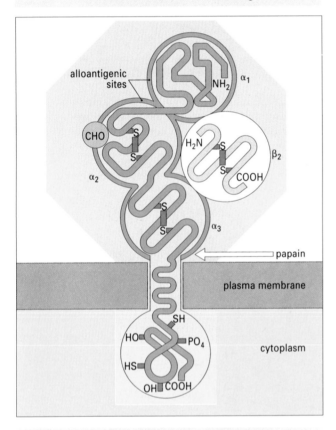

Fig. 4.30 The three globular domains of MHC (α_1, α_2 and α_3) are shown in green. The α_3 domain is closely associated with the non-MHC-encoded peptide, β_2-microglobulin (grey). β_2-microglobulin is stabilized by an intrachain disulphide bond (red) and has a similar tertiary structure to an immunoglobulin domain. Alloantigenic sites (carrying determinants specific to each individual) occur on the α_1 and α_2 domains and there is a carbohydrate unit attached to the α_2 domain (CHO). Papain cleaves the molecule close to the outer margin of the plasma membrane.

The extracellular domains of an MHC class I molecule

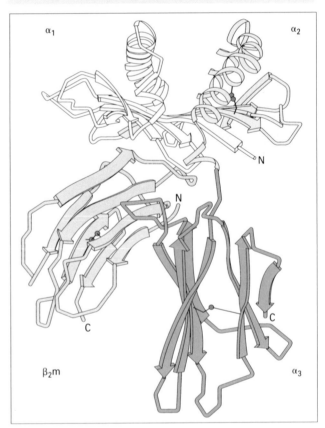

Fig. 4.31 The peptide backbone of HLA-A2 is shown. The three domains of the heavy chain each make interactions with α_1m. The groove formed by the α_1 and α_2 domains is clearly visible.

have immunoglobulin-like folds, although they interact in a manner not found between pairs of antibody constant domains, the $\beta_2 m$ molecule sitting at an angle under the α_1 and α_2 domains.

The α_1 and α_2 domains constitute a platform of eight anti-parallel β strands on top of which run two anti-parallel α helices (Fig. 4.32). The disulphide bond in the α_2 domain connects the N-terminal β strand to the α helix of the α_2 domain.

A long groove separates the α helices of the α_1 and α_2 domains. The original crystal structure of the HLA-A2 molecule revealed the presence of diffuse 'extra electron density' in the groove, suggesting that it was the binding site for processed antigen. This contention is strengthened by the observation that the majority of polymorphic residues and T-cell epitopes on class I molecules are located in or near the groove (see Fig. 4.32).

Comparison of the structures of HLA-A2 and HLA-Aw68 have further refined the structural basis for the binding of peptide to class I antigens. The differences

between HLA-A2 and HLA-Aw68 result from amino acid side-chain differences at 13 positions, six of which are in α_1, six in α_2 and one in the α_3 domain (residue 245, which contributes to interactions with CD8). Ten of the α_1 and α_2 differences are at positions lining the floor and side of the peptide-binding groove (Fig. 4.33). These differences give rise to dramatic differences in the shape of the groove and on the peptides that it will bind. Interestingly, the groove is not a smooth structure, but has a number of subsites formed from ridges and pockets with which amino acid side chains could interact (Fig. 4.34). For example, two pockets extend under the helix of the α_1 domain into which side chains or the ends of peptides could extend. Amino acid variations within the groove can vary the positions of the pockets (see Fig. 4.34), providing a structural basis for differences in peptide binding affinity that in turn govern responsiveness versus non-responsiveness in the immune response.

THE STRUCTURE OF CLASS II MOLECULES

The products of the class II genes (A and E in the mouse, DR, DQ and DP in humans) are heterodimers of heavy (α) and light (β) glycoprotein chains. The α chains have molecular weights of 30–34 kDa and the β chains range from 26–29 kDa depending on the locus involved. A number of lines of evidence indicate that the α and β chains have the same overall structures. An

The top surface of HLA-A2

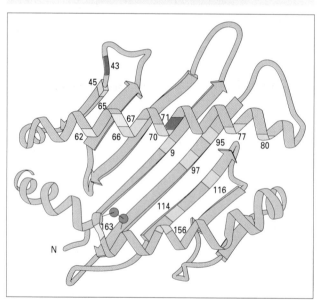

Fig. 4.32 The view of the peptide antigen-binding groove in HLA-A2 as 'seen' by the TCR, is shown. The α_1 and α_2 domains each consist of four antiparallel β strands followed by a long helical region, and the domains pair to form a single eight-stranded β sheet topped by α helices. The locations of the most polymorphic residues are highlighted. Five residues on the central β strands of the α_1–α_2 β sheet point up between the two helical regions and may make contact with bound antigenic peptides. Six residues face into the site from the sides of the helices (red). Three residues are on the top face of the helices and are candidates for making direct contacts with the TCR (yellow). Residues coloured green are not in a position to affect the binding of antigenic peptides. (Modified from Bjorkman et al [1987].)

HLA-A2 and HLA-Aw68

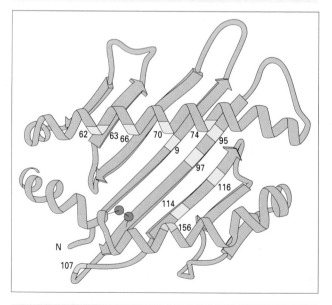

Fig. 4.33 HLA-A2 and HLA-Aw68 differ at 13 amino acid residues. Twelve of these are in the α_1 and α_2 domains. The ten amino acid differences that line the peptide groove are coloured yellow. (Modified from Parham [1989].)

extracellular portion comprising two domains (α_1 and α_2, or β_1 and β_2) is connected by a short sequence to a transmembrane region of about 30 residues and a cytoplasmic domain of about 10–15 residues. A schematic structure for class II antigens is shown in Fig. 4.35.

The α_2 and β_2 domains are similar to the class I α_3 domain and β_2m, having the structural characteristics of immunoglobulin constant domains. The β_1 domain contains a disulphide bond generating a 64 amino acid loop. The difference in molecular weights of the class II α and β chains is primarily due to differential glycosylation, the α_1, α_2 and β_1, but not β_2, domains are N-glycosylated, the β_2 domain is not.

Although at a superficial level the class II α_1 and β_1 domains show only weak overall sequence similarity to the class I α_1 and α_2 domains (which create the peptide binding groove), the presence of key conserved residues suggests that many structural features may be shared. Molecular modelling studies have been carried out on the assumption that the four extracellular domains of the class II antigens (α_1, α_2, β_1, β_2) associate in a similar fashion to the class I molecule. When class II molecules are modelled onto the HLA-A2 structure (see Fig. 4.31), an analogous groove appears, formed from the C-terminal α helices of the α_1 and β_1 domains. The base underlying the groove is formed by the N-terminal β strands of each domain. Class II structural polymorphism turns out to be concentrated in and around this groove, just as it is in class I. If the supposed structural analogy with class I antigens is correct, this groove constitutes the antigen binding site of the class II molecule. However, formal proof of this requires high-resolution analysis of class II crystals.

GENOMIC ORGANIZATION OF THE MHC
Murine class I loci

There are about 30 class I genes in the murine haploid genome but this number varies amongst haplotypes of different inbred strains. These encode the classical, serologically defined H–2 loci, H–2K, H–2D and H–2L. Most of the remaining genes, which map to the Qa, Tla and M regions, are of unknown significance (Fig. 4.36) although it is possible to trigger T-cell activation via the Qa-2 molecule.

The organization of the H–2K region is similar in all strains that have been studied. It contains two class I genes, termed K and K2 (see Fig. 4.36). The H–2K gene encodes the appropriate H-2K antigen, whereas the H–2K2 gene exhibits varied patterns of expression in different strains.

The number of class I genes in the H–2D/H–2L region varies between the H–2^d and H–2^b haplotypes (see Fig. 4.36). Five class I genes map to the D/L region of BALB/c H–2^d mice, two genes encoding the serologically detectable H–2D^d and H–2L^d antigens. Only one B10 H–2D^b gene has been identified. Three additional class I genes are found in the 170 kb of DNA between the proximal H–2D^d and distal H–2L^d genes. These genes, called D2^d, D3^d and D4^d are of unknown function.

The Qa locus comprises about 200 kb of DNA distal to H–2D/L (see Fig. 4.36). This region encodes the serologically detectable specificities Qa-2, 3, 4 and 5 and encompasses a cluster of eight (BALB/c) to ten (B10) class I genes.

Comparison of the binding sites of HLA-Aw68 and HLA-A2

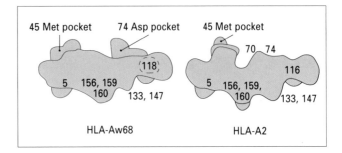

Fig. 4.34 Schematic outlines of the peptide binding grooves of HLA-Aw68 and HLA-A2 are shown . The pockets into which residues of the bound antigenic peptides are thought to fit are labelled.

Schematic representation of a class II antigen

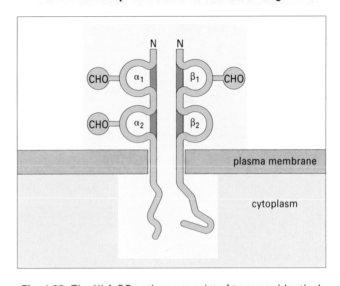

Fig. 4.35 The HLA-DR antigens consist of two non-identical peptides (α and β), non-covalently bound, which traverse the plasma membrane towards the C terminus. Both chains have two globular domains outside the cell. The domain closest to the membrane in each chain is structurally related to immunoglobulin domains. All except the α_1 domain are stabilized by interchain disulphide bonds (red). Both chains have carbohydrate units attached. The shorter β chain (mol. wt 28 000) contains the alloantigenic sites although there is also some structural polymorphism in the α chain of some class II molecules.

The murine Tla region, although defined initially as encoding the TL (thymus leukaemia) antigen, has subsequently been shown to contain the largest number of class I genes and the greatest number of differences in organization between the B10 and BALB/c haplotypes (see Fig. 4.36).

The M region is located distal to the Tla region and contains a number of new class I genes, termed M1–M7. These genes exhibit a low degree of polymorphism. One of these genes is associated with the maternally transmitted antigen (Mta). It is now known that Mta comprises two components: MTF, a hydrophobic peptide from the N-terminal end of the mitochondrially encoded ND1 protein, and the product of the class I-like gene from the M region.

Human class I loci
The human class I region contains three loci, called HLA-A, HLA-B and HLA-C. These loci encode the classical major transplantation antigens and extend over 1.5 million bases of DNA (Fig. 4.37). However, further analysis of this region has revealed multiple additional class I genes. The HLA-E, -F and -G genes can potentially direct the synthesis of class I protein and the HLA-G gene product has been demonstrated in extravillous cytotrophoblast-derived choriocarcinoma cell lines and in the tamarins (a group of New World primates). A non-classical class I gene called cda12 has been mapped to within 50 kb of HLA-A. Other class I genes that may be the human counterparts of the murine Qa, Tla and M genes reside near the HLA-G and HLA-A genes.

Murine class II loci
The α and β chains of murine class II molecules are encoded by separate genes located in the I region of the H–2 complex and are shown in Fig 4.38, where the comparison with human MHC genes is made. The Ab and Aa genes encode the A molecule and Eb and Ea genes encode the E molecule. Several other α- and β-chain genes have been cloned, for which no protein product is known. One of these, Pb, is a pseudogene whereas two others, called Ob and Eb2, are potentially functional. These latter genes contain a low level of polymorphism and are transcribed, but it is not known whether they are translated. Almost the whole H–2I region has been mapped and has been linked to the class I H–2K subregion.

Genes within the murine class I region

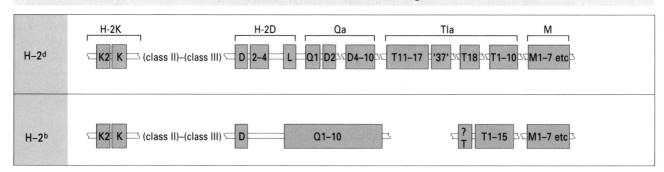

Fig. 4.36 The organization of the MHC class I region of two haplotypes, BALB/c (H–2^d) and B10 (H–2^b) is shown. The class II–class III region splits the H–2K and H–2D regions. The brackets denote gaps added to align alleles between the two haplotypes. The Tla region contains the largest number of class I genes.

Genes within the human class I regions

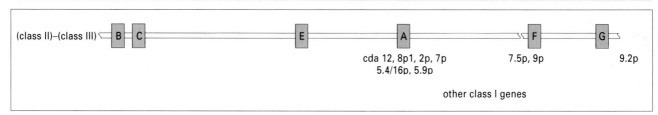

Fig. 4.37 The human class I region lies telomeric to the class II–class III region. In addition to the genes encoding the classical transplantation antigens (HLA-A, HLA-B and HLA-C), several other class I-like genes have been identified that may be the equivalent of the murine Tla/Qa region. Brackets denote areas where the orientation is not known.

Mice of the b, s, f and q haplotypes fail to express I-E class II products. The b and s haplotypes fail to transcribe the Ea gene but make normal cytoplasmic levels of Eβ chain. Mice of f and q haplotypes fail to make both Eα and Eβ chains.

Human class II loci

Human class II genes are located in the HLA-D region that encodes at least six α and ten β chain genes (see Fig. 4.38). Three loci, DR, DQ and DP, encode the major expressed products of the human class II region, but additional genes have also been identified. The DR family comprises a single α gene (DRA) and up to four β genes (DRB1–4), whereas DQ and DP families each have one expressed α and β gene, and an additional pair of genes which may or may not be functional. As with their murine counterparts the DR, DQ and DP α chains associate in the cell primarily with β chains of their own loci. The DPA1 and DPB1 gene products associate to generate the HLA-DP class II molecules detected using specific antibodies. Similarly, DQA1 and DQB1 encode the HLA-DQ antigens. Within the DR locus, DRA, DRB1 and DRB3 or DRB4 are generally expressed and DRB2 is a pseudogene. The organization and length of the DRB region varies in different haplotypes. The DPA2, DPB2, DVB and DRB2 genes are generally pseudogenes and are therefore not expressed. In contrast, the DNA, DOB, DQB2 and DQA2 genes may be functional.

The order of all the known HLA class II genes has been established using long-range genetic mapping techniques. The region spans about 1000 kb of DNA and the order of the various loci is similar to that of the homologous loci in the murine class II region.

MHC POLYMORPHISM

A hallmark of the MHC is the extreme degree of polymorphism encoded within it. Polymorphism is not evenly spread throughout the MHC. The class I-like Qa, Tla and M antigens are much less polymorphic than the classical class I and class II antigens. The list of current specificities, with the allelic variants detected for HLA class I and class II antigens, is shown in Fig. 4.39.

Within a particular class I or class II molecule, the structural polymorphism is clustered in particular regions of the molecule. The amino acid sequence variability in class I antigens is clustered in three main regions of the α_1 and α_2 domains. The α_3 domain appears to be much more conserved. In class II molecules, the extent of variability depends on the subregion and on the polypeptide chain. For example, within human class II molecules, most polymorphism occurs in DR and DQβ chains while DPβ chains are slightly less polymorphic. DQα is polymorphic whereas DRα chains are virtually invariant and DRα chains are represented by two alleles. In outbred populations where individuals have two MHC haplotypes, hybrid class II molecules, with one chain from each haplotype, can be produced. This generates additional structural diversity in the expressed molecules.

As discussed above, most of the polymorphic amino acids in class I and class II antigens are clustered on top of the molecule in the large groove that acts as the peptide binding site. Thus, variation is almost exclusively centred in the base of the antigen binding groove or pointing in from the sides of the α-helix region. The implications of this concentration of polymorphic residues for T-cell antigen recognition are discussed more fully in Chapter 6.

Genes within the human and murine class II regions

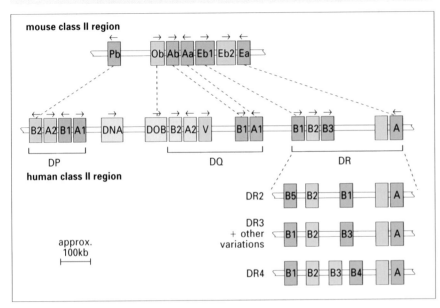

Fig. 4.38 The arrangement of the genes within the human and murine MHCs is shown. Homologous genes between the two species are indicated. Expressed genes are indicated (orange) and pseudogenes are represented (yellow). Pink areas denote genes for which a protein product has not been found, but which do not appear to be pseudogenes. Different arrangements of DR haplotypes are shown.

FURTHER READING

Bjorkman PJ, Parham P. Structure, function and diversity of Class I major histocompatibility complex molecules. *Annu Rev Biochem* 1990;**59**:253–88.

Bjorkman PJ, Saper MA, Samraoui B, Bennett WS, Strominger JL, Wiley DC. The structure of the human Class I histocompatibility antigen HLA-A2. *Nature* 1987;**329**:506–12.

Bjorkman PJ, Samraoui B, Bennett WS, Strominger JL, Wiley DC. The foreign antigen binding site and T-cell recognition regions of Class I histocompatibility antigens. *Nature* 1987;**329**:512–16.

Bodmer JG, Marsh SGE, Parham P, *et al.* Nomenclature for factors of the HLA system, 1989 *Hum Immunol* 1990;**28**:327–42.

Brenner MB, MacLean J, Dialynas DP, *et al.* Identification of a putative second T-cell receptor *Nature* 1986;**322**:145–49.

Brown JH, Jardetzky T, Saper MA, Samraoui B, Bjorkman PJ, Wiley DC. A hypothetical model of the foreign antigen binding site of Class II histocompatibility molecules. *Nature* 1988;**332**:845–50.

Burton DR. Antibody: the flexible adaptor molecule. *Trends Biochem Sci* 1990;**15**:64–69.

Capra D, Edmundson AB. The antibody-combining site. *Sci Am* 1977;**236**:50.

Clevers H, Alarcon B, Wileman T, Terhorst C. The T-cell receptor/CD3 complex: a dynamic protein ensemble. *Annu Rev Immunol* 1988;**6**:629–62.

Davis AC, Schulman MJ. IgM – molecular requirements for its assembly and function. *Immunol Today* 1989;**10**:118–22 & 127–28.

Davies DR, Metzger H. Structural basis of antibody function. *Annu Rev Immunol* 1983;**1**:87–117.

Duncan AR, Winter G. The binding site for Clq on IgG. *Nature* 1988;**332**:738–40.

Duncan AR, Woof JM, Partridge LJ, Burton DR, Winter G. Localization of the binding site for the human high-affinity Fc receptor on IgG. *Nature* 1988;**332**:563–64.

Feinstein A, Richardson N, Taussig MJ. Immunoglobulin flexibility in complement activation. *Immunol Today* 1986;**7**:169–73.

Flanagan BF, Owen MJ. T cell antigen receptor. In: Farid NR, ed. *The Immunogenetics of Autoimmune Diseases*. Vol 1. Oxford: CRC Press, 1991:19–42.

Garratt TPJ, Saper MA, Bjorkman PJ, Strominger JL, Wiley DC. Specificity pockets for the side chains of peptide antigens in HLA-w68. *Nature* 1989;**342**:692–96.

Germain RN. The ins and outs of antigen processing and presentation. *Nature* 1986;**322**:687–89.

Green NM. The semiotics of charge. *Nature* 1991;**351**:349.

Guillemot F, Auffray C, Orr HT, Strominger JL. MHC antigen genes. In: Hames BD, Glover DM, eds. *Molecular Immunology*. Oxford: IRL Press, 1988:88–143

Hahn GS. Antibody structure, function and active sites. In: Ritzmann SE, ed. *Physiology of Immunoglobulins: Diagnostic and Clinical Aspects*. New York: Alan Liss Inc, 1982.

Hedrick SM, Nielsen EA, Davis MM. Sequence relationships between putative T-cell receptor polypeptides and immunoglobulin. *Nature* 1984;**308**:153–158.

Helm B, Marsh P, Vercelli D, Padlan E, Gould H, Geha R. The mast cell binding site on human immunoglobulin E. *Nature* 1988;**331**:180–183

Kappes D, Strominger JL. Human Class II major histocompatibility complex genes and proteins. *Annu Rev Biochem* 1988;**57**:991–1028.

Lefranc M-P, Rabbitts TH. The human T-cell receptor γ (TRG) genes. *Trends Biochem Sci* 1989;**14**:214–18.

Manolios N, Letourneur F, Bonifacino JS, Klausner RD. Pairwise cooperative and inhibitory interactions describe the assembly and probable structure of the T-cell antigen receptor. *EMBO J* 1991;**10**:1643–51.

Mestecky J, McGhee JR. Immunoglobulin A (IgA): molecular and cellular interactions involved in IgA biosynthesis and immune response. *Adv Immunol* 1987;**40**:153–245.

Möller G, ed. Immunoglobulin D: structure, synthesis, membrane representation and function. *Immunol Rev* 1977;**37**.

Möller G, ed. Immunoglobulin E. *Immunol Rev* 1978;**41**.

Nisonoff S. *Introduction to Molecular Immunology*. 2nd ed. Baltimore: Sinauer Associates Inc, 1984.

Parham P. Getting into the groove. *Nature* 1984;**342**:616–17.

Shakib F, ed. *The human IgG subclasses. Molecular analysis of structure, function, and regulation*. Oxford: Pergamon Press, 1990.

Townsend A, Bodmer H. Antigen recognition by Class I-restricted T lymphocytes. *Annu Rev Immunol* 1989;**7**:601–24.

Trowsdale J, Campbell RD. Physical map of the human HLA region. *Immunol Today* 1988;**9**:34–35.

Turner MW. Structure and function of immunoglobulins. In: Glynn LE, Steward MW, eds. *Immunochemistry: An advanced textbook*. Chichester: John Wiley & Sons, 1977.

Turner MW. Immunoglobulins. In: Holborrow EJ, Reeves WG, eds. *Immunology and Medicine. A comprehensive guide to clinical immunology*. 2nd edition. London: Grune & Stratton, 1983.

Underdown BJ, Schiff JM. Immunoglobulin A: strategic defence initiative at the mucosal surface. *Annu Rev Immunol* 1986;**4**:389–417.

Vercelli D, Helm B, Marsh P, Padlan E, Geha RS, Gould H. The B cell binding site on human immunoglobulin E. *Nature* 1989;**338**:649–51

Weiss A, Imbodan J, Hardy K, Manger B, Terhorst C, Stobo J. The role of the T3/antigen receptor complex in T-cell activation. *Annu Rev Immunol* 1 986;**4**:593–619.

Williams AF, Barclay AN. The immunoglobulin superfamily – domains for cell surface recognition. *Annu Rev Immunol* 1988;**6**:381–405.

Zÿlstra M, Bix M, Sinister NE, Loring JM, Raulet DH, Jaenisch R. β_2-microglobulin deficient mice lack CD4$^-$8$^+$ cytolytic T cells. *Nature* 1990;**334**:742–46.

chapter 5

The Generation of Diversity

The ability of the immune system to recognize antigens depends on the antibodies generated by B cells and on the antigen receptors expressed by T cells. Although the ways in which T cells and B cells recognize antigen are quite different, both cell populations are capable of recognizing a wide range of antigens. This chapter is concerned with the ways in which the immune system generates a great diversity of antibodies and T-cell antigen receptors (TCRs), of different antigenic specificities. In spite of the differences between antibodies and T-cell receptors, the cellular and molecular processes which generate diversity are very similar for each type of molecule.

Antibodies are remarkably diverse; not only do they provide enough different combining sites to recognize the millions of antigenic shapes in the environment, but also each class of antibody has a different effector region so that, for instance, IgE can bind to Fc receptors on mast cells, whereas IgG can bind to phagocytes. It has been estimated that an individual produces more different forms of antibody than all the other proteins of the body put together. In fact, we produce more types of antibody than there are genes in our genome. How can all this diversity be generated? Ideas about the formation of antibodies have changed considerably over the years, but it is perhaps surprising how close Ehrlich came with his side-chain hypothesis at the beginning of this century (Fig. 5.1). His idea of antigen-induced selection is close to our present view of clonal selection except that he placed several different receptors on the same cell.

THEORIES OF ANTIBODY FORMATION

After Ehrlich the situation became complicated. The problem was that many new organic chemicals were now being synthesized and Landsteiner was showing that the immune system could react with the production of specific antibody for each new compound. It was simply not thought possible that the immune system could, by natural selection, have maintained genes for all these antibodies directed at novel, artificial compounds. This led to the development of the instructive hypothesis, which suggested that a flexible antibody molecule is acted on by antigen to form a complementary binding site. With the spectacular progress in molecular biology in the 1950s and 1960s, the instructive hypothesis became untenable, since it had become clear that the mechanism for the proposed 'instruction' simply did not exist. The circle turned, and selective theories came back into favour with Jerne and Burnet

independently putting forward the idea of clonal selection – each lymphocyte produces one type of immunoglobulin only, and the antigen selects and stimulates cells carrying that immunoglobulin type.

This still left the problem of antibody diversity. One solution was the existence of a separate gene for each antibody specificity. This immediately presented a problem: looking at the structure of a light chain, half the chain is variable in amino acid sequence but the other half is constant. Similarly with heavy chains, a quarter of the chain is variable while the rest is constant. How, if there were many genes, was it possible to maintain this constancy of sequence in the constant

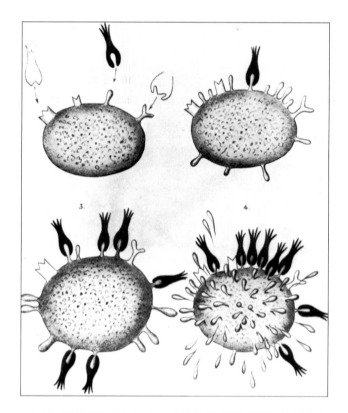

Fig. 5.1 Ehrlich's side-chain theory. Ehrlich proposed that the combination of antigen with a preformed B cell receptor (now known to be antibody) triggered the cell to produce and secrete more of those receptors. Although the diagram indicates that he thought a single cell could produce antibodies to bind more than one type of antigen it is evident that he anticipated both the clonal selection theory and the idea that the immune system could generate receptors before contact with antigen.

regions? Dreyer and Bennett proposed a solution to this problem by suggesting that the constant and variable portions of the chains are coded for by separate genes, with one or only a few genes coding for the constant region and many genes coding for the variable region. The theory now only had to account for the multiple variable regions! A solution to this aspect of the diversity problem was suggested by the idea of somatic mutation. A relatively few germ line genes would give rise to many mutated genes during the lifetime of the individual. Furthermore, it had been suggested that a number of gene segments could recombine to give a complete V gene. This gave three possible solutions to the problem of generating diversity:

1. multiple V region genes in the germ line
2. somatic recombination between elements forming a V region gene
3. somatic mutation.

It is now known that mammals use all three mechanisms to generate diversity (Fig. 5.2). Interestingly, however, sharks rely on having a large number of antibody genes, and do not use somatic recombination, while birds have small numbers of antibody genes which undergo a very high level of gene conversion (see Chapter 14).

Generation of antibody diversity

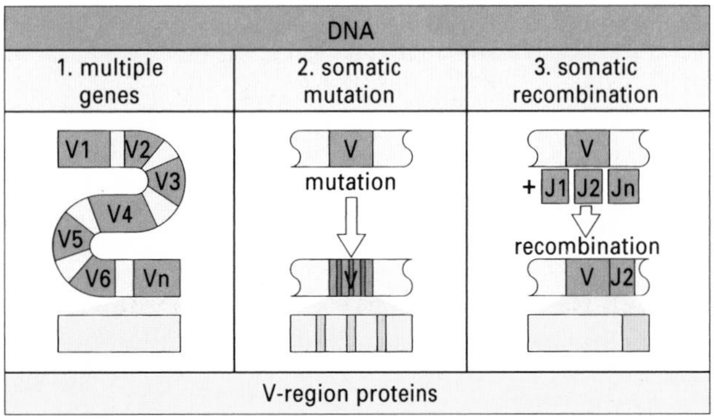

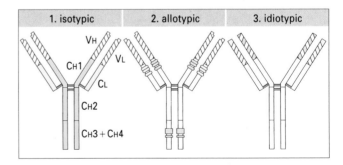

Fig. 5.2 Three mechanisms are proposed by which the immune system could generate different V regions on the immunoglobulin H and L chains.
1. Multiple genes. There are a large number of separate genes (V1–Vn), each encoding one V region domain.
2. Somatic mutation. A primordial V gene mutates during B cell ontogeny to produce different genes in different B cell clones.
3. Somatic recombination. A number of gene segments (J1–Jn) recombine to join the main part of the V region gene. This occurs during B cell ontogeny and results in a protein containing elements encoded by different gene segments. It is known that all three mechanisms are involved in the generation of antibody diversity in mammals.

 IMMUNOGLOBULIN VARIABILITY

Immunoglobulins are composed of heavy and light chains, the light chains being either κ or λ. Since virtually any light chain can combine with any heavy chain, the number of possible antigen-binding sites is the product of the number of heavy and light chains. Part

Chromosome location of MHC and antigen receptor genes

peptide	mouse	human
IgH	12	14
λ	16	22
κ	6	2
TCRα	14	14
TCRβ	6	7
TCRγ	13	7
TCRδ	14	14
MHC	17	6
β₂-microglobulin	2	15

Fig. 5.3 The numbers refer to the chromosomal location of the genes for the various peptides in man and mouse. Note that all of the loci are completely separate, with the single exception of the T cell receptor (TCR) δ chain which lies within the TCR α gene loci.

Variability of immunoglobulin structure

Fig. 5.4 All immunoglobulins have the basic four-chain structure. There are three types of immunoglobulin variability.
1. Isotypic variation is present in the germ line of all members of a species, producing the heavy (μ, δ, γ, ε, α) and light chains (κ, λ) and the V region frameworks (subgroups).
2. Allotypic variation is intraspecies allelic variability.
3. Idiotypic variation refers to the diversity at the antigen-binding site (paratope) and in particular relates to the hypervariable segments.

of the variability in immunoglobulin structure is derived from the interaction of these separate polypeptide chains. For example, if there are 10^4 different light chains each capable of binding with any of 10^4 different heavy chains, then theoretically, 10^8 different antibody specificities may be produced. Separate diversification mechanisms exist for each of the chains as they are encoded on separate chromosomes (Fig. 5.3).

Polymorphic forms of immunoglobulins derive from variation in many parts of the molecule (Fig. 5.4). It is the idiotypic variability, which pertains to the generation of the antigen-binding site, with which we shall first be concerned. Kabat and Wu analysed the variable regions from the amino acid sequences of many light and heavy chains. For a source of identical antibodies, they relied on myelomas (monoclonal B cell tumours producing antibody). It was clear that the variability in amino acid sequence was concentrated in three hypervariable regions surrounded by relatively invariant framework residues. These hypervariable regions were shown to be the regions which made contact with the antigen (complementarity-determining regions, or CDRs). Initially they studied the mouse, a species where less than 5% of the antibodies possess λ light chains and diversity is correspondingly less. (This was later shown to be due to the very small number of Vλ genes in the mouse.) Out of 19 λ1 light chain sequences examined, 12 were found to be identical, with the other 7 differing from each other and the prototype sequence by only a few residues (Fig. 5.5).

The variability in the heavy chain is similarly concentrated in three hypervariable regions, with background variability on each side of the CDRs (Fig. 5.6). The heavy chain frameworks (between the CDRs) can be arranged into groups on the basis of similarity, or identity, of framework sequences (see Fig. 5.7).

LIGHT CHAIN GENE RECOMBINATION

With the advent of recombinant DNA techniques in the 1970s it became possible to attempt analysis of the genes responsible for coding for antibodies. Because of its lesser heterogeneity, work started on the λ1 system (first of the four sets of λ genes in the mouse), using restriction endonucleases to digest the DNA. It was found that two separate segments of DNA coded for the constant and variable regions and that, in cells not producing antibody, these gene segments are far apart on the chromosomes, whereas in antibody-forming cells they are brought closer together. Even in a fully differentiated B cell these two gene segments do not join directly, but remain about 1500 base pairs apart. Between the V and C segments, and joined onto the V segment in the rearranged chromosomes, is an extra short section of DNA known as the J segment.

Variability of lambda light chains

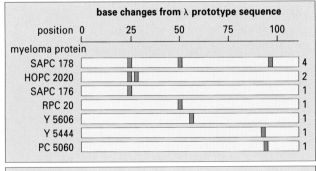

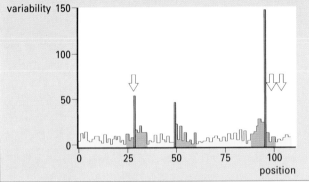

Fig. 5.5 The amino acid sequences of seven mouse λ₁ myeloma proteins are represented. Positions in yellow indicate identity to the prototype sequence (MOPC 104E), positions in red indicate differences. The number of base changes in the DNA required to produce the given alteration in amino acid structure is given on the right. Below is a Kabat and Wu plot of light chain variability. Arrows indicate extra bases in some sequences.

Variability of heavy chains

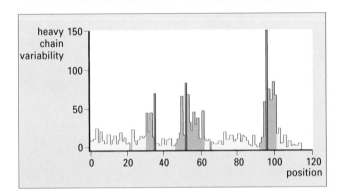

Fig. 5.6 This Kabat and Wu plot shows variability concentrated in three regions of the variable region of heavy chains. The method for determining variability is described in Chapter 4.

Basically the V gene segment codes for the V region of the antibody light chain, up to and including amino acid 95, and the J segment gene codes for the rest of the V region (Fig. 5.8). In mouse, but not in man, the total number of gene segments contributing to the λ light chain system is limited compared with the other immunoglobulin or T-cell receptor (TCR) loci. Three V segments, and four Jλ–Cλ clusters have been described (Fig. 5.8). One of these J segments, Jλ4, is a pseudogene. Recombination nearly always takes place within a V–J–C cluster so that only four combinations are possible – Vλ2Jλ2, VλXJλ2, Vλ1Jλ3 and Vλ1Jλ1. Each V segment gene is preceded by a signal or leader sequence coding for a short hydrophobic sequence, which is responsible for the transport of the antibody molecule through the membrane of the endoplasmic reticulum during translation. This leader sequence is then cleaved away after synthesis of the chain. The J segments which form part of the V domains are completely different from the J chain present in IgM and dimeric IgA.

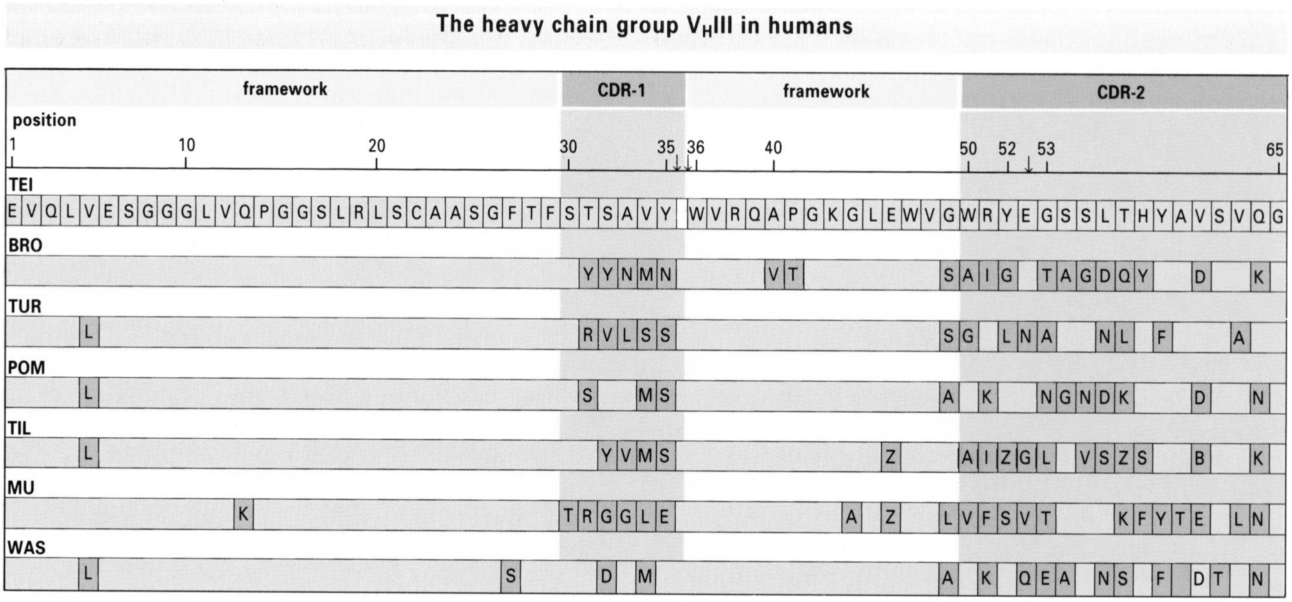

The heavy chain group V_HIII in humans

	framework	CDR-1	framework	CDR-2
position	1 ... 10 ... 20 ... 30	35 36	40	50 52 53 ... 65
TEI	E V Q L V E S G G G L V Q P G G S L R L S C A A S G F T F S	T S A V Y	W V R Q A P G K G L E W V G	W R Y E G S S L T H Y A V S V Q G
BRO		Y Y N M N	V T	S A I G · T A G D Q Y · D · K
TUR	L	R V L S S		S G · L N A · N L · F · A
POM	L	S · M S		A · K · N G N D K · D · N
TIL	L	Y V M S	Z	A I Z G L · V S Z S · B · K
MU	K	T R G G L E	A Z	L V F S V T · K F Y T E · L N
WAS	L	S · D M		A · K · Q E A · N S · F · D T · N

Fig. 5.7 The 65 N-terminal amino acids of six human myelomas falling into the V_H III group are compared diagrammatically to the prototype sequence TEI . Amino acids identical to those in TEI are shown in yellow, amino acids which differ from those at the same position in TEI are orange. The majority of differences within a single group occur in the complementarity-determining regions CDR-1 and CDR-2. The third hypervariable region is not shown.

Lambda chain production in the mouse

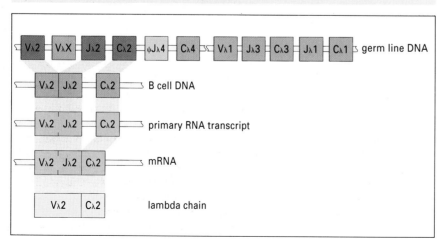

germ line DNA: Vλ2 – VλX – Jλ2 – Cλ2 – ψJλ4 – Cλ4 – Vλ1 – Jλ3 – Cλ3 – Jλ1 – Cλ1

B cell DNA: Vλ2 Jλ2 – Cλ2

primary RNA transcript: Vλ2 Jλ2 – Cλ2

mRNA: Vλ2 Jλ2 Cλ2

lambda chain: Vλ2 Cλ2

Fig. 5.8 During B cell differentiation one of the germ line Vλ genes recombines with its J-associated segment to form a V–J combination. The rearranged gene is transcribed into a primary RNA transcript complete with introns (non-coding segments occurring between the genes), exons (which code for protein) and a poly-A tail. This is spliced to form messenger RNA (mRNA) with loss of the introns, and then translated into protein. Gene segments which encode the final polypeptide are indicated in a darker shade, DNA is in orange, RNA in green and immunoglobulin peptides in yellow.

The κ chain system is more heterogeneous because there are more V segment genes but only one constant region gene (Fig. 5.9). In an embryonic or non-lymphoid cell the Vκ segment genes, of which there are about 350, are again at some distance on the chromosome from the C gene. In the mouse these V segment genes appear to be organized in sets, each set comprising about seven genes. In between and closer to the C gene are five J genes; one of the J genes is a pseudogene and is never expressed. During differentiation of lymphoid cells there is a rearrangement of the DNA such that one of the V segment genes is joined to a J segment gene. Thus the number of possible κ chain variable regions that can be produced is approximately 1400 (350 × 4). There is still a gap or intron between the J segment genes and the gene for the C region. This whole stretch of DNA (from the leader to the end of the C gene, including introns) is then transcribed into heterogeneous nuclear RNA, i.e. unprocessed messenger RNA (mRNA). A process of RNA splicing then removes the introns, leaving mRNA which can be translated into protein. This splicing out of introns can be revealed by heteroduplex analysis, where the mRNA is mixed with denatured single-stranded DNA from the antibody-forming cell, allowed to reanneal and then examined by electron microscopy. Hybridization of V and C regions readily occurs revealing the intron that lies between them (Fig. 5.10).

HEAVY CHAIN GENE RECOMBINATION

The heavy chain is also encoded by V and J segment genes. Additional diversity is provided by a third gene segment, the D segment gene (Fig. 5.11). If one examines the family of monoclonal antibodies which bind dextran, the gene segment for the VH domain appears to end at codon 99 while the gene segment for the JH segment starts at codon 102. This leaves two codons in between not accounted for by either V or J segments, and these form the additional D (diversity) segment. This section is highly variable both in the sequences of the codons and in their number. In antibodies binding dextran this section comprises two amino acids, but in those binding phosphorylcholine up to eight amino acids are inserted, while in anti-levan antibodies this section is completely missing. More than one D segment may join to form an enlarged D region. The D region may be read in three possible reading frames without generating stop codons, so adding to diversity.

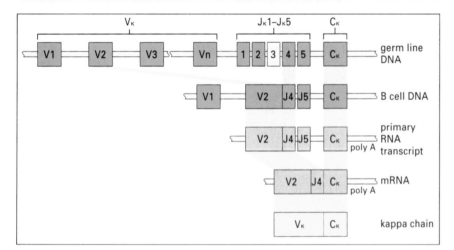

Fig. 5.9 During differentiation of the pre-B cell one of several Vκ genes on the germ line DNA (V1–Vn) is recombined and apposed to a Jκ segment (Jκ1–Jκ5). The B cell transcribes a segment of DNA into a primary RNA transcript which contains a long intervening sequence of additional J segments and introns. This transcript is processed into mRNA by splicing the exons together and is translated by ribosomes into kappa (κ) chains. Note that the J3 gene lacks the necessary base sequences to allow it to recombine and is therefore effectively an intron. The rearrangement illustrated is only one of the many possible recombinations.

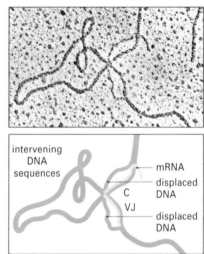

Fig. 5.10 Heteroduplex analysis of a kappa V–C region. The mRNA for a kappa gene is incubated with denatured single-stranded germ-line DNA of a plasmacytoma producing the heteroduplex above, as seen under the electron microscope. There is a large intron in the DNA between V–J and C but no intron between V and J in this active B cell.

So far, thirty germ line D segments have been identified with 100–200 different V$_H$ segments and six functional J segments plus three J pseudogenes, but solution analysis has now indicated that there may be more than 1000 murine V$_H$ segments. The combination of V, D, and J segments in the heavy chain make up the third complementarity-determining region, which forms an essential part of the antigen-binding site. In fact in some systems, such as the family of anti-dextran antibodies, the differences between antibodies are nearly all situated in this region.

RANDOM OR PROGRAMMED V-REGION READOUT?

When animals are immunized with selected antigens during fetal life or soon after birth, the ability to respond to each antigen develops in a precise order suggesting that there is a programmed pattern of development. The V regions nearest to the J regions are utilized first, and it is interesting that the V$_H$ gene V1, the nearest V gene, is a single conserved sequence. In all primate species examined only a single copy is present and no sequence variation occurs within a species. Between humans and other primates, only 2% of the nucleotides vary.

This fetal repertoire is over-represented in autoantibodies, indicating that autoimmunity might, in part, be the result of dysregulation of these early sequences. There is similar over-representation of particular V segments in tumours of early B cells, 20 V segments accounting for 85% of chronic lymphocytic leukaemias.

RECOMBINATION SEQUENCES

A key feature then of the generation of a functional gene for both light and heavy chain variable regions is the recombination of gene segments. The precise mechanism by which this recombination occurs is unknown, but specific base sequences that appear to act as joining signals have been identified (Fig. 5.12). On the J or downstream side of each V and D segment gene (in the direction of the J gene) are found two signal sequences, each of which is highly conserved.

The first is composed of seven nucleotides, a heptamer CACAGTG or its analogue, followed by a spacer of unconserved sequence, and then a nonamer ACAAAAACC, or its analogue. Immediately preceding all germ line D and J segments are again two signal sequences, first a nonamer and then a heptamer, again separated by an unconserved sequence. The heptameric and nonameric sequences following a V$_L$, V$_H$ or D segment are complementary to those preceding the Jλ, D or J$_H$ segments with which they recombine. All functional Vκ, Jλ and D spacers are 12 base pairs long, while all functional Vλ, V$_H$ and J$_H$ spacers are 22–24 base pairs long. This has led to the suggestion that the recombination may be brought about by a recombinase enzyme containing two DNA binding proteins, one recognizing the heptamer and nonamer with a 12 base pair spacer and the other recognizing them with a 23 base pair spacer. Alternatively, base pairing may occur directly between heptamers and nonamers, and the recombining enzyme(s) then recognize the overall paired structure. It is of interest to note that 12 base pairs represents one turn of the DNA helix, and 23 base pairs, two turns.

ADDITIONAL DIVERSITY

VARIABLE RECOMBINATION

As if the diversity generated by simple recombination were not enough, the precise place at which V and J segment genes join may vary slightly. The 95th residue of the κ light chain is coded for by the last codon of the V segment gene; the 96th is frequently coded by the first Jκ triplet. Sometimes, however, the 96th amino acid is coded for by a composite triplet formed by the second and third, or third base alone, of the first Jκ triplet, with the other bases of the triplet coming from the intron 3' to the V segment gene (Fig. 5.13). This will lead to variations in amino acid sequence at this point. Obviously, to produce a functional light chain the correct reading frame must be preserved, but it is possible for the gene segments to join out of phase leading to non-functional lymphocytes.

V–D–J recombination in the mouse

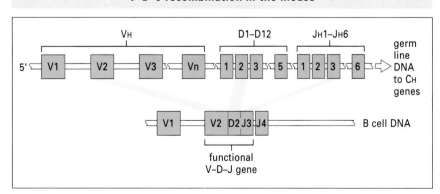

Fig. 5.11 The heavy chain gene loci combine three segments to produce the exon (V–D–J gene) which codes for the V$_H$ domain. One of several hundred V genes recombines with one of thirty D segments, and one of six J segments, to produce a functional V–D–J gene, in the B cell. The rearrangement illustrated is only one of the many thousands possible.

Similar imprecision in joining occurs on the heavy chain chromosome between the D and JH segment genes and can extend over as many as 10 nucleotides (Fig. 5.14). Furthermore, a few nucleotides may be inserted between D and JH and between VH and D without the need for a template by means of the enzyme, terminal deoxynucleotidyl transferase. The addition of these novel nucleotides called N-region diversity. In mice, terminal deoxynucleotidyl transferase activity increases with age, giving rise to long 'N' segments in adult animals. The recombinational variability of the D region can be so great that no recognizable D gene segment remains.

Severe combined immune deficiency (SCID) mice do not generate functional T or B cells because of a defect in V–(D)–J recombination.

SOMATIC MUTATION

The idea that somatic mutations during the lifetime of an individual could increase the diversity of antibodies has been strongly argued for many years. As seen earlier (Fig. 5.5) most Vλ sequences are identical, with a few variations in the complementarity-determining regions giving eight sequences in all. However, as only one

Recombination sequences

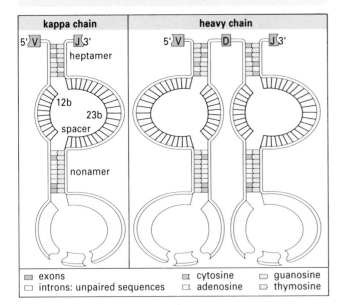

☐ exons	☐ cytosine
☐ introns: unpaired sequences	☐ adenosine
	☐ guanosine
	☐ thymosine

Fig. 5.12 This diagram shows the sequences of introns next to the V and J genes (kappa light chains) and V, J and D genes (heavy chains) which are involved in recombination of these genes. The recombinational events involved in V–J splicing and V–D–J splicing are facilitated by the base sequences of the introns following the 3' end of V and D matching up with the bases preceding the 5' end of J and D. Base pairing between these sequences apposes the exons. Note that individual base-pair sequences may vary slightly from the stated ones but the heptamer–spacer–nonamer pairing patterns remain. It is thought that enzymes related to those involved in DNA repair effect the join.

Light chain diversity created by variable recombination

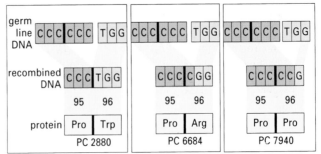

Fig. 5.13 The same Vκ21 and J1 sequences of the germ line create three different amino acid sequences in the proteins PC2880, PC6684 and PC7940 by variable recombination. PC2880 has proline and tryptophan at positions 95 and 96, caused by recombination at the end of the CCC codon. Recombination one base down produces proline and arginine in PC6684. Recombination two bases down from the end of Vκ21 produces proline and proline in PC7940.

Heavy chain diversity created by variable recombination

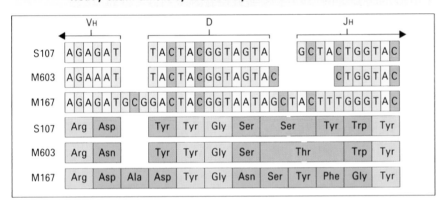

Fig. 5.14 The DNA sequence (upper) and amino acid sequence (lower) of three heavy chains of anti-phosphorylcholine are shown. Variable recombination between the germ line, V, D, and J regions causes variation (red) in amino acid sequences. In some cases (e.g. M167) there appear to be additional inserted codons. However, these are in multiples of three, and do not alter the overall reading frame.

VλI gene segment has been found per haploid genome, and as this corresponds to the main shared prototype sequence, all variant sequences must be generated by somatic mutations. All the variants could be produced by single base changes. Similar somatic mutants have been identified in κ light chains and in heavy chains.

The family of antibodies binding the antigen phosphorylcholine has been extensively investigated. Nineteen VH segments from antibodies binding phosphorylcholine have been fully sequenced. Ten of these have an identical sequence while the other nine differ by one to eight residues. The germ line genome from sperm was examined to see if each of these sequences was encoded by a separate DNA sequence. In fact, only DNA coding for the main prototype sequence could be found, indicating that the other sequences must have arisen by somatic mutation (Fig. 5.15). Strikingly, all the mutated forms were in the IgA and IgG classes, suggesting that the mutation might even be associated with immunoglobulin class switching. Presumably those somatic variants with a better fit for antigen are selected for, and certainly the somatic variants binding phosphorylcholine are of higher affinity than the germ-line encoded antibodies.

There is some evidence that the region of DNA encoding the variable region may be particularly susceptible to mutation. For example, examination of the nucleotide sequences of two anti-phosphorylcholine antibodies (T15 idiotype) shows them to have numerous mutations from the germ line sequence (3.8% of bases are mutated in the protein M167). These mutations occur in both introns and exons of the region implying that the whole region of DNA is particularly mutable, by comparison with adjoining DNA, where mutations have not been found (Fig. 5.16).

Antibody diversity thus arises at several levels. First there are the multiple variable-region genes recombining with J and D segments. Then, above this, the imprecision with which recombination occurs achieves further variation. At this level the structures of the first and second hypervariable regions are coded for entirely by germ line genes, while the third complementarity-determining region is largely the result of recombination. Additionally, point mutations occur throughout the variable region, giving fine variations in specificity. As virtually any light chain may pair with any heavy chain the combination binding of heavy and light chains amplifies the diversity enormously (Fig. 5.17). Somatic hypermutation probably contributes less than 5% of total sequence variability, but up to 90% of B cells express VH genes which have undergone somatic mutation.

DIVERSITY IN SHARKS, BIRDS AND RABBITS
Sharks

The development of an extensive antibody repertoire has been of great importance in vertebrate evolution, yet the various groups have arrived at different solutions to the problem. In the elasmobranchs, which include the sharks and skates, the heavy chain genes are developed along the pattern of the mouse λ light chains. A basic unit of VH–DH1–DH2–JH–CH is multiply repeated but, as recombination can occur only within each repeat unit, there is no scope for recombination between different gene segments. This results in a rather limited repertoire.

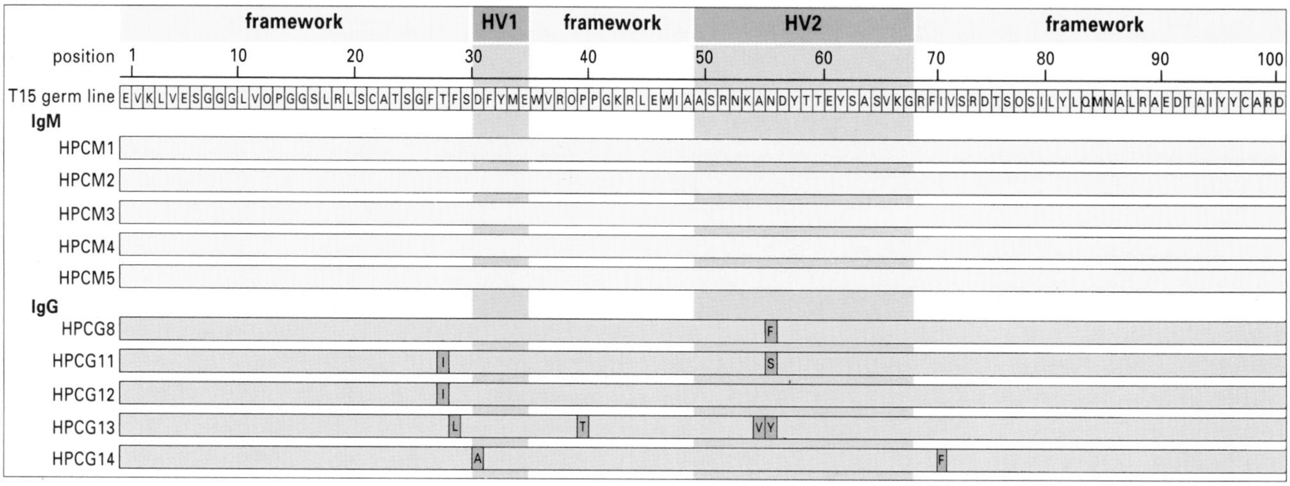

Fig. 5.15 The amino acid sequences of five IgM and five IgG hybridoma anti-phosphorylcholine antibody VH regions are compared to the primary amino acid structure of the T15 germ line DNA, as identified by sequencing sperm cell DNA. Positions which correspond to the germ line sequences are shown in yellow; points at which different amino acids occur are shown in red. Areas of hypervariability (HV1, HV2) are also indicated. Mutations have only occurred in the IgG molecules and the mutations are seen in both hypervariable framework segments.

Birds

In contrast to sharks, chickens possess extremely limited numbers of genes coding for immunoglobulins. In the light chain system there is only one V, one J and one C segment gene. The heavy chains are similarly restricted with single V and J segments. Although there are about 15 D_H segments, these are all very similar in sequence and add little to diversity. Despite this severe limitation chickens are perfectly able to mount a wide range of antibody responses and produce sequentially diverse antibody molecules.

Upstream of the V_L gene is a region containing 25 sequences similar to V_L regions, but each lacking a leader exon and a promoter region. They also lack the characteristic heptamer–spacer–nonamer sequences needed for V–J rearrangement. These pseudogenes are not wasted but are used in a process of gene conversion, with sections of the pseudogene being inserted into the viable V_L region. This is a continuous process which carries on after the B cells have left the bursa and multiple conversion events can occur during the lifetime of the B cell.

Mutations in the DNA of two V_H T15 genes

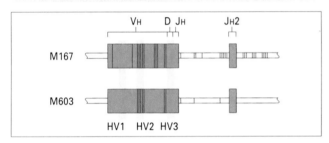

Fig. 5.16 DNA of two anti-phosphorylcholine antibodies with the T15 idiotype. (Black lines indicate positions where the genome has mutated from the germ line sequence.) There are large numbers of mutations in the introns and the exons of both genes, but particularly in the second hypervariable region, HV2. By comparison, no mutations are detectable in genes coding for the constant regions.

Five mechanisms for the generation of antibody diversity

1. multiple germ line V genes
2. V–J and V–D–J recombinations
3. recombinational inaccuracies
4. somatic point mutation
5. assorted heavy and light chains

Fig. 5.17 Since each mechanism can occur with any of the others, the potential for increased diversity multiplies at each step of immunoglobulin production.

Similar processes occur with the heavy-chain gene locus, where up to a 100 V_H pseudogenes act to increase the diversity by similar conversion mechanisms.

Rabbits

Rabbit immunoglobulins have always presented a puzzle, particularly in the way in which allotypes are regulated. Although the rabbit has many V_H genes, the V_H gene nearest to the D segment is used in most rabbit B cells. Recent evidence suggests that the rabbit may also use a gene conversion mechanism to diversify this single V_H gene.

PSEUDOGENES IN HUMAN DIVERSIFICATION

Several V and J segment genes are also in the form of pseudogenes. Whether gene conversion is involved in generating human V regions is a matter of speculation and interest.

HEAVY CHAIN CONSTANT REGION GENES

All classes of immunoglobulin use the same set of variable region genes. When the class is changed, by a B cell that has matured into an antibody-forming cell and is therefore committed to a particular antigen, all that is switched is the constant region of the heavy chain. This is also shown by the analysis of double myelomas, where two monoclonal antibodies are present in the serum at the same time. IgM and IgG antibodies from a patient with multiple myeloma have been found to have identical light chains and V_H regions; only the constant regions were switched from μ to γ. Often IgM and IgD are found on the lymphocyte surface at the same time. Capping these receptors with antigen has revealed that the IgM and IgD from the same B cell have the same specificity for antigen, indicating similarity of V_H regions on the two classes (Fig. 5.18).

All the constant region genes are arranged downstream from the J segment genes. In the mouse there is one gene for each of the μ, ϵ and α isotypes and one γ gene for each of the four different IgG isotypes (Fig. 5.19). In man the constant region genes are more complicated, and it appears that one section of this region has undergone gene duplication and diversification. In man the ordering of genes is μ, δ, [$\gamma3$, $\gamma1$, $\epsilon1$ $\alpha1$], γ, [$\gamma2$, $\gamma4$, ϵ, $\alpha2$]. The two sets within square brackets indicate the possible area of reduplication. The genes $\epsilon1$ and γ are pseudogenes and are not expressed. Just upstream (5') to the μ genes is a switch sequence (S) which is repeated upstream (5') to each of the other constant region genes (Fig. 5.20). Class switching is important in the maturation of the immune response and may be accompanied or preceded by somatic mutation. Initially a complete section of DNA, including the recombined V_H region through the δ and μ constant regions, is transcribed; then by differential splicing, two mRNA molecules are produced, each with the same V_H but having either μ or δ constant regions. It is suggested that sometimes much larger stretches of DNA are also

Co-capping of IgM and IgD with antigen

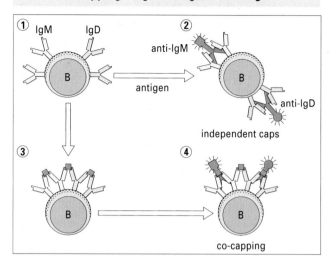

Fig. 5.18 Some B cells have both IgM and IgD on their surface (1). This can be demonstrated by treating the cells with rhodaminated anti-IgM (red) and fluoresceinated anti-IgD (green). The anti-IgM causes the IgM antibodies to aggregate on the surface, while the anti-IgD causes the IgD to aggregate, producing separate red and green caps on the cell (2). If the experiment is repeated by first treating the cells with antigen (blue) as in (3) and then with the anti-IgM and anti-IgD, the red anti-IgM and green anti-IgD caps appear together on the cell, that is, they co-cap. This implies that the IgM and IgD on the cell surfaces are cross-linked by antigen (4). This could only occur if the IgM and IgD had the same antigen-binding specificity, and is therefore evidence that different constant regions (μ and δ) can be linked to the same V region.

Fig. 5.19 The constant region genes of the mouse are arranged 6.5 kb downstream from the the recombined V–D–J segment. Each C gene (except Cδ) has one or more switching sequences at its start (red circles) which correspond to a sequence at the 5' end of the μ gene. This allows any of the C genes to recombine with V–D–J. δ genes appear to use the same switching sequences as μ but the μ gene transcript is lost in RNA processing to produce IgD. The C genes (expanded below for μ and γ2a)

Constant region genes in the mouse

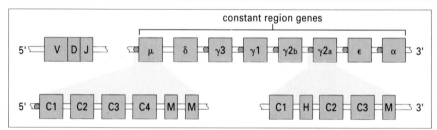

contain introns separating the exons for each domain (C1, C2, etc.). The γ genes also have a separate exon coding for the hinge (H), and all the genes have one or more exons coding for membrane-bound immunoglobulin (M).

Maturation of the immune response and class switching

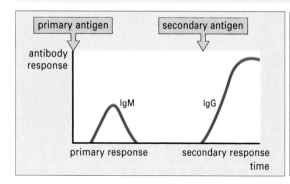

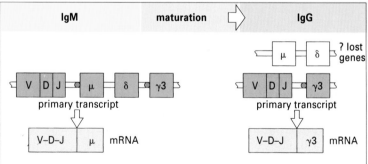

Fig. 5.20 Following a primary antigen injection there is an antibody response which consists mostly of IgM; the response following a secondary challenge is mostly IgG. The underlying mechanism for the class switch is shown (right). In the primary response the V–D–J region is transcribed with a μ gene. After removal of introns during processing,

mRNA for secreted IgM is produced. During maturation (involving T-cell help and possibly activation of a mutation mechanism for the V–D–J segment) another C gene (Cγ3 in this case) is brought up to exchange with the μ gene at its switch region (red). The μ and δ genes are probably lost; transcription and processing produce mRNA for IgG3.

Isotype switching by differential RNA splicing

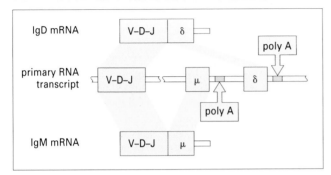

Fig. 5.21 Single B cells produce more than one antibody isotype from a single long primary RNA transcript. A transcript containing μ and δ is shown here. Polyadenylation can occur at different sites (black), leading to different forms of splicing, producing mRNA for IgD (top) or IgM (bottom). Even within this region there are additional polyadenylation sites which determine whether membrane immunoglobulin or secreted immunoglobulin is formed.

Lost genes

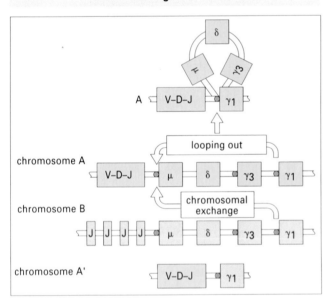

Fig. 5.22 A and B are chromatids of the chromosome section of the Ig genes. A contains the rearranged V–D–J segment. In the looping out hypothesis, a section of C genes (μ, δ, γ3) loop out and are lost. In the chromosome exchange hypothesis, similarities in the switching sequences permit unequal somatic recombination between maternal and paternal chromosomes. The A chromosome recombines with another part of the unrearranged B chromosome. The loss of gene segments gives rise to the IgM–IgG1 switch, shown as A'. The 'lost' C genes are on the other, non-functional chromosome B' (not shown), which now contains two copies of several C genes.

transcribed together, with differential splicing giving other immunoglobulin classes sharing VH regions (Fig. 5.21). This has been observed in cells simultaneously producing IgM and IgE. More often, class switching appears to be mediated by a recombination between S recombination sites, allowing a looping out and deletion of DNA and bringing another C region close to the VDJ gene (Fig. 5.22). A further possibility has been suggested involving exchange between chromosomes.

MEMBRANE AND SECRETED IMMUNOGLOBULIN

Membrane immunoglobulin (antigen receptor) is identical to secreted immunoglobulin (antibody), except for a stretch of amino acids at the C terminus of each heavy chain. Membrane immunoglobulins are larger than their

Membrane and secreted IgM: mouse

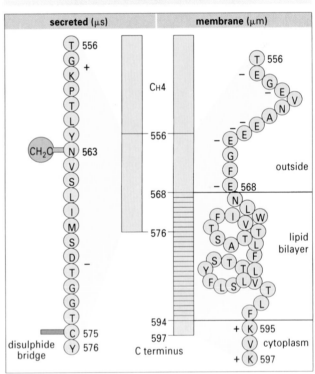

Fig 5.23 C-terminal amino acid sequences are shown for both secreted and membrane-bound IgM, and are identical up to residue 556. Secreted IgM has 20 further residues. Residue 563 (asparagine) has a carbohydrate unit attached to it while residue 575 is a cysteine involved in the formation of interchain disulphide bonds. Membrane IgM has 41 residues beyond 556. A stretch of 26 residues between 568 and 595 contains hydrophobic amino acids sandwiched between sequences containing charged residues. This hydrophobic portion may traverse the cell membrane as two turns of α helix. A short, positively-charged section lies inside the cytoplasm.

secreted counterparts; their additional amino acids traverse the cell membrane to anchor the molecule. In membrane IgM, for example, a section of hydrophobic (lipophilic) amino acids are sandwiched between hydrophilic amino acids, which lie on either side of the membrane (Fig. 5.23). The hydrophobic residues are thought to form a stretch of α helix within the membrane. Membrane immunoglobulins only exist as the basic four-chain unit, and do not polymerize further.

Production of two forms of immunoglobulin occurs by differential transcription of the germ line C region gene, which is transcribed in two different ways (Fig. 5.24). It is thought that the poly A sequence is important in determining which RNA transcript is produced, but exactly how this is controlled is uncertain.

Evidently the way the cell regulates which immunoglobulin it produces is complicated. The first step is the heavy chain rearrangement of D to J, followed by

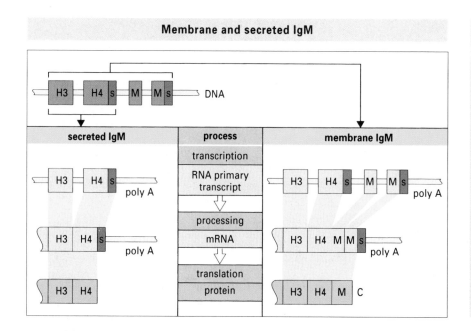

Membrane and secreted IgM

Fig. 5.24 Part of the DNA coding for IgM is shown diagrammatically. The exons for the μ3 and μ4 domains (H3 and H4) and the transmembrane segment of membrane IgM (M) are indicated. Translation stop sequences (S) are present at the end of the H4 and second membrane segments. The DNA can be transcribed in two ways. If transcription stops after H4 the transcript with a poly-A tail is processed to produce mRNA for secreted IgM. If transcription runs through to include the membrane segments, processing removes the codons for the terminal amino acids and the stop signal of H4, so that translation yields a protein with a different C terminus.

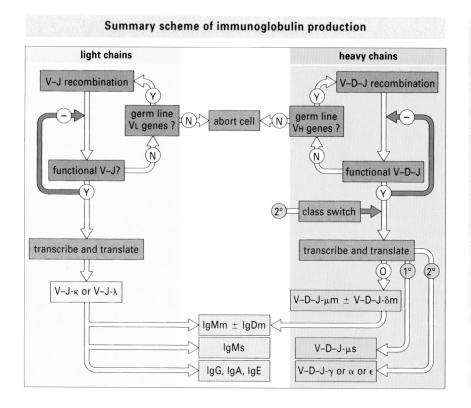

Summary scheme of immunoglobulin production

Fig. 5.25 Stages of immunoglobulin production. Pre-B cells attempt to recombine a V–J from the germ line genes (left). If functional (Y) it is transcribed and translated to form a light chain. Once a cell has produced a functional recombination, negative feedback (−) prevents further rearrangements. If the V–J is not functional (N) the cell makes another attempt. If a cell exhausts its store of germ line gene segments then it is aborted. The same occurs for heavy chains; the early B cell (right) expresses mIgM and/or mIgD. This occurs with no antigen stimulation (0). After primary antigen stimulation (1°), transcription changes so that secreted IgM is released. After secondary antigen stimulation (2°) and with T cell help, there is DNA rearrangement, resulting in a class switch, possibly also with mutation in VH and VL. The end products are cells bearing and secreting IgG, IgA or IgE.

addition of V; μ chain stimulates the κ locus to attempt V–J rearrangement, followed by the lambda locus if necessary. It is postulated that this occurs repeatedly in both maternal and paternal chromosomes until a functionally recombined gene is produced or the genetic material is exhausted and the cell is aborted. Once the V regions of that cell are determined they remain essentially unaltered thereafter (except for any somatic mutation). However, there is still switching in the C_H

genes to produce different isotypes and a change to production of secreted immunoglobulin following cell activation. A compilation of facts and hypotheses is shown in Fig. 5.25.

PRODUCTION OF IMMUNOGLOBULIN

Before the antibody is synthesized it is first necessary to splice the introns out of the primary RNA transcript. It is found that the beginning and end of each intron have particular forms of RNA base sequences, referred to as donor and acceptor junctions. It is thought that the junctions interact with each other and with ribonucleoproteins in the nucleus to remove the introns and splice the joins back together again to form mRNA. It is, of course, essential that this is done accurately so that the reading frame of the mRNA is unaltered.

Messenger RNA for immunoglobulins is translated across the membranes of the endoplasmic reticulum, after which the heavy and light chains associate (Fig. 5.26). Cellular immunoglobulins and secreted immunoglobulins are processed differently to arrive at their correct locations, by mechanisms which are unknown.

GENES OF THE T-CELL ANTIGEN RECEPTOR

The antigen–MHC binding portion of the TCR is generated by four different sets of genes. The α and β gene sets are expressed in the majority of peripheral T cells, whereas the γ and δ genes are expressed in a subpopulation of thymic T cells and also in a minor population of peripheral T cells. These chains become associated with the γ, δ, ε and ζ chains of the CD3 molecule to form the complete TCR (see Chapter 4).

The general arrangement of TCR genes is remarkably similar to that of immunoglobulin heavy chains. Interestingly, the δ genes for the TCR lie in the middle of the α genes, with their own sets of D, J, and C segments (Fig. 5.27).

RECOMBINATION OF T-CELL RECEPTOR GENES
Diversification of the TCR gene occurs by recombination between V, D, and J segments, with minor variations in detail for each locus.

The α chain is superficially simple, except for the complication of the δ chain embedded between V and J loci. As in the κ locus, a complete variable region is produced by rearrangement of a Vα segment to a Jα segment. Diversity is markedly increased by the unusually large number of J segments.

The β locus includes two sets of D, J, and C genes. Most of the Vβ genes are grouped together, but one (Vβ14) is present at the extreme 3' end of the locus. The tandem duplication of Dβ, Jβ and Cβ must have occurred early in the evolution of mammals since it is present in both mice and humans. Extensive diversity is generated in the joining process as not only are V–D–J

Production of secreted immunoglobulin

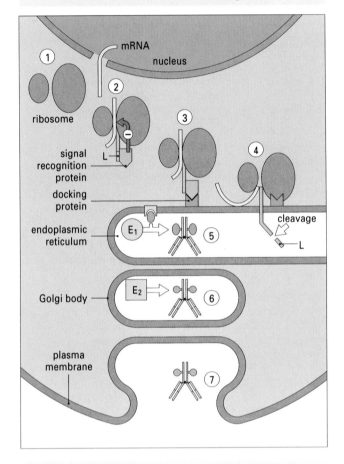

Fig 5.26 Messenger RNA for a secreted heavy chain leaves the nucleus and enters the cytoplasm where it is bound by a ribosome (1). The leading sequence (L) is translated and binds to signal recognition protein (SRP) which blocks further translation (2). The SRP ribosome complex migrates to the endoplasmic reticulum (ER) where the SRP binds to the docking protein at a vacant site on the ER (3). Translation may now proceed and the synthesizing chain traverses the membrane into the ER (4). The leader sequence is removed and the chain combines with other H and L chains to form the immunoglobulin subunit (5). Enzymes (E₁) add carbohydrate (purple) as the ER pinches off to form the Golgi body (6). In the Golgi body further enzymes (E₂) modify the carbohydrate before the completed molecule is secreted to the outside by reverse pinocytosis (7).

T-cell receptor genes

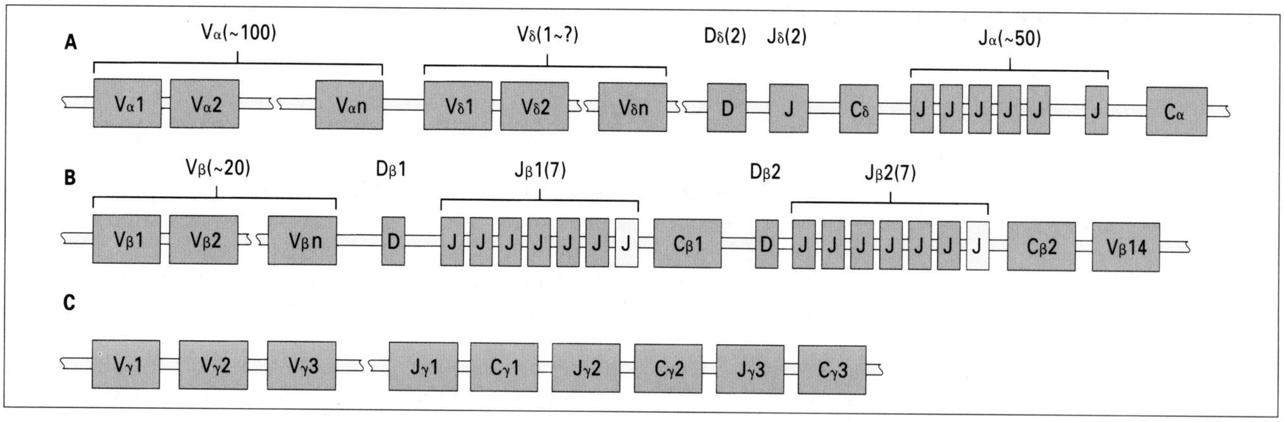

Fig. 5.27 The general management of TCR genes is similar to that of immunoglobulin heavy chains. The genes of the murine T-cell receptor α and β polypeptides are shown. Note the location of the δ loci embedded within the α loci, and the tandem duplication which has occurred in the β chain loci. The last of each set of Jβ genes is a pseudogene.

arrangements possible, but also V–J and V–D–D–J joins. The D segments are used in all three reading frames, adding even further to β chain diversity.

The arrangement of the γ-chain loci in mice and in humans is rather different. The murine locus bears a striking similarity to the antibody light-chain locus, with four Cγ genes (including a pseudogene), each associated with one Jγ gene, and one to four Vγ genes. There are no D genes. In man there are eight Vγ genes, followed upstream (5') by three Jγ and the first Cγ; then there are two additional Jγ genes before Cγ2. Imprecise joining of V with J, together with insertions in the joins, is important in generating diversity.

The δ locus was discovered during studies on the α locus. Although relatively simple, with only five Vδ two Dδ and six Jδ genes, it has been calculated that 10^{14} different δ chains could be generated by imprecision in joining, insertion of additional residues and use of the D genes in all three reading frames.

The mechanisms by which TCR gene recombination occurs appear to be similar to those of B cells, since the genes have similar patterns of heptamer–12 or 23 base-pair spacer–nonamer sequences flanking them. Similar or identical rearrangement enzymes operate in B and T cells, as experiments show that transfected TCR, Dβ and Jγ can rearrange appropriately in B-cells. N-region development is particularly marked and contributes extensively to the diversity.

Although somatic mutation is an important mechanism in generating immunoglobulin diversity, it does not occur in TCR genes. This is probably linked with the necessity to maintain tolerance to self and recognition of MHC by T cells.

■ MAGNITUDE OF DIVERSITY

Diversity depends on the simple combinations of V, D and J regions plus N-region diversification, joining-site variation and multiple D regions. The precise distance between the end of germline V and germline J is variable; it corresponds to about 6–15 amino acid residues for Vβ and 3–7 residues for Vα. Hunkapiller & Hood have estimated that it is possible to make about 4.4×10^{13} different forms of Vβ and 6.5×10^{12} forms of Vα. These authors estimate that if only 1% of the sequences code for viable proteins this would still give 2.9×10^{18} receptors. Making the assumption that 99% of these are rejected owing to coding for autoantigens or other defects, this would still give 2.9×10^{20} potential TCRs. Since, during the lifetime of a mouse, less than 10^9 thymocytes leave the thymus, this raises the question: how random is the generation of receptors? A similar problem arises with immunoglobulins, where the potential repertoire is many orders of magnitude greater than the numbers of B cells ever produced.

FURTHER READING

Blackwell TK, Alt FW. Mechanism and developmental program of immunoglobulin gene rearrangement in mammals. *Annu Rev Genet* 1989;**23**:605.

Brack C, Hirama M, Lenhard-Schuller R, Tonegawa S. A complete immunoglobulin gene is created by somatic recombination. *Cell* 1978;**15**:1.

Davis MM, Bjorkman PJ. T-cell antigen receptor genes and T-cell recognition. *Nature* 1988;**334**:395.

Hunkapiller T, Hood L. Diversity of the immunoglobulin gene superfamily. *Adv Immunol* 1990;**44**:1.

Owen MJ, Lamb JR. *Immune Recognition.* Oxford: IRL Press, 1988.

Pascual V, Capra JD. Human immunoglobulin heavy-chain variable region genes: organization, polymorphism and expression. *Adv Immunol* 1991;**49**:1.

chapter 6

Antigen Recognition

Antibody and the T-cell antigen receptor have many features in common. They both have variable (V) and constant (C) domains, and the processes of gene recombination which produce the variable domains (from V, D and J gene segments) for each type of receptor are also similar. Nevertheless, the ways in which B cells and T cells recognize antigens are quite different: antibody recognizes antigens in solution or on cell surfaces, but always in their native conformation, whereas the T-cell receptor only sees antigen in association with MHC molecules on cell surfaces. Frequently, antigens recognized by T cells have been degraded or processed in some way, so that the determinant recognized by the T-cell antigen receptor is only a small fragment of the original antigen.

Another difference between antibody and the T-cell antigen receptor is that antibody may be produced in two forms, whether as the B-cell antigen receptor or as secreted antibody, whereas the T-cell antigen receptor is always an integral membrane protein. Secreted antibody is essentially a bifunctional molecule; the V domains are primarily concerned with antigen binding and the C domains interact with receptors on host tissues.

This chapter describes the ways in which the antibody's V domains and the T-cell antigen receptor form an antigen binding site, and how they interact with their specific antigens or antigen–MHC. These interactions underlie the specificity of the adaptive immune response.

ANTIGEN–ANTIBODY BINDING

X-ray crystallography studies of antibody V domains show that the hypervariable regions are clustered at the end of the Fab arms; particular residues in these regions interact specifically with antigen (Fig. 6.1). The framework residues do not usually form bonds with the antigen. However, they are essential for producing the folding of the V domains and maintaining the integrity of the binding site.

The binding of antigen to antibody takes place by the formation of multiple non-covalent bonds between the antigen and amino acids of the binding site. Although the attractive forces involved (namely, hydrogen bonds, and electrostatic, Van der Waals and hydrophobic forces) are individually weak by comparison with covalent bonds, the multiplicity of the bonds leads to a considerable binding energy.

Intermolecular attractive forces

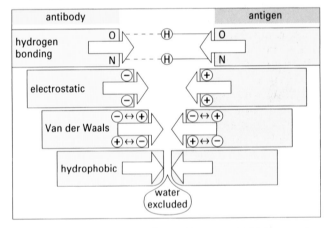

Fig. 6.2 The forces binding antigen to antibody require the close approach of the interacting groups. *Hydrogen bonding* results from the formation of hydrogen bridges between appropriate atoms. *Electrostatic forces* are due to the attraction of oppositely charged groups located on two protein side chains. *Van der Waals* bonds are generated by the interaction between electron clouds (here represented as induced oscillating dipoles). *Hydrophobic bonds* (which may contribute up to half the total strength of the antigen–antibody bond) rely upon the association of non-polar, hydrophobic groups so that contact with water molecules is minimized. The distance of separation between the interacting groups which produces optimum binding varies depending on the type of bond.

The antibody combining site

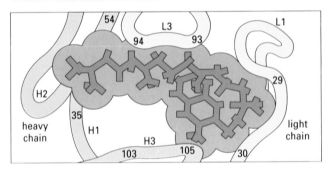

Fig. 6.1 The antigen molecule nestles in a cleft formed by the heavy and light chains, called the antibody combining site. The example shown is based on X-ray crystallography studies of human IgG (the myeloma protein NEW) binding γ-hydroxyl vitamin K. The antigen makes contact with 10–12 amino acids in the hypervariable regions of both heavy and light chains. The numerals refer to amino acids identified as actually making contact with the antigen.

The non-covalent bonds are critically dependent on the distance (d) between the interacting groups. The force is proportional to $1/d^2$ for electrostatic forces and to $1/d^7$ for Van der Waals forces; thus the interacting groups must be close in molecular terms before these forces become significant (Fig. 6.2). In order for an antigenic determinant (epitope) and the antibody combining site (paratope) to combine (see Fig. 6.1), there must be suitable atomic groupings on opposing parts of the antigen and antibody, and the shape of the combining site must fit the epitope, so that several non-covalent bonds can form simultaneously.

If the antigen and the combining site are complementary in this way, there will be sufficient binding energy to resist thermodynamic disruption of the bond. However, if electron clouds of the antigen and antibody overlap, steric repulsive forces come into play which are inversely proportional to the twelfth power of the distance between the clouds: $F \propto 1/d^{12}$. These forces play a vital role in determining the specificity of the antibody molecule for a particular antigen, and its ability to discriminate between antigens, since any variation from the ideal complementary shape will cause a fall in the total binding energy through increased repulsive forces and decreased attractive forces (Fig. 6.3).

Recent studies have shown how protein antigens interact with specific antibodies. For example, an examination of the interaction between lysozyme and the Fab of an antibody to lysozyme shows that the antigen epitope on the lysozyme molecule and the binding site have complementary surfaces and that these extend even beyond the hypervariable regions. In this example, 17 amino acid residues on the antibody were in contact with 16 residues on the lysozyme molecule (Fig. 6.4). All of the hypervariable regions contributed to the antibody binding site, although the third hypervariable region, formed by the V–D–J join in the heavy chain gene, appeared to be most important. This may be related to the greater variability generated by recombination of the V, D, and J segments.

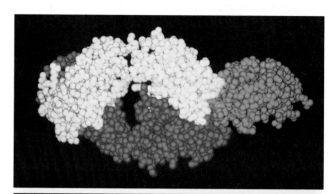

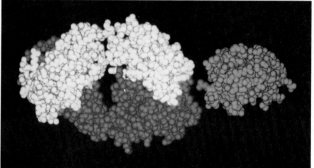

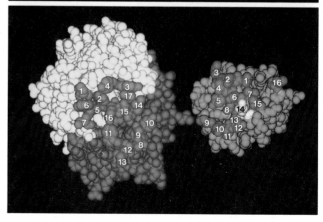

Fig. 6.4 The Fab–lysozyme complex The upper figure shows lysozyme (green) binding to the hypervariable regions of the heavy (blue) and light (yellow) chains of the Fab fragment of antibody D1.3. The centre panel shows the complex separated with Glu 121 (red) visible. This residue fits into the centre of the cleft between the heavy and light chains. The lower panel shows the molecules rotated forward 90° to show the contact residues which contribute to the antigen–antibody bond. (Courtesy of Dr R. J. Poljak, from *Science* 1986:**233**;747–753, with permission.)

Good fit and poor fit

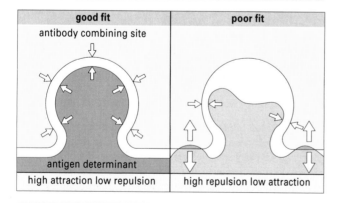

good fit	poor fit
antibody combining site	
antigen determinant	
high attraction low repulsion	high repulsion low attraction

Fig. 6.3 A good fit between the antigenic determinant and the binding site of the antibody will create ample opportunities for intermolecular attractive forces to be created and few opportunities for repulsive forces to operate. Conversely, when there is a poor fit the reverse is true, that is, when electron clouds overlap high repulsive forces are generated, which dominate any small forces of attraction.

ANTIBODY AFFINITY

The strength of a single antigen–antibody bond is the antibody affinity; it is produced by summation of the attractive and repulsive forces described above (Fig. 6.5). Interaction of the antibody combining site with antigen can be investigated thermodynamically. To measure the affinity of a single combining site it is necessary to use a monovalent antigen or even a single isolated antigenic determinant – a hapten. Since the non-covalent bonds between antibody and epitope are dissociable, the overall combination of an antibody and antigen must be reversible; thus the Law of Mass Action can be applied to the reaction and the equilibrium constant, K, can be determined. This is the affinity constant (Fig. 6.6).

AFFINITY AND AVIDITY

Since each antibody unit of four polypeptide chains has two antigen binding sites, antibodies are potentially multivalent in their reaction with antigen. In addition, antigen can also be monovalent or multivalent. A hapten has only one epitope and can therefore react with only one antigen combining site; thus it is monovalent. Many molecules however, have more than one antigenic determinant. Microorganisms have a large number of antigenic determinants exposed on their surfaces, hence they are all multivalent. When a multivalent antigen combines with more than one of an antibody's combining sites, the binding energy between the two is considerably greater than the sum of the binding energies of the individual sites since all the antigen–antibody bonds must be broken simultaneously before the antigen and antibody dissociate.

The strength with which a multivalent antibody binds a multivalent antigen is termed avidity, to differentiate it from the affinity of the bond between a single antigenic determinant and an individual combining site. The avidity of an antibody for its antigen is dependent on the affinities of the individual combining sites for the determinants on the antigen; it is greater than the sum of these affinities if both antibody binding sites can combine with the antigen (Fig. 6.7). In normal

Antibody affinity

good fit	poor fit
high attraction – low repulsion	high repulsion – low attraction
affinity ≡ Σ attractive and repulsive forces	

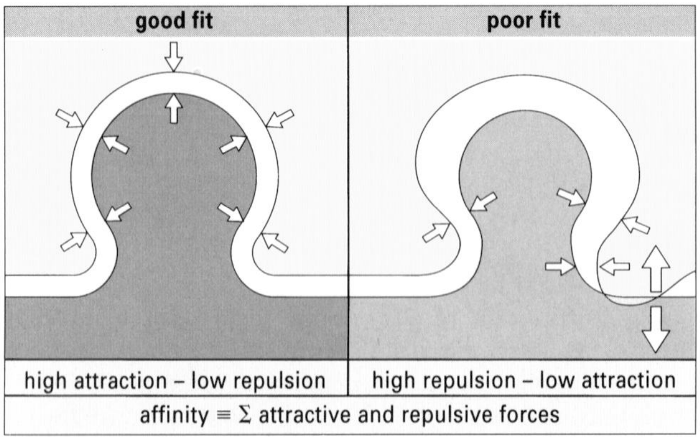

Fig. 6.5 The affinity with which antibody binds antigen results from a balance between the attractive and repulsive forces. A high affinity antibody implies a good fit and conversely, a low affinity antibody implies a poor fit.

Calculation of antibody affinity

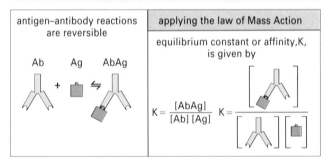

antigen–antibody reactions are reversible	applying the law of Mass Action
Ab + Ag ⇌ AbAg	equilibrium constant or affinity, K, is given by $$K = \frac{[AbAg]}{[Ab][Ag]}$$

Fig. 6.6 All antigen–antibody reactions are reversible and the Law of Mass Action has been applied, from which antibody affinity (given by the equilibrium constant, K) can be calculated at equilibrium. (Square brackets refer to the concentrations of the reactants.)

Affinity and avidity

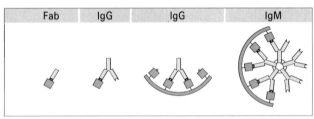

antibody	Fab	IgG	IgG	IgM
effective antibody valence	1	1	2	up to 10
antigen valence	1	1	n	n
equilibrium constant (L/M)	10^4	10^4	10^7	10^{11}
advantage of multivalence	–	–	10^3-fold	10^7-fold
definition of binding	affinity	affinity	avidity	avidity
	intrinsic affinity		functional affinity	

Fig. 6.7 Multivalent binding between antibody and antigen (avidity or functional affinity) results in a considerable increase in stability as measured by the equilibrium constant, compared to simple monovalent binding (affinity or intrinsic affinity, here arbitrarily assigned a value of 10^4 L/M). This is sometimes referred to as the 'bonus effect' of multivalency. Thus there may be a 10^3-fold increase in the binding energy of IgG when both valencies (combining sites) are utilized and a 10^7 increase when IgM binds antigen in a multivalent manner.

Specificity, cross-reactivity and non-reactivity

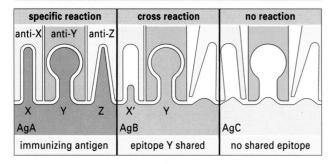

specific reaction			cross reaction		no reaction
anti-X	anti-Y	anti-Z	X'	Y	
X	Y	Z	AgB		AgC
AgA					
immunizing antigen			epitope Y shared		no shared epitope

Fig. 6.8 Antiserum specificity results from the action of a population of individual antibody molecules (anti-X, anti-Y, and anti-Z) directed against different determinants (epitopes) (X, Y, Z) on different antigen molecules. Antigen A (AgA) and antigen B (AgB) have epitope Y in common. Antiserum raised against AgA (anti-XYZ) not only reacts specifically with AgA but cross-reacts with AgB (through recognition of epitopes Y and X'). The antiserum gives no reaction with AgC because there are no shared epitopes.

Specificity and cross-reactivity

radical (R)	sulphonate	arsonate	carboxylate
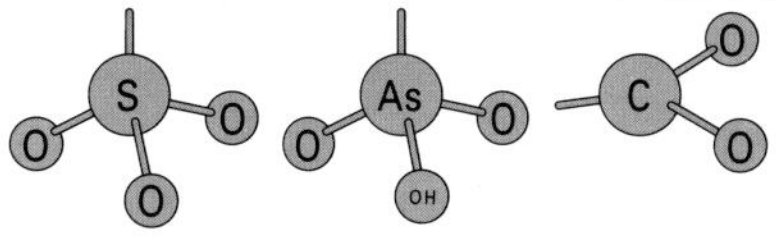	tetrahedral	tetrahedral	planar
ortho 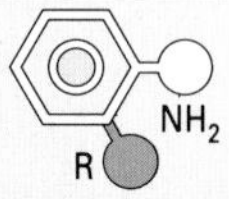	+ +	–	–
meta 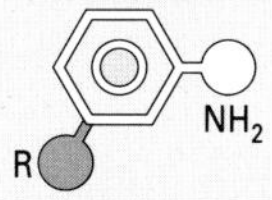	+ + +	+	±
para 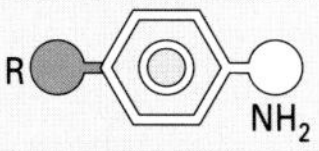	±	–	–

Fig. 6.9 Antiserum raised to the meta isomer of aminobenzene sulphonate (the immunizing hapten), is reacted with ortho and para isomers of aminobenzene sulphonate, and also with the three isomers (ortho, meta, para) of two different but related antigens: aminobenzene arsonate and aminobenzene carboxylate. The antiserum reacts specifically with the sulphonate group in the meta position but will cross-react (though more weakly) with sulphonate in the ortho position. Further, weaker, cross-reactions are possible when the antiserum is reacted with either the arsonate group or the carboxylate group in the meta, but not in the ortho or para position. Arsonate is larger than sulphonate and has an extra H atom, while carboxylate is the smallest. These data suggest that an antigen's configuration is as important as individual chemical groupings.

physiological situations avidity is likely to be more relevant than affinity since naturally occurring antigens are multivalent; however, the precise measurement of hapten–antibody affinity is more likely to give an insight into the immunochemical nature of the antigen–antibody reaction.

KINETICS OF ANTIBODY–ANTIGEN REACTIONS

Measurements of antibody affinity relate to equilibrium conditions, and affinity indicates the tendency of the antibodies to form stable complexes with the antigen. However, for many biological activities of antibodies, it is possible that the kinetics of the reaction may have significance. By kinetics we mean the measurement of the forward rate (on-rate) constant $K_{1,2}$ (mol^{-1}·s^{-1}) and the reverse rate (off-rate) constant $K_{2,1}$ (s^{-1}). At equilibrium the ratio of the two constants gives the equilibrium constant or affinity of the antibody. It has been claimed that differences in affinity are a result primarily of differences in off-rates, but more recently it has been shown that affinity can also be influenced by differences in on-rates.

Recent work has suggested that B-cell selection and stimulation during a maturing antibody response depend both upon selection for the ability of antibodies to bind to antigens rapidly (kinetic selection) and selection for the ability to bind antigens tightly (thermodynamic selection).

ANTIBODY SPECIFICITY

Antigen–antibody reactions can show a high level of specificity. For example, antibodies to a virus like measles will bind to the measles virus and confer immunity to this disease, but will not combine with, or protect against, an unrelated virus such as polio. The specificity of an antiserum is the result of the summation

Configurational specificity

antiserum	antigen		
	lysozyme 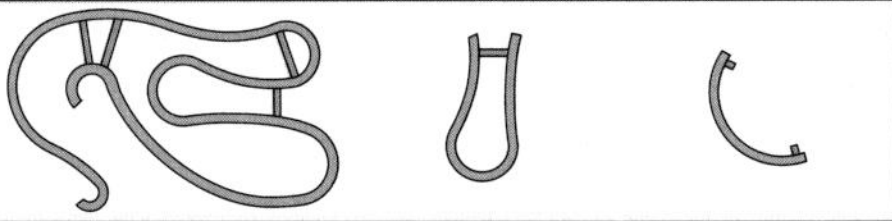	isolated 'loop' peptide	reduced 'loop'
anti-lysozyme	+ +	+	–
anti-'loop' peptide	+	+ +	–

Fig. 6.10 The lysozyme molecule possesses an intrachain bond (red) which produces a loop in the peptide chain. Antisera may be raised against either whole lysozyme (anti-lysozyme) or the isolated loop (anti-'loop' peptide) and are found to distinguish between the two. Neither antiserum reacts with the isolated loop in its linear, reduced form. This demonstrates the importance of tertiary structure in determining antibody specificity.

of the actions of the various antibodies in the total population each reacting with a different part of the antigen molecule and even different parts of the same determinant (Fig. 6.8). However, when some of the determinants of an antigen, A, are shared by another antigen, B, then a proportion of the antibodies directed to A will also react with B. This phenomenon is termed cross-reactivity.

There is evidence that antibody recognizes the overall configuration of an epitope rather than particular groups (Fig. 6.9). Antibodies are capable of expressing remarkable specificity, and are able to distinguish between small differences in the primary amino acid sequence of protein antigens, as well as differences in charge, optical configuration and steric conformation (Fig. 6.10). One consequence of this specificity is that many antibodies will only bind to native antigens or fragments of antigens which retain sufficient tertiary structure to permit the multiple interactions required for bond formation. This specificity can create a problem when one wishes to produce antibodies for immunological assays. For example, it is often easier to raise antibodies to short synthetic polypeptides from antigens of known primary structure (which can be obtained in large quantities), rather than purify sufficient amounts of the native antigen for immunization. However, antibodies to such polypeptides often do not bind well or predictably to the native antigen.

DESIGNER ANTIBODIES

Molecular biology has paved the way for the production of monoclonal antibodies of defined specificity, affinity and immunoglobulin isotype. It is possible to make antibody genes which have, for example, mouse V domains on human C regions. This allows immunologists to develop antibodies of a particular specificity in the mouse and then to attach that specificity to a human antibody, which is of low antigenicity in man, for use in patients *in vivo*. Working at an even smaller level, sets of complementarity determining regions (CDRs) from one species can be grafted into a framework V domain from another. At the lowest level, it is possible to alter individual residues in the combining site to increase the affinity of that antibody (Fig. 6.11).

POLYFUNCTIONAL BINDING SITES

Over the past few years, research has suggested that an antibody molecule may be complementary to several dissimilar antigens. The binding of these antigens is competitive, and it appears that there are specially separated positions within the combining site (Fig. 6.12).

The specificity of a population of antibodies is not due to each antibody reacting exclusively with the induction antigen. However, if a large number of different polyfunctional antibodies all have a site which can combine with a particular antigen A, the net reactivity of these antibodies is high to A but low to all other

Designer antibodies

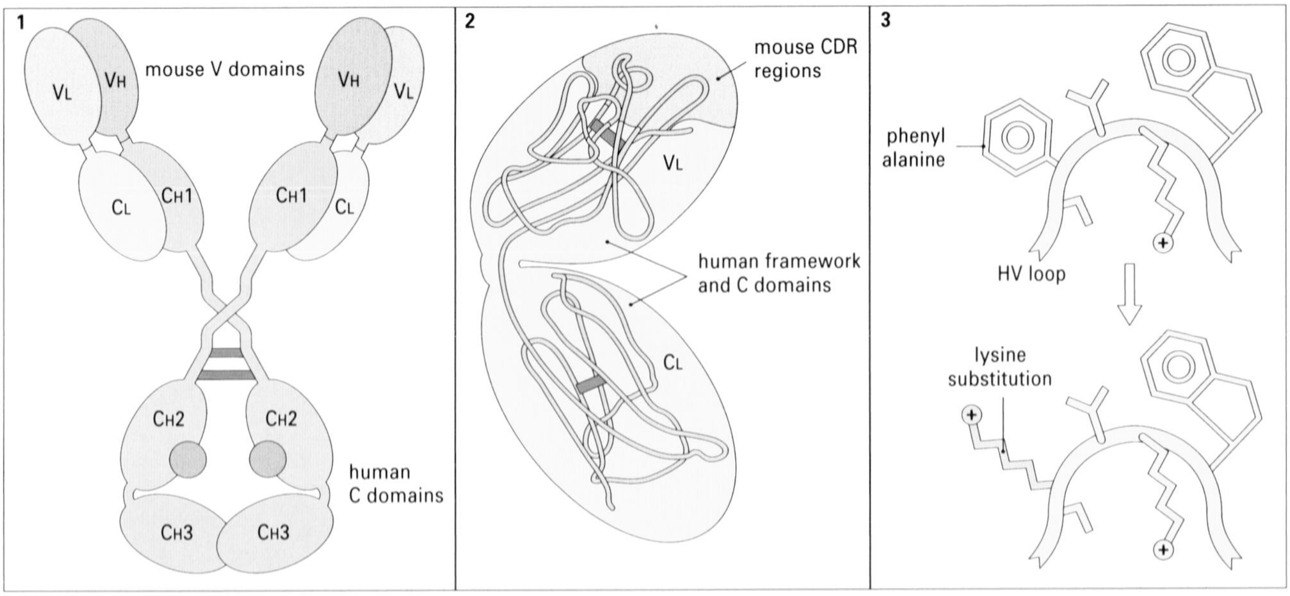

Fig. 6.11 It is possible to splice the genes for a mouse V domain on to human C genes, and transfect this into a cell which then makes chimeric mouse/human antibodies (1). Alternatively, just the required CDR regions can be spliced into another framework (2). The affinity of a binding site can also be modified by point mutation of the DNA of the hypervariable loops – here illustrated as a Phe → Lys change (3).

antigens. Thus specificity can be a population phenomenon, an average characteristic of all the antibodies in an antiserum (Fig. 6.13).

THE PHYSIOLOGICAL SIGNIFICANCE OF HIGH AND LOW AFFINITY ANTIBODIES

Binding affinity is not merely a matter of theoretical interest, since affinity and avidity affect the physiological and pathological properties of the antibodies. High affinity antibody is superior to low affinity antibody in a number of biological reactions (Fig. 6.14). In experimental animals, antigen–antibody complexes containing low affinity antibody persist in the circulation, localize on the glomerular basement membrane of the kidney and impair renal function. High affinity complexes are more rapidly removed from the circulation, localize in the mesangium of the kidney, and have little effect on renal function.

Antibody affinity to most T-dependent antigens increases during an immune response, and a similar effect can be produced by certain immunization protocols. For example, high affinity antibody sub-populations are potentiated following immunization with antigen and IFN$_\gamma$ (Fig. 6.15). A number of adjuvants are capable of enhancing levels of antibody but few have this characteristic of also potentiating affinity. As affinity markedly influences the biological effectiveness of antibodies, IFN$_\gamma$ could be an important adjuvant for vaccine use.

DETERMINATION OF AFFINITY AND AVIDITY

A number of methods are available for the determination of affinity and avidity. In each procedure a system is set up in which antigen and antibody are allowed to come to equilibrium: Ab + Ag $\leftrightarrows$ AbAg. The quantities of free antigen and complexed antigen are then measured without disturbing the equilibrium. There are several ways of doing this. Some separate the free antigen from bound antigen by physical methods such as dialysis, gel filtration, centrifugation and selective precipitation. Others use changes in the fluorescent properties of the complexed antigen or antibody. Data from these systems can be analysed by application of the Law of Mass Action to give the equilibrium constant, K, which is a measure of antibody affinity since:

$$K = \frac{[AbAg]}{[Ab].[Ag]}$$

where [AbAg] is the concentration of complexed antigen, [Ag] is the concentration of free antigen and [Ab] is the concentration of free antigen-binding sites at equilibrium. When half the binding sites are occupied by antigen, [Ab] = [AbAg], and it follows that K = 1/[Ag]. In other words, a high affinity antibody (one with a high K) only requires a low antigen concentration to achieve binding of antigen to half its combining sites, whereas a low affinity antibody requires a much higher concentration of antigen to achieve this.

Competitive binding

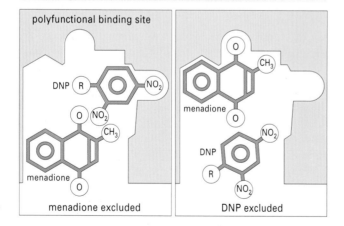

Fig. 6.12 The antibody combining site may bind more than one antigenic determinant. For example, antibody 460 has two different sites in the binding cleft which are 1.2–1.4 nm apart. The antibody binds the hapten menadione or the hapten DNP. The binding is competitive, that is, the binding of one excludes binding of the other. Binding sites capable of specifically binding more than one antigenic determinant are termed polyfunctional binding sites.

Polyfunctional binding sites

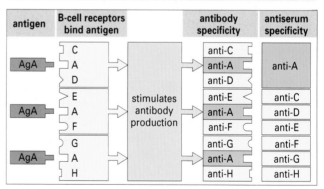

Fig. 6.13 Specificity as a population phenomenon. A single antigen (AgA) may bind to the antibody molecules of different B cells which are specific not only for A but also for other antigens (C, D, E, F, etc), that is, the B-cell receptors possess polyfunctional binding sites. Each B cell stimulated by AgA produces antibody specific not only to AgA, but also to the other antigens. Since all the B cells stimulated are AgA specific, but not all are specific to the other antigens, the concentration of antibody would be high to AgA but low to the other antigens.

ANTIBODY AFFINITY HETEROGENEITY

When enzymes interact with their substrate, the equilibrium constant (K value) for the reaction at different substrate concentrations is invariant. The reaction between antigen and antiserum differs from this: K varies with antibody concentration, reflecting the heterogeneity of the antibody population. For many years it was assumed that in any particular population of antibodies, the affinities would have a Gaussian (normal)

Advantages of high affinity antibody

haemagglutination
haemolysis
complement fixation
passive cutaneous anaphylaxis
immune elimination of antigen
membrane damage
virus neutralization
protective capacity against bacteria and viruses
enzyme inactivation

Fig. 6.14 Biological reactions in which high affinity antibody is superior to low affinity antibody.

Affinity maturation *in vivo*

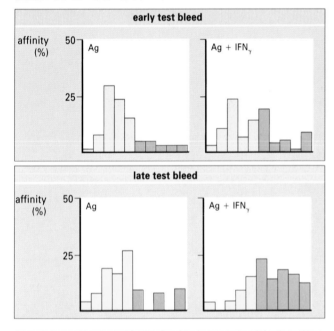

Fig. 6.15 Mice were immunized either with antigen alone (Ag) or with antigen plus 30 000 units of IFN_γ (Ag + IFN_γ). The affinity of the antibodies was measured either early or late after immunization. Mice receiving IFN_γ show more high affinity antibody (darker bars) in both the early and late bleeds than those which received antigen only.

distribution. However, this is not in fact so. Average affinity of a population of antibodies in a serum (K_0) is defined as the reciprocal of the free antigen concentration at equilibrium when half of the total antigen binding sites are occupied: $K_0 = 1/[Ag_{free}]$. When the equilibrium constant for the reaction between an antiserum and antigen is analysed (using different antigen concentrations) a non-Gaussian range of K values (affinities) is obtained (Fig. 6.16).

Affinity heterogeneity is difficult to assess experimentally, particularly since no precise mathematical description of this parameter is possible. This is because we are not sure whether the distribution of affinities in a particular serum is normal, skewed, biphasic or polyphasic. Complicated computer analyses of binding curves have been used to define heterogeneity but have made assumptions that the distribution is normal. A simple experimental approach to getting an assessment of heterogeneity which does not rely on such assumptions has been described. In this technique, an appropriate dilution of the antibody and serial dilutions of free antigen in solution are added to antigen-coated microtitre plates. (The free antigen blocks binding to the antigen on the plates.) The percentage inhibition at each concentration of free antigen is calculated and the molar concentration for 50% inhibition determined ($I_{0.5}$). The percentile inhibition contributed at each concentration of free antigen is calculated and the values used to analyse heterogeneity by histogram. A mathematical value describing heterogeneity (the Shannon index) can be calculated from these values. High values indicate a large spread of affinities, and low values indicate the converse.

Affinity heterogeneity

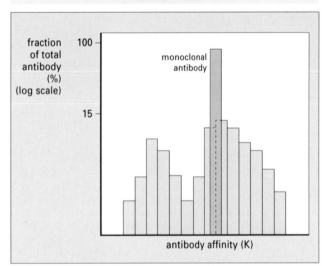
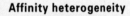

Fig. 6.16 This histogram shows a typical distribution of antibody affinities (K) in an antiserum to an antigenic determinant, compared to the single affinity with which a monoclonal antibody binds its antigenic determinant. Note that the antibody affinities do not have a normal distribution.

THE STRUCTURE OF ANTIGENS

The number of different antibodies which may be produced to an antigen is high, because antigens are three-dimensional structures and present many different configurations to the B cells. Different antibodies to an antigen often bind to epitopes which overlap on the antigen surface. In this way different antibodies can bind to a particular antigenic region of the molecule, without binding to exactly the same epitope.

Although it is possible to produce antibodies to almost any part of an antigen, this does not normally happen in an immune response. It is usually found that certain areas of the antigen are particularly antigenic, and that the majority of antibodies bind to these regions. These regions, which are referred to as the immunodominant regions of the antigen, are often at exposed areas on the outside of the antigen, particularly where there are loops of polypeptide that lack a rigid tertiary structure.

In some cases, the immunodominant regions of the antigen correspond to the most mobile surface areas of the molecule. This observation has led immunologists to suspect that the interaction between antibody and antigen is not a rigid fit with perfect complementarity between the shape of the antibody and antigen, but that there is some flexibility, both in the antigen epitope and the hypervariable loops of the antibody, which allows the optimum binding energy to be achieved. This proposal has been amply confirmed by X-ray crystallographic analysis of the complex between Fab and the antigen neuraminidase. The various factors involved in complementarity have been summarized elsewhere (see Figs 6.3, 6.4 and 6.5)

T CELL–ANTIGEN RECOGNITION

T cells recognize cell-bound antigen in association with MHC molecules. MHC class I and class II antigens act as guidance systems for T cells, and this process is called MHC restriction. The key experiment, that initially demonstrated the principle of MHC restriction, involved the murine cytotoxic T cell response to virally infected target cells (Fig. 6.17). It showed that cytotoxic T (Tc) cells from an animal infected with a virus are primed to kill cells of the same H–2 haplotype infected with that virus, but will not kill cells of a different haplotype infected by the same virus. One possible reason for the evolution of this joint recognition system is that by recognizing viral antigen in association with MHC antigen, receptors on Tc cells do not become saturated with free virus: saturation would prevent the Tc cells from killing virally infected cells. Similar principles of MHC-restricted recognition were subsequently shown to apply to helper T (TH) cells which recognise antigen on cells such as macrophages and B cells in association with MHC class II molecules. In this case, the class II region molecules act as recognition signals between antigen-presenting cells (such as macrophages) and the TH cell.

Killing of virally infected cells

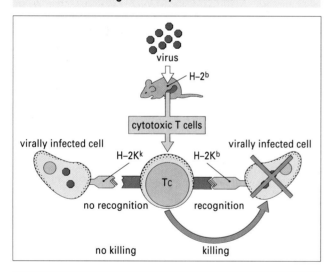

Fig. 6.17 Killing of virally infected target cells and haplotype restricted killing. A mouse of the H–2^b haplotype is primed with virus, and the Tc cells thus generated are then isolated. These T cells are then tested for their ability to kill cells of the H–2^b and H–2^k haplotypes infected with the same virus. The Tc cells kill H–2^b cells but not cells of a different haplotype, H–2^k. It is concluded that the T cell is recognizing a specific structure resulting from the association between the class I H–2K (or H–2D) product and viral antigen (e.g. a virus/H–2K complex). As a control measure, both groups are treated with anti-viral antibody, which does not exhibit haplotype restriction: infected cells of both haplotypes are killed by anti-viral antibody and complement.

T cell and B cell epitopes are distinct

glucagon	N 1	17 18	29
antibody response	+++		+
lymphocyte stimulation	–		+++
DTH response	+		+++

Fig. 6.18 The immune response to two peptides of the antigen glucagon are shown. Antibody (B-cell response) is primarily directed to epitopes at the N terminus, while the C–terminal peptide 18–29 stimulates T-cell responses, including lymphocyte stimulation *in vitro* and the delayed type hypersensitivity (DTH) response *in vivo*.

ANTIGEN PROCESSING AND PRESENTATION

Antibody responses and cell-mediated immune reactions are generally directed against different determinants on the antigen. For example, mouse B cells recognize an epitope at the N terminus of glucagon, whereas T cells recognize determinants near the C terminus (Fig. 6.18). The basis for this dichotomy lies in the fact that antigens are not presented by MHC antigens as intact proteins, but rather as processed forms at the cell surface. The cells that process antigen in this way may be either specialized antigen-presenting cells (APCs), capable of stimulating T cell division, or any virally infected cells within the body, which then become a target for Tc cells. Antigen processing involves degrading the antigen into peptide fragments.

Thus, the vast majority of epitopes recognized by T cells are linear fragments from a peptide chain, and they are often sterically hindered in the intact protein. Only a minority of peptide fragments from a protein antigen are able to bind to a particular MHC molecule. Furthermore, different MHC molecules bind different sets of peptides. For example, using a viral antigen that is recognized by mouse strains of different haplotypes (that is, having different MHC molecules) it was found that TH cells of different haplotypes recognized distinct peptides from that antigen, depending largely on the ability of a particular peptide to bind to a particular MHC class II (Fig. 6.19). Another example of this principle of epitope selection by different MHC molecules is the immune response of rodents to myelin basic protein, or MBP (Fig. 6.20). Different strains of rodent respond to different areas of the MBP.

T cell sites in the λ repressor protein

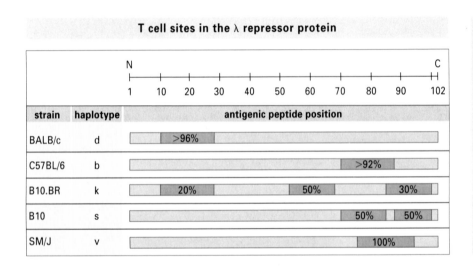

Fig. 6.19 Diversity of antigenic peptides in relation to MHC class II. Mice were immunized with λ repressor protein. T cell hybridomas generated from mouse cells were tested against a panel of overlapping peptides which spanned the entire protein. Positions of antigenic peptides are shown in dark blue, with the percentage of T cells which recognized both the protein and the fragment. One peptide was always immunodominant, although more than one peptide was antigenic in some mouse strains. Adapted from data by Roy *et al.* (1989).

T cell response to antigen peptides

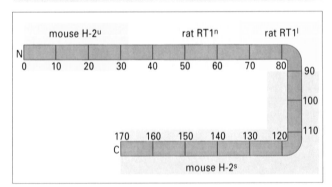

Fig. 6.20 Response in rats and mice to myelin basic protein. H-2u mice respond to determinants at the N terminus (0–32), while SJL mice (H–2s) respond to peptide 90–170. The peptides recognized by Lewis (RT-1l) and Brown Norway (RT-1n) rats are also indicated. (RT-1 is the rat MHC).

Antigen processing

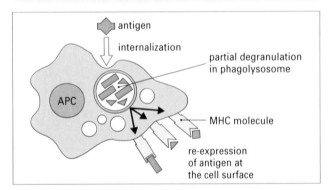

Fig. 6.21 Antigens are internalized by antigen-presenting cells and are then degraded by proteolytic enzymes in specialized intercellular compartments. Antigenic peptides, which are linear fragments, associate with class II MHC molecules that intersect the endocytic pathway as they are moved to the cell surface.

PROCESSING OF ANTIGENS

The processing of antigens, to generate peptides that can bind to MHC molecules, occurs in intracellular organelles (Fig. 6.21). The internal degradation by APCs can be circumvented by the use of synthetic peptides. The ability to synthesize peptides chemically has enabled the epitopes recognized by T cells with different specificities to be identified (Fig. 6.22). The relative importance of different amino acids within a defined epitope can also be investigated by amino acid replacements at different sites. Using defined peptides, direct binding to both MHC class I and class II antigens has also been demonstrated. A comparison of the effects of an amino acid substitution on MHC binding and T-cell reactivity has enabled tentative conclusions to be drawn on which amino acids contact the MHC molecule and which contact the T-cell receptor. For example, a peptide representing residues 52–61 of hen egg-white lysozyme has been shown to be recognized by H–2-IA^k restricted T cells. This peptide binds with a dissociation constant of about 3 μmol/10^{-6} to IA^k molecules. Direct MHC binding and functional data have implicated three amino acid residues within this peptide as interacting with Ia, and another three residues as contacting the TCR. The TCR- and MHC-contacting residues are segregated at opposite faces if the peptide is modelled as an α helix (Fig. 6.23). However, the conformations adopted by antigenic peptides when bound to MHC molecules are contentious. This point is discussed further below in relation to the structure of the MHC binding groove.

STRUCTURE OF CLASS I ANTIGENS

Knowledge of the three-dimensional structure of MHC class I antigens and the location of the peptide binding region as a groove formed from the α$_1$ and α$_2$ domains, has helped to explain these observations (Fig. 6.24). The structure of the peptide binding groove of class I and, by inference, class II antigens has been discussed more fully in Chapter 4. The peptide binding site is a structure with a variety of pockets, clefts, ridges, intrusions and depressions. Its precise topology depends partly on the nature of the amino acids within the groove, and these vary from one haplotype to another. Thus, whether a peptide binds to a particular MHC molecule depends on the nature of the side chains of that peptide and their complementarity with the MHC molecule's binding groove. Some amino acid side chains of the peptide will be oriented out of the groove and would be available to contact the TCR.

Recent studies have shown that experiments with synthetic peptides are not perfect models for *in vivo* T-cell recognition. Advances in techniques of protein purification and in the sensitivity of protein sequencing have made it possible to study peptides that have been produced by the cell and then bound by MHC molecules at the cell surface. The peptides expressed at the cell surface include not just foreign peptides from internalized antigens or viral particles, but also self molecules produced within the cell or endocytosed from extracellular fluids. When self peptides eluted from MHC class I molecules were purified and

T cell sites in proteins	
peptide	**amino acid sequence**
myoglobin	69–78 102–118 132–145
flu haemagglutinin	109–119 130–140 302–313
hepatitis B surface Ag	38–52 95–109 140–154
hepatitis B pre-S	120–132
FMDV VPI	141–160
rabies spike precursor	32–44
* 6 other proteins also studied in this way: 18 of 23 known sites predicted	

Fig. 6.22 The table shows peptides that are known to stimulate T cells. The peptides come from a number of proteins. Synthetic peptides corresponding to the entire amino acid sequence of a protein antigen can be used to stimulate specific T cells. Usually, only one or few peptides from a protein are stimulators.

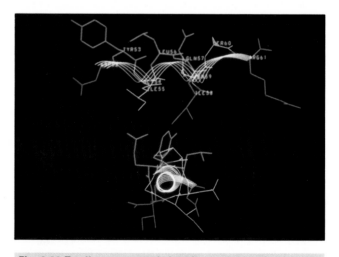

Fig. 6.23 T-cell receptor and class II contact residues. Peptide 52–61 of hen egg-white lysozyme modelled in an α helix viewed from the side (above) and end (below) with the N terminus to the left. (T-cell receptor contact residues are in red, class II contact residues in blue, other residues in yellow. The α helix is shown as a white ribbon.) Residues of the epitope tend to occur on one side of the antigen and of the agretope on the other. (Courtesy of Professor P. M. Allen, from *Nature* 1987:**327**;714. With permission from Macmillan Magazines Ltd.)

sequenced, they were shown to be nine amino acids in length. This contrasts with the size of about 12–15 amino acids that were shown to be the optimal epitope defined using synthetic peptides. Interestingly, these 'natural' peptides eluted from MHC molecules were more precisely defined than expected. Thus, from sequencing peptides bound by particular MHC molecules, characteristic residues were identified – one at the C terminus and another close to the N terminus of the peptide. These distinguish sets of binding peptides for different class I molecules (Fig. 6.25). These characteristic motifs are thought to act as anchoring residues for the peptide within the groove. Recent analysis of the three-dimensional structure of the HLA-B27 molecule has generated a particularly clear picture of the peptide residing in the binding groove. It is an extended (not α-helical) chain of nine amino acids with its ends tethered at opposite ends of the groove, and the side chains of some amino acids extending into the pockets formed within the variable region of the class I heavy chain. This structural picture is consistent with the characteristic motifs found at the ends of peptides eluted from class I molecules. It is not known at present whether the same constraints apply to the binding of peptides to class II molecules.

MHC–PEPTIDE ASSOCIATION

Using a combination of biochemical and X-ray crystallographic studies, a picture emerges of the long groove at the top of the MHC molecule selecting out a specific set of peptides. The set selected would depend on the precise structure of the groove, which is dictated by the polymorphic amino acids clustered around the groove.

How and where do peptides become associated with MHC molecules? Evidence is emerging that peptide/MHC association occurs in specific intracellular organelles and that interaction of peptides with class I and class II antigens occurs at different sites within the cell.

It is now apparent that cells can present not just foreign antigen, but also peptide fragments of their own molecules. However, the individual does not react against these self molecules because of the mechanisms which produce tolerance to self. Of these, the most important is the education of T cells during maturation in the thymus, leading to deletion of those which react to self-peptides on self-MHC molecules (see Chapter 11).

CLASS I–PEPTIDE ASSOCIATION

A number of experiments demonstrate that class I restricted T cells (Tc cells) recognize endogenous antigens synthesized within the target cell, whereas class II restricted T cells (Th cells) recognise exogenously added antigen. Experimentally, manipulation of the location of a protein determines whether it elicits a class I or class II restricted response. For example, influenza virus haemagglutinin (HA), a glycoprotein associated with the membranes of the host cell, normally elicits only a weak Tc cell response. However, influenza HA can be generated in the cytoplasm by

Binding peptides for class I molecules

restriction element	motif	position 1	2	3	4	5	6	7	8	9
H–2Dᵇ	dominant anchor residues					N				M
	strong		M L P V	I E Q V	K	L	F			I
H–2Kᵇ	dominant anchor residues					F Y			L	
	strong			Y					M	
H–2Kᵈ	dominant anchor residues		Y							I L
	strong			N I L	P	M	K F	T N		
HLA–A2	dominant anchor residues		L							V
	strong		M			E K	V	K		

Fig. 6.25 Allele-specific motifs in peptides eluted from MHC molecules. Class I molecules from different haplotypes were immunoprecipitated from extracts of cultured cell lines. The peptides bound to these molecules were purified and sequenced. Amino acid residues that were commonly found at a particular position are classified as dominant anchor residues. Residues that are fairly common at a site are shown as 'strong'. Positions for which no amino acid is shown could be occupied by several different amino acids with equal frequency. The one letter amino acid code is used.

MHC class I–peptide complex

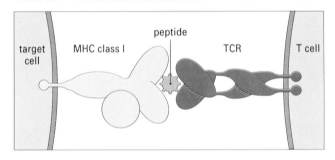

Fig. 6.24 A scheme for the structure of the ternary complex between MHC class I peptide and TCR. The peptide is located in the groove formed by the α₁ and α₂ domains of the MHC class I molecule. The region contacts the binding site of the TCR formed by the six hypervariable regions of the Vα and Vβ domains.

deleting the cDNA sequence coding for the N-terminal signal peptide to HA. When this is done there is a strong Tc cell response to HA. Similarly, the introduction of ovalbumin into the cytoplasm of a target cell, using an osmotic shock technique, generates Tc cells recognizing ovalbumin, whereas addition of exogenous ovalbumin generates exclusively a Th cell response.

PROCESSING OF CYTOPLASMIC ANTIGEN

Cytoplasmic antigens are processed into peptides by cytoplasmic proteases prior to transport of the peptides into the rough endoplasmic reticulum (RER) of the cell. This is the organelle on which membrane proteins, including class I and class II antigens, are synthesized and assembled. Once within the RER, peptides are thought to associate efficiently with newly synthesized class I molecules. The assembly of the MHC heavy chain and β_2m is thought to be driven by peptide because 'empty' class I MHC complexes lacking peptide are unstable, β_2m and heavy chain rapidly dissociating at physiological temperatures.

There is now a better understanding of the proteins that process and transport cytoplasmic peptides bound by class I molecules. Remarkably, some of these proteins are encoded within the MHC. Cytoplasmic antigens are thought to be processed, at least in part, by an organelle known as a proteasome. Proteasomes are multicatalytic proteinase complexes expressed ubiquitously and found throughout the animal kingdom. Two genes encoding components of the human and murine proteasomes have been mapped within the class II region of the MHC.

TRANSMEMBRANE TRANSPORTERS

Two genes encoding members of the so-called 'ABC' superfamily of transmembrane transporters have also been discovered not within the class I region, but within the class II region. These ABC proteins are a large family of proteins that transport a variety of substrates, including peptides, across cellular membranes in an ATP-dependent manner. The most compelling evidence

that these genes encode proteins implicated in the transport process comes from the use of mutant cell lines. These fail to express class I antigens on their surface at 37°C. Class I expression can, however, be rescued by growing the cells at 30°C or by adding a high concentration of exogenous peptide. The MHC class I molecules expressed at 30°C are 'empty' of endogenous peptides. The defect in these mutants therefore appears to be the inability to load peptide onto class I antigens. These mutants have characteristic deletions within the MHC class II region. In at least one of these mutants, class I expression can be re-established by the introduction of DNA encoding the MHC-linked transporter genes.

The positions of the murine and human MHC-encoded transporter and proteasome genes are shown in Fig. 6.26. The size of the MHC, and the likelihood that this region encodes a number of as yet undiscovered genes raises the possibility that other genes involved in antigen processing and presentation will be found within the MHC.

The current view of the processing of peptides bound by class I molecules is shown in Fig. 6.27. Viral or other proteins synthesized in the cytoplasm are processed by proteasome complexes. Peptides are transported into the RER by the ABC transporter where some associate with, and stabilize, the class I–β_2m complex. Only peptides that fulfil the steric requirements for fitting into the peptide binding groove will bind. It is not known whether peptides are transported into the RER as nonapeptides or whether larger forms can bind to class I molecules and be trimmed after binding. The ternary complex is transported to the cell surface. Class I molecules lacking bound peptide dissociate (and are presumably degraded) prior to, or at the cell surface.

Class II molecules are also synthesized and assembled in the RER and one question that arises is why class II molecules do not apparently bind cytoplasmically derived peptides within the RER? It is likely that the class II binding site is physically blocked at this stage and is, therefore, unavailable for peptide binding.

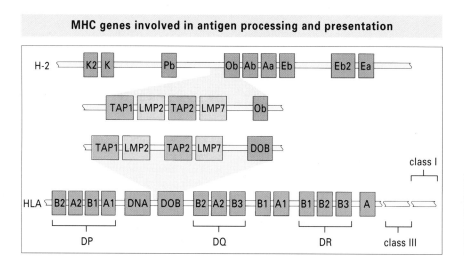

MHC genes involved in antigen processing and presentation

Fig. 6.26 Genes encoding a peptide transporter (TAP) and components of a organelle called a proteasome (LMP) are located within the murine and human class II regions.

CLASS II–PEPTIDE ASSOCIATION

Class IIα and β chains reside in the RER as a complex with an additional polypeptide called the invariant chain (Ii). This protein is encoded by a gene outside of the MHC. The αβ–Ii complex is transported to an acidic endosomal or lysosomal compartment where dissociation of Ii occurs. The αβ complex spends 1–3 hours in this compartment before reaching the cell surface and it is here that peptide loading most probably occurs. Experiments show that mutually exclusive binding of peptide and Ii to class II molecules occurs and suggest that dissociation of Ii in the acidic environment of the endosomal/lysosomal compartment permits binding of peptide.

How do antigenic peptides derived from endogenous peptides meet class II antigens in the appropriate compartment? The answer to this question lies in the intracellular traffic routes of MHC antigens. Following synthesis in the RER, both class I and II antigens are transported to the Golgi compartment, class I in association with antigenic peptide and class II bound to the invariant chain. It is in the Golgi complex that class I and class II antigens segregate; class I molecules are transported directly to the cell surface, and class II molecules arrive in the lysosomal-like compartment.

It is likely that MHC class II molecules contact exogenous antigen in this compartment. Exogenous antigens, taken up by endocytosis, would move through the cell in order to reach the acidic compartment at which dissociation of Ii from the class II molecule occurs. Proteases along the endocytic pathway could process the exogenous antigen to generate peptides for presentation. The swapping of antigenic peptide for Ii generates a stable class II molecule that is transported to the cell surface. The constraints for binding of peptide to the MHC class II groove are probably broadly the same as for class I peptide binding, although there is some evidence that their binding sites are larger and more accessible to synthetic peptides.

The intracellular transport routes of MHC antigens in B cells, and the postulated site of peptide loading to class II antigens, is presented in Fig. 6.28. The crux of this model is that the intracellular distribution of class I and class II molecules reflects the dichotomy in presentation of antigen from endogenous and exogenous origin. Further work is required to determine whether other antigen presenting cells, such as macrophages, dendritic cells and Langerhans cells use this mechanism for peptide–class II interaction.

■ ROLE OF ACCESSORY MOLECULES

The specificity of T-cell interactions with target cells clearly derives from the interaction of the TCR with class I or class II antigen loaded with peptide. However, this interaction is often of too low affinity to activate the T cell and interactions between accessory molecules are required to increase the overall avidity. There are a number of molecules, involved in antigen-non-specific interactions, that perform an adhesion function. The two most important ones on T cells are CD2, which interacts with the LFA-3 ligand on the target cell, and LFA-1, which interacts with its ligands ICAM-1 and ICAM-2. LFA-1 is a member of the integrin superfamily of adhesion molecules and is present on most leucocytes. ICAM-1 and ICAM2 are present on endothelial tissue and ICAM-1 is also expressed on activated T and B cells. In addition to its adhesion properties CD2 may contribute to T-cell activation by transducing signals into the T-cell. LFA-1 may have a similar role.

Assembly of endogenous peptides with MHC class I antigens

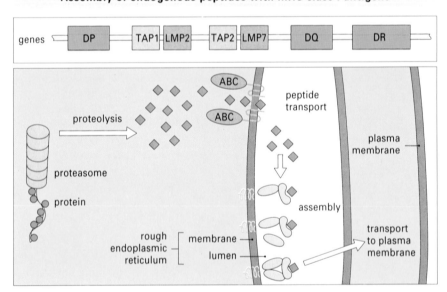

Fig. 6.27 Cytoplasmic antigens are thought to be processed by proteasomes, two subunits of which are encoded within the MHC. Peptides are thought to be transported by two members of the 'ABC' superfamily of transporters, also encoded within the MHC. Antigenic peptides associate with class I heavy chains and β₂m in the RER. Stabilized class I molecules are then transported to the cell surface (see Fig. 6.12).

Proposed routes of intracellular trafficking of MHC molecules involved in antigen presentation

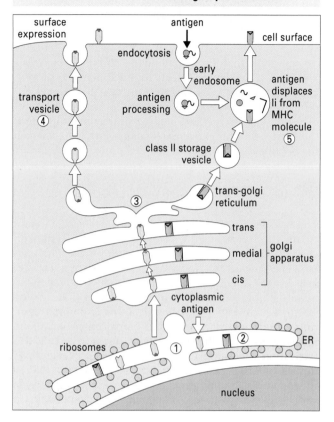

The CD4 and CD8 accessory molecules have a weak affinity for MHC class II and class I molecules, respectively. Recent studies indicate that CD4 or CD8 molecules associate with the TCR–MHC–peptide complex. The low affinity of the interaction between CD4 or CD8 and MHC molecules means that they are unlikely to contribute to the avidity of the T cell for its target cell. However, the recruitment of CD4 or CD8 molecules to the antigen-receptor complex may stimulate intracellular events that are important in the activation process. These aspects of T cell activation are discussed more fully in Chapter 7.

Fig. 6.28 Newly synthesized class I molecules are loaded with peptide (1). Class II molecules associate with Ii in the RER (2). Ii prevents loading with peptide and contains sequences that enable the class II molecule to exit the RER. Class I and class II molecules segregate after transit through the Golgi (3); class I molecules go directly to the cell surface (4) and class II molecules enter an acidic compartment, where they are loaded with peptide derived from exogenous antigen (5).

FURTHER READING

Allen PM, Matsueda GR, Evans RJ, Dunbar (Jr) JB, Marshall GR, Unanué ER. Identification of the T cell and Ia contact residues of a T-cell antigenic epitope. *Nature* 1987;**327**:713–15.

Babbitt BP, Allen PM, Matsueda G, Haber E, Unanué ER. Binding of immunogenic peptides to Ia histocompatibility molecules. *Nature* 1985;**317**:359.

Bierer BE, Sleckman BP, Ratnofsky SE, Burakoff SJ. The biologic roles of CD2, CD4 and CD8 in T-cell activation. *Annu Rev Immunol* 1989;**7**:579–99.

Bjorkman PJ, Parham P. Structure, function, and diversity of class I major histocompatibility complex molecules. *Annu Rev Biochem* 1990;**59**:253–88.

Cresswell P. Questions of presentation. *Nature* 1990;**343**:593.

Demotz S, Grey HM, Appella E, Sette A. Characterization of a naturally processed MHC class II-restricted T-cell determinant of hen egg lysozyme. *Nature* 1989;**342**:682.

Falk K, Rötzschke O, Stevanovic S, Jung G, Rammensee H-G. Allele-specific motifs revealed by sequencing of self-peptides eluted from MHC molecules. *Nature* 1991;**351**:290-296.

Glynne R, Powis SH, Beck S, Kelly A, Kerr L-A, Trowsdale J. A proteasome-related gene between the two ABC transporter loci in the class II region of the human MHC. *Nature* 1991;**353**:357.

Jardetzky TS, Lane WS, Robinson RA, Madden DR, Wiley DC. Identification of self peptides bound to purified HLA-B27. *Nature* 1991;**353**:326–29.

Lanzavecchia A. Receptor-mediated antigen uptake and its effect on antigen presentation to class II-restricted T lymphocytes. *Annu Rev Immunol* 1990;**8**:773.

Neefijies JJ, Stollorz V, Peters PJ, Geuze HJ, Ploegh HL. The biosynthetic pathway of MHC class II but not class I molecules intersects the endocytic route. *Cell* 1990;**61**:171.

Parham P. Transporters of delight. *Nature* 1990;**348**:674–75.

Parham P. Half of a peptide pump. *Nature* 1991;**351**:271–72.

Robertson M. Proteasomes in the pathway. *Nature* 1991;**353**:300.

Roche PA, Cresswell P. Invariant chain association with HLA-DR molecules inhibits immunogenic peptide binding. *Nature* 1990;**345**:615.

Roy S, Scherer MT, Briner TJ, Smith JA, Gefter ML. Murine MHC polymorphism and T cell specificities. *Science* 1989;**244**:572–75.

Schwartz AL. Cell biology of intracellular protein trafficking. *Annu Rev Immunol* 1990;**8**:195.

Teyton L, O'Sullivan D, Dickson PW, *et al.* Invariant chain distinguishes between the exogenous and endogenous antigen presentation pathways. *Nature* 1990;**348**:39–44.

Townsend A, Öhlen C, Bastin J, Ljunggren H-G, Foster L, Kärre K. Association of class I major histocompatibility heavy and light chains induced by viral peptides. *Nature* 1989;**340**:443.

chapter 7

Cell Cooperation in the Antibody Response

The organized lymphoid tissues, such as lymph nodes and spleen, consist of closely packed cells, as are the cells at an inflammatory site. This alone suggests that lymphoid cells do not function in isolation. Indeed, it is now known that they interact in a well organized sequence of events, leading up the induction of antibody, delayed hypersensitivity or other types of immune responses. In this chapter the principles of the cell interactions in the immune system are described, together with some of the consequences (e.g. affinity maturation, immunological memory) and some of the critical molecules involved, such as cytokines.

 COOPERATION BETWEEN DIFFERENT CELL TYPES

ANTIGEN-PRESENTING CELLS (APCs) AND T CELLS

The interaction between T cells and the heterogeneous group of cells collectively termed 'antigen-presenting cells' is the most extensively studied example of cell interaction in the immune system, because of its under-lying importance. It is the first cellular interaction to occur after antigen challenge, and its outcome largely dictates the subsequent events: if sufficient CD4$^+$ T-helper (TH) cells are triggered, then the activation of B cells or the development of delayed hypersensitivity almost certainly follows. If TH cells are not triggered, or are subject to a form of immunological tolerance known as 'clonal anergy', which is discussed in more detail in Chapter 10, then no other immunological events follow.

TYPES OF APC

A wide spectrum of cells can present antigen, depending on how and where the antigen first encounters cells of the immune system (Fig. 7.1). In the T-cell dependent areas of lymph nodes and spleen, there are abundant interdigitating dendritic cells (IDCs), which are considered to be the most effective cells for the initial activation of resting CD4$^+$ T cells. IDCs express high levels of MHC class II antigens, but so may macrophages or B lymphocytes, so this cannot explain the greater effectiveness of IDCs in antigen presentation.

Localization of antigen in lymph nodes in association with APCs

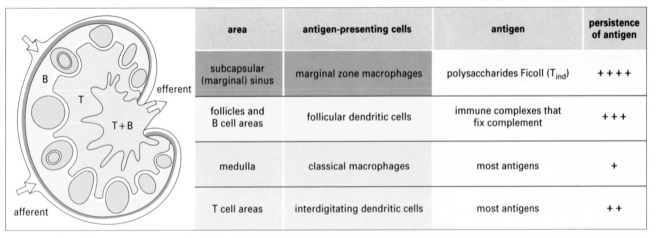

area	antigen-presenting cells	antigen	persistence of antigen
subcapsular (marginal) sinus	marginal zone macrophages	polysaccharides Ficoll (T$_{ind}$)	+ + + +
follicles and B cell areas	follicular dendritic cells	immune complexes that fix complement	+ + +
medulla	classical macrophages	most antigens	+
T cell areas	interdigitating dendritic cells	most antigens	+ +

Fig. 7.1 A lymph node represented schematically (above, left) shows afferent and efferent lymphatics, follicles, the outer cortical B cell area and the paracortical T cell area. Different antigen-presenting cells predominate in these areas (though the demarcation is not absolute) and selectively take up different types of antigen which then persist on the surface of the cells for variable periods. Thus many polysaccharides are preferentially taken up by marginal zone macrophages and may persist for months or years, whereas antigens on recirculating macrophages in the medulla may last for only a few days or weeks. Note that recirculating 'veiled' cells (Langerhans' cells), which are thought to arise from the skin, change their morphology to become interdigitating dendritic cells within the lymph node. Both these cells, and the follicular dendritic cells, have long processes which are in intimate contact with lymphocytes.

It is considered that IDCs are the major APC involved in primary immune responses, as judged by their greater effectiveness in inducing T-cell proliferation. Cell proliferation is a key step as it augments the numbers of antigen-specific T cells, but it is only one facet of effective T cell triggering – macrophages may be *more* effective than IDCs in inducing primary T helper function, but *less* efficient than IDCs at inducing proliferation. In human systems, where the blood lymphoid cells are usually studied, the blood monocytes are the most widely studied APC, and these have the capacity to induce both T-cell proliferation and helper function.

B lymphocytes have immunoglobulins on their surface which can bind to antigen, inducing the B cell to take it up. The cell then degrades the antigen into peptides which become associated with MHC class II. If antigen concentrations are very low, then B cells with high-affinity receptors (IgM or IgD) specific for that antigen are the most effective APCs, because other APCs cannot capture enough antigen. Thus for secondary responses, after the number of antigen-reactive B cells has been augmented during the primary immunization, B lymphocytes may be a major type of APC. The properties and functions of APCs are summarized in Figs 7.2 and 7.3.

Antigen-presenting cells

	phago-cytosis	type	location	class II expression
phagocytes (monocyte/macrophage lineage)	+	monocytes	blood	$(+) \rightarrow +++$ inducible
		macrophages	tissue	
		marginal zone macrophages	spleen and lymph node	
		Kupffer cells	liver	
		microglia	brain	
non-phagocytic constitutive antigen-presenting cells	–	Langerhans' cells	skin	++ constitutive
		interdigitating dendritic cells (IDCs)	lymphoid tissue	
		follicular dendritic cells	lymphoid tissue	–
lymphocytes	–	B cells and T cells	lymphoid tissues and at sites of immune reactions	$- \rightarrow ++$ inducible
facultative antigen-presenting cells	+	astrocytes	brain	inducible
		follicular cells	thyroid	inducible
	–	endothelium	vascular and lymphoid tissue	$- \rightarrow ++$ inducible
		fibroblasts	connective tissue	
		other types in appropriate tissue		

Fig. 7.2 Many APCs are unable to phagocytose antigen, but can take it up in other ways. In certain circumstances, cells not normally considered to be part of the 'immune system' act as APCs. Endothelial cells, which have been induced to express class II molecules by interferon-γ (IFN$_\gamma$), are sometimes capable of acting as APCs. Certain epithelial cells, provided they are expressing class II, may also act as APCs. The most widely studied example of this phenomenon involves the thyroid follicular cell, which acts as an APC in the pathogenesis of Graves' autoimmune thyroiditis.

Antigen presentation

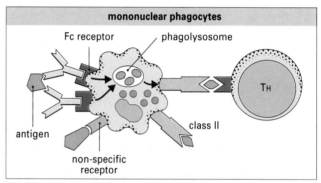

mononuclear phagocytes

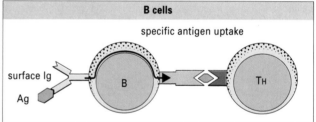

B cells

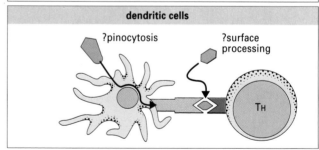

dendritic cells

Fig. 7.3 Mononuclear phagocytes (top), B cells (centre) and dendritic cells (bottom) can all present antigen to MHC class II restricted T-helper (TH) cells. Macrophages take up antigen via non-specific receptors or as immune complexes, and probably process it internally before returning fragments to the cell surface in association with class II molecules. Activated B cells can take up antigen via their surface immunoglobulin and present it to T cells alongside the class II molecules. Dendritic cells constitutively express class II MHC molecules, but are not phagocytic. Presumably they either take up antigen by pinocytosis or process it at the cell surface.

WHAT ARE THE ESSENTIAL MOLECULAR INTERACTIONS OF ANTIGEN PRESENTATION TO T CELLS?

The T-cell receptor for antigen (TCR) recognizes peptides lodged in the peptide binding groove of MHC molecules. This interaction dictates immunological specificity, since a peptide associated with an MHC molecule of one particular haplotype forms a unique structure to be recognized by the TCR. Evidence to support this came from experiments in which the complementary DNA (cDNA) encoding human MHC molecules was transfected into mouse fibroblasts, inducing these cells to produce human MHC molecules. They could then act as human APCS, but with low efficiency compared to cells that expressed other relevant molecules as well. One such molecule is intercellular adhesion molecule-1 (ICAM-1) which is known to interact with lymphocyte functional antigen-1 (LFA-1), present on all immune cells. If mouse cells are transfected with both human MHC and human ICAM-1, their capacity to act as human APCs is augmented.

The CD2 molecule on T cells is also involved in T-cell activation, in conjunction with the TCR. CD2 is a receptor for lymphocyte functional antigen-3 (LFA-3) which is widely distributed on cells and is present on all APCs. The presence of LFA-3 on sheep red cells is responsible for the sheep red cell rosetting reaction (the E rosette), widely used to purify T cells before the advent of monoclonal antibodies. Molecules involved in APC function are summarized in Fig. 7.4.

It is likely that other cell surface molecules are of major importance in antigen presentation, but we do not know what they are. It has been proposed that a currently unknown molecule is needed to reinforce the signal from TCR and induce positive activation of the T cells; this has been termed the 'second signal'. Without this signal, T cells cannot respond, and once they have recognized their antigen in a non-stimulating manner they become inactivated, producing a state of immunological tolerance. This tolerance is specific, only affecting TH cells that respond to a particular antigen, hence the term 'clonal anergy'.

Apart from the cell-surface interactions, cytokines are also involved in T-cell activation, where interest has focused on IL-1 and IL-6, molecules produced by certain APCs, for example macrophages. T cells do not always require stimulation by these molecules – if they are already dividing, it is not necessary. In resting T cells IL-1 and IL-6 induce the expression of receptors for the T-cell growth factor, IL-2.

While the interaction between CD4$^+$ T cells and APCs is reasonably well studied, that between CD8$^+$ T cells and APCs is less understood. It is known that CD4$^+$ cells help in the activation of most CD8$^+$ T cells. Since a single interdigitating dendritic cell (IDC) can bind many T cells, it has been proposed that CD8$^+$ activation takes place as part of a cell cluster, together with CD4$^+$ cells, on the surface of one or more IDCs.

ANTIGEN PROCESSING

The pioneering studies of Ada and Nossal showed that only a very small proportion (<1%) of injected antigen is involved in the immune response, the rest being rapidly degraded and excreted. This explains why antigen presentation is the rate-limiting step in immune reactions. Antigen processing refers to the degradation of antigen fragments into peptides which become bound to MHC class I or class II molecules. These are the critical antigenic fragments involved in the triggering of T cells, whose receptors recognize sequences of amino acids in peptides rather than protein shapes, or 'conformational' determinants, as B-cell immunoglobulins do. For the triggering of B cells there is a store of antigen complexed with antibody and complement in the germinal centres of lymph nodes, adherent to dendritic follicular cells. Details of antigen processing are discussed in Chapter 6.

INTERACTION OF B CELLS AND T CELLS

With the capacity to enrich antigen specific T cells by growing and cloning them with antigens, APCs and IL-2, it has become possible to directly visualize the T–B interaction, in clusters *in vitro*. The cells become polarized, with the T-cell receptors concentrated to the B cell side. The B cell also becomes polarized and expresses most of the class II antigen in proximity to T cells. These clusters do indeed look like an intense exchange of information, which leads to two important events in the B cell life cycle, induction of proliferation, and differentiation into antibody-forming cells.

The interaction between T cells and B cells is a two-way process, in which B cells present antigen to T cells and receive signals from the T cells for division and differentiation. The central interaction is that between MHC class II–antigen and the TCR; it is augmented by interactions between LFA-3 and CD2, and ICAM-1 and

Critical molecules involved in antigen presentation

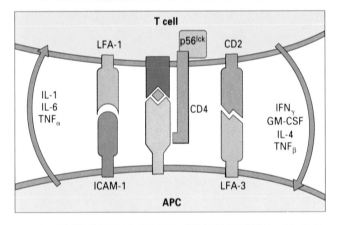

Fig. 7.4 The molecules involved in the interaction between T cells and APCs. The various cytokines and their direction of action are also shown.

LFA-1 (Fig. 7.5). A number of other cell surface molecules are also involved. The B7/BB1 surface antigen on B cells interacts with CD28, which causes stabilization of mRNA for IL-2 and other cytokines in the T cells, thereby prolonging the delivery of the activation signals. Additionally, CD5 (T cell) interacts with CD72 (Lyb2 in the mouse) on the B cell surface. IL-1 and IL-6 released by some B cells enhance expression of IL-2 receptor on the T cells, but since only some B cells make these cytokines, it is likely that most B cells can only efficiently activate preprimed or memory T cells.

CYTOKINE SECRETION AND ACTION

During the interaction, T cells can secrete a number of cytokines which have a powerful effect on B cells. These include IL-2, a proliferation inducer for B cells as well as T cells, IL-4 which acts early in B cell activation of proliferation, IL-5 which in the mouse (but not man) is a powerful B cell activator, and IL-6 which is the strongest signal for B cell differentiation (Fig. 7.6). T cells also produce tumour necrosis factors α and β. These molecules have also been reported to be important for B cell growth. Despite this long catalogue of molecules which act to trigger B cells, there are other signals which remain to be identified. One of the strongest signals for long-term proliferation of B cells is the antibody which recognizes the B cell CD40 antigen. CD40 has the structure of a cell surface receptor resembling the TNF receptor, but the ligand which it recognizes is not yet known. This will be a molecule of importance in B cell activation, and may be the signal responsible for the initial B cell activation.

Cell-surface molecules involved in the interactions between B cells and T$_H$ cells

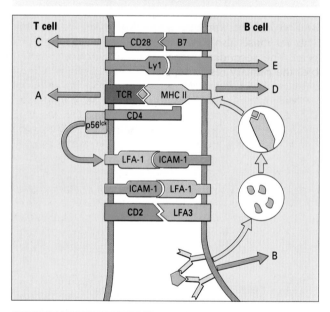

Fig 7.5 The yellow arrow represents membrane-immunoglobulin directed (mIg-directed) delivery of antigen (Ag) to an intracellular compartment where it is degraded and peptides can combine with MHC class II molecules. Other arrows show the discrete signal-transduction events that have been established. A and B are the antigen-receptor signal-transduction events involving tyrosine phosphorylation and phosphoinositide breakdown. The antigen receptors also regulate LFA-1 affinity for ICAM-1, possibly through the signal transduction events. In the T cell, CD28 also sends a unique signal to the T cell (C). In the B cell, class II MHC molecules and Lyb2 (CD72 in man) appear to induce distinct signalling events (D and E). Not shown is the exchange of soluble interleukins and binding to the corresponding receptors on the other cell. (Adapted, with permission, from DeFranco (1991) *Nature* **351**: 603.

Stages in B-cell activation and development

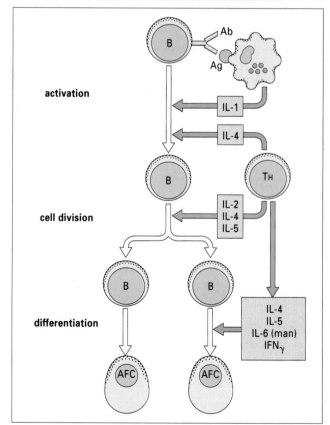

Fig. 7.6 B cells are activated by antigen on antigen-presenting cells (APCs) such as macrophages in the presence of IL-4 and IL-1. This causes expression of receptors for IL-2 and other cytokines. IL-2, IL-4 and IL-5 (in the mouse) drive cell division. Only one cycle of cell division is illustrated although many cycles will usually occur. Differentiation into antibody-forming cells (AFCs) is effected by IL-4, IL-5, IL-6 (in man) and IFN$_\gamma$.

CONSEQUENCES OF B–T INTERACTION

The above description of B–T interaction is incomplete. It suggests that the only possible outcome to B–T interaction is activation of the B cell. However this is not the case. In the same way that APC–T cell interaction may yield two diametrically opposing results, (T-cell activation or inactivation – clonal anergy), B cells frequently become anergic. This is important because affinity maturation of B cells during the immune response, due to rapid mutation in the genes encoding the antibody variable regions, could easily result in high-affinity autoantibodies. Hence, clonal anergy in the periphery is an important device for silencing these potentially damaging clones. However, the details of this process are still unknown.

T-independent antigens

antigen	polymeric	polyclonal activation	resistance to degradation
lipopolysaccharide (LPS)	+	+ + +	+
Ficoll	+ + +	−	+ + +
dextran	+ +	+	+ +
levan	+ +	+	+ +
poly-D amino acids	+ + +	−	+ + +
polymeric bacterial flagellin	+ +	+ +	+

Fig. 7.7 The major common properties of some of the some of the main T-independent (T_{ind}) antigens are listed. T_{ind} antigens induce the production of cytokines IL-1, TNF and IL-6 by macrophages. (Note: both poly-L amino acids and monomeric bacterial flagellin are T_{dep} antigens, demonstrating the role of antigen structure in determining T_{ind} properties.)

The respective roles of IgM and IgD, the two cell surface receptors for antigen on B cells, is also not understood in terms of activation or inactivation. Both IgM and IgD appear to be capable of transmitting signals for both functions.

T-DEPENDENT AND T-INDEPENDENT ANTIGENS

The response to most antigens depends on both T cells and B cells recognizing that antigen. This type of antigen is called T-dependent (T_{dep}). There are, however, a small number of antigens capable of activating B cells without T-cell help, referred to as T-independent antigens (T_{ind}). T_{ind} antigens share a number of common properties (Fig. 7.7). In particular they are all large polymeric molecules with repeating antigenic determinants. Many possess the ability, at high concentrations, to activate B-cell clones that are specific for other antigens (polyclonal B cell activation); however, at lower concentrations they only activate B cells specific for themselves. Many T_{ind} antigens are particularly resistant to degradation. Primary antibody responses to T_{ind} antigens *in vitro* are generally weaker than those to T_{dep} antigens and peak fractionally earlier (Fig. 7.8).

SECONDARY RESPONSE *IN VITRO*

This response also differs between T_{dep} and T_{ind} antigens. The secondary response to T_{ind} antigens resembles the primary response, by being weaker and almost entirely confined to IgM production, whereas the secondary IgG response to T_{dep} antigens is far stronger and appears earlier (Fig. 7.9). It seems therefore that T_{ind} antigens do not usually induce the maturation of a response that is seen with T_{dep} antigens, leading to class switching to IgG and increase in affinity. Memory induction is also relatively poor. The mechanism by which T_{ind} antigens trigger B cells without requiring T_H cells is not fully understood. It is likely that their polymeric structure enables T_{ind} antigens to crosslink B-cell

Comparison of primary immune responses to T_{dep} and T_{ind} antigens *in vitro*

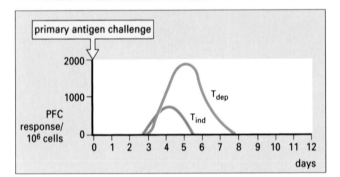

Fig. 7.8 The differing primary responses (assessed by plaque-forming cell [PFC] assay) to T_{dep} antigen and T_{ind} antigen. The responses differ in that the T_{ind} peaks slightly earlier, and is much weaker, than the T_{dep}.

Comparison of secondary immune responses to T_{dep} and T_{ind} antigens *in vitro*

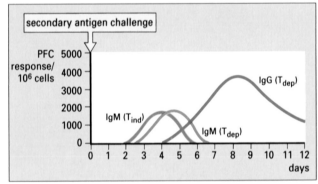

Fig. 7.9 The IgM plaque-forming cell (PFC) response is similar for T_{dep} and T_{ind} antigens, but only T_{dep} antigens produce an IgG response.

receptors, and this process would be facilitated by their resistance to degradation. Many T_{ind} antigens are products of bacteria, for example endotoxin, dextrans and levans, found in bacterial walls, and the polymerized flagellin, found in the flagellae. There are potential survival advantages if the immune response to bacteria does not depend on complex cell interactions, as it could be more rapid. Many bacterial antigens can bypass T-cell help because they are very effective inducers of cytokine production by macrophages – they induce IL-1, IL-6 and TNF_α from macrophages. The short-lived response and lack of IgG may be due to the lack of IL-2, IL-4 and IL-5, which T cells produce in response to T_{dep} antigen. T_{ind} antigens often activate a subset of B cells expressing CD5.

HAPTENS AND CARRIERS

In the late 1960s and early 1970s, studies with chemically modified proteins by Mitchison and others led to significant advances in our understanding of what was being recognized by lymphocytes, and of the specialized functions of T and B cells.

To induce an optimum secondary response to a small chemical group or hapten (which is only immunogenic if bound to a protein carrier) it was found that the experimental animal must be immunized and then challenged using the same hapten–carrier conjugate, not just the same hapten (Fig. 7.10). This was referred to as the 'carrier effect' and it implies that B cells and T cells recognize at least two different parts of the antigen.

Further experiments showed that the response to secondary challenge was not dependent on the primary carrier protein if the animal was previously primed to the secondary carrier protein alone, or had received spleen cells from a donor primed to the secondary carrier (Fig. 7.11). By repeating the experiment, but first removing T cells from the donor spleen cells, it was shown that TH cells are responsible for recognizing the carrier while the B cells recognize hapten.

One consequence of this system is that an individual B cell can receive help from T cells specific for different carrier determinants provided that the B cell can present those determinants to each T cell. In an

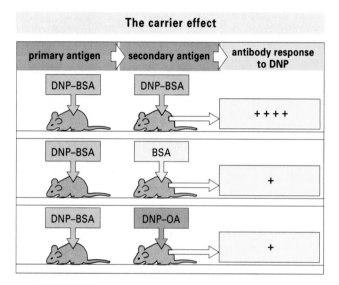

The carrier effect

primary antigen	secondary antigen	antibody response to DNP
DNP–BSA	DNP–BSA	+ + + +
DNP–BSA	BSA	+
DNP–BSA	DNP–OA	+

Fig. 7.10 Three groups of mice were immunized (primary antigen) with the hapten dinitrophenyl (DNP) bound to bovine serum albumin (BSA). They were later challenged (secondary antigen) with either BSA, dinitrophenylated ovalbumin (DNP–OA) or the original hapten carrier complex (DNP–BSA). The antibody response to the DNP hapten was then measured. The optimal antibody response to DNP was obtained with animals immunized twice with the same antigen. The BSA acts as a specific carrier for the antibody response to DNP.

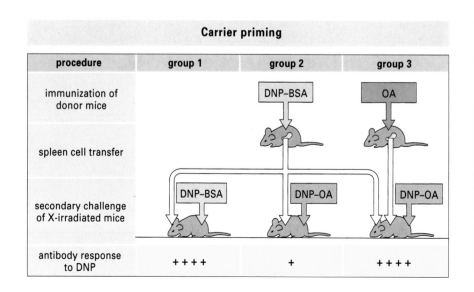

Carrier priming

procedure	group 1	group 2	group 3
immunization of donor mice		DNP–BSA	OA
spleen cell transfer			
secondary challenge of X-irradiated mice	DNP–BSA	DNP–OA	DNP–OA
antibody response to DNP	+ + + +	+	+ + + +

Fig. 7.11 Three groups of X-irradiated mice were given antigen-primed spleen cells and challenged with antigen. (1) received DNP–BSA primed cells and were then challenged with DNP–BSA; a strong antibody response to DNP. (2) received DNP–BSA primed cells and, when challenged with DNP–OA, gave a weak antibody response; no carrier effect. (3) received DNP–BSA primed cells and OA primed cells and were then challenged with DNP–OA; a strong response to DNP. This shows that the need for carrier priming can be circumvented by supplying carrier-primed spleen cells.

immune response *in vivo* it is thought that the interactions between T cells and B cells which drive B cell division and differentiation, involve T cells which have already been stimulated by contact with the antigen on other APCs (e.g. dendritic cells) (Fig. 7.12). It is also clear that two types of signal are required to activate a B cell to respond to a T_{dep} antigen.

These results have led to the basic scheme for cell interactions in the antibody response set out in Fig 7.12 It is proposed that antigen entering the body is processed by cells which present the antigen in a highly immunogenic form to the TH cells and B cells. The T cells recognize separate determinants on the antigen to those recognized by the B cells. They deliver help to the appropriate B cells which are stimulated to differentiate and divide into antibody-forming cells. This has

led to the concept that two types of signal are required to activate a B cell:
1. antigen interacting with B cell immunoglobulin receptors
2. stimulating signal(s) from TH cells.
A variety of T cell stimuli are needed for optimal growth and differentiation of B cells (see Fig. 7.5).

CELL ACTIVATION

In immune responses activation of T and B cells, and of APCs, takes place in different parts of the immune system and at varying times.

Activation of APCs is rapid, and it can be induced by the immunogenic entity itself, in the case of bacteria, or by the adjuvant component of a vaccine. However, the majority of APC activation is by cytokines from T cells. The best known macrophage-activating factors are interferon-γ (IFN$_\gamma$), granulocyte–macrophage colony stimulating factor (GM–CSF), and tumour necrosis factor (TNF$_\alpha$). (As these molecules illustrate, the cytokine nomenclature, based on the first workable assay for the molecule, is rarely a good description of its actual functions.) When APCs are activated, they express more MHC class I and II, more receptors for the Fc portion of immunoglobulin and more adhesion molecules. They also produce numerous cytokines (e.g. IL-1, IL-6, TNF$_\alpha$) and enzymes.

Activation of lymphocytes leads to two partially competing processes: cell proliferation, and differentiation into effector cells. Cells at the end stage of differentiation may become so specialized, like the highest-rate antibody-forming cells, the plasma cells, that they lose surface molecules such as class II, and are unable to respond to regulatory signals or to proliferate.

The fate of lymphocytes responding to antigen is varied. Some can persist for a long time as memory cells. The lifespan of memory cells can be over 40 years in man, as judged by the chromosome abnormalities (e.g. crosslinking of DNA which would prevent mitosis) found in the blood cells of Hiroshima survivors. Others have a short life span, which explains why moderate antigenic stimulation does not lead to lymphoid enlargement. However, a short life span is sufficient for generating effective cell-mediated and antibody responses.

ANTIGEN-SPECIFIC TRIGGERING OF LYMPHOCYTES
As discussed in Chapter 4, the TCR variable chains α and β, or γ and δ, have molecules attached to them which transmit signals to the inside of the cell. These are the CD3 γ, δ, ϵ molecules, the ζ and η chains, and the CD4 or CD8 proteins linked to the tyrosine kinase enzyme known as p56^{lck} (this abbreviation stands for a protein of 56 kDa, which is a lymphocyte-specific kinase, an enzyme which phosphorylates). B cells are now recognized to also have a family of molecules attached to the surface IgM and IgD, involved in signal transduction (see Chapter 6).

Cell cooperation in the antibody response

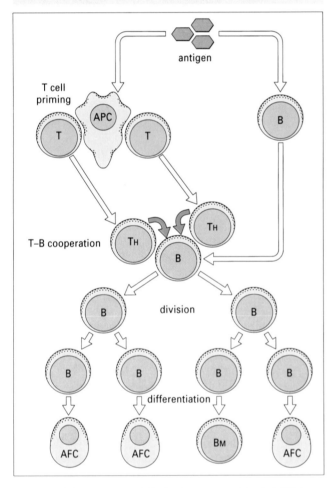

Fig. 7.12 Antigen is presented to virgin T cells by APCs such as dendritic cells. B cells also take up antigen and present it to the T cells, receiving signals from the T cells to divide and differentiate into antibody-forming cells (AFCs) and memory B cells (BM).

It is still not clear exactly what is an effective antigenic signal. For a T cell, interaction at a single TCR is not sufficient, but exactly how many interactions are necessary may depend on what other lymphocyte stimulatory signals are present, and the type and activation state of the T cell being stimulated. Murine T-cell hybrids (derived from the fusion of a normal T cell with a T-cell tumour cell), are known to be easily triggered, and for them an effective APC (e.g. a macrophage) must carry over 60 class II antigen fragment complexes to stimulate the T cell. However a weak APC, such as a class II transfected fibroblast, needs 5000 of these complexes. This would suggest that, in normal circumstances, a few tens to a few hundred TCR need to be activated for effective triggering. This type of information is not available for B cells, except for triggering by T_{ind} antigens, where binding to a single receptor is not sufficient, but binding to tens or hundreds probably is.

Mitogens are a class of molecule which can activate T or B cells in a non-antigen-specific manner. These are useful experimentally for studying T or B cell activation. The majority of T cells can be stimulated by phytohaemagglutinin (PHA) extracted from red kidney beans, and concanavalin A (Con A) extracted from castor beans. The mechanism by which they do so has been extensively studied, and it is known that these molecules bind to T cell surface molecules involved in activation – TCR and CD2, for example.

Another group of molecules which can activate T cells non-specifically are the 'superantigens', mostly of bacterial origin. They include the staphylococcal enterotoxins (responsible for some types of acute food poisoning), toxic shock syndrome toxin (responsible for tampon-sepsis induced shock), exfoliative dermatitis toxin, as well as some viral proteins. Superantigens bind to class II molecules on APCs and are recognized by TCRs, but not in the same way that class II–antigen peptide complexes are recognized. Binding is to the Vβ chain of the TCR alone, but this is sufficient to activate the T cells. Depending on experimental conditions, the effects are the same as with antigen, either an immune response is induced, or clonal anergy occurs (Fig. 7.13).

CO-STIMULATORY SIGNALS

Interaction at the TCR or membrane immunoglobin alone cannot mediate a positive activation signal for T or B cells. It may be sufficient for a 'negative' or tolerogenic signal, but even that is doubtful. Lymphoid activation is currently believed to involve a number of interactions, each with a potential signalling function. Costimulatory signals are the name given to interactions that do not involve antigen-specific receptors.

These interactions may involve either secreted molecules, such as cytokines, or cell-surface molecules, which increase binding affinity, collectively called 'adhesion molecules'. These adhesion molecules are not just responsible for binding: their cytoplasmic domains are involved in signalling. This was shown by experimental deletion of the intracytoplasmic domain, which interfered with activation, even though the adhesion function was unaltered.

The best documented 'costimulatory signals' for T cell activation are the cytokines IL-1 and IL-6, made by certain APCs. One curious anomaly is that no-one has yet been able to demonstrate production of these cytokines by the APCs considered most active in primary T cell activation, the interdigitating dendritic cells. It is likely that there are other costimulatory cytokines. For example IL-7 is more potent than IL-1 or IL-6 in inducing T cells to express IL-2 receptor, but it is not known whether IL-7 is produced by any APCs.

CYTOKINES

Cytokines are proteins (usually glycoproteins) of relatively low molecular mass (rarely more than 8–25 kDa) and often consisting of just a single chain. They regulate all the important biological processes – cell growth, cell activation, inflammation, immunity, tissue repair, fibrosis and morphogenesis. Some cytokines are also chemotactic for specific cell types.

Although cytokines are considered to be a 'family', this is a functional rather than a structural concept, as these proteins are not all chemically related. However, there are pairs of cytokines which share about 30% of their sequences, e.g. IL-1$_\alpha$ and IL-1$_\beta$, TNF$_\alpha$ and TNF$_\beta$, EGF and TGF$_\alpha$. There are also subfamilies that are highly (about 80%) homologous. IFN$_\gamma$, with about 20 members, is an example of a large subfamily. The properties of the best studied cytokines are summarized in Fig. 7.14.

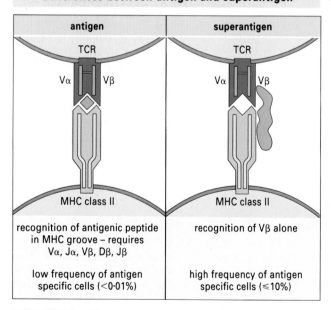

Differences between antigen and superantigen

antigen	superantigen
TCR	TCR
Vα Vβ	Vα Vβ
MHC class II	MHC class II
recognition of antigenic peptide in MHC groove – requires Vα, Jα, Vβ, Dβ, Jβ	recognition of Vβ alone
low frequency of antigen specific cells (<0·01%)	high frequency of antigen specific cells (≤10%)

Fig. 7.13 Antigenic peptides must be processed in order to trigger the TCR. In contrast, superantigens such as staphylococcal enterotoxins are not processed, binding directly to class II and Vβ. Each superantigen activates a distinct set of Vβ-expressing T cells.

Interferons

These proteins were first characterized by antiviral assays, but they are also potent immune regulators and growth factors. They fall into three groups: IFN$_\alpha$, the largest (20 variants), made by leucocytes in response to viruses or nucleic acids; IFN$_\beta$, a single protein made by fibroblasts in response to viruses or nucleic acids; and IFN$_\gamma$, a single protein made by lymphocytes (T and LGL) in response to immune stimuli. The interferons all have antiviral activity (IFN$_\gamma$ much less than IFN$_\alpha$ or IFN$_\beta$). The inhibition of cell growth by IFN$_\alpha$ or IFN$_\beta$ is clinically useful in certain rare cancers such as renal cell cancer and hairy cell leukaemia.

IFN$_\gamma$ is produced by activated T cells and natural killer (NK) cells. A degree of immune activation therefore leads to the production of IFN$_\gamma$ and an increase in APC function (partly by inducing class II molecules), and the potential to activate T cells further. Thus, IFN$_\gamma$ acts as a positive feedback signal. IFN$_\gamma$ also activates macro-phages in general, and probably enhances their capacity to act as APCs. The properties of IFN$_\gamma$ are summarized in Fig. 7.15. IFN$_\gamma$ is probably responsible for regulating APC function in many cell types, including astrocytes, microglia, endothelium, and thymocytes. Excessive production of IFN$_\gamma$ can play a part in the induction of autoimmunity, as proven in experimental animal models and transgenic mice.

INTERLEUKINS

Interleukins (represented by the abbreviations IL-1 to IL-11) were first given this name in 1981. They were defined as molecules made by leucocytes which acted on leucocytes. Although subsequent research has revealed that some of these molecules are also made by non-leucocytes, and that some (the interferons) act on non-leucocytes, the nomenclature has stuck. The main targets for their action vary from T and B cells to fibroblasts and endothelium. A summary of the most important properties of these molecules follows.

The main features of the best-studied cytokines

cytokine	mol. wt	cell source(s)	main cell target(s)	main actions
IFN$_\gamma$	40–50 000 (dimer)	T cells, NK cells	lymphocytes, monocytes, tissue cells	immunoregulation, B cell differentiation, some antiviral action
IL-1$_\alpha$ IL-1$_\beta$	33 000 17 500	monocytes, dendritic cells, some B cells, fibroblasts, epithelial cells, endothelium, astrocytes, macrophages	thymocytes, neutrophils, T and B cells, tissue cells	immunoregulation, inflammation, fever
IL-2	15 000	T cells NK cells	T cells, B cells, monocytes	proliferation, activation
IL-3	15 000	T cells	stem cells, progenitors	pan-specific colony stimulating factor
IL-4	15 000	T cells	B cells, T cells	division and differentiation
IL-5	? 15 000 (153 amino acids)	T cells	B cells, eosinophils	differentiation
IL-6	20 000	macrophages, T cells, fibroblasts, some B cells	T cells, B cells, thymocytes, hepatocytes	differentiation, acute phase protein synthesis
IL-8 (family)	8000	macrophages, skin cells	granulocytes, T cells	chemotaxis
TNF$_\alpha$	50 000	macrophages, lymphocytes	fibroblasts, endothelium	inflammation, catabolism (cachexia), fibrosis; production of other cytokines (IL-1, IL-6, GM-CSF) and adhesion molecules
TNF$_\beta$ (lymphotoxin)	50 000 (trimer)			

Fig. 7.14 Summary of the main features of the best studied cytokines. In some cases the molecular weight is derived from study of cDNA sequences. Only the most important targets and actions are shown.

Actions of IFN$_\gamma$

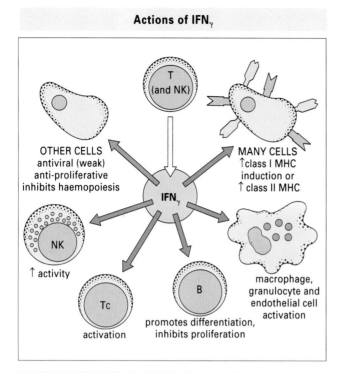

Fig. 7.15 Interferon-γ (IFN$_\gamma$) has numerous immuno-regulatory actions. Its antiviral and antiproliferative activities are less potent than those of IFN$_\alpha$ and IFN$_\beta$. Furthermore, it is not as effective as IFN$_\alpha$ at inducing natural killer (NK) cells. It is, however, the most potent inducer of macrophage activation, and of class II molecules on tissue cells. In this and other functions it synergizes with TNF$_\alpha$ and TNF$_\beta$.

IL-1 (previously known as endogenous pyrogen, lymphocyte activating factor, or catabolin) is made by many cells (e.g. endothelial cells, B cells, fibroblasts) but most abundantly by macrophages. It stimulates T and B cells and induces inflammatory responses, such as the production of prostaglandins and degradative enzymes such as collagenase. This is believed to be of special importance for the destruction of cartilage and bone. It travels to the brain where it induces fever, and acts to augment corticosteroid release. In the liver it induces the production of 'acute phase' proteins, liberated in response to injury. Virtually all cells of the body have receptors for IL-1 and can respond to it (Figs 7.16 and 7.17).

IL-2 (previously known as T-cell growth factor). This is produced by T cells, chiefly by CD4+ cells, but also by CD8+ cells and LGLs. It acts on a restricted range of cells, chiefly T cells (all types) where it is the most powerful growth factor and activator (Fig. 7.18). It also acts on LGLs and B cells to induce growth and differentiation, and it activates macrophages and oligodendrocytes. IL-2 is used in experimental cancer therapy, especially for renal cell cancer. The benefit here may be related to the activation of many cells that can produce a cytotoxic anti-cancer effect, e.g. lymphokine-activated killer (LAK) cells.

IL-3 (previously known as multispecific haemopoietin) stimulates the growth of precursors of all the haemopoietic lineages (red cells, granulocytes, macrophages and probably lymphocytes). A minor population of T cells (CD4−CD8− T cells with the αβ TCR) also responds to IL-3.

Actions of IL-1 on non-immune cells

tissue/cell type	prostaglandin synthesis	proliferation	protein synthesis	other effects
brain	+	astrocyte tumours	–	fever, somnolence, anorexia
synovial cells	+	–	collagenase	proteolytic enzyme release
bone/osteoclasts	–	–	collagenase	–
cartilage/ chondrocytes	+	–	collagenase, plasminogen activator	–
muscle cells	+	–	–	proteolytic enzyme release
fibroblasts	+	+	collagenase	–
endothelium	+	+	procoagulant activity	boosts macrophages and neutrophil adhesion
epithelial cells	–	+	type IV collagen	–
liver/ hepatocytes	–	–	acute phase proteins	–

Fig. 7.16 IL-1 acts on many cell types other than those of the immune system in its role as an inflammatory mediator. On many cell types IL-1 induces the production of other cytokines, for example TNF, GM–CSF and IL-6, which in turn have a secondary effect on skin cells. The classic effect of IL-1 is as a pyrogen, which accounts for its effect in the brain. It also induces prostaglandin synthesis in cells of the musculoskeletal system. Proliferative effects are seen especially in astrocyte tumours, but also in vascular endothelium and fibroblasts. Protein synthesis, of enzymes such as collagenase for example, are a characteristic feature of IL-1 induced reactions, as is the production of acute phase proteins by hepatocytes.

IL-4 (previously known as B-cell activating or differentiating factor-1) acts on B cells to induce activation and differentiation, leading in particular to production of IgG1 and IgE. It also acts on T cells as a growth and activation factor. With macrophages, it induces MHC class II expression, but inhibits cytokine production. Excess IL-4 plays a part in allergic disease, resulting in augmented IgE production.

IL-5 in man is chiefly a growth and activation factor for eosinophils. In the mouse it also acts on B cells, to induce growth and differentiation. IL-5 is responsible for the eosinophilia of parasitic disease.

IL-6 (previously known as B-cell differentiating factor or hepatocyte stimulating factor) is produced by many cells, including T cells, macrophages, B cells, fibroblasts and endothelial cells. It acts on most cells, but is particularly important in inducing B cells to differentiate into antibody-forming cells (AFCs). In the liver it stimulates the production of acute phase proteins. IL-6 is considered to be an important growth factor for multiple myeloma, a malignancy of plasma cells.

IL-7 was initially described as a pre-B-cell growth factor, made by bone marrow stroma. IL-7 made by thymic stroma acts on thymocytes and is a T-cell growth and activation factor, and a macrophage activation factor.

IL-8 belongs to a large family (over 15 members) of low molecular weight (about 8 kDa) cytokines. They are produced by macrophages and endothelial cells and are involved in inflammation and cell migration, particularly IL-8 itself which is a powerful inducer of neutrophil and T-cell chemotaxis. The related RANTES is an inducer of chemotaxis of memory T cells and monocytes.

IL-10 (also known as cytokine synthesis inhibitory factor) inhibits the production of IFN_γ, inhibits antigen presentation and macrophage production of IL-1, IL-6 and TNF_α, and plays a role in the regulation of IgE.

Actions of IL-1 on cells of the immune system

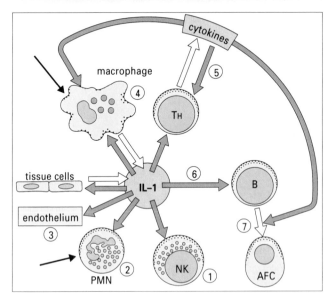

Fig. 7.17 IL-1 is produced by many cell types in response to damage, infection or antigens. It influences many cells and processes: (1) NK cell cytocidal activity increases. (2) PMNs are metabolically activated and move towards the site of IL-1 production by chemotaxis (black arrow). (3) In the endothelium, adhesion molecules and procoagulants are induced, and permeability is increased. (4) Prostaglandin production and cytocidal activity increase in macrophages. Chemotaxis is also stimulated (black arrow). (5) TH cell proliferation, IL-2 receptor expression and cytokine production are all enhanced. (6) B cell proliferation and differentiation into AFCs is stimulated and regulated (7) by other cytokines.

Actions of IL-2

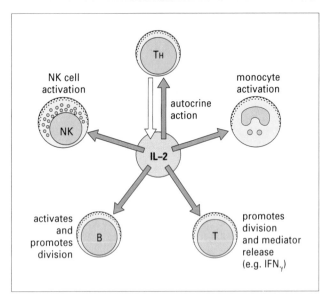

Fig. 7.18 IL-2 is generated by TH cells. In addition to its essential role in promoting T cell division and the release of mediators such as IFN_γ, IL-2 also potentiates B cell growth. The activation of monocytes and natural killer (NK) cells is important in amplifying the immune response. In patients with renal cell carcinoma, autologous NK precursors can be activated in vitro by high doses of IL-1 (1000 IU/ml) to produce lines of so-called lymphokine-activated killer (LAK) cells which are used in experimental cancer therapy.

Haemopoiesis

Haemopoiesis is regulated by a wide spectrum of cytokines. IL-1 and IL-6 are involved in activating resting stem cells (self-renewing cells) to enter the cell cycle. IL-3 is involved in the growth of precursors of all haemopoietic lineages, as is granulocyte–macrophage colony stimulating factor (GM–CSF). As cells differentiate, lineage-specific cytokines play the major role; erythropoietin (EPO) for the red cells, macrophage colony stimulating factor (M–CSF) for macrophages, granulocyte colony stimulating factor (G–CSF) for granulocytes. As yet, little is known about the control of platelet production. GM–CSF, M–CSF and G–CSF also act on mature cells as activation factors.

Inhibitory cytokines

Only a few cytokines are currently known which have inhibitory properties in the immune system. IL-10 has already been described. Transforming growth factor-β (TGFβ) is a family of 5 closely related molecules which stimulate connective tissue growth and collagen formation, but are inhibitory to virtually all immune and haemopoietic functions.

IFN$_\alpha$, IFN$_\beta$ and IFN$_\gamma$ can interfere with immune cell proliferation. IFN$_\alpha$ and IFN$_\beta$ inhibit class II induction by IFN$_\gamma$. IFN$_\gamma$ can interfere with B cell class II induction by IL-4.

CYTOKINE RECEPTORS

Cytokines are effective at very low concentrations, often at a few pg/ml (10^{-12} gm/ml). This is due to their mode of action which involves binding to high-affinity receptors on the cell surface, which transmit the cytokine signals to the nucleus.

While developments in biochemistry, and especially in gene cloning, have helped reveal the structure of many cytokine receptors, our knowledge of how they transmit signals lags far behind. This is probably because what has been elucidated so far is only the cytokine binding chain. The associated chains which transmit signals mostly remain to be defined.

Whereas the cytokine proteins do not have any structural resemblances, many of the cytokine receptors belong to families with distant similarities, at least in their extracellular domains (Fig. 7.19). The biggest is the haemopoietin family. This has two main characteristics: four invariant amino acids, consisting of two doublets of tryptophan and serine near the transmembrane domain, and certain conserved cysteines. Receptors for erythropoietin (EPO), G–CSF, GM–CSF, IL-3, IL-4, IL-2 (β chain), IL-5, IL-6 and IL-7 belong to this family.

Receptors for IL-1, IL-6 and M–CSF belong to the immunoglobin superfamily of molecules, which also

Cytokine receptor families

family	members	features
Ig	M–CSF, IL-6, IL-1	Ig-V or Ig-C like domains, IL-6 also has some haemopoietin features
haemopoietin	IL-2$_\beta$, IL-3, 4, 5, 6, 7, EPO, GM–CSF, G–CSF	Trp–Ser ×2, conserved cysteines
TNF/NGF	TNF, NGF, CD40	4 cysteine-rich (6 cys) regions in extracellular domain

Fig. 7.19 Some cytokine receptors show sequence homology with others, which allows grouping into families. The IL-6 receptor has features of 2 families.

Structure of the high affinity IL-2 receptor

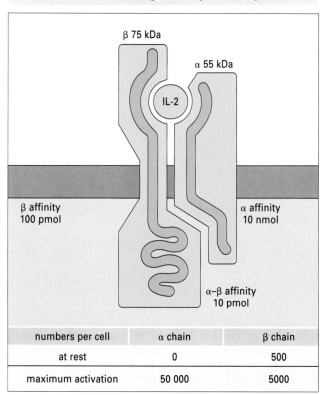

numbers per cell	α chain	β chain
at rest	0	500
maximum activation	50 000	5000

Fig. 7.20 The high affinity IL-2 receptor consists of two chains, each of which, alone, can bind IL-2 only weakly. Resting T cells do not express the α chain, but following activation, they may express up to 50 000/cell (maximum). Some of these associate with the β chain to form the high affinity IL-2 receptor.

includes many other important molecules such as MHC, TCR and the immunoglobulins themselves.

Receptors for nerve growth factor (NGF) and TNF, as well as some surface antigens (e.g. CD40), belong to another family.

In contrast, the intracytoplasmic domains are not homologous, suggesting that there are many mechanisms of signal transduction to the cell. Knowledge of two receptors, for IL-2 and IL-6, is more advanced, and the IL-2 receptor is schematically represented in Fig. 7.20. The IL-6 receptor has a cytokine binding chain whose affinity is augmented by gp130, a transmembrane protein involved in signal transduction.

CYTOKINE ANTAGONISTS

Recently two groups of cytokine inhibitory proteins have been described. One consists of molecules that act as receptor antagonists, but do not activate the cell. For example, the IL-1 receptor antagonist (IL-1ra) is a protein of 18 kDa produced by IgG-adherent monocytes. The protein binds to the IL-1 receptor, has no agonist activity and does not bind to the cytokine itself. Experiments in which human recombinant receptor antagonist has been given to mice after a lethal injection of *Escherichia coli* endotoxin (lipopolysaccharide – LPS), have shown effective protection. This provides direct evidence that the lethal effects of LPS may be mediated through the action of IL-1. IL-1ra may therefore provide a new treatment strategy for diseases mediated by this cytokine.

The great majority of cytokine inhibitors bind not to the receptor but to the cytokine itself. With the cloning of the cDNAs for receptors, and hence the determina-

tion of their amino acid protein sequence, it was found that the soluble serum inhibitors of cytokines were often fragments derived from the extracellular domain of the receptors by enzymic cleavage (Fig. 7.21). Among the soluble receptors detected in serum are those for IL-2 (p55 low affinity chain only), IL-4, IL-6 (not known to be inhibitory), IL-7, IFN$_\gamma$ and both TNF receptors (Fig. 7.22). There are soluble forms of receptors for hormones, for example growth hormone, and for adhesion molecules such as ICAM-1.

INTRACELLULAR PATHWAYS OF ACTIVATION

T-cell activation appears to use similar mechanisms to those seen in other cell types. TCR ligation causes the activation of phospholipase C, leading to the generation of inositol triphosphate (IP$_3$) and diacyl glycerol (DAG). IP$_3$ leads to release of Ca^{2+} from intracellular stores while DAG is involved in the activation of protein kinase C (PKC). The activation process involves a complex series of phosphorylations of components of the TCR (CD3) as well as CD4 (or CD8) and the leucocyte common antigen CD45, which is associated with CD4 and is itself a phosphatase. In addition to PKC, two other kinases (p56^{lck}, associated with CD4 or CD8, and p59^{fyn}) are involved in these steps.

TNF receptors

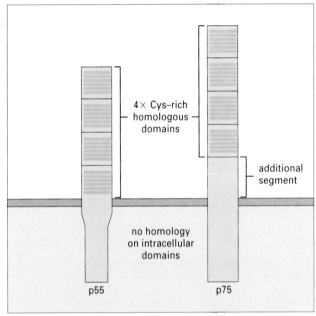

Fig. 7.22 There are two receptors, each of which binds TNF$_\alpha$ and TNF$_\beta$ (lymphotoxin) with high affinity. Their extracellular domains are homologous, each with four subdomains of 40 amino acids, containing six cysteines. They are believed to have evolved by gene duplication. In contrast the intracytoplasmic domain is not homologous, suggesting that their mechanism of signal transduction is distinct.

Structure of receptors for TNF

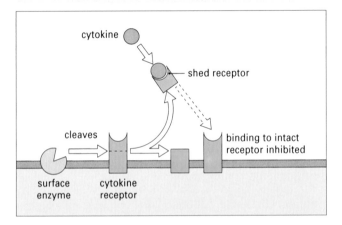

Fig. 7.21 Enzyme cleavage of the extracellular domain of a receptor (for example, TNF, IFN$_\gamma$, IL-6 or IL-2 [p55] receptor) releases the binding fragment. For TNF (and probably others) this soluble receptor retains its high-affinity binding properties. It is capable of neutralizing the ligand by blocking its access to intact receptors in the membrane.

CELL PROLIFERATION

Lymphocyte proliferation is a complex and indirect process. Stimulation of, for example, a T cell by an APC, does not automatically lead to lymphocyte proliferation. Effective interaction at the TCR leads to the production of the p55 chain of the receptor for the T-cell growth factor (IL-2), which together with the existing p75 chain forms a high affinity receptor. In all T cells TCR activation also induces the production of cytokines. In most $CD4^+$ and some $CD8^+$ T cells, there is transient production of IL-2 for 1–2 days. During this time, the interaction of IL-2 with the high affinity IL-2 receptor results in T-cell growth and activation (Fig. 7.23).

IL-4 is a weaker growth factor for T cells, and its production is also inducible. Surface IL-4 receptor is also augmented by TCR activation. IL-7 is also a growth factor for T cells and it is likely that these three T-cell growth factors permit the fine tuning of the growth and activation of T cells during an immune response. The

T cell proliferation

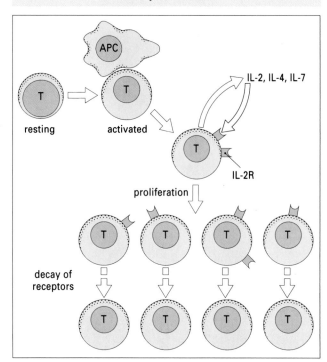

Fig. 7.23 Resting cells do not make T-cell growth-factor cytokines (IL-2, IL-4 or IL-7) and do not express large numbers of receptors for these molecules. Some receptors for IL-4 and IL-7 are present, but not for IL-2. Only the p75 chain of the IL-2 receptor is present, which has intermediate affinity. Activation induces the p55 chain and this combines with p75 to give high affinity IL-2 receptor. Activation induces production of mRNA and protein for IL-2 and IL-4. Secretion of IL-2 and IL-4, and interaction with receptors induces growth. This is 'autocrine' (acting on the same cell) or 'paracrine' (acting on the neighbouring cell). In the absence of antigen stimulation the IL-2 receptor population declines, leading to an end of the proliferative phase of the response.

transient expression of the high-affinity IL-2 receptor for only a week or so after stimulation of the TCR, helps to limit T-cell growth.

ANTIBODY RESPONSES *IN VIVO*

The earliest studies on antibody responses followed the development of specific antibodies in animals immunized with T_{dep} or T_{ind} antigens. With our improved knowledge of B-cell development and maturation, it is now possible to understand the features of immune responses *in vivo* in terms of the underlying cellular events. Features of antibody responses *in vivo*, which are related to the cellular events described above include:
1. the enhanced secondary response
2. isotype class switching
3. affinity maturation
4. the development of memory.
However, some of these events can only be understood by viewing the B cell population as a whole, rather than as a collection of individual cells. The elements of the antibody response *in vivo* are detailed below.

Following primary antigenic challenge, e.g. with sheep erythrocytes injected into a mouse, there is an initial lag phase when no antibody can be detected. This is followed by phases in which the antibody titre rises logarithmically to a plateau and then declines again. The decline occurs because the antibodies are either naturally catabolized or they bind to the antigen and are cleared from the circulation (Fig. 7.24).

An examination of the responses following primary and secondary antigenic challenge shows that the responses differ in four major respects.
1. Time course. The secondary response has a shorter lag phase and an extended plateau and decline.
2. Antibody titre. The plateau levels of antibody are much greater in the secondary response, typically 10-fold or more than plateau levels in the primary response.
3. Antibody class. IgM antibodies form a major proportion of the primary response, whereas the secondary response consists almost entirely of IgG, with very little IgM.
4. Antibody affinity. The affinity of the antibodies in the secondary response is usually much greater. This is referred to as 'affinity maturation'.

The characteristics of primary and secondary antibody responses are compared in Fig. 7.25.

It is possible to detect AFCs in the spleen following antigen challenge, using plaque-forming cell assays (see Chapter 25). Studies show that the appearance of AFCs in the spleen precedes the rises in serum antibody titres by about one day.

CLASS SWITCHING

During a T-dependent immune response there is a progressive switch in the predominant immunoglobulin class of the specific antibody produced, usually to IgG. This is in contrast to T-independent responses, when the predominant immunoglobulin usually remains IgM.

Isotype switching from IgM to IgG is not a random event. The IgG subclasses produced by the plasma cells vary depending on the stimulus. Thus in the mouse, complete Freund's Adjuvant yields predominantly IgG2

antibodies, whereas alum-precipitated protein antigens result in a predominantly IgG1 response. Switching to IgA or IgE also occurs and cells producing these isotypes are concentrated in the mucosa-associated lymphoid tissues.

Evidence has accumulated which explains the molecular mechanisms of isotype switching (see Chapter 6), and although there is universal agreement that T cells are important in controlling this phenomenon, the signals which control the switch are not fully understood. IL-4, which is produced by T-cells, is important in the production of IgG1 and IgE. IL-5 is important in the switch to IgA production, and IFN$_\gamma$ favours the production of IgG2a in mice.

AFFINITY MATURATION

The antibodies produced in a secondary response to a T-dependent antigen have higher average affinity than those produced in the primary response. This is associated with the switch from IgM to IgG production, since there is no maturation in the affinity of the IgM response.

The degree of affinity maturation is inversely related to the antigen dose administered: high antigen doses produce poor maturation compared to low antigen doses (Fig. 7.26). A plausible hypothesis to account for this observation is as follows: in the presence of low antigen concentrations, only B cells with high affinity receptors bind sufficient antigen and are triggered to divide and differentiate. However, in the presence of

The four phases of a primary antibody response

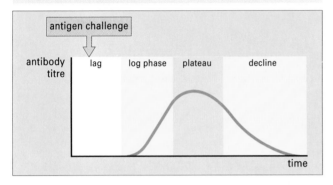

Fig. 7.24 Following antigen challenge the antibody response proceeds in four phases:
1. a lag phase when no antibody is detected
2. a log phase when the antibody titre rises logarithmically
3. a plateau phase during which the antibody titre stabilizes
4. a decline phase during which the antibody is cleared or catabolized.
The actual time course and titres reached will depend on the nature of the antigenic challenge and the nature of the host.

Primary and secondary antibody responses

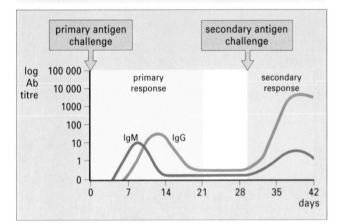

Fig. 7.25 In comparison with the antibody response following primary antigenic challenge, the antibody level following secondary antigenic challenge in a typical immune response:
1. appears more quickly and persists for longer
2. attains a higher titre
3. consists predominantly of IgG.
In the primary response the appearance of IgG is preceded by IgM.

Affinity maturation

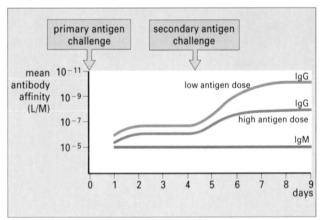

Fig. 7.26 The average affinity of the IgM and IgG antibody responses following primary and secondary challenge with a T-dependent antigen are shown. The affinity of the IgM response is constant throughout. The affinity maturation of the IgG response depends on the dose of the secondary antigen. Low antigen doses (low [Ag]) produce higher affinity immunoglobulin than high antigen doses (high [Ag]).

high antigen concentrations, there is sufficient to bind and trigger both high and low affinity B cells (Fig. 7.27).

Although individual B cells do not usually change their overall specificity, the affinity of the antibody produced by a clone may be altered as a result of somatic hypermutation acting on the recombined antibody genes as mentioned above. It appears then, that two processes are involved in affinity maturation.

1. The generation of higher-affinity clones of B cells by slight alterations in the antibody structure of daughter cells. Such changes occur late in the primary response to a T-dependent antigen.

2. Selective expansion of high-affinity clones, driven by antigen.

Somatic hypermutation is a common event in AFCs during T-dependent responses and is important in the generation of high affinity antibodies. In this context it is a normal and beneficial event. However, the same process could occasionally yield high-affinity IgG auto-antibodies, such as anti-DNA, and may be highly deleterious. This type of mutation has been demonstrated experimentally in long-term tissue culture, but its role in the development of common autoimmune diseases is not known. It has been demonstrated in mouse anti-DNA hybridomas.

IMMUNOLOGICAL MEMORY

The capacity to mount a secondary response is based on 'immunological memory', which is also exploited by the process of vaccination.

The cellular basis of memory is the expansion of populations of antigen-specific lymphocytes during the primary response, so that there is an increased frequency of resting B and T cells capable of responding to that antigen in the future. Memory B cells differ qualitatively from unprimed B cells, as they are prone to make IgG earlier and they usually have higher affinity antigen receptors, due to selection during the primary response.

It is not known whether memory T cells have higher affinity receptors than unprimed T cells, as methods for measuring the affinity of TCRs are not available. However, memory T cells can respond to lower doses of antigen, implying that their receptors are more efficient. It is now known that 'memory' is not just due to increased numbers of the same cells. There are changes in properties, manifest at the cell surface and by the secretory activities. Thus memory CD4$^+$ T cells also have differences in CD45 compared to unprimed T cells, and are capable of synthesizing cytokines more readily and more rapidly.

Clonal selection by high and low antigen doses

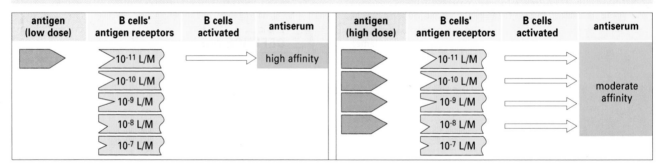

Fig. 7.27 Low antigen doses (left) bind to and trigger only those B cells with high affinity receptors, whereas high antigen doses (right) allow triggering of more B cell clones and therefore produce antibody responses with lower average affinity.

FURTHER READING

Balkwill FR. *Cytokines in Cancer Therapy.* Oxford: Oxford University Press, 1989.

Cerottini J-C, Robson MacDonald H. The cellular basis of T cell memory. *Annu Rev Immunol* 1989;**7**:77.

Chantry D, Feldmann M. The role of cytokines in autoimmunity. *Biotech Ther* 1991;**I(4)**:361–409.

Feldmann M, Lamb JR, Owen MJ, eds. *T cells.* Chichester: J Wiley and Sons, 1989.

Finkelman FD, Holmes J, Katona IM *et al.* Lymphokine control of *in vivo* immunoglobulin isotype selection. *Annu Rev Immunol* 1989;**8**:303.

Kupfer A, Singer SJ. Cell biology of cytotoxic and helper T cell functions. *Annu Rev Immunol* 1989;**7**:309.

Ullman K, Northrop JP, Verweij CL, Crabtree GR. Transmission of signals from T lymphocyte antigen receptor to the genes responsible for cell proliferation and immune function. *Annu Rev Immunol* 1989;**8**:421.

chapter 8

Cell-Mediated Immune Reactions

The term 'cell-mediated immunity' (CMI) was originally coined to describe localized reactions to organisms, usually intracellular pathogens, mediated by lymphocytes and phagocytes rather than by antibody (humoral immunity). However it is now often used in a more general sense for any response against organisms or tumours in which antibody plays a subordinate role. It is not possible however to consider cell-mediated and antibody-mediated responses entirely separately. Cells are involved in the initiation of antibody responses, and antibody acts as an essential link in some cell-mediated reactions. Moreover no cell-mediated response is likely to occur in the total absence of antibody, which can

modify cellular responses in numerous ways. For instance, formation of antigen–antibody complexes during an immune response leads to the release of chemotactic complement fragments which enhance accumulation of cells, and local inflammation. Antigens which would otherwise be targets for cytotoxic cells, may be modulated or stripped from cell membranes by antibodies. Antibody may also be involved in linking antigens to cells, via the cells' Fc receptors, thus modulating the cells' responses. In the case of phagocytic cells and killer cells, antibodies can link them to their targets.

Similarly it should not be assumed that all cell-mediated immunity is dependent on T cell function. It is often forgotten that much of the initial defensive reaction to microorganisms depends on recognition of common microbial components by receptors which are unrelated to the antigen-specific receptors of T cells and B cells. In SCID mice, which have no mature T cells, these rapid T-cell-independent mechanisms can result in surprisingly effective immunity against some pathogens.

T-CELL-INDEPENDENT CELL-MEDIATED DEFENCE MECHANISMS

PHAGOCYTOSIS
Chemotaxis
Numerous microbial components will cause chemotaxis of phagocytes towards the site of infection (Fig. 8.1). Some, such as bacterial endotoxin, do this by activating the alternative pathway of complement, so releasing C5a and C3a. Other microbial components are chemotactic in their own right. For instance formyl peptides are chemotactic, and also directly stimulatory for phagocytes, which have receptors for these common bacterial products.

Binding and uptake of microorganisms
The next stage in the phagocytosis of an organism is its binding to the surface of the cell. This binding is facilitated if complement has been activated by the classical or alternative pathways. This leads to deposition of C3b on the organism, and the interaction between this and the CR3 receptor is an efficient way of triggering antimicrobial mechanisms in the phagocyte. Similarly if antibody has bound to the pathogen, Fc receptors on the phagocyte may contribute to the uptake. Some organisms have evolved ways of binding to these surface structures which normally result in uptake, but without triggering microbicidal pathways. These points, and the nature of the microbicidal pathways, are discussed in greater detail in Chapter 15.

T-cell-independent cell-mediated functions – I
Phagocytosis

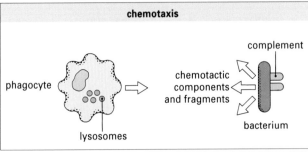

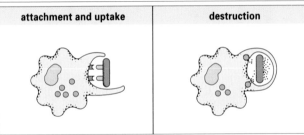

Fig. 8.1 Most of the effectors of T-cell-independent cell-mediated immunity are functional even in animals with no T cells, and in normal animals they play a protective role before the T-cell-mediated response gets under way. Subsequently these functions may be enhanced by T-cell-derived mediators known as cytokines. Most microbial organisms release factors which are chemotactic for phagocytes. They are then taken up by phagocytosis, and killed without a requirement for further activation of the phagocyte. This process is assisted by the alternative complement pathway, which does not rely on antibodies.

CYTOKINE RELEASE

Another mechanism which is independent of T-cell or antibody responses, and plays a vital role in the initial stages of an infection, is the triggering of cytokine release from macrophages. All organisms appear to contain or release molecules that have this effect (see Chapter 15). Cytokines are peptide or glycopeptide mediators released from appropriately stimulated cells. The first cytokines to be identified came from lymphocytes and were termed lymphokines. The term cytokines now includes lymphokines (some of which are given interleukin [IL] designation), interferons (IFNs), colony stimulating factors (CSFs), and tumour necrosis factors (TNFs). This topic is dealt with in detail towards the end of this chapter. The most important of the mediators released by the macrophages in response to these microbial components is TNF_α. This, in synergy with other mediators, has several rapid protective effects.

Rapid protective role of cytokine release

1. TNF_α enhances the microbicidal capacity of macrophages and neutrophils.
2. TNF_α, together with unidentified bacterial components, causes NK cells to release IFN_γ. This further augments the microbicidal activity of macrophages (Fig. 8.2).
3. TNF_α causes changes in endothelial cells and phagocytes which result in greater adhesion of the phagocytes to blood vessel walls, thus increasing the entry of the cells into sites of inflammation.

These pathways may explain the paradoxical resistance of SCID mice, which totally lack functional T cells, to certain bacterial infections.

Immunoregulatory role of cytokine release

The pattern of different cytokines released at this early stage probably influences the subsequent pattern of immune effector systems. This is a potentially important area, about which little is known. However, an injection of TNF_α can block development of contact sensitivity, and injection of TNF_α into the same site as an antigen can alter the type of helper T cell which is subsequently generated.

 T-CELL-DEPENDENT CELL-MEDIATED RESPONSES

Fig. 8.3 illustrates the most important functions of immunologically active cells (individual cells may perform more than one function) and emphasizes the central organizing role of helper T (TH) cells . This figure does not include the secondary effects of the activities of these cell types, for example delayed hypersensitivity and granuloma formation (see Chapter 22) or tissue-damaging immunopathology (discussed below and more fully in Chapter 15).

THE REGULATORY ROLE OF TH CELLS

TH cells play several central roles in cell-mediated immunity:
1. They direct the fine specificity of the response, i.e. they determine which antigens and which epitopes are recognized
2. They are involved in the selection of the effector mechanisms to be directed against the selected target antigens
3. They aid proliferation of the appropriate effector cell types
4. They enhance the functions of phagocytes and other effector cells.

These points are indicated in Fig. 8.3, and explained below. It is important to distinguish TH cells, which control and modulate the development of immune responses, from cytotoxic T cells (TC cells – also known as cytotoxic T lymphocytes or CTLs) which are effector cells able to recognize and kill target cells either because they are infected or because they are allogeneic. TC cells are considered later.

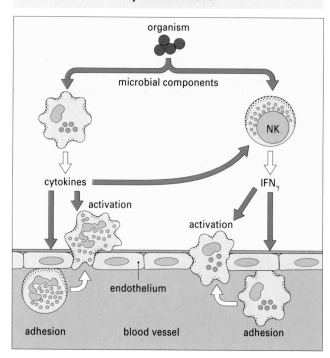

T cell-independent cell-mediated functions – II
Cytokine release

Fig. 8.2 A second early protective pathway is the triggering of cytokine release from macrophages and NK cells (discussed later) by microbial components, or by microbial components in synergy with TNF_α. These rapidly increase the microbicidal potential of phagocytes, and increase their adherence to endothelial cells. The spectrum of cytokines released may also help to determine the nature of the T-cell-mediated response which subsequently develops.

THE ROLE OF TH CELLS IN THE SELECTION OF EFFECTOR MECHANISMS DIRECTED AGAINST TARGET ANTIGENS

TH cells, via their interaction with antigen-presenting cells bearing antigenic peptides associated with MHC Class II, clearly play a major role in determining which epitopes become targets of the immune response. This is discussed in detail in Chapter 7. However, when confronted with an invading organism, the immune system must make a second, perhaps even more important 'decision'. It must select effector mechanisms appropriate for the infection in question. Not all the effector systems illustrated in Fig. 8.3 are activated equally in any one immune response.

The three most easily recognizable patterns of effector mechanism which can be selected (and there may be many others) are:
1. cytotoxic T cells
2. antibody plus mast cells and eosinophils
3. macrophage activation and delayed hypersensitivity.

This 'decision' is so important that activation of inappropriate effector mechanisms can lead to enhanced susceptibility to the pathogen rather than protection. For instance, in a model of influenza virus infection, mechanism 1 protects, whereas 3 increases susceptibility. Similarly, in BALB/c mice, mechanism 3 protects from *Leishmania major*, while 2 is detrimental.

The regulatory role of cytokines

The way in which this selection of effector mechanism is first made remains obscure (though the initial pattern of cytokine triggering by the pathogen may play a role; see Fig 8.2), but it is ultimately associated with TH cells which release different subsets of cytokines. These subsets of TH cells probably represent different patterns of differentiation from the same precursors, but it is conceivable that they arise from different cell lineages. In the mouse it is suggested that virgin (THP) cells, which have not previously been stimulated, release only IL-2. Short term stimulation leads to the development of TH0 cells which can release a wide range of cytokines (Fig. 8.4). After chronic stimulation, the specialized TH1 and TH2 types arise. Some cytokines are released by both types (IL-3, GM-CSF, and TNFα) while others are not.

The central role of TH cells in cell-mediated immunity

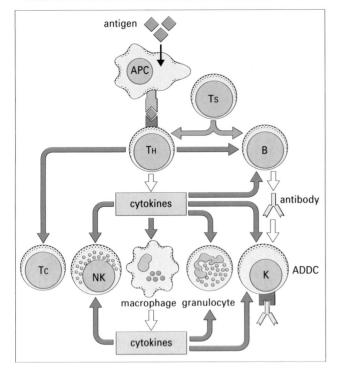

Fig. 8.3 Antigen-presenting cells (APCs) present processed antigen to helper T cells (TH), which are central to the development of immune responses. These cells recognize particular epitopes and thus select those which act as targets for the relevant effector functions. They then select and activate the appropriate effector cells. They can help B cells to make antibody and modulate the actions of a variety of other effector cells, including TC cells, natural killer (NK) cells, macrophages, granulocytes and antibody-dependent cytotoxic (K) cells. Many of these effects are mediated by lymphokines, but cytokines from other cells, particularly macrophages, are also important. Both T and B cells may in turn be influenced by TS cells.

Differentiation of murine TH cells

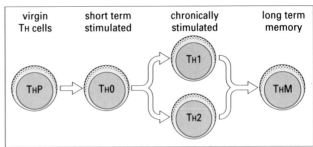

cytokines released				
THP	TH0	TH1	TH2	THM
	IFNγ	IFNγ		
IL-2	IL-2	IL-2		IL-2
	IL-4		IL-4	
	IL-5		IL-5	
			IL-6	
	IL-10		IL-10	

Fig 8.4 The suggested differentiation of murine TH cells into subsets with distinctive patterns of lymphokine release. Similar subsets are found in man when cells are taken from sites of chronic inflammation rather than from the blood.

Thus TH1 cells release IL-2 and IFN$_\gamma$ while TH2 cells release IL-4, IL-5, IL-6, and IL-10. Fig. 8.5 shows how these differing patterns of cytokine secretion may direct the response towards particular effector mechanisms. For instance TH1 cells will tend to activate macrophages, and there is some evidence that they respond particularly well to antigen presented by these cells. On the other hand TH2 cells tend to increase production of eosinophils and mast cells, and to enhance production of antibody, including IgE. These cells respond well to antigens presented by B cells.

Once established, each of these patterns of response is able to suppress the other, because the IFN$_\gamma$ from TH1 cells inhibits proliferation of TH2 cells, while IL-10 from TH2 cells reduces cytokine secretion from TH1 cells, and perhaps also from cytotoxic T cells and NK cells (Fig. 8.5).

This specialization of TH cells was first recognized in the mouse, but is now clearly demonstrated in man. Thus T-cell clones from the eyelids of patients with severe pollen allergy, leading to vernal conjunctivitis, resemble TH2 cells, as do clones from the skin of patients with atopic dermatitis. Clones from the CSF of patients with multiple sclerosis, a primarily cellular response, are like murine TH1 cells. However, it seems likely that there will be several more types of TH cell in man (and perhaps even in the mouse), since many patterns of inflammation recognizable clinically (for instance, in the joints of patients with rheumatoid arthritis) fail to fit the TH1/TH2 classification. Moreover

it is not clear what TH cell type, or cytokine combination, is required to select a predominantly Tc cell pattern of response.

CELL-MEDIATED CYTOTOXICITY

The effector cells at the bottom of Fig. 8.3 are all able to lyse target cells to which they are sufficiently closely bound. Cell-mediated cytotoxicity is therefore a property not only of Tc cells, but also of certain other subpopulations of lymphoid cells and, under some circumstances, of myeloid cells. However these cell types do not necessarily operate in the same way and confusion has arisen because the term 'cell-mediated cytotoxicity' covers several distinct phenomena. Thus different receptors can be involved in the binding of the cytotoxic cell to the target, and in the triggering of the killing pathways. Moreover there seem to be several killing mechanisms. The main types of receptor–ligand interaction involved (illustrated in Fig. 8.6) are:

1. Specific antigens (e.g. viral antigens on infected cells) recognized by MHC-restricted T-cell receptors of Tc cells
2. Determinants (e.g. those on tumour cells) recognized by receptors on NK cells
3. Antibody, already bound to antigen (e.g. viral antigen on an infected cell), recognized by Fc receptors of K cells (antibody-dependent cell-mediated cytotoxicity [ADCC]).

Selection of effector mechanisms by TH1 and TH2 cells

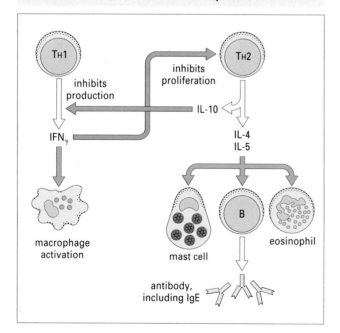

Fig 8.5 Not only does their lymphokine output drive different effector pathways, but TH1 cells tend to switch off TH2 cells, and vice-versa.

Cell-mediated cytotoxicity

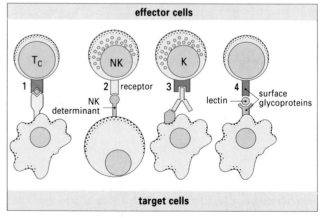

Fig. 8.6 Four different types of cell binding in cell-mediated cytotoxicity.
1. Tc cells bind their target while recognizing antigen and MHC determinants.
2. NK cells recognize determinants expressed on neoplastic cells.
3. K cells recognize the Fc of IgG antibody bound to antigen on the target cell surface.
4. Experimentally, glycoproteins on the surface of effector and target can be cross-linked by lectins.

These possible types of cell binding are, in reality, somewhat more complex; this is because these types of interaction represent functional categories, rather than being strictly limited to particular types of immune cell as recognized morphologically. More than one type of target cell interaction may be manifested by a particular morphological cell type. Moreover, other receptor–ligand interactions, such as those shown in Fig 8.7, can also help to stabilize the bond between the cytotoxic cell and the target, and can even help to trigger the killing event. Thus experimentally, by adding antibodies to CD3, CD2 or CD16 (an IgG Fc receptor) to Tc

Interactions between Tc and target cells

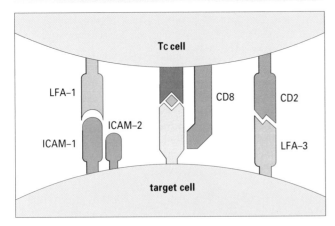

Fig 8.7 Ligands which may be involved in the interaction between cytotoxic cells and their targets.

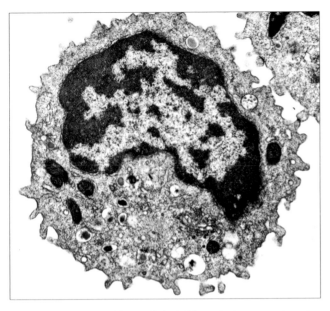

Fig 8.8 A large granular lymphocyte. Large granular lymphocytes, which can be isolated by density gradient centrifugation, contain the majority of peripheral blood NK effector activity.

cells, it is possible to trigger their killing of cells bound to them. It is probable that binding of physiological ligands to these molecules also triggers the cytotoxic cells.

ANTIBODY-INDEPENDENT CELL-MEDIATED CYTOTOXICITY
MHC-Restricted Cytotoxic T Cells
MHC-restricted cytotoxic T-cells are a subpopulation of small lymphocytes. They are known to be derived from non-lytic, radiosensitive precursor cells. The majority are CD8$^+$ and recognize antigens in association with class I MHC molecules, or foreign class I alone on allogeneic/xenogeneic cells, since foreign class I may mimic syngeneic class I associated with antigens. About 10% of MHC-restricted cytotoxic T cells are functionally distinct; being CD4$^+$ and class II restricted. It is the CD4 or CD8 molecule which interacts with the appropriate MHC molecule, and this interaction probably helps to stabilize the cell–cell recognition: antibodies to any of these cell surface molecules can inhibit killing. The most important role of Tc cells may be elimination of virus-infected cells (see Chapter 15). It therefore 'makes sense' that Tc cells tend to recognize antigen presented by Class I MHC molecules, since these are expressed on essentially all nucleated cells.

Non-specific, MHC-unrestricted cytotoxic cells
Several, partly overlapping cell populations have been shown to possess the property of non-specific, MHC-unrestricted killing. These include:
1. Cells naturally present in spleen or peripheral blood populations, usually known as Natural Killer (NK) cells
2. Cells activated by culture in relatively high concentrations of IL-2, known as Lymphokine Activated Killer (LAK) cells
3. Mixed populations with non-specific killing activity developing in mixed lymphocyte cultures, or in cultures stimulated with the lectin phytohaemagglutinin (PHA).

NK Cells These cells are mostly derived from the 'large granular lymphocytes' (LGLs) which comprise about 5% of human peripheral blood lymphoid cells (Fig. 8.8). The majority of NK cells are CD3$^-$CD16$^+$CD56$^+$ (CD16 = IgG Fc receptor), and do not contain productive rearrangements of the T cell receptor genes. In rodents, NK cells express asialo-GM1 which is also found on macrophages and granulocytes, though the tissue distribution of NK cells is different from that of macrophages. Cloned NK cells are heterogeneous in the range of targets which they will lyse. However it is still not clear whether this is because NK cells are several distinct lineages, or a distinct cell lineage with different receptors on different clones of cells. It is also possible that the apparent diversity is really due to variation in both the degree of activation, and in the contribution of several other receptors to the binding between the NK cell and the target cell. Other receptors may also contribute to the triggering of killing, as outlined above.

LAK Cells   There is increasing evidence that the enhanced cytotoxic activity of peripheral blood or spleen cell populations that have been precultured with IL-2 is largely derived from precursor cells which are indistinguishable from NK cells. Thus LAK cells probably do not represent a separate lineage, but rather a consequence of activation. The differences in specificity may also be attributable to activation, and to the changing contribution of other receptors. This type of cell is undergoing trials for the treatment of cancer in man. The patient's own T cells are stimulated *in vitro* with IL-2, and then returned to the patient.

Mixed populations with non-specific killing activity

Stimulation of peripheral blood cells by autologous tumour cells, or by mixed lymphocyte culture, or by phytohaemagglutinin, gives rise to many $CD3^+CD8^+$ cells which show typical class I-restricted cytotoxicity. However, clonal analysis of these complex cultures reveals some $CD3^+$ cells that express either the α and β, or the γ and δ chains of the T cell receptor, and

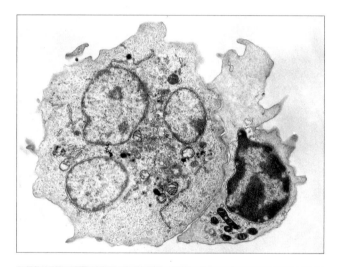

Fig. 8.9 K cell activity. Electron micrograph of a lymphocyte (right) engaging a target cell sensitized with antibody (left). × 2500. (Courtesy of Dr P. Penfold.)

whose cytotoxic effects show little or no apparent MHC restriction. These are particularly common when PHA has been used as a stimulus. It is possible that such cells merely recognize determinants which are present on a wide range of target cells, or are recognizing unknown restriction elements. The situation is further complicated by the fact that such cultures also contain LAK cells, presumably derived from NK cells in the presence of the IL-2 released by other lymphocytes in the culture.

ANTIBODY-DEPENDENT CELL-MEDIATED CYTOTOXICITY (ADCC)

Cells with cytotoxic potential which also possess Fc receptors for IgG may bind to and lyse target cells coated with IgG (Fig. 8.9). It is customary to refer to this as killer (K) cell activity but it is now clear that K cells represent a function rather than a separate cell type. Since some Tc cells and NK cells have such Fc receptors, they can also perform this function. Observations of single cells have proved that both K and NK activity can be properties of the same cell. The models most frequently studied involve antibodies to viral antigens expressed on the membrane of the target cell membrane; determinants present on tumours or particular MHC molecules, haptens such as TNP conjugated onto the membrane; and membranes of avian nucleated erythrocytes. Myeloid cells expressing Fc receptors can also show K cell activity, but they probably use different killing mechanisms (discussed later). Thus monocytes, and according to some controversial reports, polymorphs, may also be active against antibody-coated tumour targets. Some myeloid cells (monocytes and eosinophils) are certainly important effectors of damage to antibody-coated schistosomulae (see Chapter 16).

In this reaction (which may also apply to other parasites) the important antibody classes appear to be the anaphylactic ones (IgE in all species, IgG in mice, and IgG2a in rats). This raises the intriguing possibility that IgE acts by first triggering mast cells to release eosinophil chemotactic factor, and then binding the arriving eosinophils onto the target (Fig. 8.10). This pattern of effector mechanisms is characteristically evoked when the helper T cell response is dominated by TH2

Dual role for antibody in the immune reaction to schistosomes

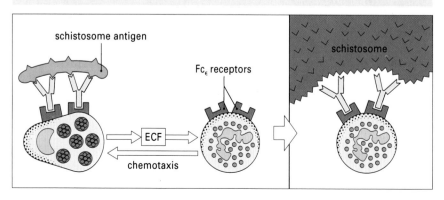

Fig 8.10 Mast cells sensitized with anti-schistosome IgE release eosinophil chemotactic factor (ECF) following contact with schistosome antigen (left). The arriving eosinophils attach to the antibody-coated worm via their Fc receptors and are important effectors in damaging the parasites (right). This is therefore a form of ADCC mediated by cells of myeloid origin.

cells (see Fig. 8.5), since the IL-4 and IL-5 released by these cells enhances the generation of eosinophils, mast cells and IgE.

THE MECHANISMS OF CELL-MEDIATED CYTOTOXICITY

It appears that the mechanisms involved in killing are similar whether Tc cells, NK cells or lymphoid K cells are involved, and whatever receptor–target interaction is responsible (Fig. 8.11). Cells of the myeloid series use different pathways. One mode of killing, by lymphoid cells, involves three distinct phases.

1. The cell binds to the target.
2. A Ca^{2+}-dependent phase, in which the vesicle contents of the cytotoxic cell are discharged – these modify the target so that it is programmed for death.
3. A late phase, when the target cell is killed.

This model is based on the observation that the vesicles of LGLs, NK cells and some Tc cells contain perforin, which is a monomeric pore-forming protein related to the lytic component (C9) of complement. The vesicles also contain a serine esterase (cf. enzymes of the complement system) which may be involved in the assembly of the lytic complex. In the presence of Ca^{2+}, the perforin monomers bind to the target cell membrane and polymerize to form transmembrane channels. The cytotoxic cell survives, and can continue to

kill further targets. It is suggested that it is protected from autodestruction by a proteoglycan (chondroitin sulphate A) which is also present in the vesicles, and may bind to the perforin.

The killing is in fact quite unlike the true lysis caused by complement. What is seen is apoptosis, with DNA fragmentation and disintegration of the cell into small membrane-bound fragments known as apoptotic bodies. Some Tc cells do not seem to contain perforin, and can lyse targets in the absence of calcium. This is particularly striking with primary Tc cells generated *in vivo*. It has been suggested that these cells must use some other mechanism (see Fig. 8.11) and that the perforin pathway is expressed only after exposure to high concentrations of IL-2.

The Tc cell vesicles can also contain tumour necrosis factor-α (TNF$_\alpha$), lymphotoxin (LT or TNF$_\beta$), and NK cytotoxic factor (NKCF) which is partially neutralized by antibody to TNF$_\alpha$. The role of these cytokines is unclear because their known cytotoxic effects take much longer than the 3–4 hours required by Tc cells.

In myeloid cells, however, TNF$_\alpha$ is certainly responsible for many examples of tumour cell killing by macrophages, and IFN$_\gamma$ (released by T cells or NK cells) is powerfully synergistic with TNF$_\alpha$ in the killing of susceptible tumours. It is not clear how these

Cell-mediated cytotoxicity

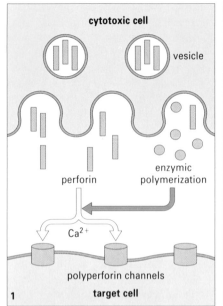 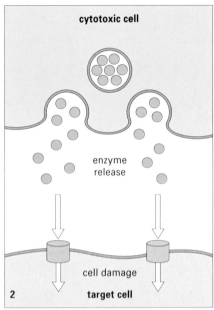 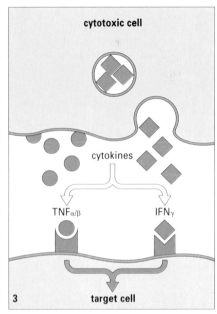

Fig. 8.11 Potential mechanisms for cytotoxic damage to target cells.

1. The cytotoxic lymphoid cell degranulates, releasing perforin and various enzymes into the immediate vicinity of the target cell membrane. In the presence of Ca^{2+} there is enzymic polymerization of the perforin, to form polyperforin channels on the target cell.

2. Degradative enzymes or other toxic substances released from the cytotoxic cell may pass through the channels on the target to cause cell damage.

3. TNF$_\alpha$ and LT (TNF$_\beta$) from the cytotoxic lymphoid cells or macrophages, and IFN$_\gamma$ either from the cytotoxic cell or from nearby lymphoid cells, trigger the target cell via its receptors. Susceptible cells die. This process takes longer than 1 and 2.

cytokines kill the target. There is increased activity of target cell cyclooxygenase and lipoxygenase, with some consequent intracellular free radical release, and this plays a role in some cases. There are also changes in protein synthesis.

TNF$_\alpha$ is not the only killing mechanism available to myeloid cells. They possess numerous other potentially cytotoxic mechanisms and it is proving difficult to define precisely which one is relevant in each experimental system. These mechanisms include nitric oxide and products of the reduction of oxygen (sometimes denoted Reactive Nitrogen Intermediates or RNIs, and Reactive Oxygen Intermediates or ROIs, respectively), cationic proteins and hydrolytic enzymes. These are discussed in detail in Chapter 15 in relation to the

killing of bacteria, but they have all been shown at some time to be cytotoxic for mammalian cells as well.

The various possible mechanisms of cytotoxicity by lymphoid and myeloid cells are illustrated in Figs 8.12 and 8.13 respectively. However, some of these mechanisms require activation of the macrophage by lymphokines, as outlined in the next section.

LYMPHOKINE-MEDIATED ACTIVATION OF MACROPHAGES

Macrophages are involved at all stages of the immune response. First, as already outlined, they act as a rapid protective mechanism which can respond before T cell-mediated amplification has taken place. Then they take part in the initiation of T cell activation by processing and presenting antigen (Chapter 6). Finally they are important in the effector phase of the cell-mediated response following T-cell mediated activation, as inflammatory, tumoricidal and microbicidal cells. This central role of macrophages within the immune response is illustrated in Fig. 8.13, and their role within inflammation and repair is outlined in Fig. 8.14.

The effector functions of macrophages which are expressed in the absence of T cells were discussed earlier (see Fig. 8.2). Thus circulating monocytes possess the ability to kill some organisms (see Chapter 16). Much of this ability is lost if they are cultured *in vitro*, but exposure to lymphokines, particularly IFN$_\gamma$, restores it, and also activates additional killing pathways which normal monocytes do not express. The destruction of many intracellular parasites, and of some tumour cells *in vitro*, requires this lymphokine-mediated 'activation' of macrophages (Fig. 8.15). The classic experiment demonstrating this showed that animals immunized to BCG and challenged with PPD, the T-cell stimulating

Mechanisms which may contribute to the cytotoxicity of myeloid cells

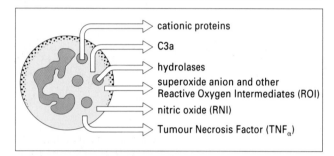

cationic proteins

C3a

hydrolases

superoxide anion and other Reactive Oxygen Intermediates (ROI)

nitric oxide (RNI)

Tumour Necrosis Factor (TNF$_\alpha$)

Fig. 8.12 Reactive oxygen intermediates (ROIs) and reactive nitrogen intermediates (RNIs), cationic proteins, and hydrolytic enzymes and complement proteins released from myeloid cells may damage the target cell in addition to cytokine-mediated attack.

The central roles of macrophages within the immune system

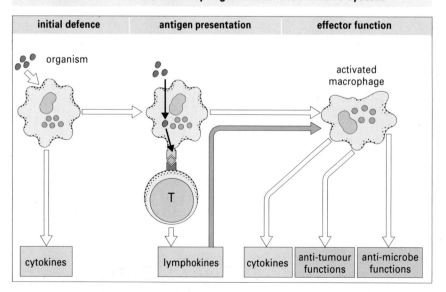

initial defence	antigen presentation	effector function

organism

activated macrophage

T

cytokines   lymphokines   cytokines | anti-tumour functions | anti-microbe functions

Fig. 8.13 Macrophages play a role in the initial response to infection before T- and B-cell-enhanced immunity can act. They then play a role as antigen processing and presenting cells. Finally, when T cells respond to antigen and release lymphokines, these act on macrophages, causing them to become activated.

antigen from BCG, were also protected against *Listeria monocytogenes*. From these experiments it was concluded that the activation of macrophages involved an antigen-specific pathway, but that the enhanced microbicidal activity was not specific for the immunizing organism. Antigen specificity was known to be a property of lymphocytes, and microbicidal activity a property of macrophages. The next step was to demonstrate *in vitro* that lymphocytes derived from a BCG-immunized mouse, when cultured with appropriate antigen (PPD for example), would release mediators which enhanced the ability of macrophages to kill or inhibit both the immunizing organism and unrelated organisms. The mediators in question were subsequently shown to be lymphokines.

HETEROGENEITY OF ACTIVATED MACROPHAGES

Macrophage activation is a complex phenomenon. Activated macrophages show enhanced ability to kill some microorganisms, but not others. Thus it is possible to activate murine macrophages so that they have an increased ability to kill *Listeria monocytogenes* without increasing their ability to kill tumour cells, or mycobacteria. Similarly, IFN$_\gamma$ used alone enables human monocytes to kill *Legionella*, but it leads to enhanced growth of *Mycobacterium tuberculosis*. There are several reasons for this complexity.

1. Activated macrophages can express numerous different effector functions. These are shown diagrammatically in Fig. 8.14; and those which are antimicrobial are discussed in greater detail in Chapter 15.

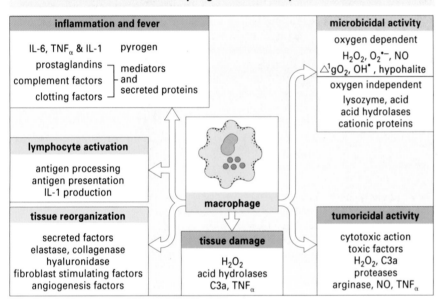

The central role of macrophages in immunity and inflammation

inflammation and fever	
IL-6, TNF$_\alpha$ & IL-1	pyrogen
prostaglandins	mediators and secreted proteins
complement factors	
clotting factors	

lymphocyte activation
antigen processing
antigen presentation
IL-1 production

tissue reorganization
secreted factors
elastase, collagenase
hyaluronidase
fibroblast stimulating factors
angiogenesis factors

macrophage

tissue damage
H$_2$O$_2$
acid hydrolases
C3a, TNF$_\alpha$

microbicidal activity
oxygen dependent
H$_2$O$_2$, O$_2^{\bullet-}$, NO
$\triangle^1$gO$_2$, OH$^\bullet$, hypohalite
oxygen independent
lysozyme, acid
acid hydrolases
cationic proteins

tumoricidal activity
cytotoxic action
toxic factors
H$_2$O$_2$, C3a
proteases
arginase, NO, TNF$_\alpha$

Fig 8.14 Macrophages and their products are important in both the induction phases of inflammation and in tissue reorganization and repair (left). Macrophage effector functions are shown on the right. The effector functions may cause tissue damage, as in delayed hypersensitivity reactions.

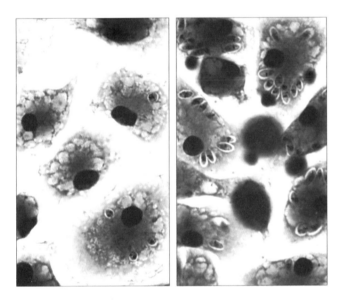

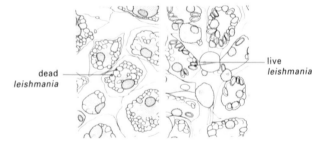

dead leishmania

live leishmania

Fig. 8.15 Killing of *Leishmania* by activated macrophages. The destruction of *Leishmania enriettii* by C57 strain mouse macrophages is enhanced by lymphokines. Parasites within the macrophages are destroyed during 48-hour culture with a lymphocyte supernatant containing lymphokines (left) by comparison with control cultures containing no lymphokine (right). Giemsa stain, × 800. (Courtesy of Dr J. Manuel.)

2. The monocyte/macrophage series is very heterogeneous and cells taken from different sites differ in such relevant characteristics as expression of class II MHC molecules and Fc receptors, lymphokine responsiveness and production of peroxidase. Most authors nevertheless believe that there is only one lineage of macrophages and that these differences are due to environmental and maturational effects.

The activation of macrophages

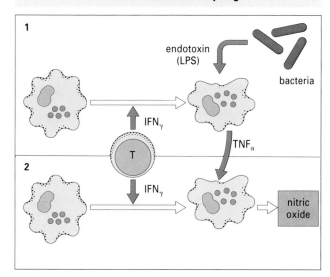

Fig. 8.16 The activation of macrophages may require interaction of several lymphokines and microbial factors.
1. Optimal release of TNF$_\alpha$ from macrophages requires activation by IFN$_\gamma$ followed by exposure to microbial components with cytokine-triggering ability, such as endotoxin. This may then provide enough TNF$_\alpha$ to trigger pathway 2.
2. IFN$_\gamma$ activates the pathway which leads to production of nitric oxide, but TNF$_\alpha$ is required in order to trigger it.

3. The functions activated may depend not only on the macrophage, but also on the precise 'blend' of lymphokines and inflammatory stimuli to which it is exposed. For instance, exposure of murine macrophages to a crude lymphokine-rich spleen cell supernatant makes them resistant to infection by *Leishmania, Candida, Trypanosoma cruzi, Rickettsia* and *Legionella*. This is an example of the synergistic interactions of lymphokines, since pure IL-2, IL-4, GM-CSF, or IFN$_\gamma$ are all unable to cause this effect. However, a combination of IFN$_\gamma$ and any of the others is active. The only mediator which was shown to be active by itself in this system was TNF$_\alpha$.

Thus several patterns of lymphokine-mediated effects can be recognized:
1. effects mediated by a single lymphokine working alone
2. quantitative effects, increased or decreased according to the status of secondary signals
3. cooperative (synergistic) effects, where one mediator has no effect unless a second mediator or bacterial product is present.

For instance the pathway which leads to formation of nitric oxide is activated by IFN$_\gamma$ but subsequent exposure to TNF$_\alpha$ greatly enhances the actual triggering of nitric oxide release (Fig. 8.16).

It is suggested that activation occurs in stages, and requires sequential stimuli, which include lymphokines, endotoxin, various mediators and regulators of inflammation (*in vitro*, plastic or glass surfaces and tissue culture media are important). Different effector functions may be expressed at each stage, and there are characteristic changes in macrophage appearance and physiology. Fig. 8.17 shows a scheme for the activation of the tumoricidal function of murine peritoneal macrophages, emphasizing the sequential action of several factors.

Stepwise activation of murine macrophages

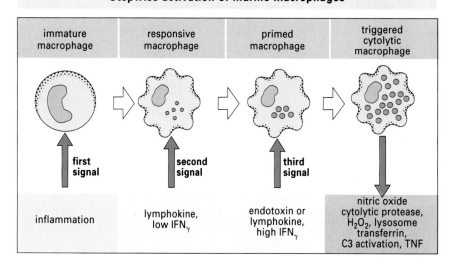

Fig. 8.17 An hypothetical scheme for the stepwise activation of murine peritoneal macrophages to develop tumoricidal activity.

THE ROLE OF CALCITRIOL IN THE ACTIVATION OF HUMAN MACROPHAGES

When human (but apparently not murine) macrophages are exposed to IFN$_\gamma$ they express a 1-hydroxylase. This enzyme enables them to convert inactive circulating 25-hydroxycholecaliferol into the active metabolite, 1,25-dihydroxycholecalciferol (also known as vitamin D$_3$, or calcitriol). Macrophages have receptors for this derivative, and it exerts additional activating effects on these cells (Fig. 8.18), and perhaps some negative feedback on lymphocytes. This pathway is of some importance in man, since production of calcitriol can be so great that it leaks from the site of macrophage activation into the peripheral circulation, where it can exert its better known effects on calcium and phosphate balance. Detectable hypercalcaemia can result.

NEGATIVE REGULATION OF MACROPHAGE EFFECTOR FUNCTIONS

There is also evidence that activated macrophages can be deactivated. Prostaglandin E may have this effect, and some effector mechanisms (but not all) are steroid sensitive. Recently a Macrophage Deactivating Factor (MDF) has been purified from a tumour cell supernatant. This factor blocks activation by IFN$_\gamma$ of increased capacity for production of ROIs and, to some extent, of nitric oxide (Fig. 8.19). So too do IL-4, CGRP (calcitonin gene related peptide), TGF$_\beta$1, TGF$_\beta$2, and TGF$_\beta$3.

GRANULOMA FORMATION

Sometimes the cell-mediated response fails to eliminate an infecting organism rapidly, or antigenic material cannot be eliminated because it is resistant to degradation or derived from self components. If, in such cases, T cells continue to accumulate and release lymphokines, this leads to granuloma formation. Granulomas are

The role of calcitriol (1,25-dihydroxycholecalciferol) in the activation of human macrophages

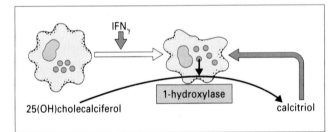

Fig. 8.18 In man, exposure to IFN$_\gamma$ leads to increased expression of 1-hydroxylase, enabling macrophages to convert inactive circulating 25-hydroxycholecalciferol into calcitriol. This is an example of an autocrine feedback loop, which further activates the macrophage.

Negative regulation of macrophage activation

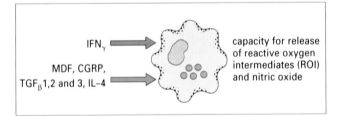

Fig. 8.19 Exposure of macrophages to IFN$_\gamma$ will increase their potential for release of both reactive oxygen intermediates, and nitric oxide. Several other factors oppose this activation.

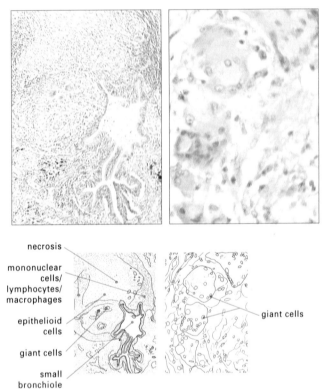

Fig. 8.20 A granulomatous reaction in pulmonary tuberculosis. The central area of caseous necrosis, in which much of the cellular structure is destroyed, is characteristic of tuberculosis in the lung, and the mechanism is discussed in Chapter 15. Apart from this necrosis, the histology is characteristic of chronic T-cell-dependent 'tuberculoid' granulomas. The lesion is surrounded by a ring of epithelioid cells and mononuclear cells. Multinucleate giant cells, thought to be derived from the fusion of epithelioid cells, are also present (left, × 170). Giant cells are illustrated at a higher magnification (right, × 270). H&E stain. (Courtesy of Dr G. Boyd.)

characteristic of infections with organisms which live at least partly intracellularly (for example, *Mycobacterium tuberculosis*, *M. leprae*, *Leishmania*, and *Listeria monocytogenes*), or organisms which are large and persistent (for example, schistosome ova).

Granulomas characteristically contain macrophage-derived cell types of somewhat obscure function, including epithelioid cells and multinucleate giant cells (Fig 8.20). Their morphology suggests secretory rather than phagocytic roles, and they are thought to result from chronic stimulation of macrophages by lymphokines.

A granuloma can be produced experimentally using soluble antigen conjugated covalently onto an insoluble particle, such as a sepharose bead. Antigen-coated beads will evoke T-cell-dependent granulomas in appropriately immunized mice, whereas control beads will not. Analysis of the T cells in granulomatous foci indicate that CD4+ cells are located at the centre and CD8+ cells around the periphery, suggesting that CD4+ cells (helper T cells) are of prime importance in inducing the accumulation and activation of other lymphocytes and macrophages (Fig. 8.21). If such granulomas are cultured *in vitro* they can be shown to release lymphokines with macrophage-activating and chemotactic properties. In mice, T-cell dependent granulomas can be evoked by schistosome ova, but they eventually wane under the influence of suppressor T cells.

IMMUNOPATHOLOGY

There are several circumstances when the cell-mediated response is itself responsible for part or all of the tissue damage resulting from infectious disease. It can also be involved in autoimmunity (Fig. 8.22). These mechanisms are described in detail in Chapters 15 and 22. Briefly:

1. Cytotoxic cells may kill virus-infected target cells which are essential to the host's survival, such as the cells of the central nervous system. If this occurs in response to a virus which does not itself cause cell death or dysfunction, the tissue damage is immunopathological.

2. Cell-mediated mechanisms may be directed towards autoantigens (or towards unidentified cryptic infections or commensal organisms), and so cause chronic tissue-damaging inflammation (as in rheumatoid arthritis, Crohn's disease, sarcoidosis, psoriasis, multiple sclerosis etc.). Often, as in the destruction of the islets of Langerhans in the pancreas leading to insulin-dependent diabetes, the relative roles of putative infectious agents and of subsequent autoimmunity are unknown.

3. The sheer size of gramulomata may compromise the function of the host tissue. Thus granulomas evoked by *M. leprae* can damage the nerves in which they form, and granulomas in the retina or brain can cause functional abnormalities.

4. Excessive release of cytokines (particularly TNF_α) can lead to shock syndromes, haemorrhagic necrosis and the Shwartzman reaction, and also contribute to necrosis within sites of cell-mediated response (the Koch phenomenon). These mechanisms are all covered in Chapter 15.

THE CYTOKINE NETWORK

Cytokines (including lymphokines and interleukins) are hormone-like peptides or glycopeptides. They have been mentioned at intervals throughout this chapter because they work in parallel with other signals arising from direct cell-to-cell contact, providing a communication network involved in every function of the immune response. The term 'lymphokine' originally referred to mediators released from lymphocytes. The word 'interleukin' was coined in the hope that by numbering these mediators (interleukin-1, interleukin-2 etc.) a universal nomenclature could be created. The term 'interleukin' may prove unfortunate since it implies that these mediators only act as signals between white cells: although many of them do have this function, most also have functions which bypass leucocytes entirely. The best term is 'cytokines' which can be used to refer to any mediator which acts as a signal between cells, whatever the cell type.

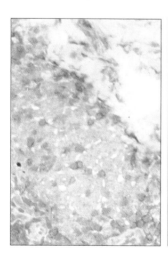 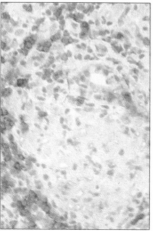

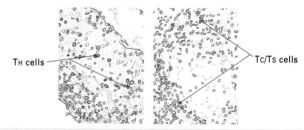

Fig. 8.21 CD4 and CD8 staining of a granuloma. Shown here is a dermal granuloma from a patient with borderline tuberculoid leprosy stained red with peroxidase-coupled antibodies to CD4 (left) and CD8 (right). CD4+ TH cells are present in and around the lesion, while CD8+ Tc/s T cells occur mainly on the periphery. (Courtesy of Dr R. L. Modlin and Dr T. H. Rea.)

Pathways of cell-mediated immunopathology

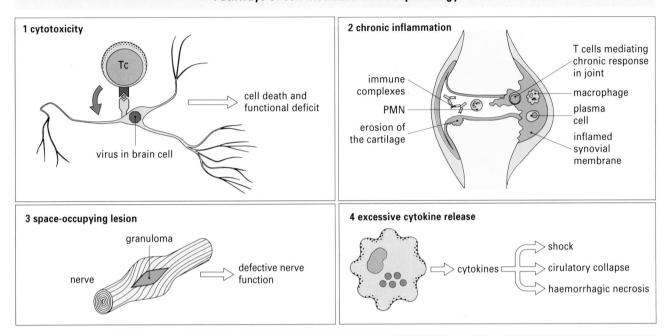

Fig 8.22 Pathways of cell-mediated immunopathology.
1. Cytotoxic cells may kill virus-infected host cells which are essential to survival.
2. The response may be directed towards autoantigens (or perhaps to unidentified cryptic infections or commensal organisms), leading to chronic inflammation.

3. A granuloma may cause a bulky space-occupying lesion, impairing the function of sensitive tissues such as brain, retina and nerve.
4. Excessive release of cytokines can lead to several tissue-damaging syndromes, discussed in detail in Chapter 15.

Effects of interleukin-6

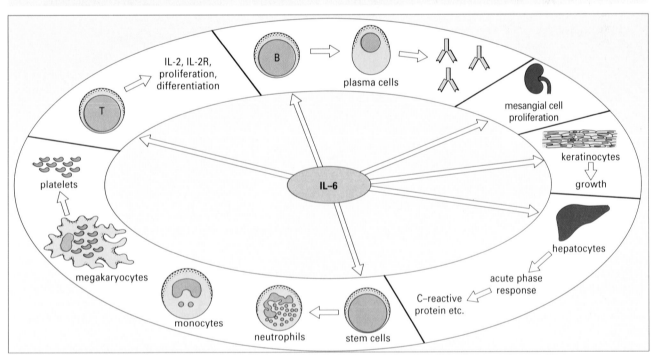

Fig. 8.23 Interleukin-6 is a typical cytokine, in that it has a range of effects on many organ systems.

Much of the confusion surrounding the nomenclature stems from the fact that cytokines are multifunctional. Thus many cytokines were discovered independently in several different laboratories, working with entirely different experimental systems. Interleukin-6 (IL-6) is a good example. It was identified as a hepatocyte stimulatory factor, a B cell stimulatory factor, a hybridoma/plasmacytoma growth factor, a monocyte/granulocyte inducer, and as β_2-interferon. Cloning of the genes has proved that these are all identical (Fig. 8.23). TNF_α was discovered almost simultaneously in two laboratories, one of which was studying weight loss in chronic infection and named this cytokine 'cachectin'.

The advent of pure recombinant cytokines has greatly facilitated the identification of cytokine functions *in vitro,* but such experiments can prove misleading when extrapolated to the *in vivo* situation. There are several reasons for this:

1. Cytokines do not operate individually *in vivo.* Perhaps each cytokine should be considered as a single 'word' in a 'sentence' of cytokines. Each cell responds to the whole sentence. Even the sequence of exposure to these mediators may be important. A mixture of cytokines can exert an effect which is not seen with any of the cytokines used alone. There can be both synergistic and antagonistic effects (Fig. 8.24), as already demonstrated when discussing their roles in the TH1/TH2 dichotomy (see Fig. 8.5) or in macrophage activation (see Fig. 8.19.).

2. There are inhibitors of cytokines *in vivo.* These can operate in three different ways (Fig. 8.25):

i) Cytokine-like mediators which bind to the cytokine receptor, but do not activate signal transduction. Thus there is an IL-1 inhibitor which is related to IL-1 itself, and competes with IL-1 for IL-1 receptors.

ii) Extracellular domains of cytokine receptors that have been shed by the cell. These can bind the cytokine and so prevent its interaction with receptors on cell membranes. Soluble TNF_α receptors do this.

iii) One cytokine can switch off the response to another, though acting via a different receptor.

Cytokines often exert autocrine effects (i.e. effects on the cell of origin). This make sense if one bears in mind the presence of inhibitors *in vivo*, since the autocrine feedback can be 'intercepted' and modulated by inhibitory products of other cells.

In vivo experiments partially resolve the problem of determining the true biological role of these multifunctional cytokines. Cytokines can be injected, or released slowly from surgically implanted osmotic minipumps.

Examples of interactions between cytokines

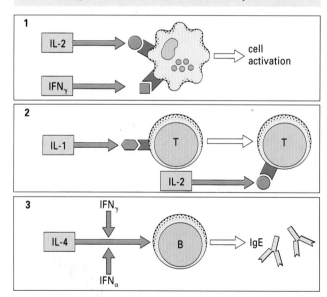

Fig 8.24 Interactions between cytokines vary.
1. Synergy. Some cytokines, e.g. IL-2 and IFN$_\gamma$, act synergistically to increase cell activation.
2. Receptor induction. Some cytokines act by inducing another receptor, a form of sequential synergy (a cascade effect).
3. Antagonism. Some cytokines are directly antagonistic, as shown by the contrasting effects of IL-4 and IFN$_\gamma$ on IgE production.

Three types of cytokine inhibitor

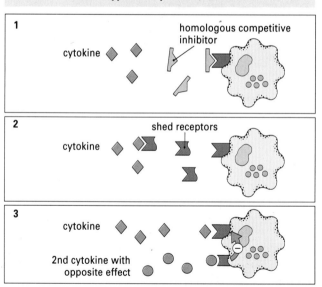

Fig 8.25 1. Molecules homologous to the cytokine and able to bind to its receptor without leading to signal transduction, act as competitive inhibitors. The gene for an IL-1 inhibitor of this type has been cloned. There may also be inhibitory glycosylation variants of some mediators.
2. The extracellular domain of the TNF receptors, and of IL-1 receptors, can be shed. They bind their cytokine in the fluid phase, and so stop the cytokine from reaching receptors on cell membranes.
3. Other mediators, acting through quite separate receptors, can exert opposite effects on the cell (see also Figs 8.5 and 8.21).

Alternatively transgenic animals can be created which overexpress the chosen cytokine. Finally, the animals can be treated with neutralizing antibodies to the cytokine. A particularly successful approach has been the weekly injection of rabbit IgG antibodies to murine cytokines, in mice previously rendered tolerant to rabbit IgG.

Such experiments have led to quite unexpected results which had not emerged from *in vitro* experiments, for instance with IL-6. Although this was known to be multifunctional, it was not until the development of transgenic mice which overexpressed the human IL-6 gene that it was realized that IL-6 has striking effects on production of both megakaryocytes and platelets. Nevertheless these *in vivo* experiments are also difficult to interpret fully. An effect can be a secondary one, due not to the injected or overexpressed cytokine but to another, possibly unidentified one ('cascade effect').

THE ROLE OF THE CYTOKINE NETWORK

It has often been pointed out that in its evolution and function, the immune system parallels the nervous system in many ways. For instance both systems have learning and memory functions based on cell-to-cell communication, and they share many mediators, receptors and antigens. In the present context it is relevant that both systems need an internal communication network, and also a communication network which can control and interact with other organs. The nervous system is directly 'wired' to most other organs via nerves, but also uses the hypothalamus-pituitary-adrenal axis to send signals to the periphery. In contrast the immune system is composed mostly of free, mobile cells: cell-to-cell interactions are intermittent and mostly concerned with internal communication. Thus communication with other organs is largely cytokine mediated. The immune system shares with the nervous system an ability to signal via the hypothalamus–pituitary–adrenal axis, since several cytokines such as IL-1, IL-6 and TNF have direct effects on the hypothalamus or pituitary. Fig. 8.26 shows how these systems are linked.

The known functions of the characterized cytokines are summarized elsewhere (see Appendix). The comments above should have made clear to the reader the need to interpret such data with caution. Not all the functions listed will turn out to be physiologically relevant, since many have been reported following *in vitro* experiments with single recombinant cytokines.

The physiological roles of the cytokine network

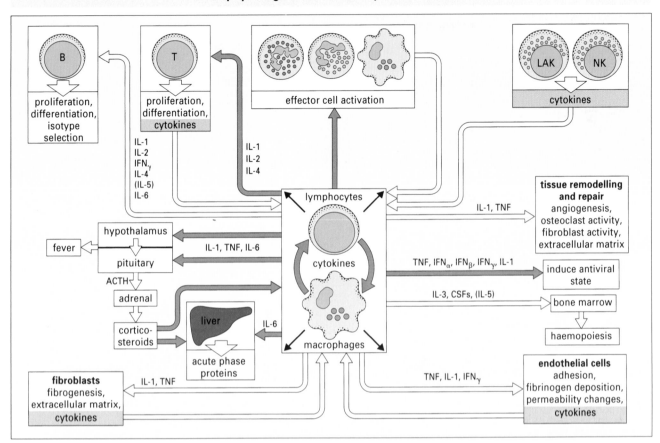

Fig. 8.26 Cytokines as communication links within the immune system, and between the immune system and other organs.

FURTHER READING

Adams D. Molecules, membranes, and macrophage activation. *Immunol Today* 1982;**3**:285.

Bloom BR, Salgame P, Diamond B. Revisiting and revising suppressor T cells. *Immunol Today* 1992;**13(4)**:131–136.

Carrick L, Boros DL. The artificial granuloma 1. *In vitro* lymphokine production by pulmonary artificial hypersensitivity granulomas. *Clin Immunol Immunopath* 1980;**17**:415.

Cerami A, Beutler B. The role of cachectin/TNF in endotoxin shock and cachexia. *Immunol Today* 1988;**9**:28.

Eckels DD, Lamb P, Lake P, Woody JN, Johnson AH, Hartzman R. Antigen-specific human T lymphocyte clones. Genetic restriction of influenza virus-specific responses to HLA-D region genes. *Hum Immunol* 1982;**4**:313.

Filley EA, Rook GA. Effect of mycobacteria on sensitivity to the cytotoxic effects of tumor necrosis factor. *Infect Immun* 1991;**59**:2567–72.

Goldberg AL, Rock KL. Proteolysis, proteasomes and antigen presentation. *Nature* 1992;**357**:375–79.

Nathan CF, Murray HW, Wiebe ME, Rubin BY. Identification of interferon-γ as the lymphokine that activates human macrophage oxidative metabolism and antimicrobial activity. *J Exp Med* 1983;**158**:670.

Janeway CA. The imune system evolved to discriminate infectious self from noninfectious self. *Immunol Today* 1992;**13(1)**:11–16.

Kohl S, Loo LS. Protection of neonatal mice against herpes simplex virus infections: probable *in vivo* antibody-dependent cellular cytotoxicity. *J Immunol* 1982;**129**:370.

McMichael AJ, Gotch F, Noble GR. Cytotoxic T cell immunity to influenza. *New Engl J Med* 1983;**309**:13.

Moretta L, Ciccone E, Moretta A, Höglund P, Öhlén C, Kärre K. Allorecognition by NK cells: nonself or no self. *Immunol Today* 1992;**13(8)**:300–306.

Mosmann TR, Coffman RL. Different patterns of lymphokine secretion lead to different functional properties. *Annu Rev Immunol* 1989;**7**:145–73.

Oppenheim JJ, Gery I. Interleukin-1 is more than an interleukin. *Immunol Today* 1982;**3**:113.

Ritz J, Schmidt RE, Michon J, Hercend T, Schlossman. Characterisation of functional surface structures on human natural killer cells. *Adv Immunol* 1988;**42**:181.

Romagnani S. Human TH1 and TH2 subsets: doubt no more. *Immunol Today* 1991;**12**:256–57.

Rook GAW. The role of activated macrophages in the immunopathology of tuberculosis. *Br Med Bull* 1988;**44(3)**: 624.

Rosenstein M, Eberlein FJ, Rosenberg SA. Adoptive immunotherapy of established syngeneic solid tumours: role of lymphoid subpopulations. *J Immunol* 1984;**132**:2117.

Steinman RM, Nussenzweig MC. Dendritic cells: features and functions. *Immunol Rev* 1980;**53**:127.

Unanue ER. Cellular studies on antigen presentation by class II MHC molecules. *Curr Opin Immunol* 1992;**4**:63–69.

Vassalli P. The pathophysiology of tumour necrosis factor. *Annu Rev Immunol* 1992;**10**:411–52.

Warner JF, Dennert G. Effects of a cloned cell line NK activity on bone marrow transplants, tumour development, and metastasis *in vivo*. *Nature* 1982;**300**:37.

Young JD, Liu C. Multiple mechanisms of lymphocyte mediated killing. *Immunol Today* 1988;**9**:140–44.

Zinkernagel RM, Doherty PC. MHC-restricted cytotoxic T cells. Studies on the biological role of polymorphic major transplantation antigens determining T cell restriction specificity and responsiveness. *Adv Immunol* 1979;**27**:51.

chapter 9

Regulation of the Immune Response

The immune response, like all biological systems, is subject to a variety of control mechanisms which serve to restore the immune system to a resting state when responsiveness to a given antigen is no longer required. An effective immune response is the end result of interactions between antigen and a network of immunologically competent cells. The nature of the immune response, both qualitatively and quantitatively, is determined by many factors, including the form and route of administration of the antigen, the genetic background of the individual and any previous history of exposure to this antigen or a cross-reacting antigen, or even antibody to the antigen. Some of these factors are discussed elsewhere (see Chapters 10, 15, 18 and 22) and are dealt with only briefly here.

REGULATION BY ANTIGEN

T cells and B cells are triggered by antigen following effective engagement of their antigen-specific receptors. In the case of the T cell, this engagement is not of antigen itself but of processed antigenic peptide bound to MHC Class I or Class II molecules (see Chapter 6). Following triggering, the T cell responds by producing cytokines and their corresponding receptors, thus permitting clonal expansion and expression of effector function. In the case of the B cell, cytokine receptor expression, clonal expansion and differentiation also occur as a consequence of triggering. The resulting antibody forming cell (AFC) secretes large amounts of antibody that is specific for the triggering antigen. An effective immune response removes antigen from the system and, since repeated antigen exposure is required to maintain T and B cells in an active expanding phase, the cells then return to a quiescent state.

Some antigens (for example those of intracellular parasites) may not be cleared so effectively and thus a sustained immune response arises, sometimes with pathological consequences (see Chapter 16).

REGULATION BY ANTIBODY

Antibody itself is able to exert a form of feedback control. Passive administration of IgM antibody together with antigen enhances the immune response to the antigen, whereas IgG antibody suppresses the response. Although the original experiments were carried out using polyclonal antibodies, these findings have been reproduced using monoclonal antibodies (Fig. 9.1). The ability of passively administered (rather than endogenously produced) antibody to down-regulate the immune response has several clinical consequences. Certain vaccines (e.g. mumps and measles) are not generally given to infants before one year of age, as the level of maternally derived IgG remains high for at least six months after birth. The presence of passively acquired IgG at the time of vaccination would result in the development of an inadequate immune response in the baby. However, the ability of passively administered antibody to down-regulate immune responses can also be turned to advantage. In cases of Rhesus (Rh) incompatibility, the administration of anti-D antibody to Rh$^-$ mothers prevents primary sensitization by fetally derived Rh$^+$ blood cells, presumably by removing the foreign antigen, in this case fetal erythrocytes, from the maternal circulation.

The mechanisms by which antibody modulates the immune response are not completely defined. In the case of IgM enhancement there are two possible interpretations. One of these involves the development of an anti-idiotypic response to the administered monoclonal, which amplifies the immune response (see below). The other involves an effect of passively administered antibody on the uptake, processing and presentation of antigen, due to binding of the IgM-containing immune complexes to certain antigen-presenting cells (APCs) through their Fc receptors.

Feedback control by antibody

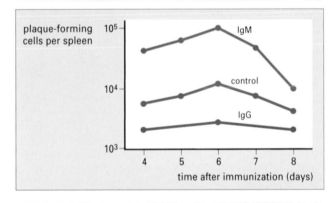

Fig. 9.1 Three groups of mice received respectively a monoclonal IgM anti-SRBC (sheep red blood cells), IgG anti-SRBC or medium alone (control). Two hours later, all groups were immunized with SRBC. The antibody response, measured over the following eight days, was enhanced by IgM and suppressed by IgG.

ANTIBODY SUPPRESSION

For IgG-mediated suppression there are also various ways in which the antibody is known to act. In one situation the passively administered antibody binds the antigen in competition with the B cells (Fig. 9.2). The impact of the IgG in this case is highly dependent on the concentration of the antibody and its affinity for the antigen, compared to the affinity of the B-cell receptors. Only high-affinity B cells would compete successfully for the antigen. This mechanism is independent of the Fc portion of the antibody. IgG antibody is also known to have an effect which is Fc dependent. The experiments showing this have been carried out *in vitro*, as it is difficult to work with F(ab')$_2$ fragments *in vivo*, because they are cleared so rapidly. The experiments demonstrate that immunoglobulin can inhibit B cell differentiation by cross-linking the antigen receptor with the B-cell receptor (see Fig. 9.2). Doses of antibody which are insufficient to inhibit completely the production of antibodies have the effect of increasing their average affinity because only those B cells with high-affinity receptors can successfully compete with the free antibody for antigen. For this reason, antibody feedback is thought to be an important factor driving the process of affinity maturation (Fig. 9.3).

REGULATION BY IMMUNE-COMPLEXES

In the previous section one of the possible ways in which antibody (either IgM or IgG) was shown to modulate the immune response involved an Fc-dependent mechanism, and immune-complex formation with antigen. Immune-complexes can inhibit or augment the immune response (Fig. 9.4).

The immune response of patients with malignant tumours is often depressed, and it has been postulated that this is the result of the presence of circulating immune-complexes composed of antibody and tumour cell antigens.

REGULATION BY LYMPHOCYTES

T cells clearly modulate the immune response in a positive sense by providing T-cell help. Furthermore, the kind of help which is generated (TH1 versus TH2) affects the nature of the immune response, favouring either humoral or cell-mediated immunity. Additionally there is clear evidence that T cells are capable of down-regulating immune responses (Fig. 9.5). Of particular interest has been the observation, made in many experimental models of autoimmune disease, that CD4$^+$ T cells, generated following administration of

---

Antibody-dependent B cell suppression

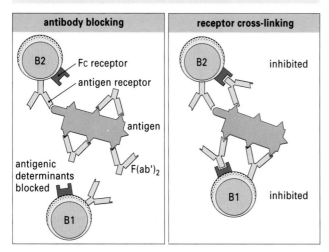

Fig. 9.2 In **antibody blocking**, high doses of antibody (or its F(ab')$_2$ fragment) block the interaction between an antigenic determinant (epitope) and B-cell receptors for that determinant, which are then effectively unable to recognize the antigen (B1). This receptor blocking mechanism also prevents B cell priming. B cells with receptors for different epitopes are unaffected (B2). In **receptor cross-linking,** low doses of antibody – but not F(ab')$_2$ – allow cross-linking by antigen of a B cell's Fc receptors and its antigen receptors. This inhibits antibody synthesis but not B cell priming. The effect is not epitope-specific.

Antibody feedback affinity maturation

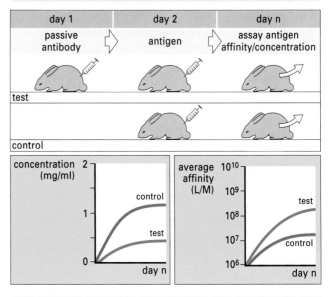

Fig. 9.3 The effect of passive antibody on the affinity and concentration of secreted antibody. One of two rabbits was injected with antibody (passive antibody) on day 1. Both rabbits were immunized with antigen on day 2 and the affinity and concentration of antibody raised to this antigen were assayed at a later time (day n). The antibody assay results show that passive antibody reduces the concentration, but increases the affinity, of antibody produced.

high doses of autoantigen (often given in a soluble or deaggregated form), prevent further induction of autoimmunity. For example, CD4⁺ T cells have been shown to prevent the development of autoantibodies to thyroglobulin (Fig. 9.6). The exact mechanism by which

T cells exert such a negative influence is not entirely clear. However, recent experiments suggest that the production by T$_H$ cells of cytokines such as TGF$_\beta$, IL-4 and IL-10 can either partially or totally suppress an immune response.

Regulatory effects of immune-complexes

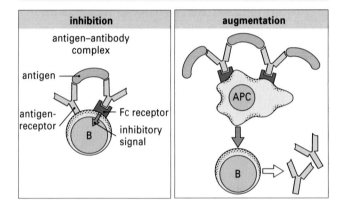

Fig. 9.4 Immune-complexes can act either to inhibit or augment an immune response.
Inhibition When the B cell's Fc receptor is cross-linked to its antigen receptor by an antigen–antibody complex, a signal is delivered to the B cell inhibiting it from entering the antibody production phase. Passive IgG may have this effect.
Augmentation Antibody encourages presentation of antigen to B cells when it is present on an antigen-presenting cell (APC), bound via Fc receptors. (Complexes can also activate complement and then bind to APCs via their C3b receptors in an analogous way.) Passive IgM may have this effect.

Suppressor cells in immunological tolerance

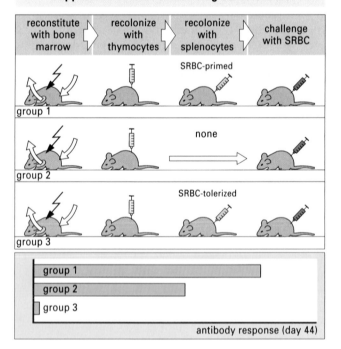

Fig. 9.5 Thymectomized and irradiated mice were reconstituted with bone marrow cells. After 30 days they were recolonized with thymocytes and spleen cells, and challenged with SRBC. At day 44, recipients given splenocytes primed with an immunogenic dose of SRBC made a strong response (1). Animals receiving no spleen cells had a moderate response (2). Animals receiving cells from mice tolerized to SRBC (with a high dose of antigen) did not respond (3), indicating that cells from tolerized animals actively suppress the response in the recipient.

Transfer of tolerance by CD4⁺ T cells

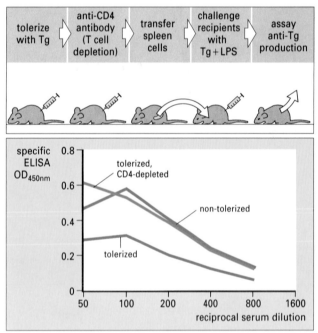

Fig. 9.6 Mice were injected with 200 μg of mouse thyroglobulin (Tg) to induce tolerance. (A control group was not tolerized.) Part of the tolerized group was further treated *in vivo* with anti-CD4 antibodies, to induce T-cell depletion. For each mouse, spleen cells were transferred into an irradiated syngeneic recipient. The recipients were then challenged with mouse thyroglobulin and LPS, and their anti-Tg antibody response was assayed using ELISA (see chapter 25). Anti-CD4 treatment removed the ability to transfer tolerance.

The production of different cytokines by different TH cell subpopulations probably provides an explanation for certain observations regarding the regulation of IgE synthesis. IgE responses are usually of short duration, as the major response to antigen is IgG. However, it has been shown that the IgE response can be augmented by a variety of treatments directed against T cells, including anti-thymocyte serum, sublethal irradiation, adult thymectomy and splenectomy. The enhanced immune responses obtained can be suppressed by the transfer of T cells (Fig. 9.7). It is known that T-cell derived cytokines, such as IL-4 or IFN_γ (see Chapter 8) influence the production of IgE, the former enhancing production while the latter suppresses it. Thus, it seems likely that the T cells mediate suppression of IgE synthesis by making IFN_γ.

Recent experiments have shown that dysregulated immune responses arise in rats when $CD4^+$ TH2 cells, which normally make IL-4 and IL-10, are removed. This strongly suggests that regulation of the immune response by $CD4^+$ TH2 cells (rather than $CD4^+$ TH1 cells) is a normal physiological process and not an artefact.

 IDIOTYPIC MODULATION OF RESPONSES

Tolerance to self-antigens is established during ontogeny (see Chapter 10). Individual antigen-specific receptors on B and T cells are only present at low levels during the neonatal period, and these levels are insufficient to generate tolerance to those epitopes which are formed by amino acids in or around the binding site. These epitopes are unique to any given receptor or antibody. Although antibodies are present in the serum, tolerance only develops to their Fc portions because only these are present in sufficient numbers. Tolerance does not develop to those unique determinants in the heavy and light chains which determine the antigen binding specificity, because each one is only present in low numbers. Individual T-cell receptors and immunoglobulins are therefore immunogenic by virtue of these unique sequences, known as idiotypes. Antibodies formed against these antigen-binding sites are called anti-idiotypic antibodies, and they are capable of influencing the outcome of an immune response.

Idiotypic determinants may be encoded in the germ line V region genes, or they may be generated by the

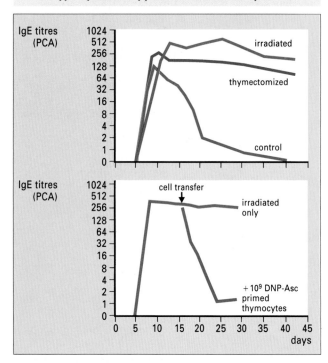

Fig. 9.7 Upper: Rats immunized with DNP conjugated to Ascaris antigen (DNP–Asc) in pertussis adjuvant develop a short-lived IgE response after five days, which wanes by day 35 (control). If the animals are irradiated or thymectomized, the IgE response persists. Lower: In a second experiment, thymocytes from an animal immunized with DNP–Asc in complete Freund's adjuvant, were transferred to an animal that had been irradiated and primed with DNP–Asc in pertussis adjuvant. The transferred thymocytes were able to turn off the IgE response. The degree of turn-off depends on the number of cells transferred. In additional experiments, splenocytes were shown to be as effective as thymocytes.

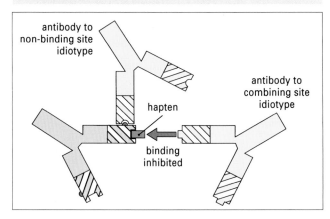

Fig. 9.8 An anti-idiotype serum may contain some antibodies directed to various sites on the immunoglobulin molecule. Those associated with the combining site are site associated idiotopes. The binding to these can be inhibited by hapten. Antibodies to non-binding site idiotopes (non-site associated) will not be inhibited by hapten.

process of recombination and mutation involved in producing functional V-region elements. Immunogenic epitopes in or around the binding site are termed idiotopes (Fig. 9.8). Jerne proposed that an immune network existed within the body which interacted by means of idiotype recognition. According to this proposition, when an antibody response is induced by antigen, this antibody will in turn invoke an anti-idiotypic response to itself. This hypothesis is conceptually very appealing, but the role of such an idiotype network in controlling a normal immune response is still hotly debated.

IDIOTYPIC INTERACTIONS IN IMMUNOREGULATION

There is good evidence that anti-idiotypes can affect the representation of recognized idiotypes in an immune response. For example, when C57Bl/6 strain mice are challenged with the hapten, NP, they produce antibodies which are largely restricted to a few defined idiotypes, for example the idiotype 146. Anti-idiotype to this antibody can enhance or suppress the production of idiotype 146 when the mice are subsequently challenged with NP on a carrier protein. The observed effect depends on the amount of anti-idiotype given (Fig. 9.9) and is idiotype-specific, as the overall level of anti-NP antibody is hardly affected. Most importantly, the amounts of anti-idiotype employed are within the

physiological range for particular idiotype-bearing antibodies, which suggests that idiotypic regulation may occur *in vivo*. This kind of observation has been made in other idiotypic systems.

Dramatic effects are observed when anti-idiotype is administered neonatally, where the effect may be lifelong. For example, the ability of neonatal mice to mount an anti-phosphoryl choline response is greatly reduced after being injected with anti-idiotype to T15 (T15 is a major idiotype in the response to phosphoryl choline). The reduction lasts many months. The response which these mice subsequently make is dominated by non-T15-immunoglobulins (Fig. 9.10).

■ NEUROENDOCRINE MODULATION OF IMMUNE RESPONSES

There is one other way in which immune responses may be modulated – by the influences of the nervous and endocrine systems.

It has long been known that stressful conditions may lead to a suppression of immune functions, such as response of lymphocytes to mitogens *in vitro*, or the ability to recover from infection. (This effect is clearest in those cases where the stressful stimulus cannot be controlled.) However, it is much more difficult to make

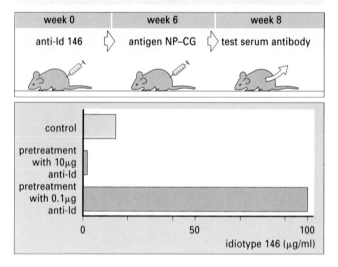

Fig. 9.9 Mice were injected at time 0 with either 10 μg or 0.1 μg of anti-idiotype (anti-Id) to the nitrophenyl (NP)-binding antibody 146. The animals were then challenged six weeks later with NP on the carrier, chicken globulin (CG). Two weeks later the serum titres of idiotype 146 (bar diagram), and total anti-NP (not shown) were assayed. Mice pretreated with 10 μg anti-Id showed suppression of idiotype 146, while mice treated with 0.1 μg showed enhanced production of idiotype 146, although the overall levels of anti-NP were similar in both groups.

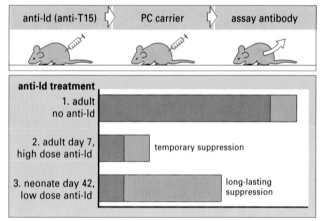

Fig. 9.10 Mice were pretreated with anti-T15.Id, either during the neonatal period or as adults. They were subsequently immunized with the hapten PC coupled to a carrier. The total antibody to PC was measured along with the T15 component of the response (darker area). Normal adult mice make a good response to PC which is dominated by T15 (1). Adult mice pretreated with anti-Id are temporarily suppressed with the loss of the T15 component, accounting for the reduction in the total anti-PC response (2). Mice treated with anti-Id in the neonatal period undergo long-term suppression of their T15⁺ B cells, but generate T15⁻ PC-specific cells to compensate (3).

direct connections at the cellular or molecular level that explain these observations. Broadly, there are two main routes by which events occurring in the CNS could modulate immune function (Fig. 9.11).

1. Most lymphoid tissues receive direct sympathetic innervation, both to the blood vessels passing through the tissues, and directly to the lymphocytes themselves.
2 The nervous system directly or indirectly controls the output of various hormones, in particular, corticosteroids, growth hormone, thyroxine and adrenalin.

Lymphocytes express receptors for many hormones, neurotransmitters and neuropeptides, including ones for steroids/catecholamines (adrenalin and noradrenalin), enkephalins, endorphins, substance P and vasoactive intestinal peptide (VIP). Expression and responsiveness varies between different lymphocyte and monocyte populations, such that the effect of different transmitters may vary in different circumstances. However, one particularly important control is mediated by corticosteroids, endorphins and enkephalins, all of which may be released during stress, and all of which are immunosuppressive *in vivo*. The precise effects *in vitro* of endorphin vary greatly with doses used, and in which system, with some levels being suppressive and some enhancing immune functions. It is certain however that the corticosteroids act as a major feedback control on immune responses. It has been found that lymphocytes themselves can respond to corticotrophin releasing factor to generate their own ACTH, which in turn induces corticosteroid release.

GENETIC CONTROL OF IMMUNE RESPONSES

There are many ways in which genetic factors may play some role in influencing the immune response. It has long been recognized that the ability to make an immune response to any given antigen varies between individuals. Familial patterns of susceptibility to *Corynebacterium diphtheriae* infection suggested that resistance or susceptibility might be an inherited characteristic. This proposal was supported by the finding that different strains of guinea pigs displayed different resistance patterns to diphtheria, and that this characteristic was inherited. In 1943 Fjord–Scheibel demonstrated, by selection of high-responder and low-responder guinea pig strains, that the production of diphtheria anti-toxin was controlled by a single gene, inherited as a Mendelian dominant trait. This study was also the first demonstration of the dominance of high responsiveness. Ninety per cent of offspring of the two high-responder animals were anti-toxin producers in the first generation, whereas it took five generations of inbreeding low-responders before ninety per cent of their offspring were low-responders.

With the development of inbred mouse strains it became possible to analyse genetic influences more rigorously and it was conclusively demonstrated that genetic factors play a role in determining immune responsiveness. It was furthermore shown that genes within the MHC (see Chapters 4 and 6) play a fundamental role in influencing the response against infectious agents.

Considerable advances have been made in recent years: the elucidation of the structures of MHC class I and, by analogy, MHC class II; the analyses of polymorphic residues in the MHC and their influence on peptide binding; the ability to monitor the T cell repertoire following the generation of reagents and molecular methods for TCR detection; the development of transgenic mice; all these have contributed to an explosion of information about genetic factors influencing the immune response. However, genetic influences on the immune response are not always linked to the MHC. For example, severe combined immunodeficiency is

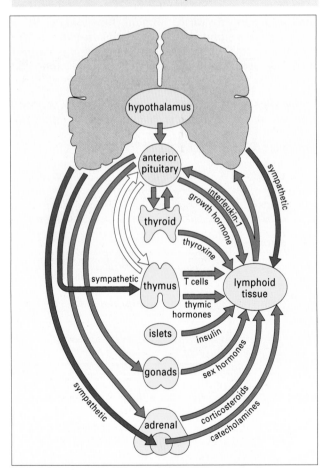

Neuroendocrine interactions with the immune system

Fig. 9.11 The diagram indicates some of the potential connections between the endocrine, nervous and immune systems. Blue arrows indicate nervous connections, red arrows indicate hormonal interactions, and white arrows indicate postulated connections for which the effector molecules have not been established.

due to the lack of a recombinase gene, and leucocyte adhesion deficiency is caused by mutations in the β_2-integrin subunit which lead to a failure of expression.

MHC-LINKED IMMUNE RESPONSE GENES

In the early studies of immune responsiveness, experiments were carried out using complex antigens and outbred animals. Although important observations were made at that time on the heritability of such responses, it was only with the development of inbred strains of mice and simple antigens, such as synthetic polypeptides, that significant advances were made. It was found that responsiveness to these simple antigens was highly specific (i.e. a high responder to one antigen would be low to another), that the genes for high responsiveness were dominant, and that they were linked to the mouse MHC (Fig. 9.12). Using recombinant mouse strains the genes governing immune responsiveness (so-called Ir genes) were mapped to the I region of the MHC (Fig. 9.13). Ir gene control could be seen with antigens which were polypeptides with limited structural diversity (e.g. TGAL, HGAL or GT) and also with responses to

complex antigens such as thyroglobulin (Fig. 9.14). Some of the more complex antigens were perceived by the mouse to be simple as a result of the development of tolerance to most epitopes (e.g. of thyroglobulin) during ontogeny (see Chapter 11).

Mapping the Ir gene

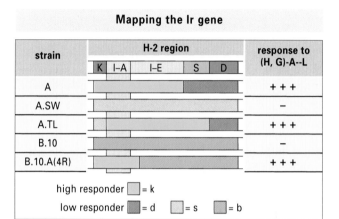

Fig. 9.13 The Ir gene controls responses to (H,G)-A--L. The H–2 regions of five strains of mice are illustrated, three strains are high responders to (H,G)-A--L and two are low responders. All three high responder strains have only the H-2^k I-A region in common, indicating that the gene present in H-2^k mice controlling the immune response to (H,G)-A--L is in the I–A region. Colours represent haplotypes.

Strain differences in the antibody response

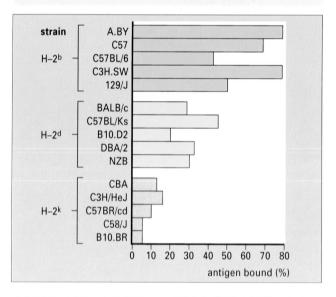

Fig. 9.12 Fifteen strains of mice were given a standard dose of the synthetic antigen (T,G)-A--L. Antibody responses are expressed as the antigen-binding capacity of the antisera. Animals with the H–2^b haplotype are high responders, H–2^d are intermediate and H–2^k are low responders. However, there is some overlap between the level of response in the different haplotypes, indicating that the H–2 linked genes are not the only ones that control the response.

High and low responder haplotypes

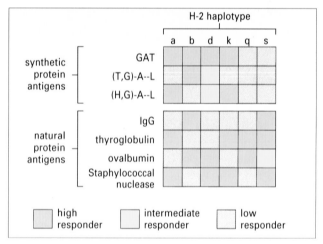

Fig. 9.14 This table shows the response of six inbred strains of mice, with different H–2 haplotypes, to seven different antigens. High responders to some antigens produce low responses to others, with no systematic pattern of response. Even with very closely related antigens, such as (T,G)-A--L and (H,G)-A--L, the response is different in H–2^a and H–2^b strains.

Effect of Ir genes on antigen presentation

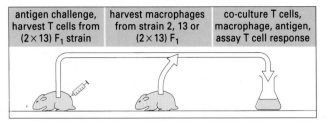

| antigen challenge, harvest T cells from (2×13) F₁ strain | harvest macrophages from strain 2, 13 or (2×13) F₁ | co-culture T cells, macrophage, antigen, assay T cell response |

(2×13)F₁ T cell response when cultured with:

macrophage strain	antigen		
	DNP-GL	GT	PPD
2	+	−	+
13	−	+	+
(2×13) F₁	+	+	+

Fig. 9.15 Strain 2 guinea pigs respond to DNP–GL but not to GT. In strain 13 animals the pattern of responsiveness is reversed. Both strains respond to PPD. T cells from a hybrid strain (2 × 13) F₁ were cultured with macrophages from the parental or F₁ strains using different antigens. The T cell response was then measured by assessing cell proliferation. Although T cells from F₁ animals are potentially capable of responding to all these antigens, they do so only in the presence of macrophages from animals of the high responder strain of the F₁. This implies that the immune response (Ir) genes are expressed on APCs. The observation that F₁ macrophages present all these antigens indicates that those Ir genes are codominantly expressed.

Anti-MHC class II blocks antigen presentation

(2×13)F₁ T cell response when cultured with (2×13)F₁ macrophages and:

antiserum	antigen		
	DNP-GL	GT	PPD
none (control)	+++	+++	+++
anti-strain 2 Ia	−	+++	+
anti-strain 13 Ia	+++	−	+

Fig. 9.16 Strain 2 guinea pigs respond to DNP–GL, and strain 13 to GT. Both strains respond to PPD. Strain (2 × 13) F₁ recognizes all the antigens. (2 × 13) F₁ T cells were cultured with (2 × 13) F₁ macrophages alone, or in the presence of antisera to MHC class II molecules of either haplotype, and T cell proliferation was assessed. With no antibody to class II present, T cells proliferate to all antigens. Anti-strain 2 Ia eliminates the response to DNP–GL and reduces that to PPD, but leaves the response to GT unaffected. Anti-strain 13 Ia eliminates the response to GT and reduces that to PPD, but leaves the response to DNP–GL unaffected. In each case, only anti-Ia antiserum directed to the responder haplotype blocks antigen presentation.

A series of classic experiments established that Ir genes acted at the level of antigen presentation and that antibodies to class II MHC molecules could prevent antigen presentation (Figs 9.15 and 9.16). Experiments using mouse strains possessing different MHC class II molecules conclusively proved that the MHC-linked Ir genes were indeed class II MHC molecules. The importance of MHC class I molecules was underlined by studies of T-cell cytotoxic responses to virally infected targets, chemically modified self antigens or a variety of minor histocompatibility antigens including the male antigen, H–Y, for which expression is determined by genes on the Y chromosome. CD8⁺ Tc cells were shown to lyse virally infected target cells only if they were matched at the H–2K or H–2D regions (Fig. 9.17); this recognition of MHC was learnt during ontogeny (Fig. 9.18). Other experiments have addressed the critical role of the thymus in the development of MHC-restricted responses. The observation that the MHC-restricted T-cell recognition of virally infected target cells was dictated by the MHC haplotype of the thymus

Genetic restriction of cytotoxic cells

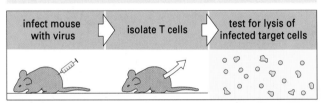

| infect mouse with virus | isolate T cells | test for lysis of infected target cells |

virus	mouse strain	H-2 region				percent lysis of infected targets of haplotype		
		K	I	S	D	H-2ˢ	H-2ᵏ	H-2ᵈ
LCM	A.TL					25	1	64
Sendai	A.TL					63	4	24
LCM	CBA					2	34	1
LCM	A/J					0	30	64

Fig. 9.17 The cytotoxic cells of virus-infected adult mice of different strains were tested for their ability to kill virus-infected target cells of different H–2 haplotype (k, s and d). The strain A.TL is H–2Kˢ, H–2Lᵏ and H–2Dᵈ and its cells kill target cells infected with lymphocytic choriomeningitis virus (LCM) only if the targets share the H–2Kˢ or the H–2Dᵈ haplotypes. Haplotype identity between the cells and targets at the H–2I locus does not produce cytotoxicity. This shows that the antiviral cytotoxic T cells are class I restricted. Note that the cytotoxicity to LCM is determined mostly by the H–2D locus. By comparison, in A.TL mice infected with Sendai virus, the cytotoxicity is principally determined by the H–2K locus. Infection of CBA mice with LCM confirms the importance of genetic restriction in these responses, while the infection of A/J mice with LCM confirms the finding that cytotoxicity to LCM is strongest to the H–2D-matched infected targets. Different viruses may associate preferentially with particular H–2K or H–2D MHC molecules to present a target for cytotoxic cells.

(Fig. 9.19), suggested that at some point during maturation in the thymus, T cells were 'educated' to recognize MHC.

As discussed in previous chapters, the immune response depends upon the activation of clones of lymphocytes. In the case of T cells, these recognize antigen only when it is presented to them as peptide complexed to Class I or Class II major histocompatibility antigens. The peripheral T-cell repertoire is influenced both by the range of endogenous polymorphic self antigens and by the MHC antigens of the individual. The ability of peptide to bind to MHC is affected by the amino acid sequences in the binding sites of the MHC molecules. The elucidation of the three-dimensional structure of human HLA-A2 and HLA-Aw68 has permitted the positions of the polymorphic residues to be assigned. These have been shown to reside in the groove in which peptide is bound and to influence affinity between a given peptide and the MHC. Thus the extensive sequence polymorphism of MHC molecules has a profound impact on peptide binding

and, as a consequence, on T cell activation. It is now established that, during development, T cells are subjected to two selection processes in the thymus:
1. positive selection, based on an interaction of the TCR with MHC on thymic cortical epithelium
2. negative selection, a result of a high-affinity interaction between the TCR and MHC–peptide presented on bone-marrow-derived cells in the thymus medulla.

POSITIVE SELECTION IN THE THYMUS

Early studies in this area used complex protocols involving thymectomy, irradiation, bone marrow reconstitution and thymus grafting. Using these techniques, it was shown that Tc cells were highly specific, and would only kill target cells which bore the same MHC antigens as those expressed on the thymus in which the T cell matured (see Fig. 9.19). This, together with other data, suggested that the maturing T cell was educated to recognize antigen only in the context of MHC originally encountered in the thymus. Experiments carried out on transgenic mice have helped to clarify this process, since it is possible to construct a transgenic animal whose T cells largely utilize a single TCR which recognizes a defined antigen. This antigen may also be expressed as a transgene.

Specificity of Tc cells

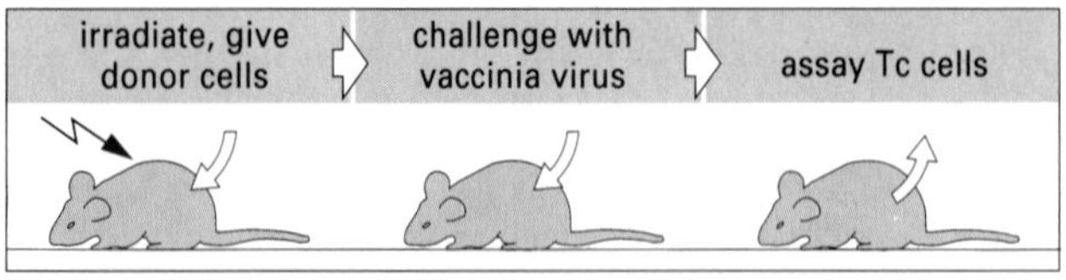

experiment	donor cells	recipient	cytotoxicity to:	
			A-vaccinia	B-vaccinia
1	A×B(BM)	A	+	−
2	A×B(BM)	B	−	+
3	A×B(spleen)	A	+	+
4	A×B(spleen)	B	+	+

Fig. 9.18 Recipient mice (type A and B) were irradiated and reconstituted with donor lymphocytes (bone marrow or spleen cells). This produced chimeric animals, in which the lymphocytes were of the donor type and other tissues were of the recipient type. The chimeras were then challenged with vaccinia virus; T cells from the spleen were removed and assayed for cytotoxicity against either type A or Type B cells infected with vaccinia (denoted as A-vaccinia and B-vaccinia). Mice reconstituted with (A×B) bone marrow cells can only kill infected targets of the same type as the recipient (1 and 2). Mature lymphocytes from the spleen of (A×B) mice can kill both A and B targets regardless of the recipient (3 and 4). The interpretation is that immature stem cells from the bone marrow (BM) undergo thymic 'education' in the recipient and can then only recognize antigen in association with the recipient's MHC haplotype. Mature cells from the donor's spleen, however, have already undergone thymic education. In most cases, for thymic education of donor cells to occur, the donor and recipient must share at least one class II region haplotype.

Importance of thymic haplotype in T cell development

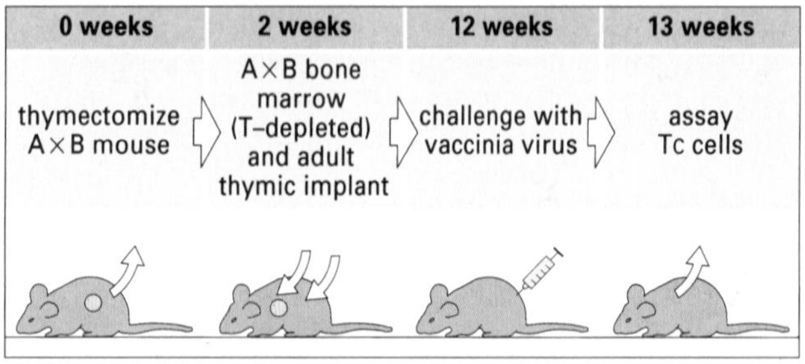

thymic donor	target cell haplotype	
	A	B
A	+	−
B	−	+

Fig. 9.19 Eight-week-old mice of MHC genotype (A×B) were thymectomized, irradiated and reconstituted with bone marrow which had been specifically depleted of T cells by treatment with anti-Thy 1.2 and complement. Each mouse was then given a subcutaneous implant of adult thymus of either type A or type B haplotype. (The grafted tissue was first irradiated to destroy mature T cells. This leaves the thymic stromal cells intact.) About 20% of animals survived this treatment and recovered immune function. Ten weeks after grafting, these mice were infected with vaccinia virus; their spleen cells were tested one week later for the ability to specifically kill virally infected target cells of haplotype A or B. Animals reconstituted with a type A thymus killed haplotype A targets, and those with a type B thymus killed haplotype B targets.

Positive selection in the thymus

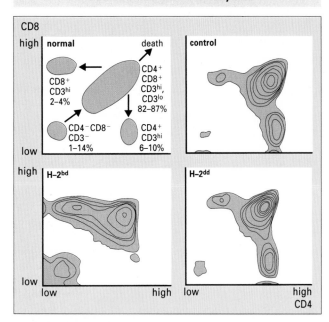

Fig. 9.20 Thymocytes were obtained from transgenic mice carrying the TCR of a CD8⁺ T cell which recognizes LCM virus on H–2ᵇ. The thymocytes were analysed for expression of CD4 and CD8 by fluorescence-activated cell sorting. In the normal developmental profile CD4⁻CD8⁻ cells become CD4⁺CD8⁺ and finally mature into CD4⁺CD8⁻, or CD4⁻CD8⁺, or die. In a control (non-transgenic mouse) the major population is CD4⁺CD8⁺, with smaller CD4⁺CD8⁻ and CD4⁻CD8⁺ populations. In a transgenic expressing an H–2ᵇ allele, the T cells are positively selected in the thymus producing a much larger CD4⁻CD8⁺ population. No such selection occurs if the relevant H–2ᵇ allele is absent.

T cell deletion by superantigens

V region	antigen recognized	T cell population expressing V region	after tolerance by clonal deletion
Vβ17a	I–E, B cell peptide	5.6%	0.9%
Vβ6	Mlsᵃ	12.4%	0.3%
Vβ8.1	Mlsᵃ	7.5%	0.3%
Vβ3	Mls-2	4.1%	0.1%
Vβ3	SEB	5.7%	1.2%
Vβ8	SEB	18.9%	0.0%
Vβ11	I–E, peptide	5.0%	0.5%

Fig. 9.21 Superantigens can cause clonal deletion of T cells expressing certain Vβ chains. The absolute number of T cells utilizing particular Vβ chains varies between mouse strains. This table provides examples of deletion values obtained in certain strains; while the absolute levels may vary from strain to strain, the overall phenomenon holds true. (SEB = staphylococcal enterotoxin B.)

This simplifies the analysis, since the T cells under investigation represent the majority and can be recognized by means of clonotypic or Vβ-specific antibodies. Thus a transgenic mouse, whose T cells largely express the TCR of a CD8⁺ Tc cell clone which recognizes a lymphocytic choriomeningitis virus (LCMV) glycoprotein presented by an H–2Dᵇ class I molecule, can be generated and then used to show positive selection. In these transgenics the TCR can be identified using antibodies specific for Vβ8, which forms part of this TCR.

Different MHC molecules have different effects on the development of mature CD8⁺ T cells expressing the transgenic TCR (Fig. 9.20). Only mice expressing the H–2ᵇ molecule show a biased development of CD8⁺ T cells using the Vβ8 chain of the transgenic TCR. This shows that this receptor is only positively selected in mice expressing the appropriate MHC haplotype. Positive selection occurs on cortical thymic epithelial cells.

NEGATIVE SELECTION IN THE THYMUS

Negative selection by clonal deletion has been demonstrated using monoclonal antibodies specific for murine TCR Vβ chains. Using this technique, it was possible to identify and count those T cells possessing TCRs with a given Vβ chain and to demonstrate that mice expressing I–E could delete Vβ17a⁺ T cells in the thymus. The presence of Vβ17a⁺CD4⁺CD8⁺ T cells but no mature Vβ17a⁺CD4⁺ T cells or Vβ17a⁺CD8⁺ T cells suggested that deletion occurred at the double positive (CD4⁺CD8⁺) stage of T-cell maturation. Deletion was shown to require expression of an endogenous ligand together with I–E, and not just I–E on its own.

T cell recognition of MLs-1ᵃ

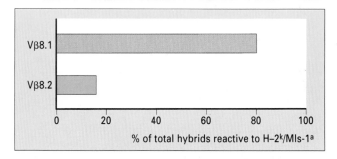

Fig. 9.22 A high frequency of T cells expressing Vβ8.1 recognize Mls-1ᵃ. T cell hybridomas were generated by fusing T cell blasts (expressing Vβ8.1 or Vβ8.2) from B10.Br (Mls-1ᵇ) lymph nodes with a variant of the T cell thymoma BW5147 (expressing neither Vα nor Vβ). These hybrids were separated by screening them with antibodies which recognized Vβ8.1 and (for comparison) Vβ8.2. They were then screened for reactivity against Mls-1ᵃ on H–2ᵏ stimulators. The great majority of the hybridomas reactive to this antigen were found to express Vβ8.1; a minority expressed Vβ8.2. This indicates the preference for use of Vβ8.1 in recognition of Mls-1ᵃ.

Comparable deletions were seen in Vβ6[+] and Vβ8.1[+] T cells in mice expressing the minor lymphocyte stimulating antigen (Mls) Mls[a] and certain MHC class II molecules (Fig. 9.21). This ability of whole families of T cells to recognize Mls explained the intense proliferative response obtained when Mls mismatched cells were cultured together. It showed that responses to certain antigens involve all the T cells expressing certain Vβ chains (Fig. 9.22). These antigens (some exogenous and some endogenous) which elicit such a powerful response are called superantigens. An example of an exogenous superantigen is Staphylococcal enterotoxin B (SEB). T cells in the mouse which respond to this antigen have TCR with Vβ3 or Vβ8 chains. One class of endogenous superantigens are those which gave rise to Mls antigens (see Chapter 7). It is now known that the Mls of a particular strain is determined by the presence of mouse mammary tumour viruses (MTVs) in the genome of that strain. The Mls antigens themselves are encoded by the open reading frames (ORFs) in the 3' LTR of these endogenous virus genomes. T cells expressing Vβ6 or Vβ8.1 respond to Mls[a] (defined by MTV-7). These endogenous superantigens are expressed in the thymus and cause deletion (negative selection) of T cells expressing TCRs with Vβ6 or Vβ8.1.

The transgenic mice described in the previous section (whose transgenes encode the α and β chains of a TCR specific for LCMV glycoprotein in the context of H–2D[b]) have also been used to demonstrate negative selection. When neonatally infected with LCMV, these mice became tolerant to, and carriers of, the virus. When the maturing T-cell populations in these neonatally infected mice are examined, there is a marked reduction in CD4[+]CD8[+] T cells, suggesting that clonal deletion of T cells has occurred at an early stage in ontogeny (Fig. 9.23). This negative selection is thought to occur as a result of antigen presentation to immature T cells by bone-marrow-derived cells within the thymus medulla. Whether thymus epithelial cells can also deliver such a negative signal remains controversial.

The expressed peripheral T-cell repertoire can therefore be shaped by both positive and negative selection (Fig. 9.24), thus affecting the immune response.

Tolerance to LCMV in transgenic mice

anti-LCMV (Vβ8.1) transgenic animal	neonatal LCMV infection	primary anti-LCMV response	thymocyte numbers	
			CD4[+]CD8[+]	CD8[+]
Mls–1[b]	–	+++	normal	normal
Mls–1[a]	–	+	normal	low
Mls–1[b]	+	–	low	low

Fig. 9.23 Tolerance induction in transgenic mice varies with the antigen. Transgenic mice expressing TCR specific for LCMV in the context of H–2D[b] were examined for their ability to mount a proliferative and cytotoxic response to CMV-infected cells. As this TCR also expresses Vβ8.1, it is possible to examine the influence of the presence of Mls–1[a] on the ability to make such a primary response to LCMV. Mice can also be infected at birth with LCMV, and so the effect of neonatal exposure to the antigen recognized by the transgenic TCR can be assessed. A partial reduction in both proliferation and cytotoxicity is seen in mice expressing Mls–1[a] and a total elimination of the response following neonatal exposure to the specific antigen. Analysis of the T-cell populations in these animals shows that LCMV-tolerant mice have markedly reduced numbers of CD4[+]CD8[+] thymocytes and mature CD8[+] T cells. On the other hand, exposure to the self-superantigen (Mls–1[a]) alone, results in the deletion of only mature CD8[+] T cells. This suggests that different antigens may tolerize T cells at different times during their development.

Positive and negative selection in the thymus

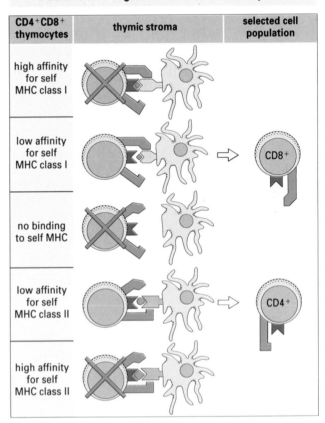

CD4[+]CD8[+] thymocytes	thymic stroma	selected cell population
high affinity for self MHC class I		
low affinity for self MHC class I		CD8[+]
no binding to self MHC		
low affinity for self MHC class II		CD4[+]
high affinity for self MHC class II		

Fig. 9.24 CD4[+]CD8[+] thymocytes interact with thymic stroma expressing MHC class I and MHC class II molecules complexed to self-peptides. Clones with high affinity for self-MHC class I or class II are deleted, as are clones which have no ability to recognize self-MHC. Clones with low affinity for self-MHC class I lose their CD4, to become CD8[+] T cells. Conversely, those that interact weakly with self-MHC class II molecules, mature into the CD4[+] population.

MHC–LINKED GENE CONTROL OF THE RESPONSE TO INFECTION

MHC-linked genes have been shown to play a role in the immune response to infectious agents and also to self antigens. In some cases the gene involved is an MHC gene itself, but in others it is thought to be a gene that is simply linked to the MHC.

The first observation that genes (*Ts-1* and *Ts-2*) within the MHC could influence the response to parasites involved the susceptibility to *Trichinella spiralis*. (It is interesting that such an effect should be noted with an antigenically complex organism, especially as these parasites express different antigens at different stages in their life cycle, with different APCs being involved in their presentation.) If different recombinant mouse strains are infected with *T. spiralis* it can be seen that resistance or susceptibility is affected by the I–E locus. Mouse strains which express I–E appear to be susceptible (Fig. 9.25). An additional MHC-linked gene has been shown to influence the response to *T. spiralis* but in this case it is not an MHC-encoding gene itself but another gene in linkage disequilibrium. This gene, which has been designated *Ts-2*, maps between *S* and *D*, close to the TNF genes.

The I–E subregion has also been shown to influence susceptibility to *Leishmania donovani*. Using H–2 congenic mice it was shown that I–E-expressing mice were unable to combat visceral leishmaniasis. Direct involvement of the I–E product in this susceptibility was shown by the ability of anti-I–E antibody, but not the anti-I–A antibody, to enhance parasite clearance.

MHC–LINKED GENE EFFECTS ON AUTOIMMUNE DISEASE

MHC associations have been found with several autoimmune diseases. For example, insulin-dependent diabetes mellitus (IDDM), an autoimmune disease in which the beta cells of the pancreas are destroyed by cells of the immune system, is associated with HLA-DR3 and HLA-DR4. The highest risk is in fact seen in HLA-DR3/4 heterozygotes. Again, because of linkage disequilibrium, although the original associations were seen with DR they are in reality with DQ. Molecular genetic analysis has permitted the association to be analysed in more detail, and it seems that the primary association in Caucasians is with DQB1*0302. In rheumatoid arthritis the predominant association is with HLA-DR4; there is little association with HLA-DQ. The way in which these disease associations contribute to susceptibility remains unclear, but possible explanations include repertoire differences through positive and negative selection on different class II genes, or preferential binding of disease-inducing epitopes on bacteria or viruses to particular MHC molecules.

Another example of linkage disequilibrium is that provided by the association of autoimmunity in the (NZB × NZW) F_1 mouse with the H–2^z of the NZW parent. It has been clearly demonstrated that this association was not with an MHC gene itself, but with the TNF_α gene closely linked to the MHC genes. The NZW TNF_α allele gives rise to the production of low amounts of TNF_α. If the concentration of this cytokine is increased, the mice are protected from the development of lupus nephritis (Fig. 9.26).

Other MHC-linked genes have recently been identified which may influence immune responses. These are genes which are involved in the generation (by proteolysis) and transport of antigen peptide fragments. These genes are polymorphic, and such polymorphism has functional consequences. For example, in the rat, different allelic forms of the *cim* locus affect peptide loading into the class I MHC, which in turn affects the ability of the class I MHC molecule to be recognized as an alloantigen. It is therefore possible that some of the

Susceptibility to *T. spiralis*

mouse strain	H–2 haplotype	I–E expression	resistance index	resistance phenotype
B10.BR	k	+	0	sus
B10.P	p	+	– 22	sus
B10.RIII	r	+	33	sus
B10	b	–	63	res/int
B10.S	s	–	100	res
B10.M	f	–	104	res
B10.Q	q	–	105	res

Fig. 9.25 Association of H-2 haplotype, expression of cell surface I–E molecules, and susceptibility to infection with *Trypanosoma spiralis*. The resistance index is measured as number of parasites present after a constant challenge, relative to strains B10.BR (susceptible = 0% resistance) and B10.S (resistant = 100% resistance).

TNF_α and lupus nephritis

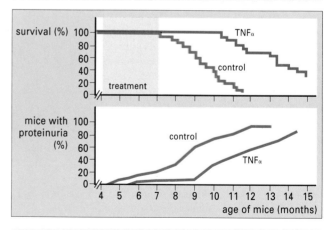

Fig. 9.26 Upper: Twenty (NZB × NZW) F_1 female mice were treated with recombinant murine TNF_α. Their survival is compared with age- and sex-matched F_1 controls.
Lower: Cumulative frequency of significant proteinuria (≥ 300 mg/dl) in (NZB × NZW) F_1 mice treated with TNF_α, and in controls.

MHC-linked disease associations which have been identified are attributable to similar genes, involved in proteolysis and transport of antigen peptides to the MHC molecules for presentation to cells of the immune system.

NON-MHC-LINKED IMMUNE RESPONSE GENES

The immune response is also governed by some genes outside the MHC region. This has been shown very clearly both in the genetic analyses of susceptibility and resistance to autoimmune diseases, and in studies of the immune responses to infectious organisms (Fig. 9.27). Individuals with defects in the complement component C3 show an increased susceptibility to bacterial infections and a predisposition towards immune-complex disease.

THE EFFECT OF NON-MHC–LINKED GENES ON THE RESPONSE TO INFECTION

Macrophages play a key role in the immune system. Genes regulating their activity may therefore determine the outcome of many immune responses. A good example of such genetic control of macrophage function is provided by the *Lsh/Ity/Bcg* gene. This gene governs the early response to infection with *Leishmania donovani*, *Salmonella typhimurium*, *Mycobacterium bovis*, *M. lepraemurium* and *M. intracellulare*. Its influence is on the the early phase of macrophage priming and activation, and it has wide-ranging effects (Fig. 9.28). The resistant allele of *Lsh/Ity/Bcg* up-regulates class II MHC antigen expression. One consequence of this activity is that it enhances the ability of the macrophages to present antigen to T cells.

Biozzi generated two lines of mice by selective inbreeding, based on their responsiveness to erythrocyte antigens. These high-responder and low-responder Biozzi mice make quantitatively different amounts of antibody in response to antigenic challenge. The basis for these differences has in part been attributed to genetic differences in macrophage activity. These high- and low-responder strains also differ markedly in their ability to respond to parasitic infections, and this does not necessarily correlate with the amount of antibody they make. (Fig. 9.29).

Eosinophils play an important role in the host response to parasitic infection. It has been shown that the degree of eosinophilia following infection is genetically determined, with marked differences being seen in different inbred strains of mice. Similar observations have been made in guinea pigs and sheep, where a consistent correlation has been found between resistance to nematode infection and the extent of eosinophilia.

NON-MHC–LINKED GENES AFFECT DEVELOPMENT OF AUTOIMMUNE DISEASE

Most autoimmune diseases have been shown to be influenced not only by MHC-linked genes, but also by genes not linked to this complex. Recently, major advances have been made in mapping the loci which govern susceptibility to the autoimmune disease insulin-dependent diabetes mellitus (IDDM). This work

Effect of the *Lsh* gene on macrophage activity

up-regulation of the oxidative burst
enhanced tumoricidal activity
enhanced antimicrobial activity
up-regulation of class II MHC expression

Fig. 9.28 The *Lsh/Ity/Bcg* gene enhances macrophage APC type activity. Other effects are also described.

Role of non-MHC genes in resistance to infection

organism	resistant		susceptible	
	strain	haplotype	strain	haplotype
Mycobacterium lepraemurium	DBA/2J	d	BALB/cJ	d
	C3H/HeJ	k	C3H/A	k
Salmonella typhimurium	DBA/2J	d	B10.D2, BALB/c	d d
M. tuberculosis	CBA, C3H	k	B10.BR	k
Listeria monocytogenes	B10.A	a	A/J	a
	B10.D2	d	DBA/2, BALB/c	d
	B10.BR	k	CBA, C3H	k
Rickettsia tsutsugamushi	AKR	k	C3H, CBA	k
	SWR	q	DBA/1	q
	BALB/c	d	DBA/2	d

Fig. 9.27 Different strains of mice vary in their resistance to the organisms listed. Since different strains with the same MHC haplotype can be susceptible or resistant, this shows that the MHC haplotype is not critical in determining resistance to infection.

Response of Biozzi mice to parasite infection

organism	Biozzi high	Biozzi low
T. cruzi	resistant	susceptible
P. berghei	resistant	susceptible
P. yoelii	resistant	susceptible
L. major	susceptible	resistant
S. mansoni	susceptible	resistant

Fig. 9.29 High- and low-responder Biozzi mice show a differential responsiveness to parasitic infections, which is not consistent within the high and low responder groups.

has been largely carried out using the NOD mouse strain which spontaneously develops an autoimmune disease similar to IDDM in man. At least 5 genetic loci have been identified in the NOD mouse (*Idd-1,2,3,4* and *5*) with only one locus (*Idd-1*) being linked to the mouse MHC on chromosome 17, and thought to encode MHC class II antigens themselves. The other genes *Idd-2,3,4* and *5* have been mapped to chromosomes 9,3,11 and 1 respectively but their identity remains to be clarified.

When the lymphoproliferative (lpr) gene is introduced into mouse strains it causes the development of a characteristic clinical syndrome. The mice develop anti-DNA antibodies, rheumatoid factor, circulating immune-complexes and glomerulonephritis. There is also a lymphadenopathy in these mice involving an expansion of CD4$^-$CD8$^-$ T cells in the periphery. These T cells are not monoclonal, but have differently arranged TCRs. It was suggested that the syndrome was due to a defect in negative selection, but it was difficult to see how a gene such as *lpr* could mediate this effect. Recently it has been shown that mice with the lpr gene have a defect in the Fas antigen which is encoded by a gene on chromosome 19. This defect results in the failure of apoptosis and, therefore, of negative selection of T cells in the thymus. It is proposed that this results in an escape of autoreactive T cells into the periphery and causes the onset of an autoimmune syndrome.

These studies further suggest that the gld gene, which has been shown to result in a similar autoimmune phenotype to that seen in *lpr* mice, may arise from a related defect. It is proposed that gld is the ligand for the Fas antigen. Mice which are *gld/gld* do not express the ligand, do not display negative selection and therefore develop autoimmunity. The gld gene is located on chromosome 1 in the mouse and thus provides yet another example of a gene which affects immune function, but which is not MHC linked.

FURTHER READING

Blalock JE, Bost KL, eds. Neuroimmunoendocrinology. *Allergy; vol 43.* Basel: Karger.

Coffman RL, Savelkoul HFJ, Lebman DA. Cytokine regulation of immunoglobulin isotype switch and expression. *Semin Immunol* 1989;**1**:55.

Cohen PL, Eisenberg RA. The lpr and gld genes in systemic autoimmunity: life and death in the *fas* lane. *Immunol Today* 1992;**13**:427.

Gershon RK, Kondo K. Infectious immunological tolerance. *Immunology* 1972;**21**:903.

Gaulton GN, Greene MI. Idiotypic mimicry of biological receptors. *Ann Rev Immunol* 1986;**4**:253.

Goodnow CC, Adelstein S, Basten A. The need for central and peripheral tolerance in the B cell repertoire. *Science.* 1990;**248**:1373.

Herman A, Kappler JW, Marrack P, Pullen A. Superantigens: mechanisms of T cell stimulation and role in immune responses. *Ann Rev Immunol* 1991;**9**:745.

Jerne NJ. Towards a network theory of the immune system. *Ann Immunol (Paris)* 1974;**1235c**:373.

Mason D, MacPhee I, Antoni F. The role of the neuroendocrine system in determining genetic susceptibility to experimental allergic encephalomyelitis in the rat. *Immunology* 1990;**70**:1–5.

Stein KE, Soderstrom T. Neonatal administration of idiotype or anti-idiotype primes for protection against *Escherichia coli* K13 infection in mice. *J Exp Med* 1984;**160**:101.

Schwartz RH. A cell culture method for T cell clonal anergy. *Science* 1990;**248**:1349.

Wakelin D, Blackwell JK. Genetic variations in immunity to parasite infection. In: *Immunology and Molecular Biology of Parasitic Infections.* Oxford: Blackwell Scientific Publications, 1991.

Zinkernagel RM, Pircher HP, Ohashi P, *et al.* T and B cell tolerance and responses to viral antigens in transgenic mice: implications for the pathogenesis of autoimmune versus immunopathological disease. *Immunol Rev* 1991;**122**:133.

chapter 10

Immunological Tolerance

Immunological tolerance refers to a state of unresponsiveness which is specific for a particular antigen, and is induced by prior exposure to that antigen. Tolerance can be induced to non-self antigens, but the most important aspect of tolerance is self-tolerance, which prevents the body from mounting an immune attack against itself. The potential for attacking the body's own cells arises because the immune system randomly generates a great diversity of antigen-specific receptors (see Chapter 5), some of which will be self-reactive. Cells bearing these receptors must be eliminated, either functionally or physically.

Self-reactivity is prevented by processes which occur during development, rather than being genetically pre-programmed. Thus animals of histo-incompatible strains A and B reject each other's skin, but F_1 hybrid offspring of matings between A and B (which express the antigens of both parents) do not reject either A skin or B skin. Yet the ability to reject such skin reappears in homozygotes of the F_2 progeny. Clearly, therefore, self–non-self discrimination is learned during development, and immunological 'self' must encompass all epitopes encoded in the individual's DNA, other epitopes being considered as non-self.

Yet the structure of a molecule does not *per se* determine the ability to distinguish self from non-self. Attributes other than the structural characteristics of an epitope must also be sensed. Among these are the time when lymphocytes are first confronted with epitopes, the site of encounter, the nature of the cells presenting epitopes, and the production by these cells of 'co-stimulatory' molecules influencing lymphocyte responsiveness.

HISTORICAL BACKGROUND

Soon after antibody specificity was established, it was realized that some mechanism must operate to prevent autoantibody formation. At the turn of the century, for example, Ehrlich coined the term *horror autotoxicus*, implying the need for a 'regulating contrivance' to stop production of autoantibodies. In 1938, Traub induced specific tolerance by inoculating mice *in utero* with lymphocytic choriomeningitis virus, producing an infection which was maintained throughout life. Unlike normal mice, these inoculated mice did not produce neutralizing antibodies when challenged with the virus in adult life. That cells carrying different antigens could develop within the same host, was reported in 1945 by Owen, who described an 'experiment of nature' in non-identical twin cattle. These exchanged haemopoietic (stem) cells via shared placental blood vessels and each animal carried the erythrocyte markers of both

calves. They exhibited life-long tolerance to the otherwise foreign cells, in being unable to mount antibody responses to the relevant erythrocyte antigens (Fig. 10.1). Following this observation, Burnet and Fenner postulated in 1949 that body cells carried 'self-marker' components which allowed recognition of their 'self' character, and that the time of encounter was the critical factor in determining responsiveness and hence recognition of non-self epitopes. The hypothesis seemed logical, as the immune system is usually confronted with most self components before birth and only later with non-self antigens. Experimental support of this notion came in 1953, when Medawar and his colleagues induced immunological tolerance to skin allografts in mice by neonatal injection of allogeneic cells (see Fig. 10.2). This phenomenon could easily be accommodated in Burnet's clonal selection theory (1957), which states that a particular immunocyte is selected by antigen and then divides to give rise to a clone of daughter cells, all with the same specificity. Antigens encountered after birth activate specific clones to proliferate and produce antibody, whereas antigen encountered before birth results in the clonal deletion of these cells, which Burnet termed 'forbidden clones'.

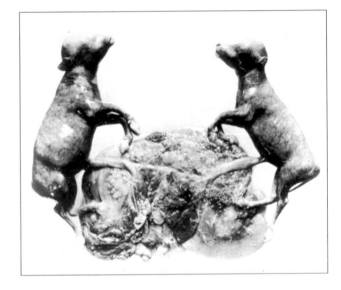

Fig. 10.1 Dizygotic cattle twins fused at the placentae.
Fusion of the placentae leads to exchange of blood cells in fetal life. Following separation, each animal permanently retains the cells of its twin. Although they are genetically different (dizygotic), each twin is permanently tolerant of the other's tissue type.

Implicit in this theory is the need for the entire immune repertoire to be generated before birth, but in fact lymphocyte differentiation continues long after birth. The key factor in determining responsiveness is thus not the developmental stage of the individual, but rather the state of maturity of the lymphocyte, at the time it encounters antigen. This was suggested by Lederberg in 1959, in his modification of the clonal selection theory: immature lymphocytes contacting antigen would be subject to 'clonal abortion', whereas mature cells would be activated. In the unborn and the neonate, most of the cells of the immune system have yet to reach maturity, so the individual is particularly susceptible to tolerance induction at this stage.

Key discoveries in the 1960s established the immunological competence of the small lymphocyte, the crucial role of the thymus in the development of the immune system, and the existence of two interacting subsets of lymphocytes, T and B cells. This set the scene for a thorough investigation of the cellular mechanisms involved in tolerogenesis. It was discovered that both T and B cells may be tolerized independently, according to the circumstances. Susceptibility varies, the threshold of tolerization for T cells being lower than for B cells.

EXPERIMENTAL METHODS

Until recently, only artificially induced tolerance was amenable to experimental study: antigens or foreign cells were inoculated into an animal and the fate of responding T or B cells was investigated under a variety of circumstances. It was not clear, however, to what extent these experimental models resembled natural self tolerance.

Transgenic methods have now made possible the direct investigation of self-tolerance. Such methods allow one to introduce a specific gene into mice of defined genetic background and analyse its effects upon the development of the immune system. If the

Induction of specific tolerance in mice

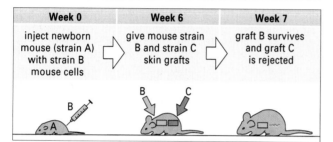

Fig. 10.2 This demonstrates the induction of specific tolerance to grafted skin in mice by neonatal injection of spleen cells from a different strain. Mice of strain A normally reject grafts from strain B. However, if newborn mice of strain A receive cells from strain B mice, at six weeks of age they show tolerance towards skin grafts from the donor strain B, but reject grafts from other strains (C).

Development pathway of murine thymocytes

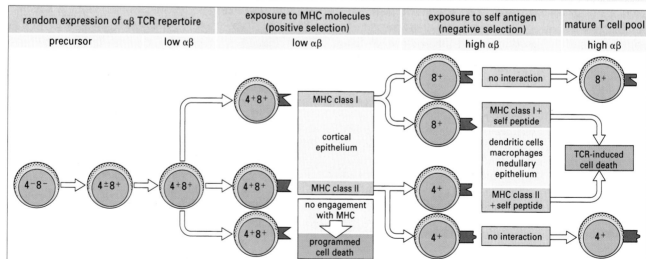

Fig. 10.3 Precursor thymocytes develop into cortical 'double positive' cells expressing low levels of the αβ TCR. These undergo positive selection for interaction with self MHC class I or class II molecules on cortical epithelium. Unselected cells (the majority) undergo programmed cell death. Cells interacting with class I MHC lose CD4 and cells interacting with MHC class II lose CD8. Finally autoreactive cells are eliminated by interaction with self peptides presented on cells at the corticomedullary junction and in the thymic medulla.

introduced gene is linked to a tissue-specific promoter, its expression can be confined to specific cell types: for example, a histocompatibility gene linked to the promoter for insulin will be expressed in the pancreatic islets where insulin-producing cells reside. The protein product encoded by the 'transgene' is treated by the immune system essentially as an authentic self antigen, and its effects may be studied *in vivo* without the trauma and inflammation associated with grafting foreign cells or tissues. In addition, the parent strain and the transgenic strain provide ideal congenic lines for control experiments and lymphocyte transfer studies.

ROUTES TO TOLERANCE

There are four possible ways in which self-reactive lymphocytes may be prevented from responding:

1. by physically deleting them from the peripheral repertoire (clonal deletion)
2. by preventing the further differentiation of the immature cell (clonal abortion)
3. by downregulating the mechanism of response (clonal anergy)
4. by continuously inhibiting cellular activity through interaction with other cells, such as cells producing inhibitory lymphokines (so-called suppressor cells, e.g. TH2 cells – see Chapter 7), or anti-idiotypic cells reactive against the antigen-receptor.

Which of these fates awaits the self-reactive lymphocyte depends on numerous factors. Among these are the stage of maturity of the cell being silenced, its distribution and developmental pattern of expression, its affinity for the autoantigen, the nature of this antigen and its concentration and the availability of costimulatory signals. As a general rule, if there is no costimulation, antigen is more likely to signal a cell negatively, switching off its ability to respond, than to stimulate an immune response. However, more work is needed to define precisely the conditions required for inducing anergy, abortion or deletion, and the biochemical and molecular mechanisms involved.

 ## T-CELL TOLERANCE TO SELF ANTIGENS

The thymus is central to the development of T cells. Within the thymus, T cells develop from precursors which have not undergone rearrangement of their T-cell receptor (TCR) genes. There too, T cells acquire the 'education' which ensures that they respond to antigens only in the context of molecules encoded by self MHC molecules (see Chapter 6). It seems likely, therefore, that self-reactive T cells are also dealt with in the thymus.

INTRATHYMIC CLONAL DELETION

As described in Chapters 3 and 11, the high proliferative rate of thymocytes is paralleled by a massive rate of cell death: the vast majority of T cells, at the double positive (CD4$^+$CD8$^+$) stage, die within the thymus. Among the factors which account for this are aberrant

TCR rearrangement, negative selection and failure to be positively selected (Fig. 10.3 – see also Chapter 11). Positive selection occurs when T cells, with some degree of binding avidity for polymorphic regions of MHC molecules, are selected for survival. The MHC molecules are encountered on thymic cortical epithelial cells, and binding is presumed to protect the cells from programmed cell death (see Chapter 11). This positive selection process ensures that the mature T cell only recognizes antigen (peptides) when associated with self MHC molecules, and so will be self-MHC restricted. Negative selection, on the other hand, eliminates self-reactive T cells, discarding those clones of T cells that are specifically reactive to self-antigens present intrathymically. For example, so-called superantigens can combine with MHC class II molecules to form ligands that stimulate whole families of T cells via certain V$_\beta$ segments of the TCR. In mice having these antigens, cells with such TCRs which can be tagged by appropriate monoclonal antibodies, were found in the immature population of thymus lymphocytes, but not in the mature intrathymic or peripheral T-cell pools (Fig. 10.4). The T cells were thus deleted during their differ-

Intrathymic clonal elimination of T cells reactive to superantigens

TCR V$_\beta$ segment used	superantigen recognized (+ MHC class II)	% T cells expressing V$_\beta$ segment in mice	
		Ag$^-$ (immature)	Ag$^+$ (post tolerization)
V$_\beta$3	Mls–2^a Mls–3^a SEA, SED	4	<0.5
V$_\beta$6	Mls–1^a	12	<0.5
V$_\beta$8.1–8.3	SEB	19	0
V$_\beta$8.1	Mls–1^a	7	<0.5
V$_\beta$11	I–E + a peptide	5	0.5
V$_\beta$17a	I–E + a peptide	6	1

Fig. 10.4 T cells bearing TCRs utilizing certain V$_\beta$ segments may be tagged by appropriate monoclonal antibodies. Some of these TCR V$_\beta$ domains confer reactivity to so-called superantigens, such as the class II MHC molecule I–E, or alleles of the minor lymphocyte stimulating (MLS) locus. In mice having these alloantigens, or injected with exogenous superantigens (e.g. staphylococcal enterotoxins, SEA, SEB, SED), TCRs were found in the immature population of thymus lymphocytes, but not in the mature intrathymic or peripheral T cell pools. The T cells were thus deleted during their differentiation in the thymus.

entiation in the thymus. Furthermore, in mice transgenic for rearranged TCR directed to the male (H–Y) antigen in the context of the class I H–2D^b MHC molecule, H–Y-autospecific T cells were deleted in male mice, but not in female mice, which do not express H–Y.

Thymic cells involved in negative selection

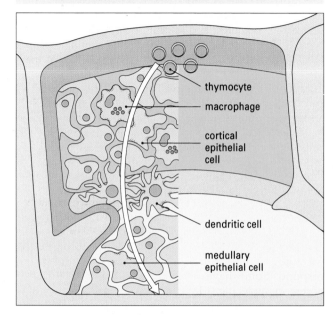

Fig. 10.5 The deleting population includes bone marrow-derived macrophages, or dendritic cells, which are situated predominantly at the corticomedullary junction. Other cells involved in deletion may be the thymocytes themselves, through their veto function, and some types of thymic epithelial cells, possibly in the medulla.

The veto effect

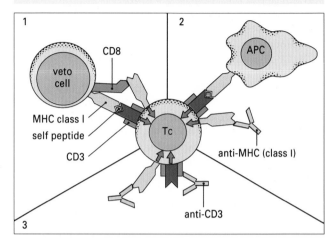

Fig. 10.6 1. Specialized veto cells bearing self-epitopes can kill a self-reactive clone.
2. The veto effect can be mimicked using an APC to present self antigen to the T cell, combined with a monoclonal antibody which binds to the class I molecule of the T cell.
3. The veto effect can also be reproduced using a monoclonal antibody, as in (2), and another monoclonal antibody in place of the APC. This antibody binds to the CD3 molecule on the T cell, suggesting that the message from the TCR is passed to the cell via the CD3.

Experimental evidence for post-thymic induction of tolerance

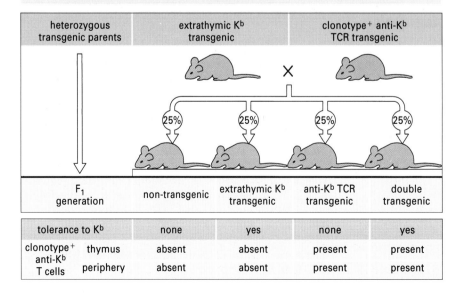

	heterozygous transgenic parents	extrathymic K^b transgenic		clonotype$^+$ anti-K^b TCR transgenic
F$_1$ generation	non-transgenic	extrathymic K^b transgenic	anti-K^b TCR transgenic	double transgenic
tolerance to K^b	none	yes	none	yes
clonotype$^+$ anti-K^b T cells — thymus	absent	absent	present	present
clonotype$^+$ anti-K^b T cells — periphery	absent	absent	present	present

Fig. 10.7 Non-b haplotype mice were given the gene for the foreign MHC class I molecule, H–2K^b, which was expressed only in extrathymic tissue. These transgenics were crossed to mice which had been given genes for a TCR directed against H–2K^b (more than 90% of the T cells were anti-H–2K^b and traceable by clonotypic antibody). Double transgenic offspring express H–2K^b in non-thymic sites and have anti-H–2K^b T cells. However, they are tolerant of H–2K^b in extrathymic tissue (K^b-bearing, but otherwise compatible skin grafts are not rejected). Clonotypic antibody tests show that they have not deleted either the thymic or the peripheral anti-H–2K^b T cells Both are present but anergic.

The timing and precise localization of negative selection depends on a variety of factors, including the accessibility of developing T cells to self-antigen, the combined avidity of the TCR and accessory molecules, CD8 or CD4 (see Chapter 2), for the self-MHC–self-peptide complex, and the identity of the deleting cells. Elimination of self-reactive cells is clearly a function of the thymic dendritic cells or macrophages which are rich in class I and II molecules and situated predominantly at the corticomedullary junction (Fig. 10.5). Some medullary or cortical epithelial cells may also impose negative selection. Other cells involved in deletion may be the thymocytes themselves. Specialized 'veto' cells bearing self epitopes would impart a negative signal, killing the self-reactive clone (Fig. 10.6). Under physiological conditions, veto signals occur when a T cell with TCRs for self antigens binds to a veto cell. The veto cell is a specialized T cell expressing self epitopes. For the veto effect to occur, the TCR has to bind to self antigen in association with MHC class I on the veto cell, while the CD8 of the veto cell binds to MHC class I on the T cell. Once binding has occurred, the T cell is killed.

B-cell response to self or foreign antigens

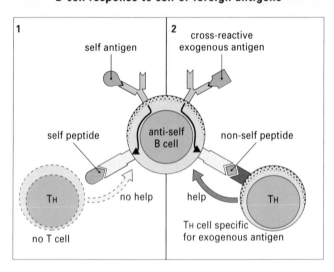

Fig. 10.8 1. If TH cells are not available, either because of a hole in the T cell repertoire (see Chapter 9), or because of deletion resulting from self-tolerance achieved intrathymically, any self-reactive B cells will be unable to mount an anti-self antibody response. 2. Autoantibodies can be produced if a self-reactive B cell collaborates with an anti-foreign TH cell in response to complexes between self and foreign antigens. Likewise the response to a foreign antigen could in some cases lead to autoantibodies because the antibodies cross-react between the foreign antigen and the self antigen. Hence there is a need to purge the B cell repertoire of self-reactive B cells.

POST-THYMIC TOLERANCE

Extrathymic antigens may not provoke an immune response if they elude the immune system. This may be the case if they are:
1. sequestered in an immunologically privileged site
2. exposed on certain cell types which do not express MHC molecules and would thus be unable to present antigens to T cells
3. present in amounts too low to be detected by T cells.

Extrathymic antigens may also escape attack if the avidity of the combined TCR and accessory molecules is not high enough for the T cell to make effective contact with the antigen. However caused, any such lack of activation is not equivalent to tolerance, since presentation of the antigen in an immunogenic form would produce a reaction.

Evasion of the immune system by extrathymic autoantigens may be one way in which autoimmune responses are avoided. Yet it is a precarious one, given that molecules may be released from dying cells and hence processed and presented by macrophages. As autoimmunity is unusual, fail-safe mechanisms must exist to induce tolerance to extrathymic autoantigens by peripheral T cells. Anergy in these self-reactive T cells has now been demonstrated: the T cells are not physically eliminated, at least initially, but fail to respond. Some have downregulated their TCR, their accessory molecule (CD8), or both (Fig. 10.7).

B-CELL TOLERANCE TO SELF ANTIGENS

Production of high-affinity IgG autoantibodies is T-cell dependent (see Chapter 7). For this reason, and since the threshold of tolerance for T cells is lower than for B cells, the simplest explanation for non-self-reactivity by B cells is a lack of T cell help. Nevertheless, circumstances exist in which B cells need to be tolerized directly. For example, there may be cross-reactive antigens on microorganisms, which include both foreign T-cell-reactive epitopes and other epitopes resembling self epitopes and capable of stimulating B cells. Such antigens could result in a vigorous antibody response to self antigens (Fig. 10.8). Furthermore, in contrast to TCRs, the immunoglobulin receptors on mature, antigenically-stimulated B cells can undergo hypermutation and may acquire anti-self reactivities at this late stage. Tolerance must thus be imposed on B cells, both during their development and after antigenic stimulation in secondary lymphoid tissues.

The fate of self-reactive B cells has been determined using transgenic technology. The transgenic models depicted in Figs 10.9 and 10.10 showed that tolerization by self-antigens could lead to one of several end results. The outcome depends on the affinity of the B-cell antigen receptor and on the nature of the antigen it encounters, whether an integral membrane protein, such as an MHC class I molecule, or a soluble and largely monomeric protein present in the circulation.

CLONAL DELETION

When B cells encounter cell-membrane-associated self-antigens (as shown in the transgenic model in Fig. 10.9) capable of cross-linking Ig receptors on the B cells with high avidity, the B cells are eliminated from lymphoid tissues. This type of tolerance occurs whether the self-antigens are expressed on cells in the bone marrow or elsewhere. In either case, the bone marrow contains residual self-reactive B cells, suggesting that immature B cells are less readily deleted than immature T cells during the early stages of differentiation.

CLONAL ANERGY

If self-reactive B cells are exposed to soluble antigen that is largely monomeric (not capable of cross-linking receptors), then the cells are not deleted from secondary lymphoid tissues, where they can be found in normal numbers, but are rendered anergic. This effect, as illustrated in Fig. 10.10, only occurs when the antigen is above a critical concentration threshold. Anergy is associated with downregulation of the membrane IgM receptor. The maturation of the self-reactive B cells is also arrested, in the follicular mantle zone, and there

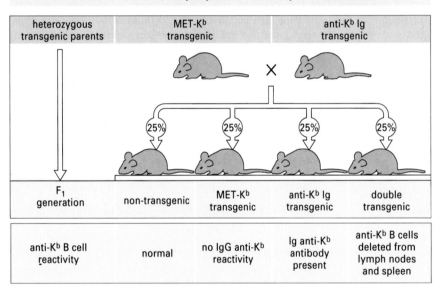

Tolerance induction in peripheral B cells by clonal deletion

heterozygous transgenic parents	MET-K^b transgenic		anti-K^b Ig transgenic
F$_1$ generation	non-transgenic	MET-K^b transgenic	anti-K^b Ig transgenic	double transgenic
anti-K^b B cell reactivity	normal	no IgG anti-K^b reactivity	Ig anti-K^b antibody present	anti-K^b B cells deleted from lymph nodes and spleen

Fig. 10.9 Non-b haplotype mice were given the gene for H–2K^b, a foreign MHC class I and a membrane protein. The gene was controlled by the metallothionein promoter, specific for sites such as the liver (MET–K^b transgenic). These mice were crossed to other non-b mice which had been given the gene for anti-H–2K^b Ig antibodies (anti-K^b Ig transgenic). Double transgenic offspring express H–2K^b in the liver and export B cells specific for H–2K^b from the marrow. However, these B cells are partially deleted in the spleen and entirely deleted in the lymph nodes, and never have the chance to produce antibodies. No idiotype identical to the anti-K^b Ig in the transgenic parents was detected.

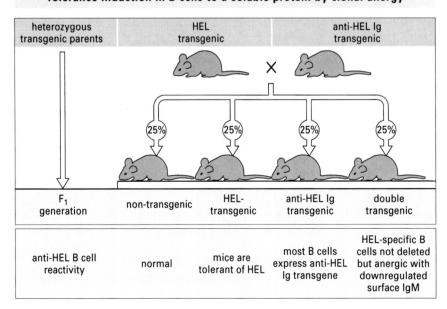

Tolerance induction in B cells to a soluble protein by clonal anergy

heterozygous transgenic parents	HEL transgenic		anti-HEL Ig transgenic
F$_1$ generation	non-transgenic	HEL-transgenic	anti-HEL Ig transgenic	double transgenic
anti-HEL B cell reactivity	normal	mice are tolerant of HEL	most B cells express anti-HEL Ig transgene	HEL-specific B cells not deleted but anergic with downregulated surface IgM

Fig. 10.10 A mouse line was given the hen egg lysozyme (HEL) gene, linked to a tissue-specific promoter. The (largely soluble) HEL led to T- and B-cell tolerance. A second transgenic line (anti-HEL Ig) carried rearranged heavy and light chain genes encoding a high-affinity anti-HEL antibody. An allotype marker (IgH^a) distinguished it from endogenous immunoglobulin (IgH^b). The majority of B cells in these transgenics carried IgM and IgD of the 'a' allotype. Double transgenic offspring were highly HEL-tolerant, producing neither anti-HEL antibody nor plaque-forming cells. HEL-binding (self reactive) B cells were not deleted but had downregulated surface IgM, but not IgD, receptors. They behaved as anergic cells.

is a striking reduction in marginal zone B cells with high levels of surface IgM. No evidence for the activity of Ts cells or of anti-idiotypic B cells was found in these transgenic models.

ARTIFICIALLY INDUCED TOLERANCE *IN VIVO*

Tolerance can be induced artificially *in vivo* by a variety of means.

1. Tolerance can be induced in neonatal hosts by inoculation of allogeneic cells. This method is also effective in adult hosts after immunosuppressive regimes, such as total body irradiation, drugs (for example, cyclosporin A), or anti-lymphocytic antibodies (for example, anti-lymphocyte globulin, anti-CD4 etc.). For tolerance to be maintained, a certain degree of chimerism must be obtained, with some allogeneic cells persisting in their host. This is best achieved if the inoculum contains cells capable of self-renewal (bone marrow cells, for example).

2. Tolerance of transplanted tissues has been achieved in adult animals by monoclonal antibodies directed to CD4 and CD8. These antibodies may or may not deplete the total numbers of T cells. In this situation, tolerance of skin allografts could be obtained even in the absence of bone-marrow chimerism.

3. Tolerance can be induced in neonatal and adult animals by the administration of soluble protein antigens in deaggregated form. At the level of the animal as a whole, T and B cells differ in their susceptibility to tolerization by these antigens. For example, tolerance is achieved in T cells from spleen and thymus with rather low doses and within a few hours. Tolerance of spleen B cells requires much longer time and higher doses (Fig. 10.11). Levels of antigen which will produce B-cell tolerance in neonates are about one-hundredth of those in adults (Fig 10.12).

4. Tolerance in T cells (and to a lesser extent in B cells), can be due to clonal exhaustion, the end result of a powerful immune response. Repeated antigenic challenge may stimulate all the antigen-responding cells to differentiate into short-lived end cells, leaving no cells that can respond to a subsequent challenge with antigen.

5. T_{ind} antigens tend to be slowly metabolized *in vivo* and therefore tend to produce long-lasting B-cell

---

The relative susceptibilities of T cells and B cells to tolerization *in vivo*

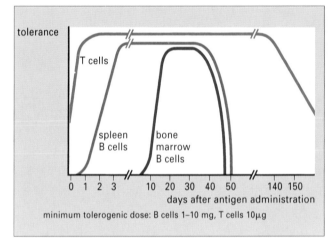

minimum tolerogenic dose: B cells 1–10 mg, T cells 10μg

Fig. 10.11 The relative susceptibilities of T cells and B cells to tolerization *in vivo*. A mouse is given antigen (human globulin – a T_{dep} antigen) at tolerance inducing (tolerogenic) doses, and the duration of tolerance is measured. T-cell tolerance is more rapidly induced and more persistent than B-cell tolerance. Bone marrow B cells may take considerably longer than splenic B cells to tolerize. Typically, much lower antigen doses are sufficient for T cell tolerization: 10 mg as opposed to 1–10 μg, a 1000-fold difference.

Tolerance susceptibility of neonatal B cells to a T_{ind} antigen *in vivo* and *in vitro*

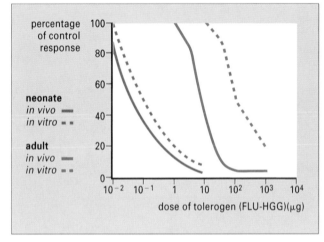

Fig. 10.12 The antibody response is represented as a percentage of the normal response. The dose required to achieve tolerance in the neonate is about one-hundredth that required in the adult, since in the neonatal period all B cells are at an early stage of their clinical ontogeny and are relatively easily tolerized. It is easier to tolerize B cells *in vivo* than *in vitro*, a phenomenon which is probably related to the different methods of antigen presentation in the lymphoid tissue *in vivo*.

tolerance, provided a large enough antigen dose is used (Fig. 10.13). A very high concentration of those antigens can actually blockade the surface receptors of fully differentiated antibody-forming cells (AFCs) and prevent them from secreting antibody (Fig. 10.14).

6. The antibody-combining site may act as an antigen and induce the formation of 'anti-idiotypic antibodies'. By cross-linking immunoglobulins on B cells, these antibodies can block the responsiveness of the cell. Tolerance to an antigen is only partial since it only affects B cells carrying one idiotype (Fig. 10.15). However, in some animals, the majority of antibodies produced in response to some antigens carry a particular idiotype, so suppression of this idiotype can significantly affect the response.

7. In some systems, tolerance appears to have been induced and to be transferable by veto cells (see Fig. 10.6) or by 'T suppressor cells' (Ts cells), which have yet to be fully characterized. One candidate for these cells is the TH2 subset of TH cells. TH1 and TH2 differ in their functions and patterns of lymphokine production (see Chapter 8). TH1 cells produce IL-2 and IFN$_\gamma$ and are involved in Type IV or delayed-type hypersensitivity (DTH). TH2 cells secrete IL-4, IL-5 and IL-10 and help B cells produce antibody. IL-10 can also suppress the activities of TH1 cells by an effect on antigen-presenting cells (APCs), and thereby the production of TH1 lymphokines active in DTH reactions (Fig. 10.16).

MAINTAINING TOLERANCE

Persistence of antigen plays a major role in maintaining the tolerance state *in vivo*. Responsiveness returns after the antigen concentration drops below a certain threshold. If tolerance results from clonal deletion or permanent anergy, recovery is related to the time required to generate new lymphocytes from the stem cell pool. Thus recovery can be prevented by measures such as thymectomy.

ARTIFICIALLY INDUCED TOLERANCE *IN VITRO*

B cells can readily be tolerized *in vitro*. Antigens which cross-link the immunoglobulin receptors, but which do not possess intrinsic mitogenic capacity, can do this. They must be at high concentration for mature B cells, but low concentrations work for immature cells. For example, a monoclonal anti-IgM antibody was used to mimic antigen cross-linking of the B-cell immunoglobulin receptors. High concentrations clonally aborted pre-B cells, preventing their further differentiation to surface membrane IgM-bearing (mIgM$^+$) B cells. Lower concentrations allowed pre-B cells to develop into morphologically normal B cells, with normal numbers of immunoglobulin receptors, but rendered them profoundly anergic (Fig. 10.17). Hence, both B cell

Dose-dependency of the response to a T$_{ind}$ antigen

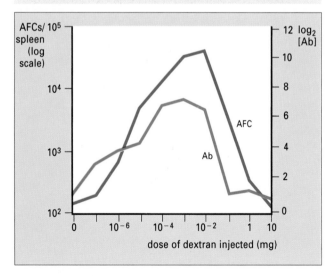

Fig. 10.13 Different groups of mice were injected with different doses of dextran B512 and the resulting levels of antibody were assessed. The dose of dextran required for tolerance induction appears to be lower with the antibody assay than with the AFC counts. This is because high levels of antigen tend to bind and remove much of the antibody in immune complexes. The AFC curve thus represents tolerance at the B cell level.

B cell clonal deletion and AFC blockade

type of tolerance	minimum effective tolerogenic dose		isotype susceptibility	tolerance attainable
	dextran (500 kDa)	levan (6 kDa)		
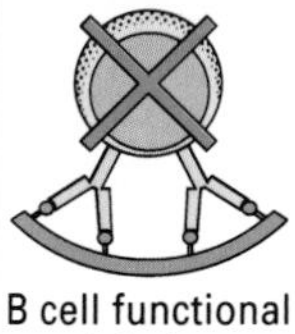 B cell functional deletion	1 mg	10 mg	IgG>IgM	complete
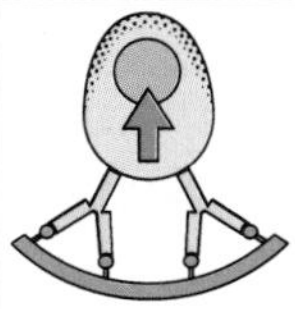 AFC blockade	0.01 mg	inactive	IgG<IgM	partial

Fig. 10.14 Binding of a T$_{ind}$ antigen to the B cell's receptors may cause functional deletion of the B cell clone, or reduce antibody production by interfering with processes involved in antibody secretion. These two tolerance mechanisms may be distinguished by the minimum effective dose of tolerogens and their molecular weight, the relative susceptibility of different classes of antibody affected and the level of tolerance attainable.

function and B cell numbers can be modulated via their surface immunoglobulin receptors, at the critical time of acquisition of these receptors (the pre-B to B cell transition).

As already mentioned, it is generally believed that antigen encounter (signal 1), in the absence of any accompanying co-stimulator activity (signal 2), is tolerogenic. The nature of the co-stimulator is unknown, although cytokines from TH cells and some forms of cell membrane perturbations, may contribute. As for the form of tolerance induced, the degree of receptor occupancy and cross-linking appears to determine whether

a particular antigen induces abortion or anergy in B cells. Factors contributing to the pathway a B cell will take include antigen valency and concentration, receptor affinity for the binding epitope of the antigen, and the state of maturity of the B cell. At one end of the spectrum is clonal abortion, likely to occur in less mature cells, especially those possessing a higher affinity epitope-binding receptor or encountering antigens of higher valency and concentration (see Fig. 10.18). At the opposite end, no effect occurs at low concentrations and affinities. Clonal anergy is induced in circumstances that lie between these two extremes.

Suppression by anti-idiotype

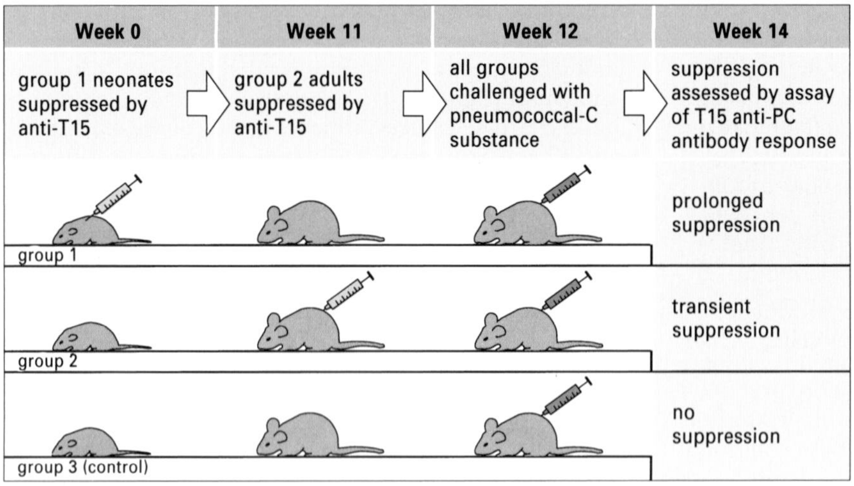

Week 0	Week 11	Week 12	Week 14
group 1 neonates suppressed by anti-T15	group 2 adults suppressed by anti-T15	all groups challenged with pneumococcal-C substance	suppression assessed by assay of T15 anti-PC antibody response

group 1 — prolonged suppression

group 2 — transient suppression

group 3 (control) — no suppression

Fig. 10.15 BALB/c mice normally produce T15 idiotype antibody to the phosphorylcholine (PC) determinant on pneumococcal-C-substance. Neonatal exposure to anti-idiotype (anti-T15 antibody) induces prolonged suppression of the T15 anti-PC response, whereas exposure in the adults leads to transient suppression. It is presumed that the prolonged suppression is due to clonal abortion, and the transient adult suppression to AFC blockade and B cell exhaustion. The suppression is passively induced in this example since the suppressive agent (anti-T15) is injected, not actively generated by the individual.

T-cell suppression of immune responsiveness

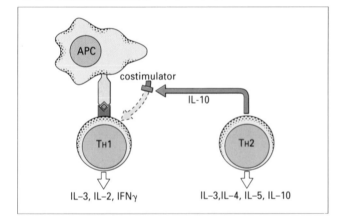

Fig. 10.16 Two subsets of TH cells, TH1 and TH2, exist. Each subset has a distinct pattern of lymphokine production. Through their production of IL-10, the TH2 cells may render TH1 cells anergic by interfering with the costimulator function of APCs.

Sensitivity of B cells to anti-IgM

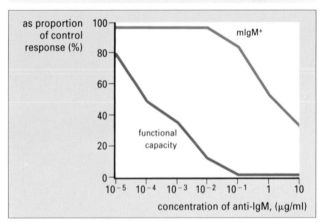

Fig. 10.17 Both surface membrane IgM (mIgM) expression and functional capacity (responsiveness to lipopolysaccharide, LPS) are represented as a percentage of the normal response. Approximately 10 000 times more anti-IgM antibody is required to reduce mIgM expression as to effect a similar reduction in functional capacity. As little as 10^{-3} μg/ml anti-IgM has a significant effect on LPS responsiveness without affecting mIgM expression.

1. Clonal abortion. Multivalent antigen can, when given in appropriate concentrations, cause immature B cells to abort by preventing their further differentiation. Tolerizability of pre-B cells is high.

2. Clonal deletion. Very strong negative signals can cause deletion of mature B cells.

3. Clonal anergy. Intermediate concentrations of multivalent antigens allow pre-B cells to develop into morphologically normal B cells, with normal numbers of Ig receptors, but render them profoundly anergic.

4. Clonal ignorance. Antigen will not have any effect on B cells if its concentration is too low or the affinity of the antigen receptors are too weak. This is not a form of tolerance.

5. AFC blockade. Excess of T_{ind} antigen interferes with antibody secretion by AFC. Tolerizability of AFC is low.

A second window of tolerance susceptibility occurs transiently during the generation of B-cell memory (see Fig. 10.18). *In vitro*, secondary B cells (derived from memory cells produced by T-dependent stimulation) are highly susceptible to tolerization by antigenic determinants presented multivalently in the absence of T cell help. Such a tolerance-susceptible stage probably ensures that any newly derived memory B cells which have acquired self reactivity (as a result of accumulated somatic mutations) are purged from the repertoire.

T cells can also be tolerized *in vitro*. For example, if an influenza-specific T cell clone is inoculated for a few hours at 37°C with a high concentration of influenza peptide but no APCs, this induces anergy and the T cells remain alive. The addition of APCs diminishes the degree of tolerance induced at any peptide concentration, so a costimulator signal derived from APC seemed to be required for immune induction. That signal may depend in part on IL-2, since this cytokine (but not IFN_γ or IL-1) inhibits tolerogenesis. Once tolerance has been established, the addition of IL-2 can reverse established tolerance. Altered regulation of the IL-2 response within T cells appears to be one outcome of the induction of tolerance in T cells.

POTENTIAL THERAPEUTIC APPLICATIONS OF TOLERANCE

A better understanding of tolerogenesis could be valuable in many ways. It could be used to promote tolerance of foreign tissue grafts, or to control the untoward immune responses of hypersensitivity or autoimmune disease. Unfortunately, there is as yet no safe means of inducing specific immunological tolerance to known antigens in adults. It is essential, therefore, to determine the mechanisms which induce 'peripheral' tolerance, and to exploit this knowledge to ensure long-term survival of foreign grafts and to limit autoimmune and allergic reactions. On the other hand, in the treatment of tumours, the ability to break peripheral tolerance to a particular self component (such as an oncogene product) might enable the body to mount an active immune response which could limit tumour growth.

The recent finding that non-depleting antibodies against the CD4 molecule can induce transplant tolerance has obvious clinical implications.

Sensitivity of B cells

Stage of B cell development	Strength of negative signal			
	very strong	strong	intermediate	weak
Pre-B → B cell	abortion	abortion	anergy	no effect
B cell	deletion	anergy	no effect	no effect
AFC	blockade	no effect	no effect	no effect
memory B cell → secondary B cell	abortion	abortion	anergy	no effect

Fig. 10.18 As an immature B cell matures into an AFC, it becomes increasingly resistant to tolerization. The type of tolerance depends on the maturity of the cell and the strength of the signal received. This in turn depends on the affinity of the antigen receptor for the relevant epitopes, and the concentration and valency of the antigen which confronts the cell. Six stages have been identified.

FURTHER READING

Basten A. Self tolerance: the key to autoimmunity. *Proc R Soc Lond (Biol)* 1989;**238**:1.

Goodnow C. *Annu Rev Immunol* 1992;**10**:in press.

Miller JFAP, Morahan G. Peripheral T cell tolerance. *Annu Rev Immunol* 1992;**10**:(in press).

Möller G, ed. Transgenic mice and immunological tolerance. *Immunol Rev* 1991;**122**.

Nossal GJV. Cellular mechanisms of immunological tolerance. *Annu Rev Immunol* 1983;**1**:33.

Nossal GJV. Immunity versus tolerance: the cell biology of positive and negative signalling of B lymphocytes. *Adv Mol Cell Biol* 1992;**6**:(in press).

Waldmann H. Manipulation of T cell responses with monoclonal antibodies. *Annu Rev Immunol* 1989;**7**:407.

chapter 11

Development of the Immune System

An efficient immune system depends on the interaction of many cellular and humoral components, which develop at different rates during fetal and early postnatal life. Many cells involved in the immune response are derived from undifferentiated haemopoietic stem cells (HSCs). These differentiate into various cell lineages, under the influence of different microenvironmental factors (Fig. 11.1).

In the chicken, HSCs originate from blood islands found within the embryonic parenchyme in the yolk sac, and later in the bone marrow. In mammals, the HSCs are found in the fetal liver, spleen and bone mar-

row, but after birth and throughout adult life they are normally found only in the bone marrow. These 'self renewing' HSCs, through the action of various growth and differentiation factors sites of haemopoiesis, give rise to most or all the cells of the immune response. The HSCs give rise to four major cell lineages: erythroid (erythrocytes), megakaryocytic (platelets), myeloid (granulocytes and monocytes/macrophages), and lymphoid (lymphocytes). The latter two lineages are critical to the functioning of the immune system. We will first deal with development of granulocytes and mononuclear phagocytes.

Origin of the cells of the immune system

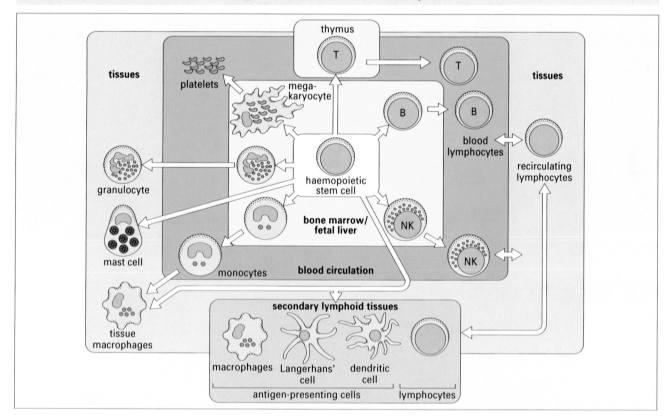

Fig. 11.1 All of these cells arise from the haemopoietic stem cell. Platelets produced by megakaryocytes are released into the circulation, granulocytes pass from the circulation into the tissues. Mast cells are identifiable in all tissues. B cells mature in the fetal liver and bone marrow in mammals, while T cells mature in the thymus. The origin of the large granular lymphocytes with NK activity is uncertain, but is probably the bone marrow. Both lymphocytes and monocytes (which develop into macrophages) can recirculate through secondary lymphoid tissue. Langerhans' cells and dendritic cells act as antigen-presenting cells in secondary lymphoid tissues.

MYELOID CELLS

Myelopoiesis commences in the fetal liver of the human fetus at about 6 weeks of gestation. *In vitro* studies where colonies have been grown from individual stem cells, have shown that the first progenitor cell derived from the HSCs is the colony-forming unit (CFU), which can give rise to granulocytes, erythrocytes, monocytes and megakaryocytes (CFU–GEMM). Maturation of these cells occurs under the influence of colony-stimulating factors (CSFs) and several interleukins including IL-1, IL-3, IL-4, IL-5 and IL-6 (Fig. 11.2). These factors, which are important in the positive regulation of haemopoiesis, are derived mainly from stromal cells of the bone marrow, but are also produced by mature forms of differentiated myeloid and lymphoid. Other cytokines (e.g. TGF$_\beta$) may down-regulate haemopoiesis.

GRANULOCYTE DEVELOPMENT

Induction of CFU–GM along the granulocyte pathway gives rise to distinct morphological stages of development. Myeloblasts develop into promyelocytes and myelocytes, and these mature further, to be released into the circulation as neutrophils, basophils or eosinophils. The one-way differentiation of cells from

Development of granulocytes and monocytes

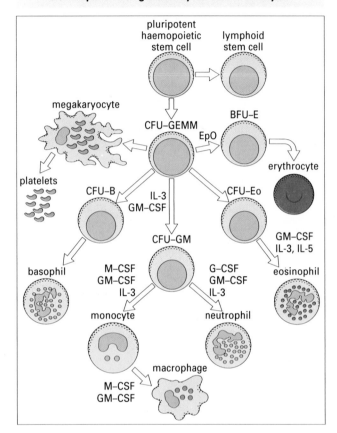

Fig. 11.2 Pluripotent haemopoietic stem cells generate CFU–GEMMs which have the potential to give rise to all blood cells except lymphocytes. IL-3 and GM–CSF are required to induce this stem cell into one of five pathways (i.e. to give rise to megakaryocytes, erythrocytes via burst-forming units, basophils, neutrophils or eosinophils) and are also required during further differentiation of the granulocytes and monocytes. Eosinophil differentiation from CFU–Eo is promoted by IL-5. Neutrophils and monocytes are derived from the CFU–GM through the effects of G–CSF and M–CSF respectively. Both GM–CSF and M–CSF, and other cytokines (including IL-1, IL-4 and IL-6), promote the differentiation of monocytes into macrophages.
(B = basophil; BFU = burst-forming unit; CFU = colony-forming unit; CSF = colony-stimulating factor; E = erythrocyte; Eo = eosinophil; BFU = burst-forming unit; M = monocytes; MM = monocytes and megakaryocytes.)

Morphology and markers on developing granulocytes and monocytes

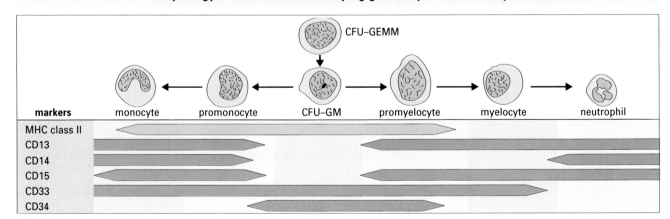

Fig. 11.3 Cells of the monocyte and granulocyte lineages develop from a common CFU–GM. Differentiation along either pathway results in loss of CD34. CD33 is maintained on monocytes but is lost from mature neutrophils, as are MHC class II molecules. CD14 is expressed on monocytes but only weakly on some granulocytes (possibly activated).

the CFU–GM into mature granulocytes is probably the result of acquiring specific growth/differentiation factor receptors at different stages of development.

Surface differentiation markers disappear or appear on the cells as they develop into granulocytes (Fig. 11.3). For example, the CFU–GM carries surface MHC class II molecules and CD38, but these are absent on mature neutrophils. Other surface molecules acquired during the differentiation process include CD13, CD14 at low density, CD15 (the Le^x hapten), the β_1 integrin, VLA-4 (CD49d, α chains), the β_2 integrins CD11a,b and c associated with CD18 β_2 chains, complement receptors and CD16 Fc receptors (see Fig. 2.43).

It is difficult to assess the functional activity of different development stages of granulocytes, but it seems likely that the full functional potential is only achieved after mature forms are produced. In fetal and neonatal life most cells of the immune system are immature, so cells from these stages of life are thought to indicate how individual cells behave as they mature. There is some evidence that neutrophil function, as measured by phagocytosis or chemotaxis, is lower in fetal than in adult life. This may be due to the lower level of opsonins in the fetal serum, rather than to a characteristic of the cells themselves. To become active, neutrophils must interact directly with microorganisms and/or with cytokines generated by a response to antigen, so this could limit neutrophil activity in early life.

Monocyte Development

CFU–GMs that take the monocyte pathway give rise initially to proliferating monoblasts. These differentiate into promonocytes and finally into mature circulating monocytes. The circulating monocytes are are thought to be a replacement pool for tissue-resident macrophages. Different forms of these macrophages comprise the reticuloendothelial system (see Chapter 2).

Like the mature neutrophils, mature monocytes and macrophages lose CD34. However, unlike neutrophils, they maintain MHC class II molecules in their membrane (see Fig. 11.3). These molecules are clearly important for the presentation of antigen to T cells. Monocytes also acquire many of the same surface molecules as mature neutrophils (see Fig. 2.30).

As with granulocytes, it is difficult to assess the functional potential of different stages of monocyte development. However, studies have been made of myeloid tumour cell lines *in vitro*, with different tumour lines believed to represent distinct stages of monocyte differentiation. These studies indicate that both phagocytic efficiency and Fc receptor-mediated cytotoxicity only become optimal in mature macrophages. Generation of the cytokine IL-1 by monocytes is equally good at birth and in adults. As with granulocytes, the function of these cells is enhanced by interaction with cytokines.

DEVELOPMENT OF ANTIGEN-PRESENTING CELLS

In addition to macrophages, most of the classical antigen-presenting cells (APCs), which include the follicular dendritic cells, Langerhans' cells and interdigitating cells, are present at birth. Their origin is still unclear but it is likely that they are all derived from bone marrow stem cells. One possibility is that they are derived from the same stem cell. Morphological, cytochemical and functional differences would then be due to local microenvironmental influences. Alternatively, APCs could be derived from different stem cells and represent separate lineages of differentiation. APCs are present in the thymus very early in development, and their function in MHC restriction and selection indicates that at least some APCs must be fully mature at this time.

However, APC activity is clearly suboptimal early in life. For example, neonatal rats fail to initiate a normal antibody response to sheep red blood cells unless they are also injected with adults' APCs (Fig. 11.4).

Development of macrophage function

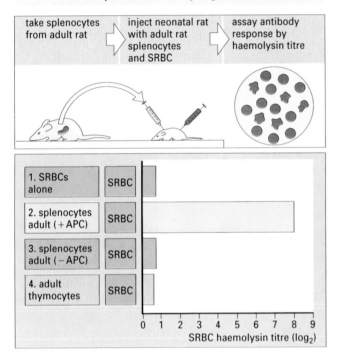

Fig. 11.4 Development of macrophage function: antigen processing and presentation. In this experiment, groups of neonatal rats were injected with sheep red blood cells (SRBCs) alone (1), or SRBCs and spleen cells (including APCs) from adult rats (2), or SRBCs and adult spleen cells depleted of APCs (3), or SRBCs and adult thymocytes (4). In all cases the adult rat was of the same strain as the neonate. The antibody response was measured in each group. Neonatal rats injected with SRBCs alone do not make antibodies to this antigen but if the rats receive adult splenocytes containing APCs with the antigen they make a response. Neither adult splenocytes (lacking APCs) nor thymocytes alone are sufficient for antibody production. Thus neonatal APCs are unable to process/present this antigen effectively.

THE COMPLEMENT SYSTEM

The complement system is another important component of the innate immune system, and plays a major role in protection against microorganisms. At least 20 distinct plasma proteins have been identified as belonging to the system (see Chapter 12). These proteins appear during fetal development, and are detectable before circulating IgM (Fig. 11.5). They are present in the neonate at 50–60% of the adult serum levels. The appearance of complement components before IgM synthesis reflects the fact that, together with phagocytic cells, complement was the main immune protection for animals before the evolutionary development of antibodies. Thus, to some extent, ontogeny recapitulates phylogeny.

LYMPHOID CELLS

Lymphocytes develop in the primary lymphoid organs: T cells in the thymus, and B cells in the bursa of Fabricius (birds) or in the fetal liver and bone marrow (mammals). These cells then migrate to the secondary lymphoid tissues, where they can respond to antigen.

T CELLS
Stem cell immigration
The thymus develops from the third (and in some species the fourth) pharyngeal pouch, as an epithelial rudiment of endodermal origin which becomes seeded with blood-borne stem cells, possibly originating in the yolk sac. Relatively few stem cells appear to be needed to give rise to the enormous repertoire of mature T cells with diverse antigen receptor specificities.

Migration of stem cells into the thymus is not a random process but results from chemotactic signals periodically emitted from the thymic rudiment. In birds, at least, it has been shown that stem cells enter in two or possibly three waves. This has been demonstrated using chicken and quail chimeras (Fig. 11.6). Once in the thymus, the stem cells begin to differentiate into thymic lymphocytes (called thymocytes), under the influence of the epithelial microenvironment. Whether

Stem cell colonization of the chick thymus

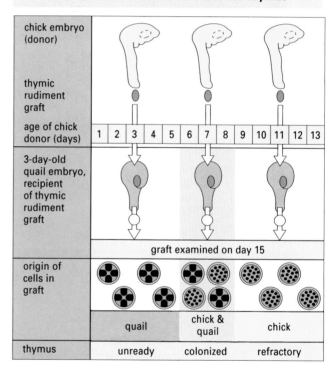

Fig. 11.6 Thymic rudiments from chick embryos of different ages were grafted onto 3-day-old quail embryos and later examined to determine the origin of cells in the thymus. Quail cells can be distinguished from chicken cells by the appearance of condensed chromatin in the resting cell. Grafts made at less than 6 days old were later found to contain quail cells only (a), showing that they had not become colonized with chick stem cells before grafting. If the graft was made after 8 days it was later found to be colonized with chick lymphocytes (c). Grafts transferred between 6 and 8 days contained both chick and quail cells (b). The interpretation is that before 6 days the chick thymus is not ready to receive stem cells. There follows a window of colonization, after which (from day 8) the thymus becomes refractory to further colonization. Further studies indicate that there may be additional windows open later in embryogenesis.

Development of the complement system

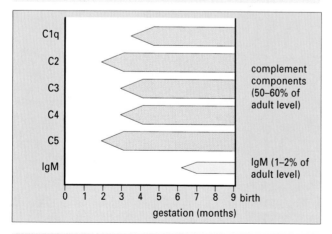

Fig. 11.5 The bar diagram shows the earliest times at which the components of the complement system can be detected in human fetal tissue. The levels of most complement components reach more than 50% of their adult value by birth. By comparison, immunoglobulins are not produced by the fetus until much later.

or not the stem cells are 'pre-T cells', committed to becoming T cells before they arrive in the thymus, is controversial. Although the stem cells express CD7, there is now substantial evidence that they are in fact multipotent.

General thymic structure

At the histological level, the thymus is organized into well-defined lobules. Each contains cortical and medullary areas (see Chapter 3) where epithelial cells, macrophages and bone marrow-derived interdigitating cells, rich in MHC class II antigens, are found. All three are important in the differentiation of the T lymphocytes (Fig. 11.7). Specialized epithelial cells in the peripheral areas of the cortex (thymic 'nurse' cells) contain intracytoplasmic thymocytes within vesicles in their cytoplasm and may be involved in the process of thymic education (see later). The subcapsular region is colonized by the pre-T cells from bone marrow; these develop into large, actively proliferating lymphoblasts which self-renew to give rise to the rest of the thymocytes. Of the developing lymphocytes in the thymus, 85–90% are found in the cortex, whilst the remainder are in the medulla. Studies of their function, and of cell surface markers, have indicated that cortical thymocytes are less mature than medullary thymocytes. Some cortical cells migrate to, and mature in, the medulla.

It has also been found that cortical cells are more sensitive to high levels of corticosteroids *in vitro* and may explain the decrease in this cell population which occurs during pregnancy in mice.

Most mature T cells leave the thymus via post-capillary venules located at the corticomedullary junction. However, other routes of exit may exist, including lymphatic vessels.

Phenotypic changes during T cell maturation

As with the development of granulocytes and monocytes, 'differentiation' antigens, of functional significance, appear or are lost during the change from the stem cells into mature T cells. Analyses have been made of the rearrangement of genes coding for the two presently known T-cell receptors, the $\gamma\delta$ (TCR-1) and the $\alpha\beta$ (TCR-2). Other studies have demonstrated changes in surface membrane antigens. Both these approaches suggest that there are at least two pathways of T cell differentiation in the thymus. It is presently unclear as to whether these pathways are distinct, but it is more likely that they diverge from an early common pathway. At any rate, less than 1% of the mature thymic lymphocytes express TCR-1. Most thymocytes differentiate into TCR-2 $\alpha\beta$ cells, which account for the majority of T lymphocytes found in the secondary lymphoid tissues and in the circulation (see Chapter 2).

Position and structure of the thymus

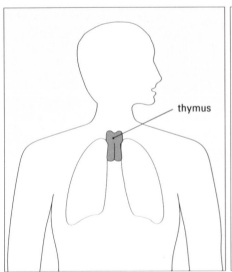
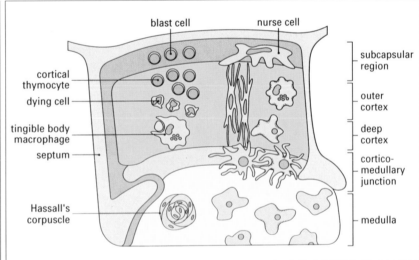

Fig. 11.7 The bilobed thymus is an encapsulated organ divided into lobules by septa. The cortex contains densely packed, dividing cortical thymocytes in a network of epithelial cells which extends into the medulla. The medulla contains fewer lymphocytes, but there are more bone-marrow-derived antigen presenting cells, both interdigitating cells and macrophages. Note the close association of the developing lymphocytes with epithelial cells and interdigitating cells, which are particularly found at the corticomedullary junction. The function, if any, of the whorled epithelial structures termed Hassall's corpuscles is unknown.

TCR-1 cells are particularly prevalent in mucosal epithelia and in the murine skin. Phenotypic analyses of surface membrane antigens have delineated a continuum of changes in surface membrane antigens during T cell maturation (Fig. 11.8). The phenotypic variations can be simplified into a three-stage model.

Stage I, or Early Thymocytes express CD7 together with CD2 (the sheep erythrocyte receptor) and CD5. Proliferation markers such as the transferrin receptor (CD71) and CD38 (a marker common to all early haemopoietic precursors) are also expressed at this stage. It is of note that none of the proliferation markers are T lineage-specific. However, the T commitment of early thymocytes is shown by the TCR β-chain gene rearrangements, and by expression of the TCR-associated complex (CD3) in the cytoplasm but not on the membrane.

Stage II, Intermediate or Common Thymocytes, which account for around 85% of the lymphoid cells in the thymus at any one time, are characterized by the appearance of additional surface markers such as CD1, and by the co-expression of CD4 and CD8 on the same cell (such cells are called 'double positives'). Genes encoding the α chain of TCR-2 are already rearranged in these intermediate thymocytes, and both chains of the TCR-2 are expressed at low density on the surface of those cells destined to be αβ, in association with the CD3–antigen complex.

Stage III or Mature Thymocytes show major phenotypic changes – namely loss of CD1, presence on the cell membrane of CD3 associated with the high density TCR-2 (in αβ cells), and the distinction of two subsets of cells expressing CD4 (T-helper or TH cells), or CD8 (T-cytotoxic or TC cells). The majority of thymocytes at this stage lack CD38 and the transferrin receptor, and are virtually indistinguishable from mature, circulating T cells. All these cells express the receptor CD44, thought to be involved in migration and homing to peripheral lymphoid tissues.

Generation of diversity of TCR in the thymus
T cells have to recognize a wide variety of different antigens. The α and β polypeptide chains of TCR-2 and the γ and δ chains of TCR-1 are each composed of variable and constant regions. The variable region peptides are encoded by a set of genes which are found in all somatic cells of the body. During the development of T cells from pre-T cells these genes undergo rearrangements so that they come closer together within the chromosome (see chapter 5 for more details). The β and δ chains are encoded by V, D and J segments, whilst the α and γ chains use only V and J segments. The first TCR genes to re-arrange during T cell development encode the γ chains and this is followed by rearrangement of the β and α chain genes. Through a random assortment of the different gene segments, a large number of productive rearrangements are made. These result in the expression of diverse variable-region peptide sequences for both chains of the TCR. Initial surface expression of the TCR is at low density. This takes place within the subcapsular and outer cortex of the thymus, where there is active cell proliferation.

Fig. 11.8 Expression of human T cell markers during development. Tdt (terminal deoxynucleotidyl transferase) is an enzyme which is present in thymic stem cells, decreases in stage II and is lost altogether in the medulla. Several surface glycoproteins appear during differentiation. CD1 is present on stage II cortical thymocytes and is lost in the medulla. CD2 and CD7 (the pan-T marker) appear very early in differentiation and are maintained through to the mature T cell stage. CD5 appears at an early stage and persists on mature T cells. CD3 is expressed first in the cytoplasm in stage I cells (cyto) and is expressed simultaneously on the surface simultaneously with TCR-1 and TCR-2. In most stage II cells, both surface CD3 and TCR-2 are expressed at low density but are present at high density on stage III cells. CD4 and CD8 are co-expressed on stage II cells (double positives) and one of these molecules is lost during differentiation into mature stage III cells.

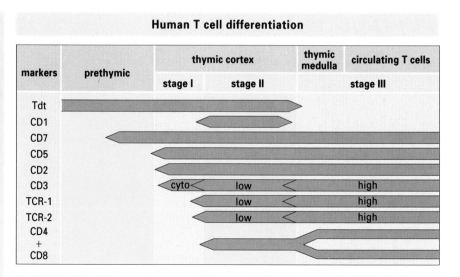

Human T cell differentiation

markers	prethymic	thymic cortex		thymic medulla	circulating T cells
		stage I	stage II		stage III
Tdt					
CD1					
CD7					
CD5					
CD2					
CD3		cyto	low		high
TCR-1			low		high
TCR-2			low		high
CD4 + CD8					

Positive and negative selection in the thymus

Whereas B cells recognize native antigen conformation directly, T cells recognize antigens only in the context of self-MHC molecules. These antigens are presented to the T cells by a variety of APCs, which include macrophages, dendritic cells, B cells and epithelial cells. In general, antigens are first processed by APCs, producing short peptides. These are present in the specialized grooves within the MHC class I and II molecules on the cell surface (see Chapter 4). T cells show 'dual recognition' of both the antigenic peptides and the polymorphic part of the MHC molecules. CD4, found on some subsets of T cells, also attaches to the class II molecule, but to the non-polymorphic portion. In the thymus, T cells which have made productive re-arrangements of their TCR genes and are expressing TCRs at low density on the cell surface, are selected for those which interact with the polymorphic components of self-MHC molecules expressed on the cortical epithelial cells. There is evidence that positive selection of T cells for self-MHC (so-called 'thymic education') does occur, and that this is mediated through APCs which are not derived from bone marrow (i.e. epithelial cells) (Fig. 11.9). The affinity of unselected TCRs for self-MHC molecules alone may vary from zero to high. T cells displaying receptor affinities at both ends of the affinity spectrum die in the cortex. These include cells not making successful TCR gene rearrangements, and those which have successfully rearranged their genes but have produced receptors with either no affinity, or very high affinity for MHC molecules. Cell death occurs by apoptosis, a pre-programmed 'suicide', achieved by activating endogenous nucleases, causing DNA fragmentation (Fig. 11.10).

T cell–MHC restriction occurs in the thymus

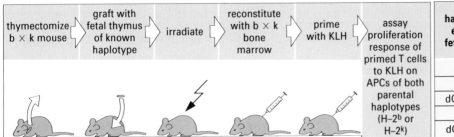

haplotype of engrafted fetal thymus	haplotype of APC's	
	H–2^b	H–2^k
b × k	++	++
b	++	−
dG-treated b	++	−
k	−	++
dG-treated k	−	++

Fig. 11.9 Host mice (F_1 [H–2^b x H–2^k]) were thymectomized, then grafted with 14-day fetal thymuses of various genotypes. They were subsequently irradiated to remove their resident T cell populations, then reconstituted with F_1 bone marrow to provide stem cells. Following priming with keyhole limpet haemocyanin (KLH), the proliferative responses of lymph node T cells to KLH on APCs from each parental strain were evaluated. In some experiment, thymus lobes were incubated before grafting with deoxyguanosine (dG), which destroys intrathymic cells of macrophage/dendritic cell lineage. The figure shows firstly that the thymic environment is necessary for T cells to learn to recognize MHC and secondly, that bone-marrow-derived macrophages/dendritic cells (removed by dG treatment) are not required for this process to occur. (Adapted from Lo D, Sprent J. *Nature* 1986:319;672.)

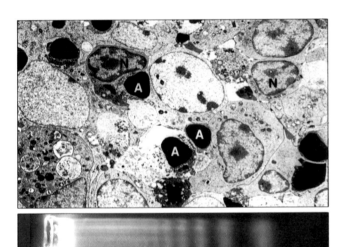

Fig. 11.10 Thymic cell apoptosis. Upper: Fetal thymic lobes in culture were treated with anti-CD3 antibodies – this simulates activation via the TCR and therefore triggers programmed cell death (apoptosis). This electron micrograph shows the heavy condensation of nuclear chromatin in apoptotic nuclei (A) as compared with the dispersed chromatin of normal cells (N). (Courtesy of Dr C. Smith.) Lower: Analysis of the DNA from apoptotic cells by agarose gel electrophoresis shows the characteristically ordered, ladder-like pattern created by bands of digested fragments.

T cells with receptors with intermediate affinities are rescued from apoptosis, survive, and continue along their pathway of maturation. Some of the positively rescued T cells may have receptors which recognize self-components other than self-MHC. These cells are deleted by a negative selection process, through interaction with antigen and APCs (interdigitating cells and macrophages). This occurs in the deeper cortex, at the corticomedullary junction and in the medulla. The existence of this negative selection process (also referred to as central tolerance) has recently received strong experimental support from murine studies where specific Vβ families are eliminated by certain endogenous superantigens during thymic development. The apoptotic double-positive, negatively selected T cells, together with those cells which are not positively selected, are phagocytosed by the tingible body macrophages in the deep cortex.

T cells at this stage of maturation go on to express TCR at high density and lose either CD4 or CD8,
becoming 'single positive' mature thymocytes. These separate subsets of CD4+ and CD8+ cells, possessing specialized homing receptors, now exit to the T cell areas of the peripheral lymphoid tissues where they function primarily as mature 'helper' and 'cytotoxic' T cells respectively. Cells leaving the thymus represent less than 5% of the total thymic population, the rest dying as the result of selective processes (Fig. 11.11).

The role of adhesion molecules and cytokines in thymic development

The maturational events outlined above depend on various aspects of the thymic environment to which both non-lymphoid cells and cytokines contribute. It has been shown that the adhesion of maturing thymocytes to epithelial and accessory cells is crucial for T-cell development. This adhesion is mediated by several complementary pairs of adhesion molecules such as CD2 with LFA3 (CD58) and LFA 1 (CD11a, CD18) with ICAM-1 (CD54).

Fig 11.11 In this model pre-thymic T cells are attracted to and enter the thymic rudiment. They proliferate below the sub-capsular region as large lymphoblasts, which replicate and give rise to a pool of cells entering the differentiation pathway. Many of these cells are associated with epithelial thymic nurse cells (TNCs) although the significance of this interaction is still debated. Cells in this region first acquire CD8 and then CD4 at low density. They also rearrange their TCR genes and may express the products of these genes at low density on the cell surface. Maturing cells move deeper into the cortex and adhere to cortical epithelial cells. These epithelial cells are elongated and branched, and thus provide a large surface area for contact with thymocytes. The TCRs on the thymocytes are exposed to epithelial MHC molecules through these contacts. This leads to positive selection. Those cells which are not selected undergo apoptosis and are phagocytosed by macrophages. There is an increased expression of CD3, TCR, CD4 and CD8 during thymocyte migration from the subcapsular region to the deeper cortex. Those TCRs with self-reactivity are now deleted through contact with autoantigens presented by
interdigitating cells and macrophages at the corticomedullary junction – a process called negative selection. Medullary epithelial cells might also contribute to this process. Following this stage, cells expressing either CD4 or CD8 appear and exit to the periphery
via specialized vessels at the corticomedullary junction. (A process of negative selection may also occur in the cortex, leading to the elimination of cells whose TCRs have high affinity for self-MHC.)

T cell differentiation and negative and positive selection in the thymus

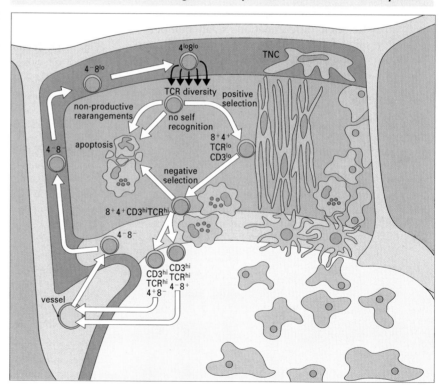

Such interactions induce the production of the cytokines IL-1, IL-3, IL-6 and GM–CSF which are required for T-cell maturation in the thymus. Thymocytes also express receptors for IL-2 and this cytokine, together with other molecules, promotes cell proliferation which mainly occurs in the subcapsular and deep cortex.

Negative selection in the periphery (peripheral tolerance)

Not all self-reactive T cells are eliminated during intrathymic development, probably due to the inability of all self-antigens to transit through the thymic tissues. The thymic epithelial barrier may also limit access to some circulatory antigens. Given the survival of some self-reacting T cells, a separate mechanism is required to prevent their attacking the body. Recent experiments with transgenic mice have suggested that peripheral inactivation of self-reactive T cells can have two causes:

1. down-regulation of TCR and CD8 (in cytotoxic cells) so that the cells are unable to interact with target autoantigens
2. anergy, due to the lack of crucial secondary activation signals provided by the target cells.

Peripheral tolerance is discussed in more detail in Chapter 10.

Extrathymic T cell development

Although the vast majority of T cells require a functioning thymus for their differentiation, small numbers of cells (often oligoclonal in nature) carrying T cell markers have been found in athymic ('nude') mice. The possibility that there are thymic remnants cannot, however, be ruled out. There is some experimental evidence suggesting that bone marrow precursors can home to mucosal epithelia and then mature to functional TCR-1 T cells, without the need for a thymus.

B CELLS

In the chicken, primary B-cell lymphopoiesis occurs in a discrete lympho-epithelial organ, the bursa of Fabricius. The bursal rudiment develops as an outpushing of the hindgut endoderm and becomes seeded with blood-borne stem cells. Studies on chicken/quail chimeras have indicated that there is a window for the immigration of stem cells into the bursa between days 10 and 14 of embryonic life (see Chapter 14). Pyroninophylic cells – the putative stem cells – are seen in contact with epithelial cells. Bursal cell proliferation gives rise to the cortex and the medulla in each bursal follicle, which may be seeded by one or a few stem cells (Fig. 11.12).

Mammals do not have a specific discrete organ for B-cell lymphopoiesis. Instead, these cells develop directly from lymphoid stem cells in the haemopoietic tissue of the fetal liver (Fig. 11.13) from 8–9 weeks of gestation in humans, and by about 14 days in the mouse. Later the site of B-cell production moves from the liver to the bone marrow, where it is continued into adult life. This is also true of the other haemopoietic lineages, giving rise to erythrocytes, granulocytes, monocytes and platelets. Recent data have indicated

that B-cell progenitors are also present in the omental tissue of murine and human fetuses. Whether or not these B-cell progenitors precede those in the fetal liver remains to be established.

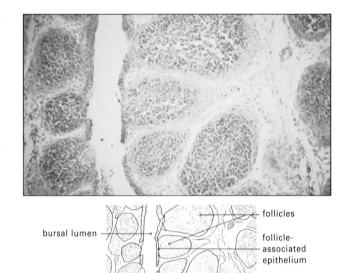

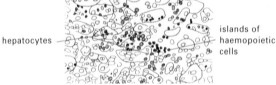

Fig. 11.12 Section of a bursa showing B cells developing in follicles. Like the fetal liver, the bursa is a site of some granulocytopoiesis, not just a site for lymphocyte development. H&E stain, ×50.

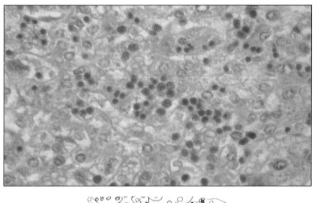

Fig. 11.13 Section of human fetal liver showing islands of haemopoiesis. Haemopoietic stem cells (HSCs) give rise to islands of differentiating lineage-specific cells, including B cells.

B-cell production in the bone marrow does not occur in distinct domains. However, it has been shown that B-cell progenitors are adjacent to the endosteum of the bone lamellae. Each B-cell progenitor, at the stage of immunoglobulin gene rearrangement, may produce as many as 64 progeny. These migrate towards the centre of each cavity of the spongy bone and reach the lumen of a venous sinusoid. In the bone marrow, B cells mature in close association with stromal reticular cells. The latter are found both adjacent to the endosteum and in close association with the central sinus, where they are termed adventitial reticular cells (Fig. 11.14). Reticular cells have mixed phenotypic features with some similarities to fibroblasts, endothelial cells and smooth muscle cells. They produce type IV collagen, laminin and the smooth-muscle form of actin. Experiments *in vitro* have shown that reticular cells sustain B-cell differentiation. Adventitial reticular cells may be important for the release of mature B cells into the central sinus. The majority of B cells (over 75%) maturing in the bone marrow do not reach the circulation but (as in the thymus) undergo a process of programmed cell death or apoptosis, and are phagocytosed by bone marrow macrophages. It has been suggested that B-cell–stromal interactions may mediate a form of positive selection that rescues a minority of B cells with productive rearrangement of their immunoglobulin genes from programmed cell death. Negative selection of autoreactive B cells may occur in the bone marrow or in the spleen, the site to which the majority of newly produced B cells are exported.

From kinetic data, it is estimated that about 5×10^7 murine B cells are produced per day. Since the mouse spleen contains approximately 7.5×10^7 B cells, a large-proportion of B cells must die, probably at the pre-B-cell stage stage where they outnumber the B cells in the marrow by a factor of two.

The characteristic markers of the B-cell lineage are immunoglobulins, which act as cell-surface antigen receptors. Lymphoid stem cells (probably expressing terminal deoxynucleotidyl transferase, Tdt) proliferate and differentiate and then undergo immunoglobulin

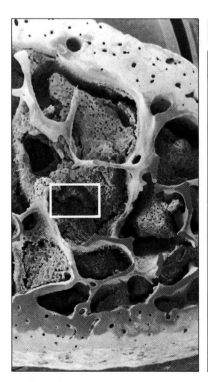

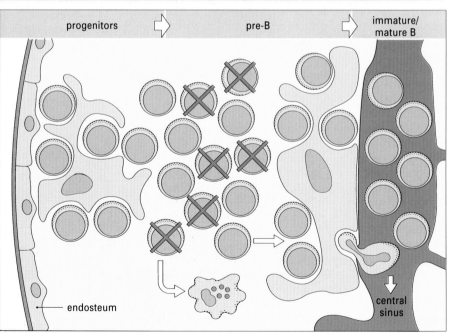

A model for B-cell differentiation in the bone marrow

progenitors ⇨ pre-B ⇨ immature/mature B

endosteum

central sinus

Fig. 11.14 Left: Low power scanning electron micrograph showing the architecture of bone and its relationship to bone marrow. A cavity has been picked out and is drawn schematically on the right. (Courtesy of Drs A. Stevens and J. Lowe). Right: Within the cavities of spongy bone, B cell lymphopoiesis takes place with maturation occurring in a radial direction towards the centre (from the endosteum to the central venous sinus). Immature progenitor cells adjacent to the endosteal cell layer mature into pre-B cells, most of which die and are phagocytosed by bone marrow macrophages containing tingible bodies (stained by haematoxylin). Cells which survive mature further and reach the central venous sinus. Association with reticular cells, and the presence of cytokines such as IL-7 is essential for all steps of B cell maturation. (Adapted from Osmond D, Gallagher R. *Immunol Today* 1991:**12**;1–3,).

gene rearrangements (see Chapter 4). Following this, they emerge as pre-B cells which express μ heavy chains in the cytoplasm. At least some of the pre-B cells express small amounts of surface μ chains associated with pseudo light chains VpreB and λ5. Allelic exclusion of either maternal or paternal immunoglobulin genes has already occurred by this time. The proliferating pre-B cells are thought to give rise to smaller pre-B cells. On synthesis of light chains, which may be either of κ or λ type, but not both, the B cell is then committed to the antigen- binding specificity of its sIgM antigen receptor. Thus one B cell can make only one specific antibody, a central tenet of the clonal selection theory for antibody production. A summary of B-cell differentiation, with expression of immunoglobulins and other relevant molecules, is shown in Fig. 11.15.

A sequence of immunoglobulin gene rearrangements and phenotypic changes takes place during B-cell ontogeny similar to that described for T cells (see above and Chapter 5). Heavy chain gene rearrangements occur in B-cell progenitors and represent the earliest indication of B-lineage commitment. This is followed by light chain gene rearrangements which occur at later pre-B-cell stages. Certain B-cell surface markers are expressed prior to immunoglobulin detection, namely class II MHC molecules, CD19, CD20, CD21 and the CD10 (CALLA) antigen. The latter marker is a highly conserved neutral endopeptidase which is transiently expressed on early B progenitors before the appearance of heavy μ chains in the cytoplasm. CALLA is re-expressed later in the B-cell life history, following activation by antigen (see Fig. 11.15). Other markers such as CD23 and CD25 (IL-2 receptor α) are mostly found on activated B cells.

A number of growth and differentiation factors are required to drive the B cells through early stages of development. Receptors for these factors are expressed at various stages of B cell differentiation. IL-7, IL-3 and low molecular weight B-cell growth factor (L–BCGF) are important in initiating the process of B-cell differentiation whereas other factors are active in the later stages (see Fig. 11.16).

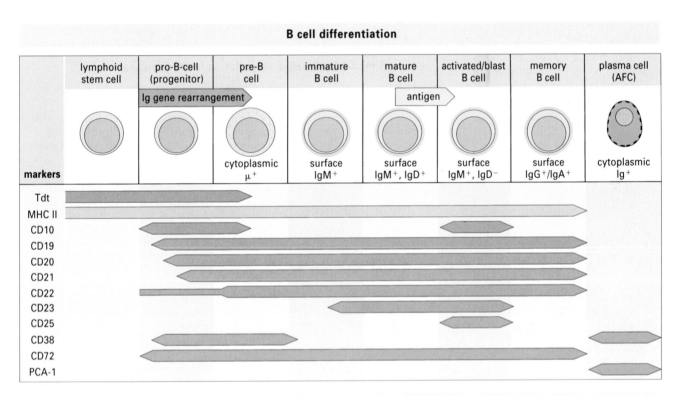

B cell differentiation

Fig. 11.15 B cells differentiate from lymphoid stem cells into virgin B cells and may then be driven by antigen to become memory cells or plasma cells. The cellular location of immunoglobulin is shown in yellow. The genes coding for antibody are rearranged in the course of progenitor cell development. Pre-B cells express cytoplasmic μ chains only. The immature B cell has surface IgM, and the mature B cell other immunoglobulin isotypes. On antigen stimulation the B cell proliferates and develops into a plasma cell or a memory cell following a phase of proliferation, activation and blast transformation. Memory cells and plasma cells are found at different sites in lymphoid tissue. Tdt is expressed very early in ontogeny. The diagram also shows the sequence of appearance of other important B cell surface markers. PCA-1 is found only on plasma cells. Note that CD38 is an example of a molecule found on early progenitors that is lost, only to reappear on the fully differentiated plasma cells.

Following their production in the fetal liver, B cells migrate and function in the secondary lymphoid tissue. Early immigrants into fetal lymph nodes (17 weeks in man) are sIgM⁺ and carry a T-cell marker (CD5). CD5⁺ B cell precursors are found in the fetal omentum. Small numbers of CD5⁺ B cells are also found in the mantle zone of secondary follicles in adult lymph nodes.

Following antigenic stimulation, mature B cells can develop into memory cells or antibody-forming cells (AFCs). Surface immunoglobulin (sIg) is usually lost by the plasma cell (the terminally differentiated form of an AFC), since its function as a receptor is finished. Immature and mature B cells respond in different ways to antigens. Treatment with anti-IgM antibodies or antigen results in loss of sIgM by capping and endocytosis in both mature and immature B cells. However, only mature B cells resynthesize sIgM in culture (Fig. 11.17). Since immature B cells can be induced to lose their antigen receptor, this could be one mechanism by which self-reactive B cells are rendered tolerant during development.

DIVERSITY OF ANTIBODY SPECIFICITY

There are tens of thousands of natural antigenic shapes. Since one B cell can make only one antigen-specific antibody, many B cells with different specific antibody receptors have to be generated from the stem cells.

The genes encoding the variable regions of antibody molecules are described in detail in Chapter 5. The variable region genes comprising V, D and J segments are present in every somatic cell in a germ-line configuration. During early development intervening sequences between D and J are deleted, bringing these genes closer together. Further rearrangements of the V, D and J segments of the variable region heavy chain genes (V_H)

occur during the progenitor stage of B-cell development (see Fig. 11.15). The various combinations of these genes (one productive rearrangement per cell) are expressed with μ heavy chain genes in the cytoplasm of the large pre-B cell. These actively proliferating pre-B cells then rearrange their $V\kappa$ genes, and later their $V\lambda$ genes, if the κ rearrangement has not been successful. When a light chain gene is productively rearranged the immature B cell expresses surface μ chains with either κ or λ light chains. Those cells not making productive rearrangements probably die (perhaps by apoptosis). This is one explanation as to why so many pre-B cells die during development (see above). There is some evidence that pseudo-light-chain genes are expressed prior to κ and λ light chains, and that these may assemble small amounts of surface IgM on pre-B cells. This might be important in selection of early pre-B cells.

Once the κ or λ light chains are being produced, the surface IgM on the immature B cell can act as a functional antigen receptor. The rearrangements of the V, D and J segments (heavy chains) and V and J segments (light chains) are thought to be randomly generated within the B cells. However, there is evidence in mice, rats and chickens for a programmed sequence of development of specific antibody specificities (Fig. 11.18). Antibody production, as distinct from antigen recognition by B cells is, however, dependent on both T cells and APCs.

The reason for this programmed development of specificities at the molecular level within B cells is unclear, but it may reflect the biased utilization of V gene segments nearest to the D or J segments, with a 3' directional movement of the relevant recombinases and/or some negative selection of particular clones (possibly for self-reactivities). Many of the first B cells to appear in ontogeny express a predominantly T cell-

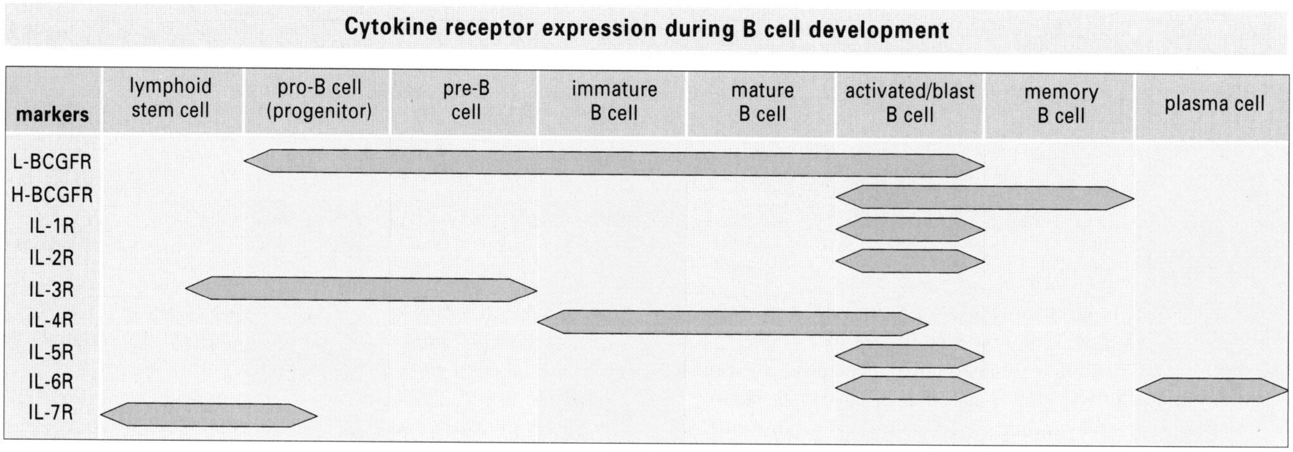

Cytokine receptor expression during B cell development

markers	lymphoid stem cell	pro-B cell (progenitor)	pre-B cell	immature B cell	mature B cell	activated/blast B cell	memory B cell	plasma cell
L-BCGFR		◁═══════════════════════════════════════▷						
H-BCGFR						◁═══════════════▷		
IL-1R						◁═══▷		
IL-2R						◁═══▷		
IL-3R		◁═══════════▷						
IL-4R				◁═══════════════════▷				
IL-5R						◁═══▷		
IL-6R						◁═══▷		◁══▷
IL-7R	◁═══════▷							

Fig. 11.16 The whole life history of B cells from stem cell to mature plasma cell is regulated by cytokines present in their environment. Receptors for these cytokines are selectively expressed by B cells at different stages of development. IL-7 plays an important role in initiating events in B cell differentiation.

associated molecule, CD5, and these B cells express their immunoglobulins from unmutated or minimally mutated germ-line genes. These CD5[+] B cells produce mostly IgM (but also some IgG and IgA) of low avidity. They produce the polyreactive 'natural antibodies' found at high concentration in adult serum. The CD5[+] cells are also involved in antigen processing and antigen presentation to T cells, and probably play a role in both negative and positive antibody responses. Functions proposed for natural antibodies include the following: the first line of defence against microorganisms; clearance of damaged self components; and 'idiotype network' interactions within the immune system.

DIVERSITY OF ANTIBODY CLASS

B cells produce antibodies of 5 major classes or isotypes, IgM, IgD, IgG, IgA and IgE. There are also 4 subclasses of IgG and 2 of IgA (see Chapter 4). Each terminally differentiated plasma cell, derived from a specific B cell, only produces antibodies of one class or subclass. It is presumed that antibody class diversity evolved to produce a versatile response at different anatomical sites, to the multitude of non-self environmental antigens. As already described, the first B cells to appear during development carry surface IgM as their antigen receptor, and this is followed by expression of other classes of immunoglobulin. That the cells carrying non-IgM classes are the progeny of the IgM-bearing B cells was shown by experiments where chickens or mice treated with anti-μ antibodies failed to develop antibodies of any immunoglobulin class. The constant region genes encoding the different heavy chains (CH) are responsible for the antibody classes and subclasses. These are clustered at the 3' end of the immunoglobulin heavy chain (IgH) locus and appear in a particular sequence along the chromosome (chromosome 14 in man and chromosome 12 in mouse). It is currently believed, on the basis of molecular analysis, that B cells switch from IgM to the other classes or isotypes by a process of recombination between highly repetitive switch regions 3' to each CH gene, and by the deletion of intervening CH genes. The details of this process are given in Chapter 5. Some B cells are found which can express more than one isotype on their surface. The mechanism is probably the differential splicing of long nuclear RNA transcripts of the CH genes.

Differentiation of B cells

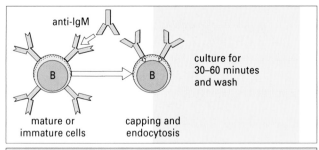

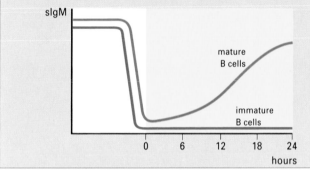

Fig. 11.17 Mature (adult) and immature (neonatal) B cells are incubated at 37°C together with antibody to their sIgM (anti-IgM) for 30–60 minutes; this causes capping of the sIgM and its internalization by endocytosis. The cells are then washed free of anti-immunoglobulin. As shown in the graph, mature B cells resynthesize their sIgM over the following 24 hours, but immature B cells do not.

Development of immune responsiveness

age (days)	*Brucella*	SRBC	DRBC	KLH	SSS$_{III}$
0	4.7	0	0	0	0
1	5.3	0	0	0	0
2		0	0		
3	7.3	2.9	0	0	0
4		5.4	0		
7			0.6	0	0
10–11			3.0	7.7	0
14–15			4.3	10.4	16%
20–22					70%
28					88%

Fig. 11.18 Five different antigens – *Brucella abortus*, sheep red blood cell (SRBC), donkey red blood cell (DRBC), keyhole limpet haemocyanin (KLH) and type III pneumococcal polysaccharide (SSS$_{III}$) – were injected into neonatal rats of different ages. The antibody responses were then measured. The responses to the first four antigens are expressed as $\log_2$ antibody titres. The response to SSS$_{III}$ is expressed as a percentage of animals responding. Blank boxes indicate not tested. Note how the ability to respond to different antigens appears at different times, indicating the programmed first appearance of antibodies of that specificity.

Isotype switching probably only occurs during proliferation and can take place prior to encounter with exogenous antigen during early clonal expansion and maturation of the B cells (Fig. 11.19). Some of the progeny of the immature cells synthesize antibodies of other immunoglobulin classes, including IgG and IgA. Further differentiation results in synthesis of surface IgD – an antibody class that is almost exclusively found on B-cell membranes. All three classes of sIg on the same cell have the same antigen specificity, that is to say they express the same V region genes, although later additional diversity within a single clone may be generated by somatic mutation following class switching.

Evidence that some class switching can occur independently of antigen comes from experiments with vertebrates raised in gnotobiotic (virtually sterile) environments, which are severely restricted in their exposure to exogenous antigens. Such animals show a sequence of expression of different isotypes on B cells similar to that of control animals.

It is well documented that certain antigens induce antibody responses dominated by different immunoglobulin isotypes. In mice for example, carbohydrates in bacterial cell walls give rise to T-cell-independent immune responses which are dominated by IgG3 antibodies whereas, in viral responses, IgG2a antibodies are more common. Following antigenic encounter, the mechanism for this isotype bias can be due to two different mechanisms. One is the 'selection' of B cell clones that have already switched classes spontaneously (see Fig. 11.19). The other is the *de novo* induction of isotype switching as the result of interaction with accessory cell-derived cytokines. There is now considerable evidence for the role of T cells and their cytokines in *de novo* isotype switching. In the mouse, T cells in mucosal sites have been shown to preferentially stimulate IgA production. IL-4 preferentially switches B cells that have been polyclonally activated (by lipopolysaccharide, LPS) to IgG1 isotype, with concomitant suppression of the other isotypes (Fig. 11.20). In a similar system, IL-5 induces a 5–10-fold increase in IgA production with no change in the other isotypes, whilst IFN_γ enhances IgG2a responses but suppresses all the other isotypes. It is interesting that IL-4 and IFN_γ, which act as reciprocal regulatory cytokines in expression of antibody isotypes, are derived from different TH subsets. TH1 cells produce IFN_γ in the mouse; TH2 cells produce IL-4, IL-5 and IL-10 (see Chapter 8). More recently, similar subsets have been described in man,

B-cell differentiation: class diversity

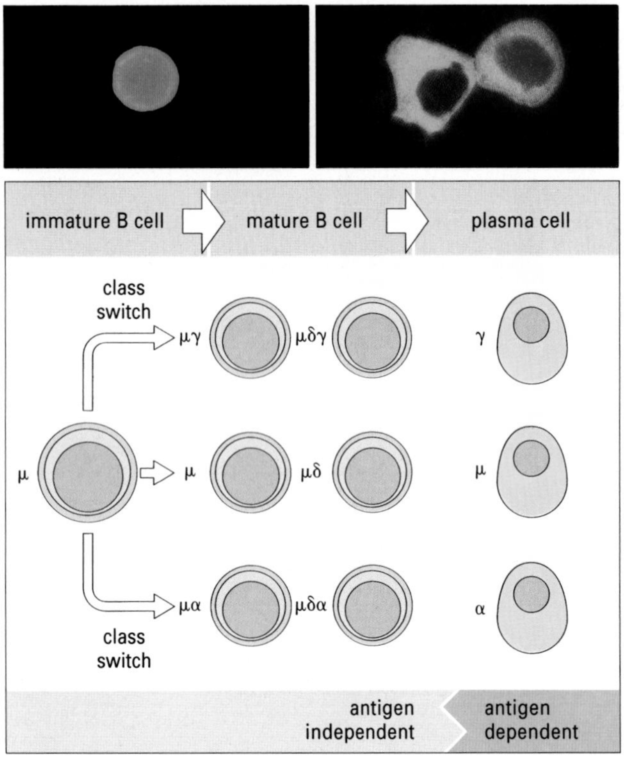

Fig. 11.19 Immature B cells produce IgM only, but mature B cells can express more than one cell surface antibody, since mRNA and cell surface immunoglobulin remain after a class switch. IgD is also expressed during clonal maturation. Maturation can occur in the absence of antigen, but the development into plasma cells (which have little surface immunoglobulin but much cytoplasmic immunoglobulin) requires antigen and (usually) T-cell help. The photographs show B cells stained for surface IgM (green, left) and plasma cells stained for cytoplasmic IgM and IgG (green and red, right). IgM is stained with fluorescent anti-μ chain, and IgG with rhodaminated anti-γ chain.

Isotype regulation by murine T cell cytokines

TH	cytokines	immunoglobulin isotypes					
		IgG1	IgE	IgA	Ig3	IgG2b	IgG2a
TH2	IL-4	↑	↑	↓	↓	↓	↓
	IL-5	=	=	↑	=	=	=
TH1	IFN_γ	↓	↓	↓	↓	↓	↑

Fig. 11.20 This figure shows the effects of IFN_γ (product of TH1 cells) and IL-4 and IL-5 (products of TH2 cells) which result in an increase (↑), a decrease (↓) or no change (=) in the frequency of isotype-specific B cells following stimulation with the polyclonal activator – lipopolysaccharide (LPS) *in vitro*. Whereas IFN_γ induces IgG2a isotype, IL-4 induces IgG1 and IgE antibodies. IL-5 enhances B cells secreting IgA.

and T-cell-derived IL-4 has been shown to be involved in the overproduction of IgE in atopic individuals.

The sequence of appearance of immunoglobulin classes on the cell surface during development is reflected in the serum immunoglobulins detected in the human fetus and neonate. IgM is synthesized before birth whilst IgG and IgA begin to appear around birth (Fig. 11.21). Serum IgG does not reach adult levels until 1–2 years after birth, whilst IgA takes even longer.

DEVELOPMENT OF MEMORY B CELLS

Following antigen activation, B cells either mature into AFCs and then into end-stage plasma cells, or they develop into memory cells. There is now substantial evidence that germinal centres in the various lymphoid tissues (see Chapter 3) are important as sites of development of memory B cells. At these sites, the B cells undergo active hypermutation of their antibody variable-region genes, a process that can lead to death by apoptosis for some cells. As described below, cells with high-affinity receptors for foreign antigen are rescued from cell death by antigen presented within the germinal centres by follicular dendritic cells.

The process outlined above will now be described in more detail. Antigen-specific B cells colonizing the primary lymphoid follicles are primed by antigen and give rise to B-cell blasts. One or a very few B cell blasts go on to form a germinal centre (Fig. 11.22). B-cell blasts proliferate at high rate and reach approximately 10^4 cells in 3–4 days. On the fourth day, the cells transform into centroblasts which have no surface immunoglobulin. These migrate to the interior-facing pole of the follicle where they form the dark zone. Centroblasts give rise to centrocytes which then re-express surface immunoglobulin and occupy the basal light zone of the germinal centre. During this period, following stimulation by antigen presented on follicular dendritic cells,

Schematic organization of the germinal centre

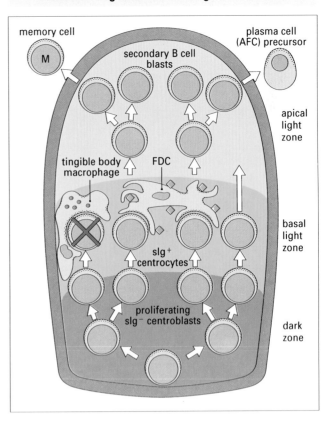

Fig. 11.22 Schematic organization of the germinal centre. In this model, the germinal centre is composed of three major zones, a dark zone, a basal light zone and an apical light zone. These zones are predominantly occupied by centroblasts, centrocytes and secondary blasts respectively. Primary B cell blasts carrying surface immunoglobulin receptors (SIg⁺) enter the follicle and leave as memory B cells or AFCs. Antigen-presenting follicular dendritic cells (FDCs) are mainly found in the two deeper zones, and cell death by apoptosis occurs primarily in the basal light zone where tingible body macrophages are also located. (Adapted from Roitt IM. *Essential Immunology* 7th ed. Oxford: Blackwell Scientific Press, 1991.)

Immunoglobulins in the serum of the fetus and newborn child

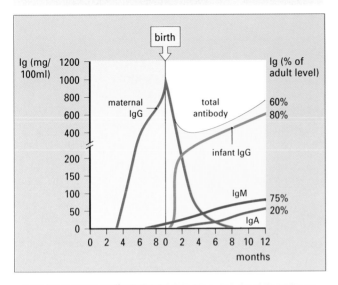

Fig. 11.21 IgG in the fetus and newborn infant is derived solely from the mother. This maternal IgG has disappeared by the age of 9 months, by which time the infant is synthesizing its own IgG. The neonate produces its own IgM and IgA: these classes cannot cross the placenta. By the age of 12 months, the infant produces 60% of its adult level of IgG, 75% of its adult IgM level and 20% of its adult IgA level.

hypermutation of the antibody variable-region genes in the B cell is thought to occur. Centrocytes are found in close association with follicular dendritic cells (FDCs), the interaction of which is mediated by LFA-1 (CD11a/CD18) on the lymphocytes and ICAM-1 (CD54) expressed by the FDC. Successful interactions of centro-cytes bearing high-affinity receptors for antigen presented by the FDCs give rise to secondary blasts which leave the secondary follicles, either as memory cells or plasma cell precursors. Lack of centrocyte–FDC interaction leads to programmed cell death by apoptosis.

FURTHER READING

Gallagher RB, Osmond DG. To B, or not to B: that is the question. *Immunol Today* 1991;**12**:1.

Hannet I I, Erkeller-Yuksel F, Lydyard PM, Denys V, DeBruyère M. Developmental and maturational changes in human blood lymphocyte subpopulations. *Immunol Today* 1992;**13**:215.

Rayewsky K, von Boehmer H, eds. Lymphocyte development. *Curr Opin Immunol* 1992;**4**:131–81.

van Ewijk W. T-cell differentiation is influenced by thymic environment. *Annu Rev Immunol* 1991;**9**:59.

Welte K, *et al*. Recombinant human granulocyte colony stimulating factor: *in vitro* and *in vivo* effects on myelopoiesis. *Blood Cells* 1987;**13(1–2)**:17–30.

Zouali M, MacLennan ICM. Molecular events in the development of the lymphocyte repertoire. *Immunol Today* 1992;**13**:41.

chapter 12

Complement

INTRODUCTION

HISTORY

The term, complement, was originally applied by Ehrlich to describe the activity in serum which, combined with specific antibody, would cause lysis of bacteria. The discovery of this heat-labile activity in serum is usually attributed to Bordet (1895), although Nuttall had described a similar activity some years earlier. In 1907, Ferrata demonstrated that complement could be separated into two components by dialysis of serum against acidified water. This yielded a euglobulin precipitate and a water-soluble albumin fraction. Complement activity could only be demonstrated in the presence of both of these fractions, which he called C1 and C2. Subsequently, Sachs and Omorokow showed that cobra venom inactivated another component (C'3), and Gordon found that a further component was destroyed by ammonia (C'4). The order of discovery of these components of complement does not correspond to their order of reaction, and this explains some of the apparent illogicality of the present-day nomenclature system.

Further analysis of complement components largely depended on the development of new techniques of protein purification. Pillemer, Ecker and colleagues in 1941 described the partial fractionation of C1 from the mixture of proteins contained in C1, and fifteen years later C1 was shown to have enzymic esterase activity by Becker, and by Pillemer and Lepow. During the 1950s, Mayer and colleagues analysed the kinetics of erythrocyte haemolysis and developed the one-hit model which suggested that a single complement lesion was sufficient to cause lysis of an erythrocyte. The next major advance, in 1960, was the purification of the major plasma protein, β1c (now known as C3), which is present at a concentration of one gram per litre. This was done by Muller-Eberhard, who also demonstrated that it corresponded to C3. Subsequently Linscott and Nishioka, and Nelson and his collaborators, were able to purify the nine active components now recognized to participate in the sequence of haemolysis by the complement classical pathway.

An antibody-independent pathway of complement activation was first suggested by Pillemer and his colleagues in the early 1950s who identified a substance they called properdin, which was involved in activation of the complement pathway by yeasts and certain bacteria. The existence of this antibody-independent pathway was not readily accepted by other scientists and caused acrimonious debate.

The role of complement proteins in mediating the adherence of certain microorganisms to leucocytes and erythrocytes was also neglected for many years. By 1930 it was known that trypanosomes treated with antibody and complement would bind to erythrocytes from primates, but it was not until the 1950s that this phenomenon was thoroughly investigated. This led to the discovery of specific cellular receptors for complement proteins.

NOMENCLATURE

Study of the complement system is not assisted by the arcane nomenclature of its proteins. The proteins of the classical pathway and membrane attack system are each assigned a number and react in the order: C1q, C1r, C1s, C4, C2, C3, C5, C6, C7, C8, C9. Many of the proteins are zymogens, i.e. pro-enzymes requiring proteolytic cleavage to become active. The enzymatically-active form is distinguished from its precursor by a bar drawn above its notation, e.g. $\overline{C1r}$. The cleavage products of complement proteins are distinguished from the parent molecules by suffix letters, a, b, etc. Conventionally the small initial cleavage fragment is designated the 'a' fragment and the large, the 'b' fragment, e.g. C3a and C3b. Unfortunately the small fragment of C2 was originally designated C2b and the large, C2a, and this nomenclature will be used here. The proteins of the alternative pathway are assigned letters preceded by the symbol, F (factor). Sometimes the 'F' is omitted, so 'Factor B' may be represented simply as 'B', for example, and 'Factor D' as 'D'.

Regulatory proteins are symbolized by abbreviations, usually derived from a name related to the functional activity of the molecule. Complement receptors are named either according to their ligand (e.g. C5a receptor) or using the Cluster of Differentiation system (CD). There is also a numbering system for receptors for the major fragments of C3: complement receptor types 1 to 4 (CR1 to CR4): This has the unfortunate consequence that some receptors have three names in current usage: the receptor for C3b is variously called 'the C3b receptor', 'CR1' and 'CD35'.

ACTIVITIES OF COMPLEMENT PROTEINS

The complement system is one of the major effector pathways of the process of inflammation. Its activities *in vivo* are best illustrated by the deleterious effects of hereditary and acquired deficiencies of individual complement proteins. Individuals with such deficiencies (discussed in Chapter 18) have increased susceptibility to two types of disease: recurrent infections by pyogenic (abscess forming) bacteria, and illnesses characterized by the production of auto-antibodies and immune complexes. These observations suggest a role for complement in both defence against bacteria and the disposal of immune complexes. This has been confirmed by *in vitro* and *in vivo* studies.

The consequences of complement activation are: i) opsonization, ii) activation of leucocytes and iii) lysis of target cells (Fig. 12.1). Opsonization involves coating of the target with certain complement proteins. Phagocytic cells carrying receptors for these complement proteins then bind and endocytose the opsonized particles. Activation of leucocytes also follows from the interaction of complement proteins with specific cell-surface receptors. The activation of complement results in the cleavage of complement proteins to yield small fragments which can diffuse readily. There are specific receptors on polymorphs and macrophages for some of these fragments which, when they bind to their

receptor, cause directed cellular movement (chemotaxis) and activation. Similar receptors on lymphocytes and antigen-presenting cells bind complement-opsonized immune complexes and enhance specific immune responses. The third physiological consequence of complement activation, lysis, is caused by the insertion of a hydrophobic 'plug' into lipid membrane bilayers, allowing osmotic disruption of the target.

FAMILIES OF COMPLEMENT PROTEINS

Many proteins can be assigned to 'superfamilies' on the basis of close structural and functional homology, for example the immunoglobulin supergene family (see Chapter 4). Within the complement system many proteins may be assigned to such families (Fig. 12.2). The molecular basis of relationships within families has become apparent with the cloning and sequencing of many genes. During evolution it seems probable that exons have been duplicated and 'shuffled' between different genes. These duplicated segments of DNA evolved in parallel and have often maintained closely related structure and functions, although in some cases activities have been lost or new activities have been acquired. Analysis of many proteins has shown that they consist of a 'mosaic' of exons derived from different families. C1s, an enzyme of complement which cleaves C4 and C2, is an example of such a mosaic, containing exons from the serine esterase and LDL receptor (LDL-B) families, plus the short consensus repeat domain from the complement control protein superfamily.

Classification of complement proteins into superfamilies provides a useful framework for understanding their structural and functional relationships. This is illustrated by a group of molecules that appear to be structurally disparate, the complement control proteins (CCP) (also known as regulators of complement activation or RCA). These share a domain of approximately 60 amino acids (called the short consensus repeat) which may appear many times in each molecule. The members of this family of proteins are:

1. Factor H: a plasma globulin with an elongated configuration
2. C4-binding protein (C4-bp): a heptameric plasma protein with a 'spider-like' configuration
3. decay accelerating factor (DAF): a membrane protein attached by an unusual glycophospholipid 'foot'
4. membrane co-factor protein (MCP): a transmembrane protein which acts as a co-factor for cleavage of C3b
5. complement receptor types 1 and 2 (CR1 and CR2): cellular receptors with transmembrane domains.

Despite apparently dissimilar structures, these six proteins share similar functions and are encoded in a closely linked gene cluster on chromosome 1. The short consensus repeats, encoded by tandemly-arranged homologous exons, provide the structural scaffold of each molecule. Certain domains provide the binding specificity of the protein.

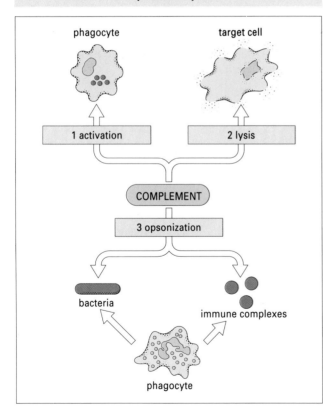

The three major biological activities of the complement system

Fig. 12.1 (1) Activation of phagocytes, including macrophages and neutrophils, (2) lysis of target cells, and (3) opsonization (coating) of microorganisms and immune complexes, so that they can be recognized by cells expressing complement receptors.

Factor H, C4-bp, DAF, MCP and CR1 all inhibit the stable formation of the C3 convertase enzymes, C4b2a and C3bBb. Some also share other functions which are overlapping, though not identical. These include:
1. inhibiting the binding of C2 to C4b, and FB to C3b
2. promoting the dissociation of C2a from C4b, and Bb from C3b
3. acting as cofactors to Factor I, the enzyme responsible for the catabolism of C3b and C4b.

The same short consensus repeat (SCR) has also been identified in the C2b portion of C2, and in the Ba portion of Factor B (C2 and FB are themselves closely homologous in structure and function, and are encoded by tandem genes located in the major histocompatibility complex). It is the C2b region that mediates the binding of C2 to C4b, while the Ba region mediates binding of FB to C3b: this observation suggests that it is the SCR domains that mediate the binding, but this awaits experimental verification. Other molecules are also known which contain this domain but which appear not to interact with proteins of the complement system; they include IL-2 receptor, β₂-glycoprotein I and Factor XIII of the blood clotting system.

 ACTIVATION OF COMPLEMENT

The essence of immunity is the discrimination between self and non-self. While antibodies and T cells play an important role in the recognition of non-self, it is not widely appreciated that the complement system also has a related discriminatory function.

The key step in distinction of self from non-self by complement is the covalent binding of C3b to particles, usually microorganisms or immune complexes. Once bound, C3b functions as an opsonin, and as a focus for deposition of the lytic membrane attack complex. Discrimination is achieved because an individual's cell surfaces carry molecules that effectively limit C3b deposition (described below), whereas non-self surfaces act as sites that allow the rapid deposition of many molecules of C3b.

C3 AND THIOESTER-CONTAINING PROTEINS

C3, the major constituent of the complement system, is present in plasma at a concentration of approximately one gram per litre. Activation of C3 occurs either by spontaneous hydrolysis of an internal bond, leaving the polypeptide chains intact, or by proteolytic cleavage by

Families of complement molecules

structural features	FI	C1r C1s	FB C2	C4bp, FH CR1, CR2 DAF, MCP	C3 C4 C5*	C6, C7 C8 C9	CR3 p150, 95	C1 inh	related molecules
serine esterase domain	+	+	+						trypsin chymotrypsin
short consensus repeats		+	+	+					IL-2 receptor β₂ glycoprotein I F XIII
internal thioester bond					+				α₂-macroglobulin
pore forming molecules						+			perforin eosinophil cationic protein
integrins							+		LFA-1
serine protease inhibitor								+	anti-thrombin III α₁-anti-trypsin α₁-anti-chymotrypsin
LDL receptor domains	+	+					+		LDL-receptor

Fig. 12.2 Structurally similar complement components are grouped together (green) and their major structural features indicated (left). Some non-complement molecules which also have these features are listed (right). *C5 has structural homologies to C3 and C4, but lacks the internal thioester group. (LDL = Low density lipoprotein.)

Comparison of the classical and alternative complement pathways

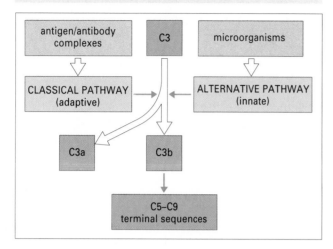

Fig. 12.3 Both generate a C3 convertase, which converts C3 to C3b, the central event of the complement pathway. C3b in turn activates the terminal lytic complement sequence, C5–C9. The first stage leading to C3 fixation by the classical sequence is the binding of an antigen to its antibody. The alternative pathway does not require antibody, since it can be promoted by the sugar component of the microorganism's cell membrane. The alternative pathway provides non-specific 'innate' immunity, whereas the classical pathway probably represents a more recently evolved adaptive mechanism.

a C3 convertase. This is the pivotal step in the process of complement activation (Fig. 12.3)

C3 belongs to a family of proteins containing an unusual post-translational modification to their structure. This is an internal thioester bond consisting of a glutamine residue whose carboxyl (-COOH) group is linked to the sulphydryl (-SH) group of a nearby cysteine residue. This bond is metastable and the electrophilic (electron-accepting) carbonyl group ($-C^+=O$) of the glutamine is susceptible to attack by adjacent nucleophilic groups (electron donors), such as hydroxyl and amine groups in adjacent proteins and carbohydrates. This reaction allows the glutamine to bind covalently to other molecules, and is the mechanism by which C3 can become linked to them (Fig. 12.4)

The thioester bond within native C3 is susceptible to very slow hydrolysis by water, generating an activated form of C3. There is a steady low level of C3 activation in plasma by this mechanism. This allows non-specific binding of C3 to nearby molecules, which can initiate the process of further C3 deposition (Fig. 12.5).

Proteolytic cleavage of the C3a peptide from the *N*-terminus of the α chain by C3 convertase enzymes results in a conformational change which makes the internal thioester bond very unstable. This now becomes a nascent binding site within C3b* (the * denotes the unstable state of the molecule in which the nascent binding site is activated), which is extremely susceptible to interaction with adjacent nucleophiles. The majority of C3b* interacts with water, but a small percentage binds proteins and sugars in the immediate

Activation of the C3 thioester bond

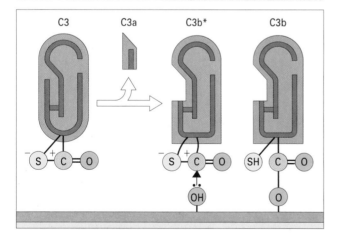

Fig. 12.4 The α chain of C3 contains a thioester bond formed between a cysteine and a glutamine residue. Following cleavage of C3 into C3a and C3b*, the bond becomes unstable and susceptible to nucleophilic attack by electrons on –OH and –NH₂ groups, allowing the C3b to form covalent bonds with proteins and carbohydrates. In this diagram and subsequently, the polypeptide chains are shown in dark green and interchain disulphide bonds in red.

C3 tick-over

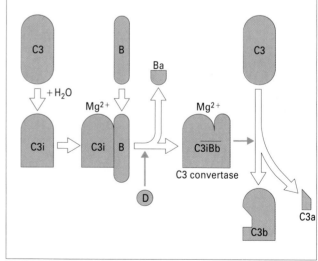

Fig. 12.5 The thioester bond of native C3 becomes hydrolysed by water forming C3i (C3(H₂0)) which binds to Factor B in the presence of Mg^{2+}. Following cleavage of B by Factor D, this complex forms a C3 convertase which can directly cleave C3 into C3a and C3b.

vicinity of the activation site. Since C3 convertases are usually generated on non-self surfaces or on immune complexes, this means that C3b deposition will be confined mostly to these places.

The complement protein C4 also contains an internal thioester bond within a sequence that is closely homologous to the one in C3. Two isotypes of C4 exist, C4A and C4B, encoded by tandem genes within the major histocompatibility complex. When activated, C4A preferentially binds to amine groups, forming an amide bond, whereas C4B mainly binds to hydroxyl groups producing an ester linkage. Thus C4A binds mainly to amino groups within proteins and C4B to hydroxyl groups within carbohydrates.

CLASSICAL PATHWAY

The classical pathway of complement is the main antibody-directed mechanism for the activation of complement. It is initiated by the binding of antibody to two or more of the 6 globular domains of C1q. C1q binds with high avidity to the C_H2 domains (part of the Fc region) of aggregated IgG molecules, as contained in an immune complex. Alternatively, C1q can bind to the C_H3 domains of a single IgM molecule whose conformation has been modified from a 'planar' to a 'staple'

configuration by binding to antigen. In an antibody-independent process, C1q is also capable of binding directly to certain microorganisms, including mycoplasmas and some retroviruses (though not HIV).

It has recently been realized that C1q belongs to a family of proteins, including mannan-binding protein (MBP), conglutinin and lung surfactant protein A. Mannan-binding protein, which is found in serum, binds to terminal mannose groups and is capable of antibody-independent activation of the classical pathway by interaction with C1r and C1s. This interaction is analogous to the interaction of C1q with C1r and C1s, which is described below. Thus certain bacteria may activate the classical pathway of complement by binding MBP.

C1 is a pentamolecular Ca^{2+}-dependent complex consisting of a single C1q molecule, two C1r and two C1s molecules (Fig. 12.6). Multiple binding of the globular domains of C1q (to IgG in an immune complex, for example) is believed to lead to a conformational change in the C1 complex. This makes one of the C1r molecules activate itself (by autocatalysis) and cleave the other C1r to yield active enzyme. These two enzymes then cleave the two C1s molecules to give active serine esterases.

Structure of C1

1	C1q subunit

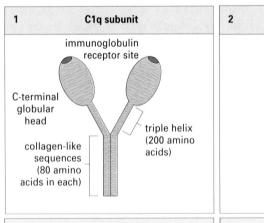

2	intact C1q

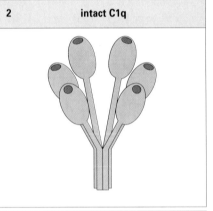

3	C1r₂ C1s₂ unit

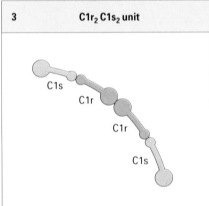

4	intact C1

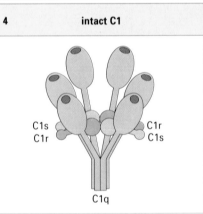

Fig. 12.6 Each subunit of C1q is Y-shaped with each branch of the Y ending in a globular head (1). C1q consists of 3 of these subunits joined together (2). There are six polypeptide chains in each subunit, giving 18 in the whole C1q molecule. The receptors for the Fc regions of IgG are in the globular heads, which form a ring in the C1q molecule. A unit consisting of two C1r molecules and two C1s molecules (3) lies across the C1q molecule (4). The catalytic sites of C1r are close together at the centre of the ring. The cohesion of the C1 complex is dependent on Ca^{2+}.

The next steps in classical pathway activation have two functions. Firstly they amplify the response. Secondly they concentrate the site of complement activation onto the particle that initiated the activation.

$\overline{C1s}$ cleaves the thioester-containing protein, C4, into C4a and the unstable intermediate, C4b*. Within a few milliseconds this is attacked by nucleophilic amine or hydroxyl groups in its immediate vicinity. These can form covalent amide bonds (mainly with C4b* from C4A) or ester bonds (mainly with C4b* from C4B). (In fact, only about 1% of C4b* binds to proteins or to carbohydrates: the rest reacts with adjacent water molecules to form the intermediate iC4b, which is rapidly catabolized. Surface-bound C4b now acts as a binding site for the zymogen C2. When combined with C4b, C2 becomes a substrate for $\overline{C1s}$, and is cleaved to C2b and C2a. The C2a segment remains bound, giving $\overline{C4b2a}$. This is the C3 convertase enzyme of the classical pathway, which cleaves C3 into C3a and C3b*. C3b* can bind to hydroxyl or amine groups (but mainly hydroxyl groups) as already described, and a small percentage binds to the surface that originally bound the C4b. The bound C3b acts as a focus for further complement activation (Fig. 12.7).

REGULATION OF CLASSICAL PATHWAY ACTIVATION

Classical pathway activation is regulated very efficiently in the fluid phase by two mechanisms. The first is the serine proteinase inhibitor (serpin), C1 inhibitor, which binds and inactivates C1r and C1s.

The second mechanism blocks the formation of the classical pathway C3 convertase enzyme, $\overline{C4b2a}$. The formation of $\overline{C4b2a}$ is inefficient in the fluid phase and this is due to the presence of plasma proteins which catabolize C4b. (The proteins that break down C4b are Factor I and C4 binding protein.) C4 binding protein also promotes the dissociation of C2a from $\overline{C4b2a}$.

The classical pathway

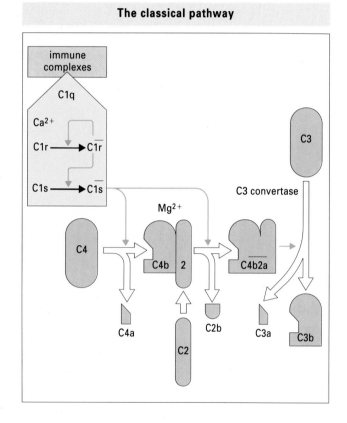

Fig. 12.7 Following binding of C1q to immune complexes, C1r catalyses its own activation and that of C1s. C1s then cleaves C4a from C4, leaving C4b, which immediately binds to adjacent proteins or glycoproteins. Surface-bound C4b now binds C2 in the presence of Mg^{2+}. C1s cleaves C2b from this complex to leave C2a. (Note that the usual nomenclature is reversed with C2, and C2a refers to the larger segment. There have been proposals to change this nomenclature, but in this book the original designations are used.) The complex of C4b and C2a is the classical pathway C3 convertase.

Regulation of C3 convertases

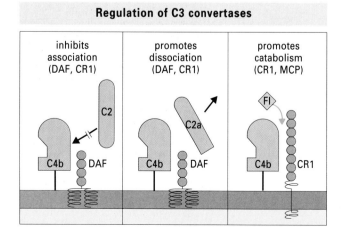

Fig. 12.8 Decay accelerating factor (DAF) and CR1 inhibit the association between C4b and C2, and promote dissociation of the $\overline{C4b2a}$ complex. CR1 and membrane cofactor protein (MCP) promote Factor I (FI) mediated cleavage of C4b. These molecules control the interactions between C3b and FB similarly.

There are also important molecules on autologous cell surfaces that regulate classical pathway activation. These are the complement control proteins (CCPs) which are members of the regulators of complement activation (RCA) gene cluster. They include: decay accelerating factor (DAF), CR1 and membrane cofactor protein (MCP). These molecules between them:

1. inhibit the binding of C2 to C4b (DAF or CR1)
2. promote the dissociation of C2a from C4b (DAF or CR1) (the process of decay acceleration)
3. promote the catabolism of C4b by Factor I (MCP or CR1) (cofactor activity) (Fig. 12.8).

ALTERNATIVE PATHWAY ACTIVATION

There are close structural and functional homologies between the proteins participating in activation of the classical and alternative pathways of the complement system (Fig. 12.9). As already described, there is continual low-level hydrolysis of the internal thioester bond of C3 in plasma. The product, C3i, acts as a binding site for Factor B (FB) (see Fig. 12.5). This is analogous to the binding of C2 to C4b. FB, bound to C3i, is cleaved by Factor D to Ba and Bb. Fluid-phase C3iBb is a C3 convertase enzyme that cleaves further C3 to C3b*, some of which covalently binds to adjacent surfaces. This surface-bound C3b can then act as a binding site for more FB and initiates the amplification loop described below. It is clear that this system of activation results in the indiscriminate binding of C3b to any adjacent surfaces; however, there are molecules on autologous cell surfaces that prevent the formation of stable C3 convertase enzymes and these are considered below.

AMPLIFICATION LOOP

On surfaces which are good activators of complement, initial binding of a few molecules of C3b, by one of the two mechanisms outlined above, is followed by an amplification step. This which results in the binding of many more molecules of C3b to the same surface.

Analogous action of the classical and alternative pathways

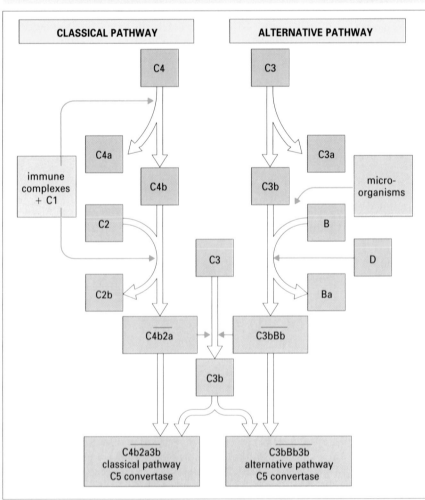

Fig. 12.9 Both pathways generate a C3 convertase: C4b2a (classical pathway) and C3bBb (alternative pathway). In the classical sequence, C1 is activated by complexed antibody and splits both C4 and C2. The small fragments, C4a and C2b, are lost and the major components form C4b2a. In the alternative pathway, pre-existing C3b binds Factor B, which is split releasing a small fragment, Ba. The major fragment, Bb, remains bound to form C3bBb. This converts more C3, so creating positive feedback. Activator surfaces, on microorganisms for example, stabilize C3b as well as facilitating its combination with Factor B and C3b. Both these activities promote alternative pathway activation. The C3 convertases of both pathways may bind further C3b to yield C5a convertase enzymes. These activate the next component of the complement system, C5. The classical pathway C5 convertase is C4b2a3b, while the alternative pathway C5 convertase is C3bBb3b.

Factor B (FB), (which is structurally and functionally homologous to C2), binds to C3b, and in this form is a substrate for the serine esterase Factor D. (This is unusual amongst complement enzymes in that it circulates at a very low concentration in an active form.) The cleavage of Factor B results in the release of a small fragment Ba, and the formation of the C3 convertase enzyme, C3bBb. This cleaves many more C3 molecules, some of which bind covalently to the activating surface (Fig. 12.10). The C3bBb enzyme dissociates fairly rapidly unless it is stabilized by the binding of properdin (P), forming the complex, C3bBbP. This amplification mechanism is a positive feedback system which will cycle until all C3 is completely cleaved unless it is regulated adequately. Indeed, the amplification pathway was originally elucidated in a patient with an hereditary deficiency of the regulatory enzyme, Factor I. Lacking FI, her amplification loop had cycled to exhaustion, so that, all the C3 in her serum was converted to C3b.

REGULATION OF ALTERNATIVE PATHWAY AND AMPLIFICATION LOOP ACTIVATION

Activation of the alternative pathway in the fluid phase (i.e. where C3b does not bind to surfaces) is an inefficient process. It is regulated by proteins similar or identical to the CCPs which inhibit classical pathway activation. Factor H, encoded by a member of the RCA gene cluster and homologous to C4 binding protein, promotes the dissociation of Bb from C3i and from C3b. Factor H also functions as a cofactor to Factor I (FI) for the catabolism of C3i and C3b (Fig. 12.11).

On cell membranes, both DAF and CR1 accelerate the dissociation of the C3bBb C3 convertase enzyme, promoting the release of C3b from the complex: CR1 and MCP both act as cofactors for the cleavage of C3b by Factor I (see Fig. 12.8). These reactions are exactly analogous to the activities of DAF, MCP and CR1 in controlling the activity of classical pathway C4b2a when it is bound to cell membranes.

Regulation of the fate of C3b bound to surfaces is the critical step enabling the non-specific distinction of self from non-self by the complement system. There are two possible outcomes for bound C3b.
1. Amplification: C3b acts as a binding site for Factor B (FB), forms a convertase enzyme, and focuses the deposition of more C3b to the the same surface.
2. Inhibition: C3b is catabolized by Factor I using one of three cofactors, FH (fluid-phase), CR1 or MCP (surface-bound).

The nature of the surface to which the C3b is bound regulates which of these two outcomes is most likely (Fig. 12.12).

It is the presence on self surfaces, particularly the cell membranes, of intrinsic molecules such as DAF, CR1, and MCP, that effectively limits the formation of C3 convertase enzymes. On the other hand, non-self surfaces, for example bacterial cell membranes, act as a protected site for C3b since factor B has a higher affinity for C3b than does Factor H at these sites. Thus the deposition of a few molecules of C3b on to a non-self surface is followed by the formation of relatively stable C3bBbP C3 convertase enzymes which focus more C3b deposition in the near vicinity.

The antibody-independent amplification loop

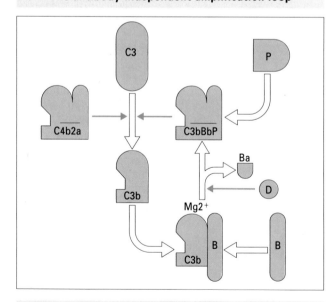

Fig. 12.10 C3b may be generated either by a classical pathway C3 convertase C4b2a or by an alternative pathway C3 convertase. C3b then binds to Factor B in a Mg²⁺-dependent complex and is acted on by Factor D. This releases Ba and generates the alternative pathway, C3 convertase C3bBb. This in turn can act on more C3 to generate further C3b. Thus there is a positive feedback loop, which may amplify the initial complement activation.

Breakdown of C3b

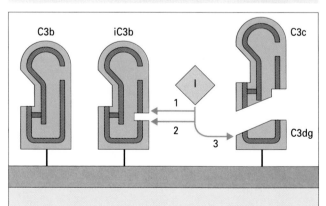

Fig. 12.11 Factor I cleaves C3b in three places to release C3c, leaving C3dg, a fragment of the α chain still bound to the substrate. The first two cleavages are promoted by Factor H and CR1 and produce an intermediate, iC3b. The third cleavage is promoted by CR1.

Aggregated immunoglobulins, for example in immune complexes, also function as 'protected sites' for C3b. Although the precise structural requirements for a 'protected surface' are not understood the carbohydrate composition seems important. The presence of acidic sugars, such as sialic acid, seem to help in protecting self membranes from amplified C3b deposition.

MEMBRANE ATTACK COMPLEX
The final phase of activation of the complement cascade is the formation of the membrane attack complex (MAC).

The first step towards MAC formation is the enzymatic cleavage of C5, which is a protein homologous to C3 and C4 but lacking the internal thioester bond. C5 must be bound to C3b before it can be cleaved by the C5 convertase enzyme.

Recent evidence suggests that the classical pathway C5 convertase enzyme is a trimolecular complex, C4b2a3b, in which the C3b is covalently bound to the C4b. The C3b that the C5 binds to is, therefore, actually part of the convertase enzyme complex (Fig. 12.13). C5 binds selectively to this complex, because it has a higher

Regulation of the amplification loop

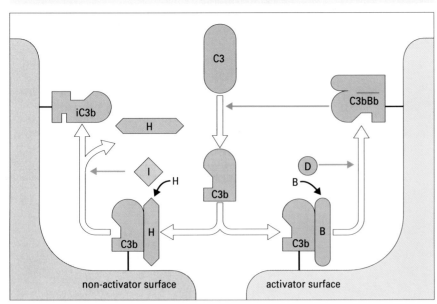

Fig. 12.12 Alternative pathway activation depends on the presence of activator surfaces. C3b which has bound to an activator surface binds factor B. This generates the alternative pathway C3 convertase, C3bBb, which drives the amplification loop. However on non-activator surfaces the binding of Factor H is favoured and C3b becomes inactivated by Factor I. Thus the binding of Factor B or Factor H controls the development of alternative pathway reactions.

Generation of C5 convertases

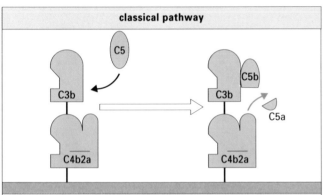
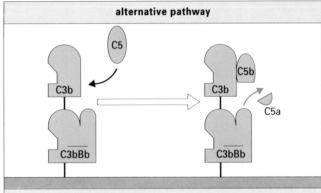

Fig. 12.13 It is thought that C3b becomes covalently attached to either a classical pathway or an alternative pathway C3 convertase, thus forming C5 convertases. The C5 convertase can then bind C5, which is acted on by either C2a or Bb. When C5 is cleaved it generates C5b, the first component of the lytic pathway.

binding constant to C3b when it is bound to C4b than for C3b which is bound to other cell surface molecules. By analogy, the alternative pathway C5 convertase enzyme will probably turn out to be a trimolecular complex, $\overline{C3bBb3b}$, in which one C3b is covalently bound to the other.

The remainder of the formation of the MAC is non-enzymatic. C5b binds C6, forming C5b6, and this then binds C7 to form a C5b67 complex (Fig. 12.14). Binding to C7 marks the transition of the complex from a hydrophilic to a hydrophobic state that preferentially inserts into lipid bilayers. C8 and C9 then sequentially bind to this complex resulting in the formation of the lytic 'plug', or pore-forming molecule, first observed in electron micrographs by Humphrey and Dourmashkin (Fig. 12.15). C9 forms a polymeric complex containing up to 14 C9 monomers. Although a small amount of lysis occurs when C8 binds to C5b67, it is the polymerized C9 that causes the majority of lysis. (Note that C5b6789 is usually abbreviated to C5b–9, and the earlier stages may be shortened in the same way, e.g. C5b–8.)

Hydrophobic molecules that polymerize to form pores may be a common mechanism for cellular cytotoxicity. T lymphocytes kill target cells by inserting a pore-forming molecule known as perforin into their membranes. Perforin has structural homology to C9 and similar molecules are found in the granules of eosinophils. Certain bacterial toxins, such as streptolysin O, are also pore-forming molecules.

REGULATION OF ACTIVATION

Once the hydrophobic C5b67 complex has formed it can insert itself into other cell membranes close to the primary surface on which complement activation is focused. This is the process of 'reactive lysis' which, if unregulated, could have damaging consequences to self/host tissues. There are a number of proteins that inhibit this process by binding to fluid phase C5b67 before it can attach to self membranes. The most abundant of these is S protein, also known as vitronectin, which is usually present in plasma. It forms the SC5b67 complex, which is unable to insert into lipid bilayers. There are specific receptors for S protein, but it is not known whether these have a physiological role in the clearance of SC5b67 from plasma. If C8 binds to C5b67 in the fluid phase this also forms a complex incapable of membrane insertion as does the binding of low density lipoprotein (LDL).

Host cells also bear membrane proteins that protect them against lysis by the MAC. This explains the old observations that erythrocytes are poorly lysed by homologous complement, but readily lysed by complement derived from other species. Two proteins have been characterized which mediate this species restriction. CD59 is a protein anchored by a glycophospholipid foot. It is widely distributed in cell membranes and inhibits the insertion and polymerization of C9 into cell membranes bearing C5b–8. A second protein, homologous restriction factor (HRF), has similar activity and distribution to CD59 but is probably a weaker

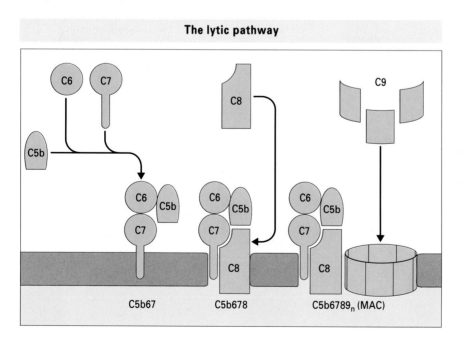

The lytic pathway

Fig. 12.14 C5b binds C6 and C7 to give C5b67, which is hydrophobic and has a membrane binding site allowing the complex to attach to plasma membranes close to the reaction site.

C8 binds to a site on C5b and penetrates the membrane, where it can polymerize a number of molecules of C9 to generate the membrane attack complex (MAC).

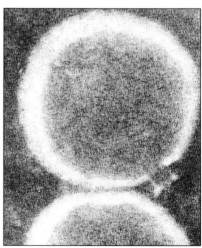

Fig. 12.15 Electron micrograph of the membrane attack complex. The funnel-shaped lesion is due to a human C5b–9 complex reincorporated into lecithin liposomal membranes. × 234 000. (Courtesy of Professor J. Tranum-Jensen and Dr S. Bhakdi.)

inhibitor of C9 insertion. HRF is a 65 kDa glycophospholipid-linked membrane protein, whose sequence has not yet been determined.

Nucleated cells are much more resistant than erythrocytes to lysis by complement. They can actively remove MAC by exocytosis and endocytosis of fragments of membrane containing MAC.

COMPLEMENT RECEPTORS

Many of the fragments of complement proteins produced during activation bind to specific receptors on the surface of immune cells. This is an important mechanism for the mediation of the physiological effects of complement, including uptake of particles opsonized by complement, and activation of the cell bearing the receptor.

Complement receptors for fragments of C3

receptor	ligands	cellular distribution
CR1	C3b>iC3b C4b	B cells, neutrophils, monocytes, macrophages, erythrocytes, follicular dendritic cells, glomerular epithelial cells
CR2	iC3b, C3dg Epstein–Barr virus interferon-α	B cells, follicular dendritic cells, epithelial cells of cervix and nasopharynx
CR3	iC3b zymosan certain bacteria	monocytes, macrophages, neutrophils, NK cells, follicular dendritic cells
CR4 (p150–95)	iC3b	neutrophils, monocytes, tissue macrophages

Fig. 12.16 CR1 binds C3b more strongly than iC3b. These receptors allow cells to take up peptides or immune complexes bearing that particular fragment.

Opsonization and phagocytosis

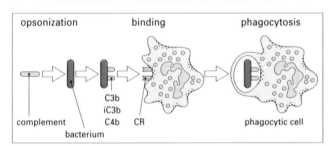

Fig. 12.17 The diagram illustrates the steps in the uptake of a particle such as a bacterium opsonized by either C3b or C4b.

C3 RECEPTORS

There are three products of C3 that bind to the membranes of target cells (sometimes called opsonic fragments). These are C3b, iC3b and C3dg. Four different receptors for these opsonic fragments are known, and they are named complement receptor types 1 to 4 (CR1, CR2, CR3 and CR4); their ligands and their cellular distribution are shown in Fig. 12.16.

CR1 (CD35) The first complement-dependent cellular binding reaction to be recognized was a phenomenon that was later named 'immune adherence'. In this reaction, trypanosomes opsonized with antibody and complement adhere to the platelets of rodents and to the erythrocytes of primates.

The receptor mediating these binding reactions is CR1, (also called the immune adherence receptor, or the C3b/C4b receptor, or CD35). CR1 is thought to have four physiological activities.

1. It is an opsonic receptor on neutrophils, monocytes and macrophages mediating endocytosis or phagocytosis by appropriately primed cells (Fig. 12.17).
2. It is a cofactor to Factor I for the cleavage of C3b to iC3b, and for the subsequent cleavage of iC3b to C3c and C3dg. (Factor H is probably more important than CR1 as a cofactor for the cleavage of C3b to iC3b, but CR1 is probably the sole cofactor for the cleavage of iC3b.) In this role, CR1 protects self cells from attack by complement.
3. On erythrocytes or platelets, CR1 may serve to pick up opsonized immune complexes or bacteria and transport them to the cells of the fixed mononuclear phagocytic system (Fig. 12.18).
4. On B lymphocytes, CR1 may serve with CR2 as a receptor mediating lymphocyte activation.

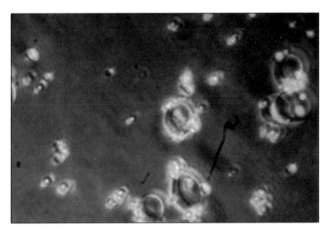

Fig. 12.18 Immune adherence. Fluoresceinated bacteria opsonized with antibody and complement are seen adhering to human erythrocytes. This reaction is mediated by C3b, iC3b and C4b on the bacteria binding to CR1. (Courtesy of Professor G. D. Ross.)

CR2 (CD21) CR2 is located on B lymphocytes, follicular dendritic cells and certain epithelial cells; its ligands are iC3b, C3dg, the Epstein-Barr virus (EBV), and IFN_α. The role of CR2 on B cells is not established with certainty, but *in vitro*, binding of CR2 to its ligand results in B cell activation in some experimental protocols. Other experiments suggest a role for C3 in the localization of immune complexes to APCs in secondary lymphoid tissues. This augments the development of antibody responses. Moreover C3 is required for the efficient induction of memory B cells which can later produce secondary antibody responses. It therefore seems likely that the main activity of CR2 on B cells is as an accessory receptor for C3b which acts to stimulate the antibody response.

The main pathophysiological activity of CR2 follows from its role as the receptor for EBV. The *in vivo* tissue distribution of this virus corresponds to the locations of CR2, and it seems likely that EBV enters cells by binding directly to CR2 without the involvement of complement.

CR3 (CD18/11b) CR3 occurs on cells of myeloid lineage and is an important receptor and adhesion molecule. It mediates phagocytosis of particles opsonized with iC3b. CR3 is also a lectin and binds certain carbohydrates. Some yeasts, including *Saccharomyces cerevisiae*, bind directly to CR3 without the mediation of complement as do other microorganisms, such as *Staphylococcus epidermidis* and *Histoplasma capsulatum*.

CR3 belongs to a family of three cell surface molecules, collectively called the leucocyte integrins. These are heterodimers containing a common β-chain (CD18) and one of three different α chains (CD11a,11b, or 11c). The other leucocyte integrins are LFA–1 (lymphocyte function-associated antigen type 1), whose composition is CD18/11a, and CR4, also called p150-95 (CD18/CD11c).

These three molecules in turn belong to a superfamily of structurally related cell surface receptors and adhesion molecules, the integrins, which includes the fibronectin and vitronectin (S protein) receptors, and the fibrinogen receptor on platelets. The different families of integrins each have their own type of β chain (β_2 in the case of the leucocyte integrins) which is combined with distinct α chains. The binding of these receptors to their ligands is calcium-dependent. Some of them have a common binding specificity for the tripeptide sequence Arg-Gly-Asp, (RGD), but there are other sequence or conformational determinants which influence their binding to particular ligands.

CR4 (CD18/11c) CR4 (p150-95) is the least well characterized of this group of receptors but has been shown to bind to iC3b in a calcium-dependent manner. It is distributed on cells of both myeloid and lymphoid lineages, and is strongly expressed on tissue macrophages, where it may be an important receptor for particles opsonized with iC3b.

ANAPHYLATOXIN RECEPTORS

Two small fragments of complement proteins, C3a and C5a, can trigger the degranulation of mast cells, and are therefore known as anaphylatoxins. This and other activities will be described in more detail later. The effects of the anaphylatoxins (C3a, C5a) are mediated by binding to specific receptors. These have been well characterized for C5a; there are between 50 000 and 112 000 receptors on neutrophils, and their molecular size is 40 kDa. The C5a receptor belongs to the rhodopsin superfamily of receptors which produce a signal (when they bind to their ligand) by interacting with intracellular GTP-binding proteins. The C5a receptor is homologous in structure to the f-met-leu-phe receptor, a receptor mediating chemotactic signals. Following receptor-binding, C5a is internalized and degraded to inactive peptide fragments; this appears to be an important mechanism for regulating and limiting C5a activity.

OTHER RECEPTORS

A 70 kDa molecule has been identified which binds to the collagen-like tail (see Fig. 12.6) of C1q. This receptor is located on polymorphs, monocytes, macrophages, B cells, platelets and endothelial cells. Its physiological function is uncertain, but it may augment the uptake of immune complexes opsonized with C1q.

Anaphylatoxin formation

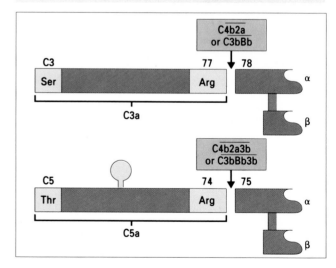

Fig. 12.19 The N-terminal ends of C3 and C5 α chains are shown. A 77-amino acid peptide, C3a, is split from the C3 molecule, revealing a C-terminal arginine, by the C3 convertase C4b2a (classical pathway) or C3bBb (alternative pathway). In the case of C5, a 74-amino acid peptide, C5a, is split from C5 also revealing a C-terminal arginine, by the C5 convertase, C4b2a3b (classical pathway) or C3bBb3b (alternative pathway). C5a contains a carbohydrate moiety indicated by the blue circle.

A receptor for Factor H has also been partially characterized. It is found on B lymphocytes, monocytes and neutrophils, and may similarly enhance immune complex uptake.

ACTIVATION OF COMPLEMENT RECEPTORS

Little is understood at present about the mechanisms of the cellular events occurring after complement receptors bind to their ligands. There is evidence that CR1, CR2 and CR3 undergo a reversible activation step of phosphorylation, which primes them to mediate activities such as phagocytosis or the generation of a respiratory burst. The cooperative ligation of other cell surface receptors (such as those for laminin or fibronectin) may stimulate this activation step.

 ## BIOLOGICAL EFFECTS OF COMPLEMENT

COMPLEMENT, INFLAMMATION AND ANAPHYLATOXINS

The complement system is a potent mechanism for initiating and amplifying inflammation. Some of the products of complement proteins stimulate chemotaxis and activation of leucocytes, notably C3a and C5a (Fig. 12.19). These two fragments are chemotactic for neutrophils, and trigger degranulation of basophils and mast cells (hence the name anaphylatoxins). The net effect of these activities is histamine- and leukotriene-mediated contraction of vascular smooth muscle, increase in vascular permeability and emigration of neutrophils and monocytes from blood vessels (Fig. 12.20). At the same time, bound C3 and C4 fragments act as opsonins (as described above) enhancing phagocytosis.

In addition to inducing phagocytosis, ligation of complement receptors on neutrophils, monocytes and macrophages may also stimulate exocytosis of granules containing powerful proteolytic enzymes, and free radical production through a respiratory burst (Fig. 12.21).

The complement cascade also interacts with other triggered-enzyme cascades: coagulation, kinin generation and fibrinolysis. There is another connection between these systems: the regulatory protein, C1 inhibitor, inhibits not only C1r and C1s but also Factor XIIa of the coagulation system, kallikrein of the kinin system and plasmin of the fibrinolytic cascade.

The production of anaphylatoxins follows not only from complement activation, but also from activation of other enzyme systems which may directly cleave C3, C4 and C5. Such enzymes include plasmin, kallikrein, tissue and leucocyte lysosomal enzymes, and bacterial proteases.

The anaphylatoxins have powerful effects on blood vessel walls, causing contraction of smooth muscle and an increase in vascular permeability. These effects show specific tachyphylaxis (i.e. repeated stimulation induces diminishing responses) and can be blocked by antihistamines; they are probably mediated indirectly via release of histamine from mast cells. C5a is the most powerful, approximately 100 times more effective than

Biological effects of C5a and C5a-des-Arg

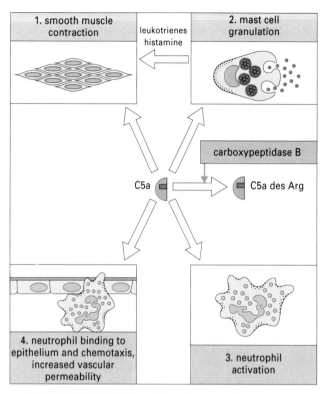

Fig. 12.20 C5a causes (1) smooth muscle contraction, (2) mast cell degranulation, (3) neutrophil activation and (4) margination and chemotaxis of neutrophils. Smooth muscle is further affected by histamine and leukotrienes released following mast cell degranulation or activation. Loss of the C-terminal arginine residue, following cleavage by carboxypeptidase B, produces C5a-des-Arg, which possesses weak cell-activating properties.

Effects of C3b and C4b

C3b and C4b facilitate:
binding of bacteria, viruses and immune complexes to neutrophils, monocytes and macrophages
endocytosis, phagocytosis and the respiratory burst, by complement receptor activation
phagocytosis and cytotoxicity via IgA (ADCC and NK activation)
erythrocyte CR1 binding to clear immune complexes
localization of immune complexes and APCs
solubilization of immune complexes by disruption of lattices

Fig. 12.21 C3b and C4b have a variety of functions, ranging from the binding of bacteria to the solubilization of immune complexes.

C3a, and 1000 times more effective than C4a or C5a-des-Arg. C5a is extremely potent at stimulating neutrophil chemotaxis, adherence, respiratory burst generation and degranulation. C5a also stimulates neutrophils to express more adhesion proteins, such as

CR3. Ligation of the neutrophil C5a receptor is followed by mobilization of membrane arachidonic acid which is metabolized to prostaglandins and leukotrienes including LTB4. This too is a potent chemotactic agent for neutrophils and monocytes. Another powerful mediator released following ligation of monocyte C5a receptors is IL-1. Thus the local synthesis of C5a at sites of inflammation has powerful pro-inflammatory properties. The role of complement in the development of inflammatory reactions and immune reactions is summarized in Fig. 12.22.

MEMBRANE ATTACK COMPLEX AND TISSUE INJURY

The single-hit model of complement lysis, developed by Mayer and his colleagues in the 1950s applies only to erythrocytes, and not to nucleated cells. These are

Summary of the actions of complement and its role in the acute inflammatory reaction

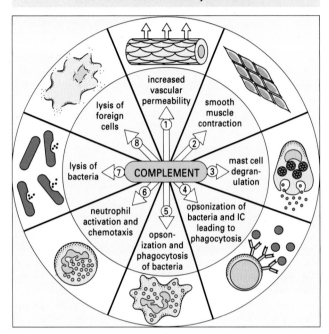

Fig. 12.22 Note how the elements of the reactions are induced: increased vascular permeability (1) due to the action of C3a and C5a on smooth muscle (2) and mast cells (3) allows exudation of plasma protein. C3 facilitates both the localization of complexes in germinal centres of spleen and lymph nodes (4) and the opsonization and phagocytosis of bacteria and immune complexes (5). Neutrophils, which are attracted to the area of inflammation by chemotaxis (6), phagocytose the opsonized microorganisms. The membrane attack complex, C5b–9, is responsible for the lysis of bacteria (7) and other cells recognized as foreign (8).

Effect of complement depletion on the IgG response

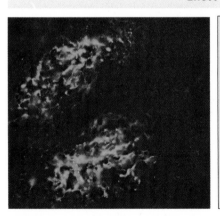

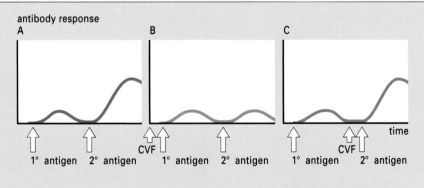

Fig. 12.23 Injection of priming (1°) and boosting (2°) doses of antigen produces a classical primary and secondary immune response (A). If the animal is complement-depleted by the addition of cobra venom factor (CVF) prior to the primary response, immunological memory fails to develop, and on subsequent antigen challenge the animal produces another primary response (B). The effect of CVF is only produced if complement is depleted prior to the primary response – depletion subsequent to the primary response does not hinder a normal secondary response (C). The effect of depletion is thought to be related to poor localization of antigen–antibody complexes in the germinal centres of complement-depleted animals. The immunofluorescence picture shows antigen localized in the germinal centres of mouse spleen (24 hours after injection of 1 mg of aggregated human IgG, here acting as antigen) and bound predominantly to the dendritic cells. This localization does not occur in complement-depleted mice. (Courtesy of Professor J Holborow.)

relatively resistant to osmotic disruption by the MAC, largely because they can endocytose and exocytose portions of membrane containing MAC. However, the perturbation of the membrane bilayer can stimulate cells (depending on their innate capabilities) to release and metabolize arachidonic acid, to undertake oxidative metabolism, or to release granules or cytokines. These responses may play an important role in amplifying inflammation following complement activation.

COMPLEMENT AND INDUCTION OF IMMUNE RESPONSES

Complement plays an important accessory role in the induction of antibody responses. It acts to enhance the localization of antigen to antigen-presenting cells and to B cells. In the case of immune complexes, their localization to the germinal centres of lymph nodes, essential for the formation of memory B cells, is a complement-dependent process (Fig. 12.23). B cells carry two receptors for C3: CR1 which binds C3b and iC3b, and CR2 which binds iC3b and C3dg. Monocytes and macrophages bear receptors, CR1 and CR3. Follicular dendritic cells are the only cells which have been shown to bear all three receptors, CR1, CR2 and CR3. Humans with hereditary deficiency of C3 have only mild impairment of antibody production. However, C2-, C3- or C4-deficiency in guinea pigs markedly impairs the primary and secondary antibody responses to low immunizing doses of T-cell-dependent antigens. Present evidence therefore suggests that complement plays an accessory, but not necessary, role in the efficient induction of antibody responses.

COMPLEMENT AND IMMUNE COMPLEXES

In the 1940s, Heidelbrger observed the complement inhibited the formation of precipitating antigen–antibody lattices. Immune complex lattice size is influenced by many factors which include:

1. the concentration of the reactants, antibody and antigen

2. the affinity of the antibody for its antigen
3. the valency of both antibody and antigen, high valency favouring large lattice formation.

The classical pathway of complement inhibits the formation of precipitating immune complexes in plasma. In the same way, activation of the alternative pathway can solubilize immune complexes that have already precipitated, including those in tissues. This is achieved by the covalent incorporation of C3 into immune-complex lattices. C3 binding may disrupt immune-complex lattices by reducing the capacity of the antibody to bind to epitopes on the antigen, thus limiting the possibilities for forming large lattices (see Chapter 21).

The activation of complement by immune complexes is normally beneficial. Immune complexes bearing C3 are efficiently removed from tissues and from the circulation by monocytes and other phagocytes. However there are circumstances in which immune complex production continues at a high level; complement activation by immune complexes may then prove deleterious. For example, inflammatory effects of immune complexes in diseases such as subacute bacterial endocarditis and SLE may be largely mediated by the complement system.

COMPLEMENT AND DEFENCE AGAINST INFECTION

Microorganisms can activate complement via the classical or alternative pathways (Fig. 12.24). The pathogenicity of many bacterial strains depends on their ability to resist destruction by complement. Many mechanisms mediating such resistance have been described, and these include:

1. the direction of C3b and MAC to specific sites on the bacterial surface where they cannot produce opsonization or lysis (conversely, bactericidal antibody may function by directing complement activation to sites on the bacteria which result in effective opsonization or lysis)
2. the possession of surface molecules which resist alternative-pathway activation, and resist the amplification of C3 deposition

Activators of complement

| | immunoglobulins | microorganisms | | | other |
		viruses	bacteria	other	
classical pathway	complexes containing IgM, IgG1, IgG2 or IgG3	murine retroviruses, vesicular stomatitis virus	–	Mycoplasma	polyanions, esp. when bound to cations, PO_4^{3-}(DNA, lipid A, cardiolipin), SO_4^{2-}(dextran sulphate, heparin, chrondroitin sulphate) arrays of terminal mannase groups (via mannan protein)
alternative pathway	complexes containing IgG, IgA or IgE (less efficient then the classical pathway)	some virus-infected cells (e.g. EBV)	many strains of gram-positive and gram-negative organisms	trypanosomes, Leishmania, many fungi	dextran sulphate, heterologous erythrocytes, carbohydrates (e.g. agarose)

Fig. 12.24 This diagram summarizes the activators of the classical and alternative pathways.

3. the complex structure of bacterial cell walls which, coupled with efficient facilities for membrane repair and rapid cell division, confers considerable resistance to complement-mediated damage.

The possession of a capsule rich in sialic acids distinguishes certain pathogenic gram-positive bacterial strains from their non-pathogenic counterparts. On such a capsule, C3b binds Factor H rather than Factor B, leading to catabolism of C3b.

The physiological role of complement as an opsonin and a bacteriolysin is elegantly illustrated by two different hereditary deficiency states in humans. Deficiency of either the classical pathway components and C3, or of the family of cell surface receptors comprising CR3 and LFA-1 produces a similar spectrum of infections by pyogenic bacteria. The fact that deficiency of either the opsonin or the receptor has similar consequences, demonstrates convincingly that complement plays an important role in the destruction of these bacteria through phagocytosis and intracellular destruction. In contrast, deficiencies of MAC components are associated almost exclusively with recurrent infections by *Neisseria meningitidis* or *N. gonorrhoeae*. Thus host defence against these bacteria, which are characterized by their ability to survive in the intracellular milieu, depends on their lysis in plasma by complement.

Complement seems to be of less importance in host defence against viral infections, where T cells play a more important role. Complement deficiency is not associated with undue susceptibility to viral infections. However there are a number of links between viruses and the complement system, of which the most striking is the use of CR2 by Epstein–Barr virus to penetrate cells. Some viruses may gain access to cells indirectly via antibody and C3b fixed to the virus. Examples of this include antibody-enhanced uptake of flaviviruses (including Dengue virus) via macrophage Fc receptors, and CR3-mediated uptake of West Nile virus (also a flavivirus) by C3 fixed to viral particles (shown in mice).

Molecules on microorganisms with Fc-receptor activities have been known for some time, e.g. Staphylococcal protein A and the Fc receptor present on many herpesviruses. A recent finding is that *Herpes simplex* also expresses a molecule with complement-receptor activity. Such molecules may protect microorganisms from the normal consequences of the binding of antibody and complement proteins to their surfaces; for example, such IgG or C3 may be blocked from recognition by opsonic receptors on host phagocytic cells.

COMPLEMENT AND THE PATHOGENESIS OF DISEASE

Under some circumstances the consequences of complement activation *in vivo* may be deleterious rather than beneficial. The state of shock that may follow bacteraemia with gram-negative organisms may, in part, be mediated by complement, which is extensively activated by endotoxin. The large quantities of C3a and C5a which result from this cause activation and degranulation of neutrophils, basophils and mast cells. These anaphylatoxins may stimulate intravascular neutrophil aggregation leading to clotting and deposition of emboli in the pulmonary microvasculature. At this site, neutrophil products, including elastase and free radicals, may cause the condition of shock lung. This condition is characterized by interstitial pulmonary oedema due to damage to small blood vessels, exudation of neutrophils into alveoli, and arterial hypoxaemia. Extracorporeal blood circulation, for example through heart–lung bypass machines, or over cuprophane dialysis membranes, may similarly cause activation of complement, accompanied by transient leucopenia, thought to be caused by aggregation of neutrophils in the lungs.

Tissue injury following ischaemic infarction may also cause complement activation. Abundant deposition of membrane attack complex may be readily seen in tissue following ischaemic injury. A possible pathophysiological role for complement activation following tissue ischaemia was demonstrated in experimental models of myocardial infarction: complement depletion reduced the size of tissue injury and infusion of soluble CR1 has recently been shown to have a similar effect.

Complement activation is also an important cause of tissue injury in diseases mediated by immune complexes. Such complexes may form in tissues, for example in glomeruli of patients with autoantibodies to glomerular basement membrane (Goodpasture's syndrome) or at motor end-plates in patients with autoantibodies to acetylcholine receptors (myasthenia gravis) (see Chapters 20 and 21). Alternatively, immune complexes may become trapped in blood vessel walls having travelled through the circulation. This occurs, for example, in systemic lupus erythematosus, and in bacterial endocarditis in which an infected heart valve provides the source of immune complexes which deposit in the kidney and other microvascular beds. Complement mediates inflammation in these diseases by two major pathways:

1. by activated leucocytes, which are attracted to sites of immune complex deposition by locally-produced anaphylatoxins, and which bind to C3 and C4 fixed to the immune complexes
2. by the membrane attack complex (MAC), which causes cell lysis and thus stimulates prostaglandin synthesis from arachidonic acid, mobilized from perturbed cell membranes.

These two mechanisms of damage are well exemplified by considering two types of glomerular disease. Autoantibodies to glomerular basement membrane cause inflammation which can be inhibited by either complement depletion or by neutrophil depletion. In contrast, membranous nephritis, (which may be induced experimentally by antibodies to subepithelial antigens), is unaffected by neutrophil depletion, but almost totally abrogated in animals deficient in C5. In this disease the basement membrane is presumed to act as a physical barrier to neutrophil exudation, so that the heavy proteinuria is caused by deposition of membrane attack complex.

FURTHER READING

Arlaud GJ, Colomb MG, Gagnon J. A functional model of the human C1 complex. *Immunol Today* 1987;**8**:106–11.

Atkinson JP, Farries T. Separation of self from non-self in the complement system. *Immunol Today* 1987;**8**:212–15.

Bhakdi S, Tranum-Jensen J. Mechanism of complement cytolysis and the concept of channel-forming proteins. *Philos Trans R Soc London (Biol)* 1984;**306**:311–24.

Campbell RD, Law SKA, Reid KBM, Sim RB. Structure, organisation, and regulation of the complement genes. *Annu Rev Immunol* 1988; **6**:161–95.

Carrell RW, Boswell DR. Serpins: the superfamily of plasma serine proteinase inhibitors. In: Barrett A, Salveson G, eds. *Proteinase Inhibitors*. Amsterdam: Elsevier, 1986: 403–20.

Colten HR, Strunk RC, Perlmutter DH, Cole FS. Regulation of complement protein biosynthesis in mononuclear phagocytes. In: Evered D, Nugent J, O'Connor M, eds. *Ciba Symposium 118: Biochemistry of Macrophages*. London: Pitman Ltd, 1986: 141–51.

Cooper NR. The classical complement pathway: activation and regulation of the first complement component. *Adv Immunol* 1985;**37**:151–216.

Couser WG, Baker PJ, Adler S. Complement and the direct mediation of immune glomerular injury: a new perspective. *Kidney Int* 1985;**28**:879–90.

Fearon DT. Cellular receptors for fragments of the third component of complement. *Immunol Today* 1984;**5**:105–10.

Gerard NP, Gerard C. The chemotactic receptor for C5a anaphylatoxin. *Nature* 1991;**349**:614–17.

Hourcade D, Holers VM, Atkinson JP. The regulators of complement activation (RCA) gene cluster. *Adv Immunol* 1989;**45**:381–416.

Kishimoto TK, Larson RS, Corbi AL, Dustin ML, Staunton DE, Springer TA. The leukocyte integrins. *Adv Immunol* 1989;**46**:149–182.

Klaus GGB, Humphrey JH. A re-evaluation of the role of C3 in B-cell activation. *Immunology Today* 1986;**7**:163–165.

Lachmann P J. A common form of killing. *Nature* 1986;**321**:560.

Lachmann PJ, Walport MJ. Deficiency of the effector mechanisms of the immune response and autoimmunity. In: Whelan J, ed. *Ciba Foundation Symposium 129: Autoimmunity and Autoimmune Diseases*. Chichester: Wiley,1987:149–71.

Morgan BP. *Complement: clinical aspects and relevance to disease*. London and New York: Academic Press, 1990.

Muller-Eberhard HJ. The membrane attack complex of complement. *Annu Rev Immunol* 1984;**2**:503–28

Muller-Eberhard HJ, Schreiber RD. Molecular biology and chemistry of the alternative pathway of complement. *Adv Immunol* 1980;**29**:1–53.

Porter RR, Reid KBM. The biochemistry of complement. *Nature* 1978;**275**:699–704.

Reid KBM, Porter RR. The proteolytic activation systems of complement. *Annu Rev Biochem* 1981;**50**:433–64.

Reid KBM, Day AJ. Structure–function relationships of the complement components. *Immunol Today*, 1989;**10**:177–80.

Ross GD, ed. *Immunobiology of the Complement System*. New York: Academic Press, 1986.

Ross GD, Medof ME. Membrane complement receptors specific for bound fragments of C3. *Adv Immunol* 1985;**37**;217–67.

Schifferli JA, Ng YC, Peters DK. The role of complement and its receptor in the elimination of immune complexes. *N Engl J Med* 1986;**315**:488–95.

Whaley K, ed. *Complement in Health and Disease*. Lancaster, UK: MTP Press, 1987.

chapter 13

Cell Migration and Inflammation

Under normal conditions, leucocytes migrate through all the tissues of the body. The purpose of this migration is to give the small numbers of lymphocytes which are specific for any particular antigen, the chance to encounter that antigen. At sites of immune reaction, there is an enhanced migration of cells into the site (Fig. 13.1). This enhanced migration includes both lymphocytes and phagocytic cells. The lymphocytes include some that are specific for the pathogen or antigen, but many that are not. Cells may be retained at the site of inflammation until the initiating antigen has been cleared, but then return to the lymphatic system.

There are two main stages in leucocyte migration. The first is the attachment of circulating cells to the vascular endothelium (Fig. 13.2), and this is followed by movement between or through the endothelial cells. After traversing the endothelium (Fig. 13.3), cells migrate towards the site of infection or inflammation, under the guidance of chemotactic stimuli. These processes are controlled partly by cell surface molecules on the migrating cells, which allow them to interact with endothelium, tissue cells or extracellular matrix, and partly by a variety of soluble signalling molecules (cytokines and chemotactic molecules).

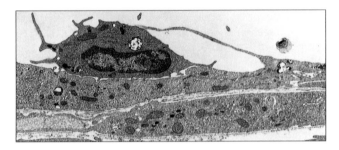

Fig. 13.1 Lymphocyte migration. Electron micrograph showing a lymphocyte adhering to brain endothelium close to the interendothelial cell junction, in an animal with experimental allergic encephalomyelitis. Adhesion precedes transendothelial migration into inflammatory sites. Courtesy of Dr C. Hawkins.

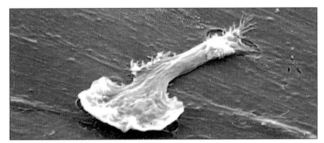

Fig. 13.2 Lymphocyte interaction with endothelium. Scanning electron micrograph showing an antigen-activated T cell binding to retinal endothelium *in vitro*. The migrating cell attaches to the endothelium and then extends pseudopodia, to probe the endothelial cell for a suitable migration point. Courtesy of Dr J. Greenwood.

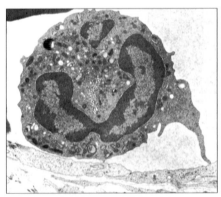 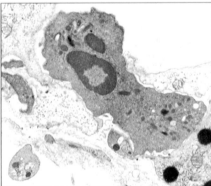 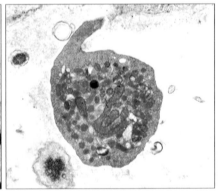

Fig. 13.3 Three phases of neutrophil migration. A polymorphonuclear leucocyte adheres to the capillary endothelium (left) before penetrating between the endothelial cells (middle). The third electron micrograph (right) illustrates a leucocyte which has traversed the endothelium. × 4000. Courtesy of Dr I. Jovis.

CELL MIGRATION AND LOCALIZATION

The cells of the immune system all originate from bone marrow stem cells, but they carry out their functions in the lymphoid tissues and at other sites throughout the body (Fig. 13.4). Consequently they must transit between these various tissues via the blood lymphatics. Neutrophils make a one-way journey from the bone marrow to the tissues where they carry out their effector functions and eventually die. In contrast, lymphocytes and some mononuclear phagocytes can recirculate between lymphoid and non-lymphoid tissues. The purpose of all this activity is to bring antigen into contact with those lymphocytes which recognize it, and to distribute effector cells to sites where they are needed. The patterns of cell migration are complex, and depend not only on the type of cell, but also on its stage of differentiation or activation. Moreover, vascular endothelium varies throughout the body, and this influences cell migration. In particular, the high endothelial venules (HEV) found in secondary lymphoid tissues are quite different from those found in non-lymphoid tissues. Among non-lymphoid tissues the small vessel endothelium varies considerably between different tissue types, and in all cases the molecules present on endothelium are modulated locally when inflammatory responses develop. All these factors affect the types of cells which migrate across different endothelial beds. In general, leucocyte migration depends on the surface charge of the interacting cells, the haemodynamic shear force in the vascular bed and the expression of complementary sets of adhesion molecules on the leucocytes and the endothelium (Fig. 13.5). Once cells have left the vasculature, they use different sets of adhesion molecules to manoeuvre through the tissues.

One can distinguish several types of leucocyte migration.
1. Virgin lymphocytes move from the primary lymphoid tissues to the blood and thence into secondary lymphoid tissues.
2. Activated lymphocytes move from the spleen and lymph nodes into the blood and may then distribute to other lymphoid tissues or cross vascular endothelium into other tissues.
3. Antigen-presenting cells (APCs) such as macrophages and dendritic cells also circulate back to lymphoid tissues and may carry antigen in from the periphery.

Different patterns of movement occur at different stages of a cell's life span. For example, resting T cells tend to migrate across high endothelial venules into secondary lymphoid tissues, while activated cells tend to migrate into sites of inflammation. Cellular localization is controlled by receptors on the leucocytes interacting with complementary ligands on endothelium.

Recirculation of lymphocytes and antigen-presenting cells

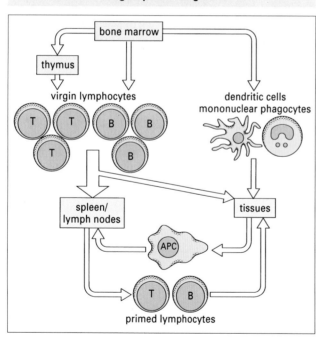

Fig. 13.4 Virgin lymphocytes from the primary lymphoid tissues migrate primarily to secondary lymphoid tissues, i.e. the spleen and lymph nodes. Antigen-presenting cells (APCs), including dendritic cells and mononuclear phagocytes, also derive from bone marrow stem cells. These APCs enter tissues, take up antigen and transport it to the lymphoid tissues to be presented to T cells and B cells. Primed lymphocytes migrate from the lymphoid tissues and accumulate preferentially at sites of infection or inflammation.

Factors controlling leucocyte adhesion

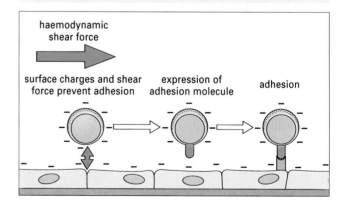

Fig. 13.5 Leucocytes adhere to vascular endothelium when the binding between pairs of intercellular adhesion molecules is sufficient to overcome the charge-based repulsion between the cells, particularly at sites where haemodynamic shear forces are low.

Subsequently, different sets of adhesion molecules interact with extracellular matrix proteins, such as collagen and fibronectin, and with the tissue cells themselves.

When immune reactions occur in tissues, in response to antigen challenge, there is usually a phased appearance of different cell populations. The types of cells which are seen, their preponderance and their time of arrival, depend primarily on the nature of the antigenic challenge and on the site where the reactions occur. In general, neutrophils are the first cells into sites of acute inflammation caused by infection. They represent the major cell type for several days. From the first day onwards mononuclear phagocytes and lymphocytes start to arrive. In contrast, during chronic autoimmune reactions, few neutrophils are seen, but there are large numbers of CD4+ T cells and mononuclear phagocytes. Reactions to parasite infections (e.g. schistosomiasis) often lead to an accumulation of eosinophils. Eosinophils, basophils and macrophages are prevalent in the wall of the bronchus following asthmatic attacks. Even different subpopulations of cells may arrive at inflammatory sites at different times. For example, in experimental allergic encephalomyelitis (an autoimmune condition initiated by sensitization to myelin), CD4+ T cells usually predominate during the acute phase of the condition, whereas CD8+ T cells are more prevalent in the later recovery phase.

Modulation of leucocyte adhesion

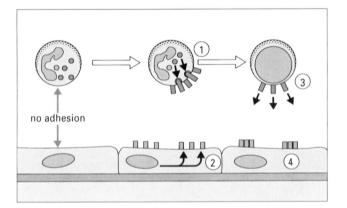

no adhesion

Fig. 13.6 There are four ways in which leucocyte binding to endothelium may become enhanced. Many cells hold stores of adhesion molecules, which can be rapidly moved to the cell surface (1). Endothelial cells at sites of inflammation may synthesize new adhesion molecules (2). Molecules such as LFA-1 can increase their affinity following cell activation (3). Reorganization of adhesion molecules on the cell surface may result in the formation of high avidity patches (4). In practice, cells may use several mechanisms and affinity changes may follow the initial interaction between the cells.

To explain these complex and varied patterns of cell migration, one must consider the large numbers of factors which modulate cell movement. These are:
1. the state of activation of the lymphocytes or phagocytes
2. the types of adhesion molecules expressed by the vascular endothelium, which is related to its anatomical site, and to the state of activation inducible by cytokines
3. the presence of chemotactic molecules, which may selectively attract particular populations of leucocytes.

INTERCELLULAR ADHESION MOLECULES

Intercellular adhesion molecules are membrane-bound proteins which allow one cell to interact with another. Often these molecules traverse the membrane and are linked to the cytoskeleton, so that the cell can use them to gain traction on other cells, or on the extracellular matrix, as they move. In many cases, a particular adhesion molecule can bind to more than one ligand, using different binding sites. Although the binding affinity of individual adhesion molecules to their ligands is usually low, the possibility of large numbers of interactions, due to the abundance or clustering of both adhesion molecules and ligands, means that the avidity of the interaction can be high. Cells can modulate their interactions with other cell types, either by increasing the numbers of adhesion molecules on the surface, or by altering their affinity/avidity (Fig. 13.6). There are two ways in which cells can alter the level of expression of adhesion molecules: many cells retain large intracellular stores of these molecules in vesicles, which can be directed to the cell surface within minutes following cellular activation. Alternatively, new molecules can be synthesized and transported to the cell surface, a process which usually takes several hours.

A bewilderingly large number of adhesion molecules have been identified, although they fall into families which are structurally related. Defining the precise function of the different adhesion molecules has proved more difficult. It now appears likely that any interaction between endothelium and circulating leucocytes involves a number of different pairs of these molecules.

FAMILIES OF ADHESION MOLECULES
The selectins or lectin cellular adhesion molecules (LECCAMS), include the molecules ELAM-1, GMP-140 and MEL-14 (homing receptor). They are transmembrane molecules, with a number of extracellular domains homologous to those seen in the complement receptors CR1 and CR2. The extracellular region also has a domain related to the EGF-receptor and a N-terminal domain which has lectin-like properties (i.e. it binds to carbohydrate residues), hence the name selectins. Unsurprisingly, their ligands (those so far identified) carry carbohydrate moieties.

The immunoglobulin supergene family includes ICAM-1, ICAM-2 and VCAM. All members of this family are expressed, or inducible, on vascular endothelium. ICAM-1 has five extracellular domains; the two N-terminal domains are structurally homologous to the two extracellular domains of ICAM-2. VCAM has six extracellular domains (Fig. 13.7).

Integrins comprise the third major group of adhesion molecules. Each member of this large family of molecules consists of two non-covalently bound polypeptides (α and β), both of which traverse the membrane. They fall into three main sub-families, depending on whether they have a β_1 chain, a β_2 chain or a β_3 chain (Fig. 13.8). Recent discoveries suggest that the assortment of α chains with β chains is not quite as precise as originally thought. Broadly speaking the β_1-integrins are involved in binding of cells to extracellular matrix, the β_2-integrins are involved in leucocyte adhesion to endothelium or to other immune cells, and the β_3-integrins (cytoadhesins) are involved in the interactions of platelets and neutrophils at inflammatory sites or sites of vascular damage. There are however several exceptions to this simple scheme.

Vascular addressins form another group of adhesion molecules. These molecules are expressed on high endothelial venules at different sites around the body, and may also be induced on other endothelium at sites of chronic inflammation (Fig. 13.9). These molecules modulate lymphocyte traffic into secondary lymphoid tissues and inflammatory sites. One addressin is present on HEVs of peripheral lymph nodes, while another is present on HEVs in mucosal lymphoid tissue, such as the Peyer's patches.

FUNCTIONS OF ADHESION MOLECULES

Although it is difficult to unequivocally associate a single pair of adhesion molecules with a particular type of cell traffic, certain principles do apply.

As noted above, neutrophils appear early at sites of acute inflammation and this is in part controlled by the induction of ELAM on the surface of endothelium in these areas. ELAM interacts with the asialo-Lewis X determinant, present on surface glycoproteins of the neutrophils. In vitro stimulation of endothelium with cytokines such as TNF_α or IL-1 induces expression of ELAM over a period of 4–12 hours, but expression wanes by 24 hours (Fig. 13.10). Cells transfected with the gene for ELAM, which express high levels of this adhesion molecule, bind neutrophils strongly. Antibodies to ELAM block this binding. This evidence implicates ELAM in the control of neutrophil accumulation.

Also important in migration of neutrophils, lymphocytes and monocytes are the β_2-integrins LFA-1 and CR3, expressed on the leucocytes. LFA-1 binds to ICAM-1 and ICAM-2 expressed on vascular endothelium. In vitro, the endothelial expression of ICAM-2 is constitutive, and it has been suggested that ICAM-2 determines the basal level of binding of lymphocytes to

Structure of three endothelial cell adhesion molecules

known ligands		
LFA-1 and CR3	LFA-1	VLA-4
⇩	⇩	⇩
		VCAM
ICAM-1		
	ICAM-2	
endothelial cell		

Fig. 13.7 The molecules ICAM-1, ICAM-2 and VCAM, are illustrated diagrammatically with their immunoglobulin-like domains. Known ligands are listed above each molecule.

Integrins

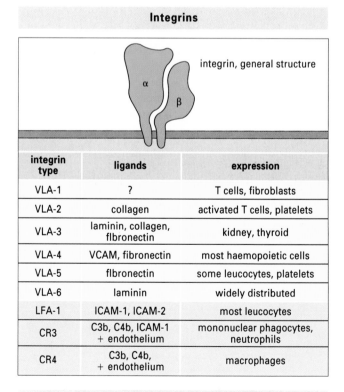

integrin, general structure

integrin type	ligands	expression
VLA-1	?	T cells, fibroblasts
VLA-2	collagen	activated T cells, platelets
VLA-3	laminin, collagen, flbronectin	kidney, thyroid
VLA-4	VCAM, fibronectin	most haemopoietic cells
VLA-5	flbronectin	some leucocytes, platelets
VLA-6	laminin	widely distributed
LFA-1	ICAM-1, ICAM-2	most leucocytes
CR3	C3b, C4b, ICAM-1 + endothelium	mononuclear phagocytes, neutrophils
CR4	C3b, C4b, + endothelium	macrophages

Fig. 13.8 The table gives the properties of the β_1- (yellow) and β_2- (red) integrins.

different types of endothelium. For example, ICAM-2 expression is relatively low on brain endothelium, and cell migration across normal cerebral endothelium is also relatively low. In contrast ICAM-1 is normally present at low levels on endothelium, but can be induced by cytokines (TNF, IL-1 and IFN$_\gamma$, depending on the species). ICAM-1 is induced over 24–96 hours *in vitro*, which corresponds to the later arrival of monocytes and lymphocytes (Fig. 13.10). The function of CR3 in phagocyte accumulation has been pinpointed by *in vivo* studies using antibodies to CR3, which inhibit phagocyte migration. Notably, a group of patients who suffer from leucocyte adhesion deficiency (LAD) syndrome, and who suffer from severe infections due to poor phagocyte accumulation, are deficient in all the β_2-integrins (LFA-1, CR3, CR4). Although CR3 and CR4 bind to the breakdown products of complement C3, this cannot explain their role in cell migration, and it is therefore thought that these molecules may have other ligands on the endothelium, possibly ICAM-1.

The possible role of LFA-1/ICAM-1 in controlling lymphocyte migration into inflammatory sites was mentioned above. Additionally, VCAM appears to be important in controlling lymphocyte migration. VCAM is induced on endothelium by cytokines, with a similar time course to ICAM-1. In fact, there are some subtle differences between the induction of these two molecules, in that IFN$_\gamma$ induces ICAM-1 but not VCAM. This suggests that different blends of cytokines at different sites could affect the spectrum of adhesion molecules present on the local endothelium. VCAM, on the endothelium, binds to the β_1-integrin VLA-4, and anti-VLA-4 antibodies block lymphocyte binding to endothelium. It has been suggested that interfering with lymphocyte–endothelial cell adhesion could be a useful way of controlling immune reactions *in vivo*. For example, it has been possible to inhibit the development of EAE using anti-VLA-4, but this kind of approach has not yet been tried in man.

One must draw a distinction between the molecules described above, which control cell movement into inflammatory sites, and those such as the addressins, which control normal lymphocyte traffic. However, there may be some overlap, as HEV-like vessels appear at chronic inflammatory sites (e.g. the joint in rheumatoid arthritis), and express HEV-specific adhesion molecules.

Once they have crossed the endothelium and entered the tissues, the cells must interact with the proteins of the extracellular matrix (collagen, laminin, fibronectin etc.), as well as the tissue cells. As neutrophils leave the blood vessel, they lose some of their surface molecules (e.g. ELAM) which are no longer required. The functional phenotype changes from that of a circulating cell to one adapted to move through tissues.

Many of the molecules which allow interaction with extracellular matrix belong to the β_1-integrin group, and are known as very late antigens (VLAs), so called because they were first identified on the T-cell surface at a late stage after T-cell activation. More recently, the whole group of β_1-integrins have been referred to as VLA molecules, even though most of them are not expressed only on lymphocytes. This group includes receptors for collagen (VLA-2 and VLA-3), laminin (VLA-3 and VLA-6) and fibronectin (VLA-3, VLA-4 and VLA-5). The fact that some of these molecules appear late after lymphocyte activation suggests that cells go through a programme of differentiation, and that the ability to interact with extracellular matrix is one of the last functions to develop.

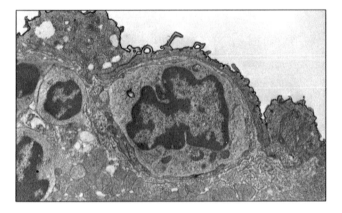

Fig. 13.9 Addressin on endothelial cell surfaces.
Immunoelectron micrograph stained to show the addressin which is normally present on high endothelial venules. In this instance the molecule is expressed on brain endothelium in chronic relapsing experimental allergic encephalomyelitis, induced by immunization of Biozzi AB/H mice with myelin basic protein. (Courtesy of of Drs J. K. O' Neill and C. Butter, with permission from *Immunology*.)

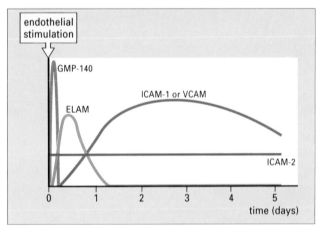

Fig. 13.10 The graph shows the time course of induction of different endothelial molecules on human umbilical vein endothelium *in vitro*, following stimulation by TNF$_\alpha$.

INFLAMMATION

Inflammation is the body's reaction to invasion by an infectious agent, antigen challenge or even just physical damage. In the same way that it is necessary to increase the blood supply to active muscles during exercise, to provide glucose and oxygen, so it is necessary to direct elements of the immune system to sites of infection or injury. Three major events occur during this response (Fig. 13.11).

1. Blood supply to the area increases.

2. There is an increase in capillary permeability, caused by retraction of the endothelial cells and possibly also by increased vesicular transport across the endothelium. This permits larger molecules to traverse the endothelium than would ordinarily be capable of doing so and thus allows antibody, complement and molecules of other plasma enzyme systems to reach the inflammatory site.

3. Leucocytes, initially neutrophils and macrophages and later lymphocytes, migrate out of the capillaries and into the surrounding tissues (see above). Once in the tissues the cells migrate towards the site of injury under the direction of chemotactic stimuli.

THE CONTROL OF INFLAMMATION

The development of inflammatory reactions is controlled by cytokines, by products of the plasma enzyme systems, and by vasoactive mediators released from mast cells, basophils and platelets (Fig. 13.12). The mediators controlling different types of inflammatory reaction differ. Fast-acting mediators, such as vasoactive amines and the products of the kinin system, modulate the immediate response. Later, newly synthesized mediators such as leukotrienes are involved in the accumulation and activation of other cells. Once leucocytes

Inflammation

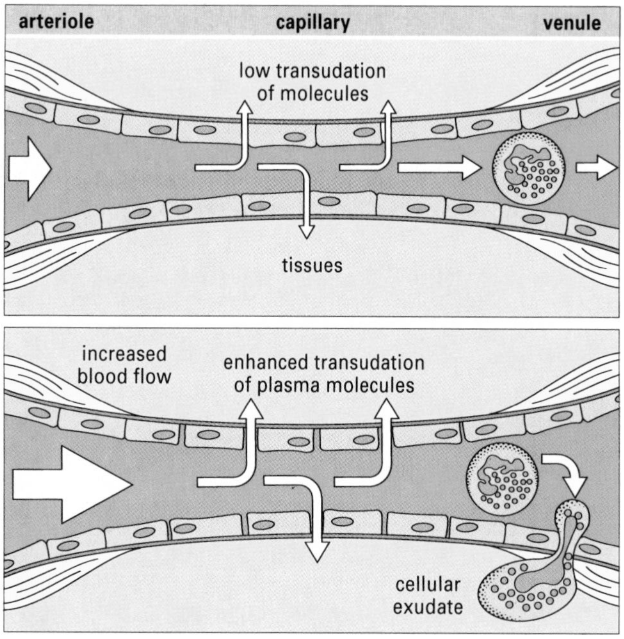

Fig. 13.11 The diagram shows normal tissue (upper), and the three main alterations which occur when inflammation develops (lower). There is an increased blood flow, increased transudation of large serum molecules in the capillary bed, and migration of leucocytes across venules.

Mediators of inflammation

mediator	origin	actions
histamine	mast cells, basophils	increased vascular permeability, smooth muscle contraction, chemokinesis
5-hydroxy-tryptamine (5HT)=serotonin	platelets, mast cells (rodent)	increased vascular permeability, smooth muscle contraction
platelet activating factor (PAF)	basophils, neutrophils, macrophages	mediator release from platelets, increased vascular permeability, smooth muscle contraction, neutrophil activation
neutrophil chemotactic factor (NCF)	mast cells	neutrophil chemotaxis
IL-8	lymphocytes	monocyte localization
C3a	complement C3	mast cell degranulation, smooth muscle contraction
C5a	complement C5	mast cell degranulation, neutrophil and macrophage chemotaxis, neutrophil activation, smooth muscle contraction, increased capillary permeability
bradykinin	kinin system (kininogen)	vasodilation, smooth muscle contraction, increased capillary permeability, pain
fibrinopeptides and fibrin breakdown products	clotting system	increased vascular permeability, neutrophil and macrophage chemotaxis
prostaglandin E_2 (PGE$_2$)	cyclooxygenase pathway	vasodilation, potentiates increased vascular permeability produced by histamine and bradykinin
leukotriene B_4 (LTB$_4$)	lipoxygenase pathway	neutrophil chemotaxis, synergizes with PGE$_2$ in increasing vascular permeability
leukotriene D_4 (LTD$_4$)	lipoxygenase pathway	smooth muscle contraction, increasing vascular permeability

Fig. 13.12 The table lists major inflammatory mediators, which control blood supply and vascular permeability or modulate cell movement. The main sources are given (centre block).

have arrived at a site of infection or inflammation, they release mediators which control the later accumulation and activation of other cells. However, in inflammatory reactions initiated by the immune system, the ultimate control is exerted by the antigen itself, in the same way as it controls the immune response itself. For this reason, the cellular accumulation at the site of chronic infection, or in autoimmune reactions (where the antigen cannot ultimately be eradicated), is quite different from that at sites where the antigenic stimulus is rapidly cleared.

There are four major plasma enzyme systems which have an important role in haemostasis and control of inflammation. These are the clotting system, the fibrinolytic (plasmin) system, the kinin system and the complement system. In many ways the complement system acts as a link between immunological events and inflammatory systems (see Chapter 12).

The kinin system generates the mediators bradykinin and lysyl-bradykinin, or kallidin. Bradykinin is a very powerful vasoactive nonapeptide, which causes venular dilation, increased vascular permeability and smooth muscle contraction. Bradykinin is generated following the activation of Hageman factor (XII) of the blood clotting system, whereas kallidin is generated following activation of the plasmin system, or by enzymes released from damaged tissues (Fig. 13.13).

Auxiliary cells, including mast cells, basophils and platelets, are important sources of the vasoactive mediators histamine and 5-hydroxytryptamine, which produce vasodilation and increased vascular permeability. Many of the proinflammatory effects of C3a and C5a result from their ability to trigger mast-cell granule release, since they can be blocked by anti-histamines.

Mast cells and basophils are also a route by which the adaptive immune system can trigger inflammation – IgE sensitizes these cells for antigen-specific triggering of granule release. The interactions of these systems are shown in Fig. 13.14. Mast cells are also an important source of slow-reacting inflammatory mediators, including the leukotrienes, prostaglandins and thromboxanes. The role of these products of arachidonic acid metabolism is outlined in Chapter 19.

Platelets may also be activated by the immune system, since they express Fc receptors and are triggered by immune complexes. This is thought to be important in Type II and Type III hypersensitivity reactions.

The immune system in acute inflammation

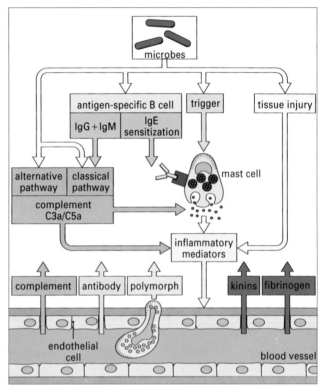

Fig. 13.14 The adaptive immune system modulates inflammatory processes via the complement system. Antigens (e.g. from microorganisms) stimulate B cells to produce antibodies including IgE, which binds to mast cells, while IgG and IgM activate complement. Complement can also be activated directly via the alternative pathway. When triggered by antigen, the sensitized mast cells release their granule-associated mediators and eicosanoids (products of arachidonic metabolism, including prostaglandins and leukotrienes). In association with complement (which can also trigger mast cells via C3a and C5a) the mediators induce local inflammation, facilitating the arrival of leucocytes and more plasma enzyme system molecules.

Activation of the kinin system

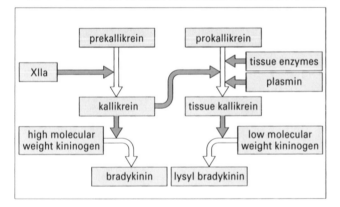

Fig. 13.13 Activated Hageman factor (XIIa) acts on prekallikrein to generate kallikrein, which in turn releases bradykinin from high molecular weight kininogen (HMWK). (Prekallikrein and HMWK circulate together, in a complex.) Various enzymes activate prokallikrein to tissue kallikrein, which releases lysyl bradykinin from low molecular weight kininogen.

Cytokines are also important in signalling between cells as inflammatory reactions develop. In the initial stages, cytokines such as IL-1 and IL-6 may be released from cells of the tissue where the inflammatory reaction is occurring. Once lymphocytes and mononuclear cells have started to enter the inflammatory site, they may become activated by antigen and release cytokines of their own (IL-1, TNF, IL-4, IFN$_\gamma$) which further enhance cellular migration by their actions on the local endothelium. Other cytokines, such as IL-8, are chemotactic.

CHEMOTAXIS

Chemotaxis is the directional migration of cells up a concentration gradient of a chemotactic molecule, in this case, towards a site of inflammation or immune reactions. Several mediators, such as histamine, are able to enhance the overall motility of cells, but do not induce directional migration: this is referred to as chemokinesis. For directional migration to occur, the cell must be responsive to gradients of the chemotactic mediator. It has been estimated that the concentration difference between the leading and trailing edges of a migrating cell may be as little as 0.1%. Nevertheless, the cells are able to recognize these small differences and move accordingly.

A large number of molecules are chemotactic for leucocytes, particularly neutrophils and macrophages (Fig. 13.15). Both of these cells have an f.Met-Leu-Phe (f.MLP) receptor. This receptor binds to peptides blocked at the N terminus by formylated methionine. Since prokaryotes (e.g. bacteria) initiate all protein translation with this amino acid, whereas eukaryotes do not, this provides a simple specific signal for the presence of bacteria, towards which phagocytes should move. These cells also have receptors for C5a and LTB$_4$, both of which are generated at sites of inflamma-tion, C5a following complement activation and LTB$_4$ following activation of a variety of cells, particularly macrophages and mast cells. In addition, molecules generated by the blood clotting system, notably fibrin peptide B and thrombin, attract phagocytes.

The first cells to arrive at a site of inflammation, if activated, are able to attract others. For example, IL-8 is a small (10 kDa) cytokine, released by activated monocytes, which can induce neutrophil and basophil chemotaxis. Similarly, macrophage activation leads to metabolism of arachidonic acid with release of LTB$_4$. There is some evidence that particular chemotactic stimuli may selectively enhance the migration of particular subpopulations of lymphocytes, although the mediators are not yet clearly defined.

Chemotactic molecules

factor	characteristic	source	action on
C5a	77 amino acid peptide	N terminus of C5 α chain	neutrophils, eosinophils, macrophages
f.Met-Leu-Phe	tripeptide with blocked N terminus	prokaryotes	neutrophils, eosinophils, macrophages
LTB$_4$	arachidonic acid metabolite via lipoxygenase pathway	mast cells, basophils, macrophages	neutrophils, macrophages, eosinophils (present in ECF)
IL-8	10kDa protein	activated monocytes	neutrophils, basophils

Fig. 13.15 The major chemotactic molecules acting on leucocytes are listed. They act over short distances at sites of inflammation.

FURTHER READING

Davies P, Bailey PJ, Goldenberg MM, Ford-Hutchinson AW. The role of arachidonic acid oxygenation products in pain and inflammations. *Annu Rev Immunol* 1984;**2**:335–58.

Dustin ML, Springer TA. Role of lymphocyte adhesion receptors in transient interactions and cell locomotion. *Annu Rev Immunol* 1991;**9**:27–66.

Hemler ME. VLA proteins in the integrin family: structures, functions and their role on leucocytes. *Annu Rev Immunol* 1990;**8**:365–400.

Hynes RO. Integrins: a family of cell surface receptors. *Cell* 1987;**48**:349–54.

Male DK. Cell traffic and inflammation. In: Male DK, Champion B, Cooke A, Owen M. *Advanced Immunology*. 2nd ed. London: Gower Medical Publishing, 1991: Chapter 16.

Proud D, Kaplan AP. Kinin formation: mechanism and role in inflammatory disorders. *Annu Rev Immunol* 1988;**6**:49–83.

Shimizu Y, Newman W, Gopal TV, *et al.* Four molecular pathways of T cell adhesion to endothelial cells. Roles of LFA-1, VCAM-1 and ELAM-1 and changes of pathway hierarchy under different activation conditions. *J Cell Biol* 1991;**113**:1203–12.

Springer TA. Adhesion receptors in the immune system. *Nature* 1990;**346**:425–34.

chapter 14

Evolution of Immunity

An evolutionary progression towards the sophisticated mammalian immune system is apparent from detailed studies of a range of vertebrate organisms. However, the phylogenetic origins of the vertebrate adaptive immune system, particularly at the molecular level, remain uncertain despite extensive research into invertebrate immunity. There is much to learn about the origins of vertebrate 'non-specific' immunity, for example phagocytosis, from examination of invertebrates. Since invertebrates comprise over 95% of all animal species and include single or colonial animals, and those that are solid-bodied (acoelomate) or have body cavities (coelomate), with or without blood systems, there is no shortage of choice of suitable experimental animals.

Fig. 14.1 shows a simplified evolutionary tree of the animal kingdom with the coelomate invertebrates divided into two main evolutionary lines, based principally upon embryological differences. One line, leading to the molluscs, annelids and arthropods (the protostomes) diverged early in evolution from the pathway forming the echinoderms, tunicates and vertebrates (the deuterostomes). Much research on invertebrate immunity has concentrated on the arthropods and molluscs because many of these have pest status, either transmitting diseases or competing for agricultural products. As a result, work with groups which are phylogenetically relevant to the vertebrates (e.g. tunicates and echinoderms) has been rather neglected. In addition, since the ancestors of vertebrates are now extinct, attempts to trace the origin of vertebrate immunity within the invertebrates, in groups such as the tunicates (Fig. 14.2), is speculative and based on the assumption that some living animals are close relatives of the vertebrate ancestor. Fig. 14.1 shows some cellular and humoral immune phenomena discovered in the invertebrate phyla.

VERTEBRATE BLOOD CELL AND IMMUNE SYSTEM EVOLUTION

Fig. 14.3 presents the main steps of possible significance in the evolution of the blood cells and immune system of vertebrates. This shows that, despite the success of the invertebrates, only vertebrates possess lymphocytes with a highly specific long-term memory component. What environmental pressures might have led to the increased sophistication of the vertebrate immune system? One can speculate that they may include the enhanced threat of cancer and of viral infections in these complex, long-lived animals. A finely tuned immune system is thus required, with circulating effector cells that recognize foreign major histocompatibility complex (MHC) glycoproteins on the surface of the mutated or infected cells.

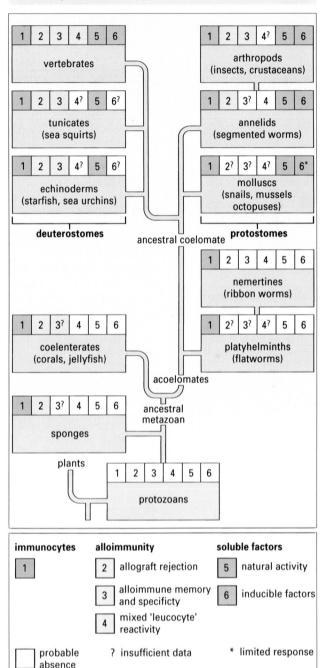

Immunopotentialities of vertebrates and invertebrates

immunocytes	alloimmunity		soluble factors	
1	2	allograft rejection	5	natural activity
	3	alloimmune memory and specificty	6	inducible factors
	4	mixed 'leucocyte' reactivity		
probable absence	? insufficient data		* limited response	

Fig. 14.1 Partial evidence for certain cellular and humoral immune phenomena in diverse vertebrate phyla is presented.

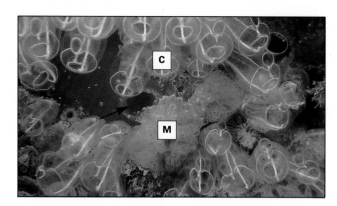

Fig. 14.2 Two colonial sea squirts (tunicates), *Clavelina lepadiformis* (C) and *Morchellium argus* (M), competing for space. An underlying solitary tunicate can be seen towards the centre (arrowed). The diameter of an individual *Clavelina* is approximately 4mm. (Courtesy of Dr P. Dyrynda.)

Evolution of the immune system

evolutionary step or selection pressure	immunological implications
single-celled animals	recognition and discrimination
multicellularity (including colonial forms)	histocompatibility system, allogeneic recognition and short-term memory
mesoderm and circulatory system, nutrition and defence as separate functions	freely circulating and more diverse blood cell types, cellular immunity and erythrocytes
cancer and viral infections associated with increasing complexity and longevity	immunosurveillance of own cells for those that are infected or cancerous
ancestral protovertebrates	increased recognition and discriminatory powers?
lower vertebrates: increased size, longer life span and reduced reproductive potential compared with invertebrates	true lymphocytes, lymphoid tissue and antibody production (IgM), longer-term memory
emergence onto land, exposure to irradiation and development of high pressure blood vascular systems	bone marrow, additional antibody classes, T- and B-lymphocytes, lymphoid organs with increased complexity, GALT
amniotes (reptiles, birds, mammals) with loss of free-living larval form	advanced differentiation of immunocompetent cells allowing increased diversity and efficiency of immune system
homoiothermy provides a more favourable environment for pathogens	increased efficiency of immune system, integrated cellular and humoral responses, germinal centres in secondary lymphoid organs, lymph nodes
viviparity with maternal–foetal interactions	additional fine-tuning of immune system to avoid rejection by mother

Fig. 14.3 Evolutionary steps of possible significance in the phylogeny of blood cells and immune system. (Adapted from Rowley AF, Ratcliffe NA, eds. *Vertebrate Blood Cells.* Cambridge: Cambridge University Press, 1988; with permission.)

INVERTEBRATE IMMUNITY

IMMUNOCYTES

Most invertebrates possess white blood cells (leucocytes), but usually lack red blood cells (erythrocytes). The leucoyctes are either fixed, free within blood vessels, or else occupy the coelom (coelomocytes) or haemocoel (haemocytes), the fluid-filled body cavities of these animals. The first blood cells probably evolved from a free-living, protozoan-like ancestor. In primitive metazoans, such as sponges, coelenterates and flatworms, wandering phagocytic amoebocytes not only function in host defence but are also involved in aspects of nutrition and excretion. In the coelomates (both protostomes and deuterostomes), as bodies increased in size and complexity, a circulatory system was required to transport food and waste substances around the body. Consequently, the amoebocyte-like cells were freed from their food-gathering role and probably migrated from the surrounding connective tissue into the circulatory system. Here, an array of cell types evolved, some of which took on specific roles in immune reactivity (Fig. 14.4).

Cells and tissues of invertebrate immune systems

cells/tissues	role(s) in immunity/physiology
mucus, cuticle, shells, tests and/or gut barrier	physicochemical barriers to invasion
five groups of free and sessile white blood cells	mediate cellular and many of the humoral defence reactions
I progenitor cells	may act as stem cells for other cell types
II phagocytic cells	phagocytosis, encapsulation, clotting, wound healing and killing
III haemostatic cells	plasma gelation and clotting by cell aggregation; non-self recognition, lysozyme and agglutinin production
IV nutritive cells	encapsulation reactions and wound healing? nutritive role?
V pigmented cells	role in defence (if any) unknown; respiratory function
fixed cells such as pericardial cells, nephrocytes or pore cells etc.	pinocytose colloids and small particulates; synthesize lysozyme (pericardial cells) and other antimicrobial factors?
haemopoietic organs – well organized in some invertebrates	haemopoiesis and phagocytosis; synthesize antimicrobial factors in a few animals
fat body (insects), mid gut and sinus lining cells (molluscs, crustaceans)	synthesize immune proteins and agglutinins (fat body), phagocytosis (mid-gut cells), clearance of foreign particles (sinus lining cells)

Fig. 14.4 Invertebrate immune systems. (Adapted from Ratcliffe NA. *Immunol Lett* 1985:**10**;253–270; Elsevier Science Publications 1985 with permission.)

Due to the huge diversity of invertebrate species and in contrast to the vertebrates, it is impossible to categorize the free leucocytes into well-defined classes by staining and morphology alone. However, a functional scheme can be devised which recognizes five main groups of cells: the progenitor cells, phagocytic cells, haemostatic cells, nutritive cells and pigmented cells (see Fig. 14.4). The progenitor cells, together with a variable array of haemopoietic tissue, may act as stem cells for the other cell types. Superficially, they resemble vertebrate lymphocytes (Fig. 14.5) although evidence for true homology is strictly limited. Phagocytic cells (Fig. 14.6) are probably the only blood cell type present throughout the animal kingdom. They correspond to the mammalian granulocyte or macrophage but lack homologous surface markers. Haemostatic cells are involved in coagulation and wound healing, and are important effectors of non-self recognition. Nutritive cells only form a minority of cells present and are assumed, but not proven, to play a nutritive role. The final cell type, the pigmented cells, may contain respiratory pigment and resemble vertebrate erythrocytes in a few species.

IMMUNE DEFENCES

Invertebrate immune systems apparently lack immunoglobulins, interactive lymphocyte sub-populations and lymphoid organs but, even so, the huge numbers and diversity of the invertebrates attests to the efficiency of their host defence mechanisms. Like vertebrates, invertebrates have extremely effective physicochemical barriers as a first line of defence (see Fig. 14.4). Mucus surrounds the body of many coelenterates, annelids, molluscs, and some tunicates, and it entraps and kills potential pathogens (Fig. 14.7). Tough external skeletons

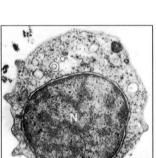
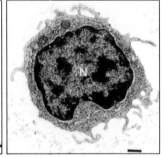

Fig. 14.5 Electron micrographs of a lymphocyte-like cell from the tunicate, *Ciona intestinalis* (left) and a lymphocyte from a fish, the blenny, *Blennius pholis* (right). Note the similarity in morphology; both cells have a large nucleus and a thin rim of undifferentiated cytoplasm. Scale bar = 0.5 μm. (Courtesy of Dr A. F. Rowley, from *Endeavour* (*New Series*)**13**;72–77, with permission. © Maxwell Pergamon MacMillan plc, 1989.)

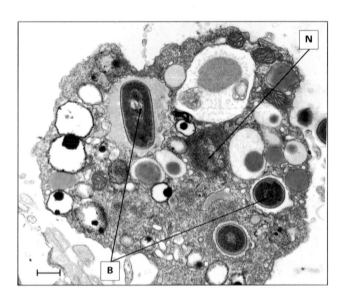

Fig. 14.6 Electron micrograph of a phagocytic cell from the tunicate, *Ciona intestinalis*. Note the ingestion of three bacteria (B) by this cell. Nucleus (N) Scale bar = 0.5 μm. (Courtesy of Dr A. F. Rowley.)

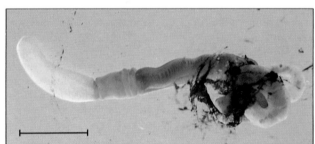
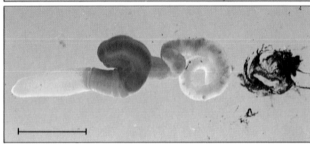

Fig. 14.7 Foreign particle entrapment and removal by the mucus layer surrounding the acorn worm, *Saccoglossus ruber*. A specimen was placed in a suspension of carbon in sea water for 2–3 minutes and then transferred to clean sea water. After 12 minutes large amounts of carbon were still enmeshed in the mucus layer surrounding the animal (upper). By 15 minutes the carbon was completely removed, wrapped in a ball of mucus (lower). Trapped microorganisms are probably dealt with in a similar fashion. Acorn worms are in a group of 'higher invertebrates' related to the tunicates. Scale bar = 5 mm. (Courtesy of Dr D. A. Millar.)

such as tests or shells are effective barriers to invasion in some coelenterates and molluscs, echinoderms and arthropods. Once these barriers are breached, would-be invaders are then exposed to a range of interacting cellular and humoral defence reactions. These include blood clotting/coagulation and wound healing, phagocytosis, encapsulation-type responses, and natural and inducible antimicrobial factors. Most of these reactions are dependent on non-self recognition and receptor molecules present in the blood and on the surfaces of the blood cells.

CLOTTING/COAGULATION AND WOUND HEALING
Both acoelomate and coelomate invertebrates rapidly seal wounds caused by injury or parasitic invasion, and so prevent the fatal loss of body fluids. The wound is closed by the extrusion of a fat body or the gut, by muscular contraction, by coagulation of body fluids, by blood cell aggregation and clotting, and/or by melanin deposition. The migration of leucocytes to the wound site is probably under the influence of cytokine-like factors (see below).

Plasma gelation or coagulation at wound sites occurs mainly in arthropods, although it has also been reported in annelids and echinoderms. Coagulation involves the haemostatic cells which aggregate at the injury site and then discharge their contents so that the plasma gelates to strengthen the cell clot. There is also a contribution from the plasma in many species. The coagulation process, as in mammals, involves a complex enzyme cascade which is activated at the wound by damaged tissue, microbial components, or changes in Ca^{2+} or pH. It has been likened to the alternative pathway in complement activation. The system is so sensitive that in horseshoe crabs it is elicited by as little as 4 ng/ml of *Escherichia coli* endotoxin. The importance of the coagulation process cannot be over-emphasized as it provides a highly sensitive method of recognizing foreign invaders through the responses of degranulating haemostatic cells. An important component of gelation is probably the enzyme prophenoloxidase (PpO), which, upon conversion to phenoloxidase (PO) by a cascade of serine proteases, may generate factors mediating later events in immunity. Interestingly, the PpO cascade has recently been shown to be present in other invertebrates such as annelids and tunicates.

PHAGOCYTOSIS AND ENCAPSULATION
Phagocytic cells are present throughout the invertebrates and, together with natural humoral factors (see below), form the first line of defence following microbial invasion (see Fig. 14.6). Chemotaxis, attachment, ingestion and killing phases are recognized, as in vertebrates. However, recognition is not mediated by Fc receptors, and C3b-like receptors have only been reported on the phagocyte surface in one species. Phagocytosis in invertebrates can occur, as in vertebrates, in the absence of opsonic factors. However, it is enhanced in molluscs, arthropods and tunicates by

plasma lectins and by components of the prophenoloxidase cascade. If the invading pathogens are too large or too numerous then they are enclosed in multicellular aggregates, termed nodules or capsules, which resemble mammalian granulomas (Fig. 14.8). Recently, it has been shown that both phagocytosis and encapsulation are dependent on cell cooperation between the haemostatic and phagocytic cells (see below). Sequestered organisms are killed, but the mechanisms involved remain largely unknown. Lysosomal enzymes and lysozyme are present in the leucocytes, and peroxidase and reactive oxygen species have been found in a few annelids and molluscs.

HUMORAL IMMUNITY
The body fluids of invertebrates probably lack immunoglobulins but they contain a range of naturally-occurring and inducible humoral defence factors. Natural substances include agglutinins, lysozyme and other lysins, non-lysozyme bactericidins, lysosomal enzymes and immobilization factors. In vertebrates, lysis of microbial and macrobial parasites is often mediated by the complement system and there is some evidence for components of this system in invertebrates. Thus, in a sea urchin, the phagocytes may bear C3b-like receptors, and a humoral lytic system similar to complement has been reported. Blood from the larvae of a lepidopteran reacts with bound cobra venom factor (cobra C3b) to produce C3-convertase activity that cleaves bovine C3 to give a molecule similar to C3b. The prophenoloxidase cascade of arthropods has also been compared with the alternative pathway of the complement system, since both are activated directly by

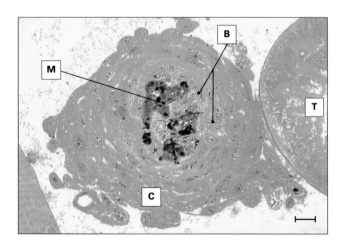

Fig. 14.8 Encapsulation of bacteria by the blood cells of a caterpillar. Final-stage larvae of the butterfly *Pieris brassicae* were injected with bacteria (heat-killed *Bacillus cereus*). After 24 hours, the capsules that had formed around the bacteria were excised and sectioned. Note the dark pigmented core of melanin (M), the multilayered sheath of blood cells (C), rod-shaped bacteria (B), and the attachment of the capsule to the Malpighian tubule (T). Scale bar = 10 μm.

microbial components and involve a series of sequentially activated proteases. Unfortunately, due to the lack of detailed molecular analysis of these factors, it is impossible to confirm that the forerunners of the alternative complement pathways arose in invertebrates.

It is known that agglutinin and haemolysin levels can sometimes be enhanced. However, only in insects have inducible antimicrobial factors been detected and studied in any great detail. There is some evidence for their presence in a few other invertebrates but their more widespread detection and characterization may await the correct immunogens and/or immunization schedule. In insects such as moths, flies and bees, up to 15 antibacterial proteins can be induced within a few hours of injection (Fig. 14.9). Many of these have been purified and sequenced; they have a broad-spectrum activity which only lasts a few days, and thus are very different from vertebrate immunoglobulins. Recently, similar antibacterial proteins have been discovered in the skin of the clawed toad, *Xenopus*, and from the small intestine of the pig. These molecules probably represent ancient, but still important, immune factors present in both invertebrates and vertebrates. One of the insect cecropins, called P4 or haemolin (see Fig. 14.9), has considerable (38%) homology with certain immunoglobulin domains. It may represent a primitive form of immunoglobulin or have evolved independently in invertebrates.

More recently, in the American cockroach, a different sort of inducible protein has been detected which is much more like vertebrate immunoglobulin. It has a molecular mass of 700 kDa, is highly specific and lasts weeks rather than days. Again, detailed comparison with vertebrate immunoglobulin awaits more detailed molecular characterization.

NON-SELF RECOGNITION AND CELL–CELL COOPERATION

There are many reports that invertebrates can discriminate, often quite specifically, between various foreign substances. The factors present in invertebrate body fluids which may act as recognition molecules include agglutinins and components of the prophenoloxidase cascade. Purified agglutinins from the blood of molluscs, insects, and tunicates have been shown to enhance the recognition of test particles *in vitro*, as well as their clearance from the circulation *in vivo*. Such agglutinins have also been detected on the surface of blood cells so that they may function as bridging molecules between the leucocyte and the foreign particle, as has also been reported in the mammalian immune system. The prophenoloxidase (PpO) system of arthropods has also been reported recently to be a likely source of recognition factors. During conversion of PpO to phenoloxidase (PO) recognition factors are released from haemostatic (granular) cells which enhance phagocytosis and encapsulation. This process of non-self recognition and subsequent phagocytosis involves cell–cell cooperation between granular (haemostatic) cells and phagocytic cells (Fig. 14.10).

Thus, although invertebrates lack interacting antigen-presenting cells and lymphocyte subpopulations, the various immunocytes cooperate during cell-mediated immune responses.

CYTOKINE-LIKE MOLECULES

There are a number of cytokine-like molecules in invertebrates, which may regulate the host defences by a network resembling that of vertebrates. The fact that molecules related to cytokines are present in protozoans indicates their universal occurrence throughout the animal kingdom. For example, a protozoan pheromone, Er-1, has structural and functional similarities to IL-2. In addition, invertebrate IL-1α and IL-1β and TNF-like activities have recently been isolated and characterized from annelids, echinoderms, and tunicates. IL-1α and IL-1β have been detected using a vertebrate assay system, the murine thymocyte proliferation assay, and shown to be inhibited by polyclonal antisera to vertebrate IL-1. Invertebrate IL-1 stimulates the 'blood' cells of these primitive animals to aggregate, phagocytose and proliferate. TNF-like activity from invertebrates has been detected with the L929 cytotoxicity assay which is normally used for vertebrate TNF.

A miscellaneous range of other molecules with cytokine-like activity has been reported from invertebrates. From insects, these include a plasmatocyte (leucocyte-type) depletion factor, a leucocyte activator (termed 'haemokinin'), and various stimulants for encapsulation and phagocytosis. A factor produced by the leucocytes of echinoderms (the sea-star factor) is mitogenic for mammalian lymphocytes and also induces the accumulation of starfish white blood cells. Finally, an inflammatory cytokine from tunicates affects antibody production, phagocytosis and cell-mediated cytotoxicity in vertebrates, and leucocyte phagocytic activity in prawns. Additional molecular characterization of these molecules is awaited in order for the cytokine network of invertebrates to be unravelled.

Inducible immune proteins of *Hyalophora cecropia*

immune protein	molecular mass	function and properties
P4 (haemolin)	48 000	main immune protein, non-self recognition?
P5 attacins A–F	21–23 000	narrow-spectrum antibacterial activity against some Gram-negative bacteria
P7 (lysozyme)	15 000	kills some Gram-positive bacteria
cecropins A–F (6 proteins)	~ 4 000	some have broad-spectrum antibacterial activity against both Gram-positive and Gram-negative bacteria

Fig. 14.9 Inducible immune proteins of the moth, *Hyalophora cecropia*, isolated from the blood 10 hours after immunization with bacteria (*Enterobacter cloacae*).

TRANSPLANTATION IMMUNITY

Vertebrate immunity is characterized by a high degree of specificity and enhanced reactivity (memory, or anamnesis) following a second exposure to antigen. These processes are governed by the lymphocytes and the major histocompatibility complex (MHC). To determine levels of specificity and memory in invertebrates, transplantation, implantation and cytotoxicity studies have also been undertaken. Such transplantation studies in invertebrates are often very difficult to perform, due to the presence of tough exoskeletons or delicate outer layers, as well as problems in deciding whether rejection has occurred. Even so, most invertebrates destroy xenografts, and allogeneic recognition is present in the sponges, coelenterates, annelids, insects, echinoderms and tunicates (see Figs 14.1, 14.11, 14.12 and 14.13). The apparent lack of allogeneic recognition in the molluscs probably reflects the technical problems in grafting these animals. Not all the groups exhibiting allograft rejection are characterized by specificity and memory and, even when present, these are usually strictly limited and short term (see Fig. 14.1). The variability in the results may stem from the temperature-dependence of the rejection process and the lack of appreciation of this by some workers.

It is not surprising that allogeneic recognition occurs in colonial invertebrates such as the sponges, coelenterates and tunicates, as the integrity of the colony may be constantly threatened by overgrowth from adjacent colonies (see Fig. 14.2). More recent work with the larvae of tunicate colonies has shown that both allorecognition and fertilization are controlled by a single gene locus with multiple alleles. Thus, there are similarities between this tunicate system and the murine histocompatibility genes.

The limited specificity and memory of invertebrate allorecognition and xenorecognition does not seem to hamper their immune system. After all, invertebrates are hugely abundant and most are capable of rapid and effective responses to pathogens and parasites.

Two hypothetical models for cell–cell cooperation in arthropod immunity

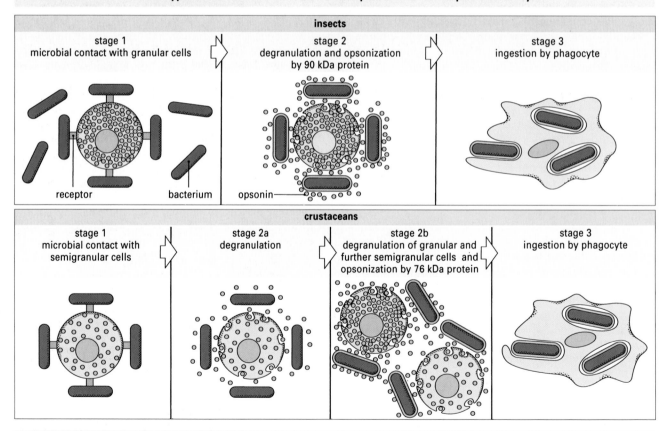

Fig. 14.10 Schemes derived from experiments which observed the reactions of purified blood cell populations to test particles. In insects, non-self recognition (Stage 1) is carried out by the granular (haemostatic) cells, and ingestion (Stage 2) by the phagocytes. The crustacean model has an extra amplification step at Stage 2, in which semigranular and granular cells interact to enhance the response. The 90 kDa and 76 kDa proteins detected in insects and crustaceans, respectively, are opsonic (recognition) molecules generated by activation of the prophenoloxidase cascade. (Adapted from Ratcliffe NA. In: Warr GW, Cohen N, eds. *Phylogenesis of Immune Functions*. Oxford: CRC Press, 1991:**62**. Data on crustaceans from the work of Professor K. Söderhäll and associates.)

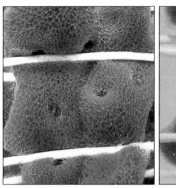
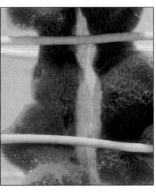

Fig. 14.11 Demonstration of cell-mediated immunity in sponges: allogeneic incompatibility and isogeneic compatibility. Two intact fingers of sponge (*Callyspongia* spp.) from the same colony and two from different colonies are parabiosed (their circulations are fused) by being held together with vinyl-covered wire. Left: The interfacial fusion between isogeneic parabionts (intracolony) persists indefinitely. × 0.5. Right: Incompatibility between allogeneic parabionts (intercolony) results in a cytotoxic interaction and necrosis after 7–9 days (24–27°C). × 0.25. (Courtesy of Dr W. H. Hildemann.)

MHC AND THE IMMUNOGLOBULIN SUPERFAMILY

The presence of allogeneic recognition in many invertebrates indicates that the ancestors of the major histocompatibility complex (MHC) could be present in these animals. This, together with the apparent absence of immunoglobulins in invertebrates, led to the proposal that the MHC is ancestral to and separate from the immunoglobulin system of the vertebrates. Thus, during evolution of the invertebrates, the MHC was retained and as the vertebrates arose the immunoglobulin system was added. This latter system would have provided a more precise recognition potential in the form of circulating antibodies and cell surface receptors. With the further evolution of the vertebrates, the MHC and immunoglobulin systems would have become more closely integrated to provide the high level of control necessary for interacting antigen-presenting cells (APCs) and T and B cells. The above proposal is hypothetical and there are those who argue that the MHC evolved within the vertebrates. This view is supported by a lack of structural or functional evidence that invertebrate cells express MHC glycoproteins or dimeric cell receptors for alloantigens. In addition, invertebrates may lack mixed leucocyte reactivity (see Fig. 14.1) which is a functional marker of the MHC in vertebrates.

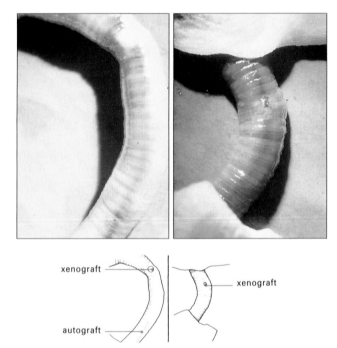
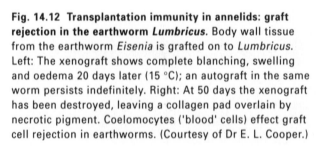

Fig. 14.12 Transplantation immunity in annelids: graft rejection in the earthworm *Lumbricus*. Body wall tissue from the earthworm *Eisenia* is grafted on to *Lumbricus*. Left: The xenograft shows complete blanching, swelling and oedema 20 days later (15 °C); an autograft in the same worm persists indefinitely. Right: At 50 days the xenograft has been destroyed, leaving a collagen pad overlain by necrotic pigment. Coelomocytes ('blood' cells) effect graft cell rejection in earthworms. (Courtesy of Dr E. L. Cooper.)

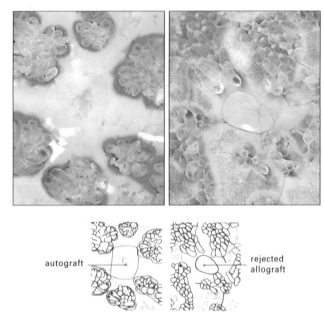

Fig. 14.13 Transplantation immunity in echinoderms: allograft rejection in starfish (*Dermasterias*). Left: In spite of the technical difficulties involved, this autograft remains in perfect condition 300 days after transplantation. Right: An allograft rejected at 287 days (14–16 °C) is blanched and contracted. Rejection involves lymphocyte-like cells and larger phagocytic cells. × 4. (Courtesy of Dr W. H. Hildemann.)

MHC and T cell evolution

Fig. 14.14 This vertebrate phylogenetic tree illustrates aspects of MHC and T cell evolution. Evidence for two functional indications of an MHC (cytotoxic T lymphocytes, CTL, and mixed leucocyte reaction, MLR) is shown, together with current biochemical evidence for the expression of class I and II MHC proteins. A blank box indicates insufficient evidence for that characteristic.

The discovery of β_2-microglobulin-like molecules in earthworms, crustaceans and insects does support the idea that MHC precursors may have arisen in the invertebrates. Although in vertebrates β_2-microglobulin is encoded by a gene not linked to the MHC, it appears to be related to both the MHC and the immunoglobulin system. β_2-microglobulin is thus associated with the heavy chain of class I MHC and has structural homology not only with class I MHC heavy chains and class II α and β chains but also with immunoglobulin constant region domains. β_2-microglobulin may be the molecular link between invertebrates and vertebrates, giving rise to MHC and immunoglobulin systems by gene rearrangement and duplication and natural selection.

Finally, there is an ever-increasing group of molecules, such as Thy-1 (present in squid brain and with some homology to β_2-microglobulin), and amalgam, fasciclin II, neuroglian and haemolin (all from insects), with immunoglobulin-like domains and present in invertebrates. These molecules belong to the 'immunoglobulin superfamily'; it has been suggested that they evolved to mediate interactions between cells and could potentially produce an immune system recognizing 'non-self'. Such a step may have already been made with haemolin, which in insects binds to bacterial cell walls where it may function in the recognition of foreignness during insect immune reactivity.

VERTEBRATE IMMUNITY

Compared with the immense variety of forms seen within the invertebrate phyla, vertebrates possess a fairly uniform basic plan of organization and are members of just one phylum – the Chordata. Although there is considerable evolutionary divergence within vertebrate stock, which includes fish, amphibians, reptiles, birds

MHCs of different species

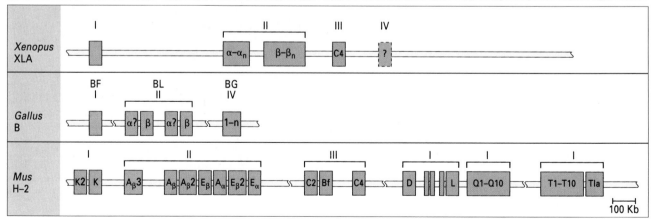

Fig. 14.15 The basic structure of the MHC appeared in a common ancestor to frogs/toads and mammals. Speculative organization of MHC loci is shown for *Xenopus* and the chicken (*Gallus*). The architecture of the mouse (*Mus*) H2 complex is well known. Distances for *Xenopus* and *Gallus* are arbitrary. (Courtesy of Dr L. Du Pasquier.)

and mammals, the basic cellular and molecular components of immunity are strikingly conserved throughout extant species. However, increased specialization of lymphoid tissues and lymphocyte functions, together with greater variety of immunoglobulin superfamily molecules (e.g. MHC antigens and immunoglobulins) appear to be associated with more complex grades of organization. The most complex structural and functional immune systems are seen in mammals.

T CELLS AND EVOLUTION OF THE MHC
Mammalian T-cytotoxic (Tc) and T-helper (TH) lymphocyte subsets, possessing αβ T-cell receptors (TCRs), recognize most foreign antigens only when presented in suitable form by appropriate MHC molecules (class I and II proteins respectively). Hence consideration of the phylogeny of certain T cell populations (e.g. cytotoxic T lymphocytes [CTLs] and those involved in mixed leucocyte reactivity [MLR]) and MHC evolution are dealt with together here (Fig. 14.14). It should be appreciated that the MHC, in addition to its involvement in pathogen presentation to T cells, may also play crucial non-immunological roles (e.g. mate selection, developmental interactions, and intracellular transport of IgG). Mammals, birds, frogs/toads and bony fish have all been shown to possess an MHC, both through molecular and genetic characterization and by functional criteria, including demonstration that MLR and acute allograft rejection are controlled by a single polymorphic genetic region, and that phenomena such as T–B cell collaboration, the generation of antigen-specific cytotoxic responses (e.g. to allogeneic cells) and thymic education of T-lineage cells are all under MHC control.

GENETIC ORGANIZATION OF THE MHC
The genetic organization of the MHC (XLA) of the clawed toad *Xenopus,* is shown in Fig. 14.15, where it is compared with the B locus of the chicken MHC and the H2 locus of the mouse. The basic structure of the MHC gene locus must have appeared by the time frogs and mammals diverged from a common ancestor (350 million years ago). Indeed recent evidence indicates that the MHC had evolved as early as the emergence of bony fish (see below). In *Xenopus,* class I α chains, encoded by MHC genes, are 40–44 kDa molecules, non-covalently bound to non-MHC-coded β_2-microglobulin. Molecular cloning studies predict amino acid sequences similar to MHC class I molecules of higher vertebrates. Class I molecules are expressed on the surfaces of all adult cells. *Xenopus* class II molecules are composed of MHC-encoded α and β chains, both of which are 30–35 kDa transmembrane glycoproteins. Class II proteins are expressed on only a limited range of adult cells, including thymocytes, B and T cells, and various APCs that include putative 'Langerhans-like' cells of skin epidermis (see Fig. 14.16). *Xenopus* MHC proteins are polymorphic: about 20 class I and 30 class II alleles are suspected. One particularly interesting feature of MHC expression in *Xenopus* is that, in contrast to the early larval appear-

ance of class II molecules (on B cells and several tadpole epithelial cells in direct contact with the external environment), class I proteins are not expressed on any cell surface prior to metamorphosis. Thus class I expression is not essential for early development or for functioning of the larval immune system: perhaps class II-restricted cellular immunity plays a crucial role during this ontogenetic period. The widespread distribution of class II MHC in tadpoles compared with adults suggests that this pattern might represent the way in which antigen was presented in a more primitive immune system. Axolotls, which display relatively poor T-cell reactivity to alloantigens, possess α and β MHC class II molecules, which are not very polymorphic. They also express MHC-encoded erythrocyte antigens, which show similarities to class I α chains (44 kDa) and to polymorphic class IV molecules found on nucleated chicken erythrocytes. These may also exist in *Xenopus.*

TCRs for antigen, and both CD4 and CD8 molecules, have been confirmed in birds. Recently, TCR molecules (α, β and γδ candidates) and a putative CD8 marker (35 kDa) have been identified on *Xenopus* T cells by use of monoclonal antibodies. Presumably such TCRs (and accessory molecules) also exist in snakes and bony fish, since *in vitro* assays demonstrate good MLR and CTL generation (i.e. T-cell functions) in these animals. Recently, class I α chains and class II β chains have been identified in bony fish, and class I α chains and heterodimeric class II molecules in various reptiles.

T-CELL FUNCTION IN 'PRIMITIVE' FISH
Evidence for T-cell function and MHC-like molecules in the most primitive group of bony fish, the chondrosteans (sturgeons and paddlefish), and in cartilaginous fish (sharks and rays) and jawless fish (hagfish and lampreys) is sparse. The distinct MLR afforded by hagfish leucocytes appears to be effected by responder populations that are immunoglobulin-positive (B cells).

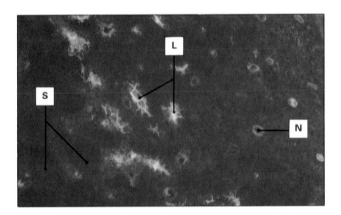

Fig. 14.16 Immunofluorescence showing class II MHC-positive dendritic cells in *Xenopus.* 'Langerhans-like' cells (L) frequent the basal epidermal layer. Also visible are class II+ neck cells of the skin gland opening through the epidermis (N), and skin glands below the epidermis (S). × 100.

Natural killer (NK) cell activity and antibody-dependent cellular cytotoxicity (ADCC) have been found in cartilaginous fish. Cells with NK activity, but identified as macrophages in cartilaginous fish, undoubtedly play a crucial role in immune responses in the 'absence' of T cell function at this level of evolution. (There is also evidence for involvement of NK cells [granular lymphocytes] in the anti-protozoan immunity of bony fish.) Temperature plays a crucial role in immune responses in ectotherms. In bony fish, low temperatures inhibit T-cell (but not B-cell) proliferation. These effects are due to the lower level in T cells of certain 'bendy' fatty acids (e.g. oleic acid). It has been suggested that diets high in appropriate fatty acids may allow fish to adapt better to low temperatures.

Evolution of immunoglobulin isotypes in vertebrates

verterbrate group	antibody synthesis	immunoglobulin heavy chains				
		M	G/Y	A	D	E
mammals	■	■	■	■	■	■
birds	■	■	■	■	□	□
reptiles	■	■	■	?	□	□
frogs/toads	■	■	■	◪	□	□
salamanders/ newts	■	■	■	□	□	□
lungfish	■	■	■	□	□	□
teleost fish	■	■	?	□	□	□
sharks/rays	■	■	■	□	□	□
jawless fish	■	◪	□	□	□	□

■ presence/ homology	◪ partial evidence	□ probable absence	? insufficient data

Fig. 14.17 Non-μ heavy chain isotypes are found in diverse groups, but the roles of many remain uncertain.

B CELLS AND IMMUNOGLOBULIN EVOLUTION

All vertebrates make antibodies to a wide range of antigens, comprised of multi-domain, heavy and light polypeptide chains. Even the jawless fish, the most primitive vertebrates, possess IgM-like heavy chains, although these lack the stabilizing disulphide bonds typical of immunoglobulins of 'higher' vertebrates'; furthermore, light chains are not found in lampreys. Polymeric IgM exists in all jawed vertebrates and is the most conserved isotype (Fig. 14.17). Each heavy μ chain comprises four constant domains and one variable domain; disulphide bonds link heavy and light chains. It appears that the μ chain family has undergone considerable phylogenetic diversity, for example, only 24% amino acid sequence homology exists between catfish and mouse μ chains.

Non-μ heavy chain isotypes are known to exist in fish, amphibians and reptiles. For example, IgG-like immunoglobulins (3 constant heavy chain domains) are found in some cartilaginous fish, while non-μ immunoglobulins, with four constant heavy chain domains, have been identified in three amphibians: *Xenopus* (IgY and IgX), *Rana,* and the axolotl (IgY). Although the precise roles of these different isotypes are not known, *Xenopus* IgY is thymus-dependent, whereas IgM and IgX are not. *Xenopus* IgX is possibly the equivalent of mammalian secretory IgA, since this isotype is found exclusively in the gut. The IgY of axolotls may also be a secretory immunoglobulin, and in the gut this immunoglobulin isotype becomes associated with 'secretory-component-like' molecules. It is interesting that fish (and amphibians) lack IgE, yet teleosts display Type I hypersensitivity reactions which may reflect tissue-bound homocytotropic antibody.

There is also light chain diversity in ectotherms. Two antigenically-distinct classes of L chains have been demonstrated in catfish and *Xenopus*, and the same situation also holds for reptiles.

The bursa of Fabricius

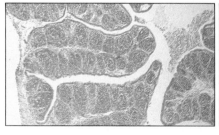

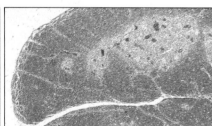

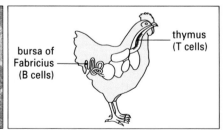

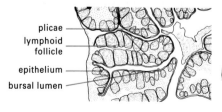

plicae
lymphoid follicle
epithelium
bursal lumen

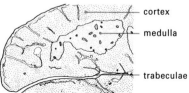

cortex
medulla
trabeculae

Fig. 14.18 The two central organs in the avian immune system are the thymus (centre) and the bursa of Fabricius (far left). Lymphocytes developing in the thymus are termed T cells and those in the bursa, B cells. H&E stain, × 20.

Frogs and toads, as well as certain urodele amphibians and bony fish, have both B cells and T cells which can be distinguished by anti-immunoglobulin and anti-T cell monoclonal antibodies, respectively. The possibility that immunoglobulin is the only type of antigen-specific receptor used by 'primitive' fish was initially suggested by studies showing that all their leucocytes stain with polyclonal anti-immunoglobulin reagents. Subsequent analysis with monoclonal anti-immunoglobulins has revealed both immunoglobulin-positive and immunoglobulin-negative leucocytes in hagfish, although the immunological role of the non-B cells awaits clarification.

In contrast to other vertebrates, birds possess a unique site for the differentiation of B cells – the cloacal bursa of Fabricius (Fig. 14.18). Transplantation experiments between quail and chicken embryos have shown that the bursa is colonized by a small number of stem cells over a few days during early embryonic development. These then proliferate and differentiate to form the B lymphocytes of the bursal follicles. The generation of antibody diversity in birds is different to that occurring in mammals. In chickens the single functional V_L gene is initially rearranged and joined to a single J–C unit (Fig. 14.19). This takes place only for only a limited period at the beginning of colonization of the bursa, whereas in mammals immunoglobulin gene rearrangements occur in the B cell precursors throughout

life. Subsequently, in the chicken, stretches of nucleotide sequences from pseudogenes (adjacent to the single V gene), replace 10–120 base-pair segments within the rearranged immunoglobulin gene sequences; this high frequency gene conversion mechanism operates throughout the time B cells proliferate in the bursa.

Immunoglobulin gene structure in teleost fish and *Xenopus* resembles that in mammals with multiple V genes and J genes, but with a lower diversity, there being only some 5×10^5 different antibody molecules in *Xenopus*. Somatic mutation contributes minimally to antibody diversity, a finding that may relate to cell economy required in an animal with less than 1×10^5 splenic lymphocytes (e.g. a larva): cell wastage due to non-productive mutants would be a threat to such a lymphoid system. It is thought that two waves of V gene rearrangements occur in *Xenopus* during ontogeny. The first wave occurs in the larva and involves relatively few B cells; more cells contribute to the repertoire after metamorphosis and offer a wider spectrum of antibody specificities than seen in the larva.

Shark immunoglobulin diversity is somewhat different to that seen in bony fish and anuran amphibians. Sharks have multiple, closely-linked V–D–J–C subunits, which limits the number of different ways these can be combined. This may explain the limited diversity of the shark antibody response (Fig. 14.20). Whether this cluster arrangement of immunoglobulin gene subunits

Genetic basis of antibody diversity in chickens

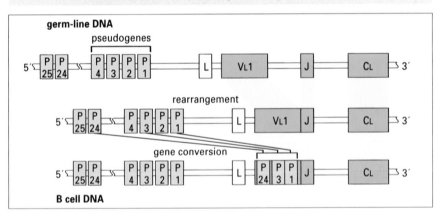

Fig. 14.19 The chicken germ-line immunoglobulin light chain locus has less than 30 kb of DNA. A single functional V gene (V_L) lies 2 kb upstream from a single J–C unit, with an adjacent cluster of 25 pseudogenes (P) in a 19 kb region. Rearrangement occurs briefly during early B cell development. Antibody diversity is achieved by gene conversion between P and the rearranged sequence. The arrangement shown (P_1, P_3 and P_{24}) is illustrative; converted segments do not necessarily lie in order in the V gene segment.

Shark immunoglobulin V_H loci

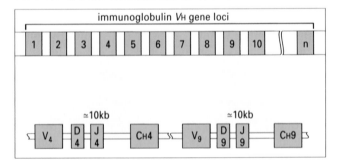

Fig. 14.20 In the shark there are a series of heavy chain gene loci, each with a single V, D, J, and C gene segment. The fourth and ninth loci are shown expanded. V_H, D_H and J_H segments are closely linked and occur within approximately 1.3 kb. Together with the C_H segment, they occupy only about 10–15 kb. Recombination appears to occur selectively only within each group of genes, which may account for the lack of inter-individual variation associated with the immune response of this species. (Based on data of Dr G. W. Litman.)

achieves clonal restriction of shark B cells is not known. The shark immunoglobulin gene arrangement may be representative of a common ancestral immunoglobulin gene family. Alternatively this arrangement may be a unique adaptation of this group.

NON-SPECIFIC MEDIATORS OF IMMUNITY

With the exception of the jawless fish, which may possess only the terminal complement components, both the classical (antibody-mediated) and the alternative pathways of complement activation have been demonstrated in all vertebrate classes. Genes coding for the full complement system and the two heavy and two light chain immunoglobulin molecule therefore appear to have arisen at about the same time in evolution.

Considerable homology appears to exist between the gene for C3 in *Xenopus* and the gene for mammalian C3. Basic properties of mammalian complement (such as thermolability, and requirements for Ca^{2+} and Mg^{2+}) are shared by fish and amphibian complement. Understandably, however, the temperature range over which ectotherm complement remains active is greater (activity remains at 4°C). Despite this, heat-inactivation can be achieved at a lower temperature; *Xenopus* serum, for example, is entirely stripped of complement activity by treatment at 45°C for 40 minutes. Guinea-pig complement may be used successfully in haemolytic antibody assays *in vitro* using antibody from adult amphibians. For most fish species and larval *Xenopus*, complement from the same species or a closely-related species, must be used.

Leukotrienes and other lipid mediators (collectively known as eicosanoids) are known to be involved in a variety of inflammatory processes in mammals. There is now evidence that leukotrienes are produced in fish (and amphibians) and play an important role in inflammatory responses in fish; for example leukotriene B_4 enhances the migration of fish leucocytes.

There is currently considerable interest in the evolution of cytokines within the vertebrates. For example, T cell growth factors (TCGF), able to promote the proliferation of T cell lymphoblasts *in vitro*, have now been identified from culture supernatants of stimulated (T) lymphocytes taken from bony fish, frogs/toads, snakes and chickens (Fig. 14.21). Molecular and genetic analysis of such 'IL-2-like' factors and their lymphocyte surface receptors are now in progress. For example, the purification of *Xenopus* TCGF indicates a 15–25 kDa protein; monoclonal antibodies against the putative *Xenopus* IL-2 receptor have recently been produced. Crude supernatants from splenocytes stimulated by T cell mitogens or alloantigens undoubtedly contain a mixture of cytokines. In *Xenopus* these supernatants can induce proliferation of B cells from normal toads and surface immunoglobulin-negative splenocytes from early-thymectomized (T-cell deficient) animals. 'IL-1-like' activity has also been detected in the macrophages of bony fish, frogs/toads and birds. 'Interferon-like' factors, with macrophage-activating and anti-viral function, are also being discovered in ectotherms (e.g. in farmed fish where there are known viral diseases that can decimate fish stocks).

T cell growth factor in Xenopus

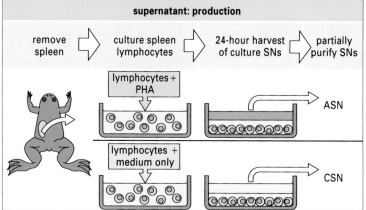

supernatant: production				supernatant: assays		
				includes ³H-thymidine incorporation in:		supports growth of T cell lines
remove spleen	culture spleen lymphocytes	24-hour harvest of culture SNs	partially purify SNs	resting splenocytes	T lymphocytes	
lymphocytes + PHA → ASN				+	+++	+++
lymphocytes + medium only → CSN				−	−	−

Fig. 14.21 Active culture supernatants (ASNs) are harvested from PHA-stimulated *Xenopus* splenocytes and compared with supernatants from control cultures (CSNs). The supernatants are partially purified by ammonium sulphate precipitation, dialysis and 'removal' of any PHA by incubation with chicken erythrocytes. The ASNs appear to contain cytokines since they induce considerable proliferation of T lymphoblasts (but are less stimulatory for resting splenocytes) and support the growth of alloreactive T cell lines; CSNs have no comparable effects. A similar but reduced level of activity can be generated in supernatants from mixed leucocyte culture and may be attributable to molecules functionally homologous to mammalian T cell growth factor (i.e. IL-2).

LYMPHOID TISSUES IN LOWER VERTEBRATES

The lymphomyeloid system produces and stores lymphocytes, granulocytes and other blood cells. In mammals, lymphoid tissues, (e.g. thymus, lymph nodes, spleen and mucosal-associated lymphoid tissue [MALT]), containing predominantly lymphocytes, are anatomically separate from myeloid tissues, (e.g. bone marrow), where granulocytes and a variety of other blood cell types predominate. However, in 'lower' vertebrates, for example fish and amphibians, lymphoid and myeloid compartments are more intermingled.

Fish lack bone marrow, lymph nodes and nodular MALT (Fig. 14.22). However, they have a well-developed thymus and spleen, and lymphomyeloid tissue associated with kidney and liver (Fig. 14.23). It should be noted that hagfish do not possess a true thymus and have only a rudimentary spleen.

Evolution of lymphomyeloid tissues in vertebrates

vertebrate group	lymphomyeloid tissue					
	thymus	spleen	bone marrow	lymph nodes	galt-associated	kidney/liver
mammals	presence	presence	presence	presence	presence	presence
birds	presence	presence	presence	presence	presence	presence
reptiles	presence	presence	presence	partial	presence	presence
frogs/toads	presence	presence	presence	partial	presence	presence
salamanders/newts	presence	presence	presence	absence	partial	presence
lungfish	presence	presence	absence	absence	presence	presence
teleost fish	presence	presence	absence	absence	partial	presence
sharks/rays	presence	presence	presence	absence	presence	presence
jawless fish	absence	partial	absence	absence	partial	presence

Key: ▨ presence/homology ◪ partial evidence ☐ probable absence

Fig. 14.22 Lymphoid and myeloid compartments are intermingled in fishes and amphibians.

Lymphomyeloid tissues in different types of fish

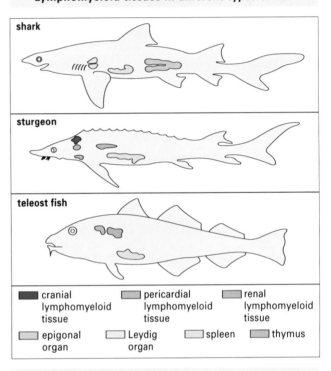

shark

sturgeon

teleost fish

■ cranial lymphomyeloid tissue   ▨ pericardial lymphomyeloid tissue   ▨ renal lymphomyeloid tissue

☐ epigonal organ   ☐ Leydig organ   ☐ spleen   ▨ thymus

Fig. 14.23 Note that the intestines of sharks and sturgeons are also rich in lymphomyeloid tissue (in the spiral valve). (Courtesy of Dr R. Fänge.)

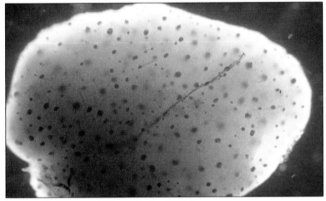

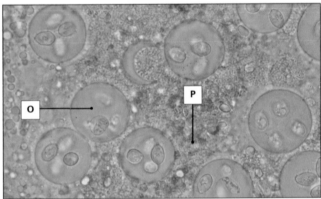

Fig. 14.24 Melano-macrophage centres (MMCs) in fish liver. Gross and microscopic views of liver of a cyptinodontid fish (*Rivulus marmoratus*) experimentally infected with the coccidian parasite *Calyptospora funduli*. At 60 days post-infection, distinct MMCs have appeared (left, × 60). The squash preparation (right, × 600) shows that these MMCs consist of degenerating oocysts (O) of the parasite and associated host pigment (P). The mononuclear phagocytes play a dominant role in MMC formation. (Courtesy of Dr W. K. Vogelbein.)

One notable feature of fish lymphomyeloid tissue is the abundance of melano-macrophage centres within the liver of 'primitive' forms and also within the spleen and kidney of teleost fish (Fig. 14.24). These centres are heavily laden with pigments, for example haemosiderin, ceroid, melanin and, in particular, lipofuscin. It has been suggested that these melano-macrophage centres represent a primitive analogue of the germinal centres found in bird lymphoid tissues. Pigment accumulation in the fish 'macrophage aggregates' may be partly related to the animals' high levels of unsaturated fats, which maintain membrane fluidity at low temperatures; these fats are particularly prone to peroxidation and formation of lipofuscin.

Two anuran amphibians – the leopard frog, *Rana pipiens,* and the clawed toad, *Xenopus laevis* – are used to illustrate general histological features of lymphoid tissues found in ectothermic vertebrates.

THYMUS

The adult *Xenopus* thymus lies just under the skin, behind the middle ear. Detachment of the thymus from the pharyngeal epithelium occurs early in development, as in most other vertebrates except teleost fish. The thymus is differentiated into an outer cortex and a central (paler-staining) medulla. The rapidly-proliferating cortical lymphocytes are particularly sensitive to irradiation (Fig. 14.25).

There is considerable evidence that the ectotherm thymus, like its counterpart in endotherms, produces lymphocytes with T-cell functions. The ultrastructure of thymic lymphocytes and neighbouring epithelial cells is

shown in Fig. 14.26. Several other stromal cell types are found within the thymic medulla, though some, for example the granular cells, appear only after metamorphosis. Myoid cells have been found in the thymus of mammals, reptiles and several amphibian species (see Fig. 14.26); it has been suggested that they are involved in promoting circulation of tissue fluids within the thymus, or that they may provide a source of self-antigen. These cells, along with thymic epithelial cells and interdigitating cells, may be involved in 'educating' T-lineage cells to become tolerant of self-antigens and to be preferentially restricted to interacting with cells expressing self-MHC. B cells have also been found in the thymus of diverse vertebrate species, including amphibian thymus, though this organ does not seem to be involved with their production.

SPLEEN

The spleen is a major peripheral lymphoid organ in all jawed vertebrates. Together with 'lymph nodes' and kidney, it traps antigen, houses proliferating lymphocytes after their stimulation by antigen, and provides for the appropriate release of these cells and their products. Thymus-dependent and -independent lymphoid zones within the spleen have been demonstrated in *Xenopus* (Fig. 14.27). The white pulp follicles are rich in B cells (Fig. 14.28), shown by selective staining of this region with anti-immunoglobulin monoclonal antibodies. Splenic T cells, found especially in the perifollicular (marginal zone) regions, lack surface immunoglobulin, but a population will bind with a monoclonal antibody (XT-1) raised against thymocytes (Fig. 14.28).

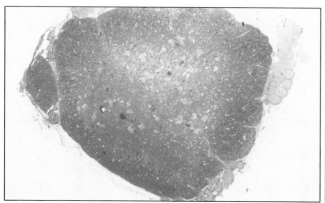
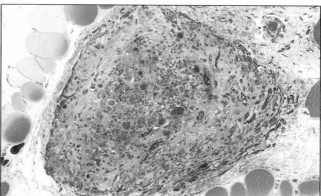

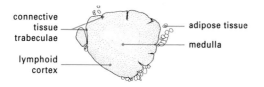
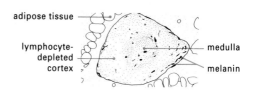

Fig. 14.25 Thymus of young adult *Xenopus*: effect of irradiation. Normal thymus (left, ×35) has an extremely lymphoid cortex and a paler-staining, less cellular medulla. Gamma-irradiated thymus (9 days after 3000 rad irradiation) is shown on the right (× 90). Note the dramatic loss of lymphocytes from the cortex following irradiation, but retention of some lymphocytes in the medulla. The irradiated thymus is reduced in size. Toluidine-blue stain.

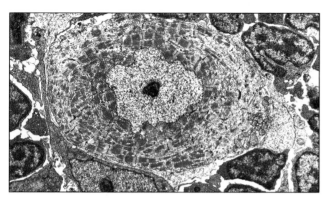

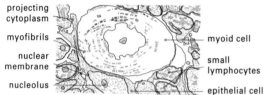

projecting cytoplasm
myofibrils
nuclear membrane
nucleolus
myoid cell
small lymphocytes
epithelial cell

Fig. 14.26 Electron micrograph of thymus medulla of larval *Xenopus*. The myoid cell nucleus is surrounded by concentric rings of striated myofibrils resembling those of skeletal muscle. The nuclear chromatin of the small lymphocytes is organized into a series of electron-dense zones; the cytoplasm is scant with few organelles. The epithelial cell nuclei have evenly-dispersed chromatin and prominent nucleoli; the cytoplasm is extensive and projections extend in an interdigitating fashion between lymphocytes and other cell types to form a supportive network. × 700. (Courtesy of Dr J. J. Rimmer.)

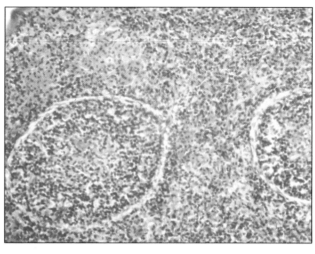

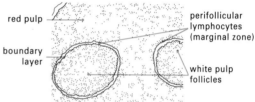

red pulp
boundary layer
perifollicular lymphocytes (marginal zone)
white pulp follicles

Fig. 14.27 Spleen section of adult *Xenopus*. Thymus-dependent (perifollicular red-pulp) and thymus-independent (white-pulp) areas are shown. In *Xenopus* (unlike many other ectotherms) the white pulp is clearly separated from the surrounding red pulp by lightly-staining boundary layer cells. Concentrations of lymphocytes are also seen in the red pulp. H&E stain, × 80.

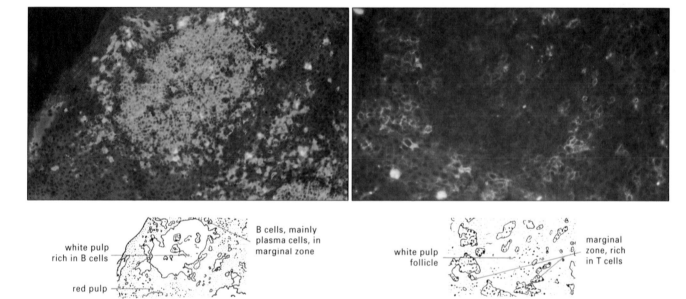

white pulp rich in B cells
red pulp
B cells, mainly plasma cells, in marginal zone

white pulp follicle
marginal zone, rich in T cells

Fig. 14.28 Adult *Xenopus* spleen, showing B and T cell-rich zones. Left: B cells frequent the white pulp follicle; they are also seen in the marginal zone and red pulp, mainly as densely-staining plasma cells. Anti-B-cell (anti-IgM) mAb stain, × 100. Right: T cells are seen concentrated in the marginal zone, just outside the white pulp follicle. They are seen especially in the perifollicular (marginal) zone and lack surface immunoglobulin. Anti-T-cell mAb stain, × 200.

Blood vessels enter the spleen through the white pulp central arteriole, from where capillaries leave and empty into the surrounding red pulp marginal zone; capillary walls contribute to the boundary layer. Experimental studies with India ink-stained and fluoresceinated antigens reveal that it is the red pulp that initially receives material circulating in the blood. Circulating antigens are later trapped within the white pulp follicles, that is, they are closely associated with potential antibody-producing cells (Fig. 14.29). Antigen is held on the surfaces of large dendritic cells, whose cytoplasmic processes extend pseudopods through the boundary layer and into the marginal zone, which is rich in T cells. The overall arrangement of the amphibian spleen is similar to that of the mammalian spleen. The spleen of anuran amphibians plays an important role in B-cell development in both the larva (along with the liver) and in the adult, where it constitutes the main site of B cell differentiation.

LYMPHOMYELOID NODES
Lymphomyeloid nodes, bearing superficial functional resemblance to the lymph nodes of endothermic vertebrates, are seen for the first time in vertebrate evolution in certain anuran amphibians. Histologically however, these anuran nodes are very different from their mammalian counterparts (Fig. 14.30). The lymphomyeloid nodes are mainly blood-filtering organs (cf. mammalian lymph nodes) although trapping of material from surrounding lymph is also believed to occur. These lymph glands do not have the clearly defined architecture of mammalian lymph nodes but appear as aggregations of lymphoid and myeloid cells, lying within the lymph channels. In the adult frog, 'lymph nodes' of similar structure to the larval lymph gland (Fig. 14.30) are found in the neck and axillary regions.

GUT-ASSOCIATED LYMPHOID TISSUE
Nodular gut-associated lymphoid tissue (GALT), analogous to the mammalian GALT system, occurs throughout the small intestine in frogs (Fig. 14.31). Smaller accumulations of lymphocytes loosely associated with the gut are found throughout the vertebrates, a first line of defence against antigens in the gut. In *Xenopus*, IgX is exclusively associated with GALT, and may represent the equivalent of mammalian IgA.

KIDNEY AND LIVER
The kidney is a major lymphomyeloid organ in fish and amphibians, but this function wanes in the kidneys of reptiles, birds and mammals. In frogs and toads, the kidney and/or liver appear as the initial site of B cell development in ontogeny. These organs are, in fact,

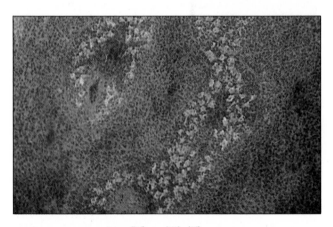

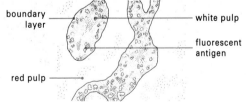

boundary layer — white pulp
fluorescent antigen
red pulp

Fig. 14.29 Immunofluorescence of adult *Xenopus* spleen showing antigen trapping. The toad was injected with human IgG. Three weeks later frozen sections were prepared and incubated with fluorescein-labelled anti-human IgG. The bright apple-green fluorescence shows the presence of antigen within white pulp follicles. The antigen is trapped in a dendritic pattern, similar to that seen in mammals and birds, where it appears to be held on reticular cell surfaces. × 35.

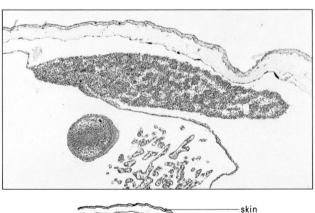

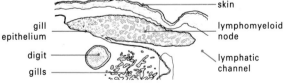

skin
gill epithelium — lymphomyeloid node
digit
gills — lymphatic channel

Fig. 14.30 Lymph gland section of larval *Rana*. The elongated (paired) lymphomyeloid node is seen attached ventrally to the epithelium of the gill chamber and projects into a large lymphatic channel. Gills, and a digit of the anterior limb lying in the gill chamber are seen medially, the larval skin lies laterally. The lymph gland consists of an extensive lymphoid parenchyma with phagocytes and intervening sinusoids (pale-staining). The lymph gland is mainly a blood-filtering organ. H&E stain, × 25

intimately involved with the early differentiation of erythroid, lymphoid and myeloid cells in diverse vertebrates. A section of *Rana* kidney (Fig. 14.32) shows the haemopoietic tissue.

BONE MARROW

Bone marrow makes its first appearance in amphibians. Its immunological role at this level of evolution still awaits clarification, but in adult *Rana pipiens* bone-marrow lymphomyeloid tissue is readily evident (Fig. 14.33) and this is an important source of antibody-producing cells. In *Xenopus*, on the other hand, bone marrow appears to be more rudimentary; the femoral marrow is mainly a site for the differentiation of neutrophilic granulocytes (Fig. 14.33).

ASPECTS OF AMPHIBIAN IMMUNOLOGY

Frogs and toads, particularly *Xenopus*, are proving to be excellent models for studying ontogenetic aspects of immunity, some of which are reviewed below. Histocompatible strains of several amphibian species have been developed and, in recent years, several isogeneic and inbred families of *Xenopus* have become available for immunological research. Different *Xenopus* families, that are either MHC compatible (but express minor histocompatibility differences), or possess one or two MHC haplotype differences, are proving invaluable for a whole range of immunological investigations, such as transplantation of skin and *in vitro* studies.

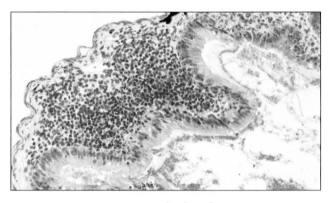

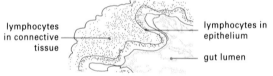

Fig. 14.31 Section of nodular gut-associated lymphoid tissue in adult *Rana*. Lymphocytes are seen in the subepithelial connective tissue and in the overlying gut epithelium. H&E stain, × 50.

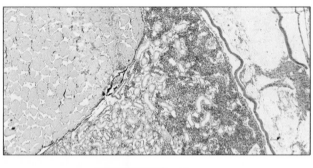

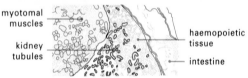

Fig. 14.32 Kidney section in larval *Rana* showing haemopoietic tissue. Haemopoietic tissue is extensive in the intertubular regions where lymphocytes, granulocytes and other developing blood cell types are found. Myotomal muscles and a loop of the intestine lie adjacent to the mesonephros. H&E stain, × 25.

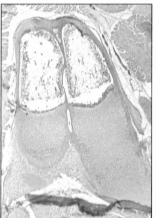
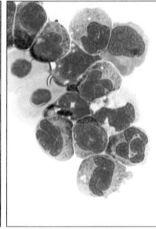

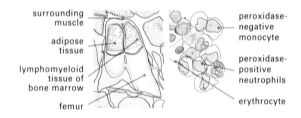

Fig. 14.33 Bone marrow. Left: Lymphomyeloid tissue, an important source of antibody-producing cells, in bone marrow from *Rana*. H&E stain, × 20. Right: A bone marrow cytocentrifuge preparation from *Xenopus*, showing peroxidase-positive neutrophilic granulocytes. × 700. (Cytocentrifuge preparation, courtesy of Dr I. Hadji-Azimi.)

THYMUS DEVELOPMENT AND THYMECTOMY EXPERIMENTS

Xenopus is ideally suited for investigating the role of the thymus in the development of the amphibian immune system, since the free-living larva can be thymectomized very early in life when the thymus is still immature (Figs 14.34 and 14.35). Different pairs of gill pouches yield the thymic buds in different vertebrates. In frogs and toads the paired thymus develops from the dorsal epithelium of the second pharyngeal

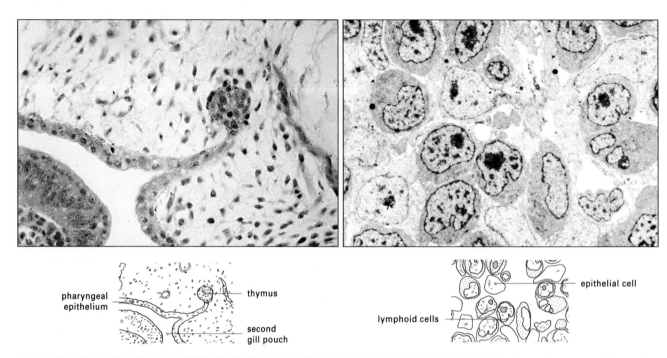

Fig. 14.34 *Xenopus* thymus at 3 days and 7 days. Left: At 3 days, developing thymus is still attached to the pharyngeal epithelium and comprised mostly of epithelial cells. H&E stain, × 100. Right: At 7 days, the thymus consists of less than 1000 cells of two major types. The epithelial cells have a prominent nucleolus, dispersed chromatin and pale-staining cytoplasm. Lymphoid cells possess large amounts of densely-staining cytoplasm with an abundance of free ribosomes and mitochondria. At 7 days, the XT-1 marker begins to appear on the thymic lymphoid cell population, and MHC class II proteins are first expressed on epithelial cells. Electron micrograph, × 500.

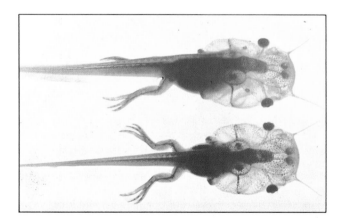

Fig. 14.35 *Xenopus* thymus at 38 days. The pigmented paired thymus lies behind the eyes (upper); its absence is readily apparent in the sibling thymectomized at 7 days (lower).

Effect of thymectomy in *Xenopus*

	antibody response to:		graft rejection	mitogen response to:	
	LPS (T_{ind})	SRBC (T_{dep})		LPS (B cells)	PHA (T cells)
normal	+	+	fast	+	+
thymectomized	+	−	slow	+	−

Fig. 14.36 *Xenopus*, thymectomized at 4–8 days, are assessed for antibody response, cell-mediated response and mitogen response *in vitro*. (LPS = lipopolysaccharide; SRBC = sheep red blood cells; PHA = phytohaemagglutinin.)

pouches. Experimental studies reveal that lymphoid precursor cells first enter the thymic epithelial rudiments at 3–4 days of age. A T-cell differentiation antigen (the XTLA-1 marker [120 kDa], recognized by an anti-thymocyte mouse monoclonal antibody named XT-1) begins to appear on the thymic lymphoid cell population at 7 days, before the emergence of XT-1$^+$ T cells in the periphery. The thymus involutes at metamorphosis when a new wave of colonization by stem cells occurs; following metamorphosis, thymocyte numbers increase, reaching maximal levels at 15–16 months.

Thymectomy of *Xenopus* from 4–8 days of age has clearly demonstrated the existence of T-dependent (T_{dep}) and T-independent (T_{ind}) components of immunity (Fig. 14.36). Following this early thymectomy, XT-1$^+$ T cells are no longer found in larval and young adult lymphoid organs, whereas surface-Ig$^+$ B cells are plentiful (Fig. 14.37). There may be an extrathymic matura-

tion pathway for alloreactive cells in *Xenopus*, however, since toads thymectomized when only 4–7 days old sometimes chronically reject MHC-disparate skin grafts. Following rejection, their splenocytes become positive when tested in mixed lymphocyte culture, but not when stimulated with the T-cell mitogen, PHA. Furthermore, splenocytes expressing T-cell markers begin to emerge in older thymectomized *Xenopus*.

Thymectomy of anuran larvae at different times during development suggests that different T-cell functions require the presence of the thymus for varying periods in order to become established in the periphery (Fig. 14.38). Studies in intact animals reveal that alloimmune reactivity (*in vivo* and *in vitro*), together with the ability of splenocytes to respond to T cell mitogens, develops early in the tadpole's larval life, whereas good IgY antibody responses are only seen in the froglet.

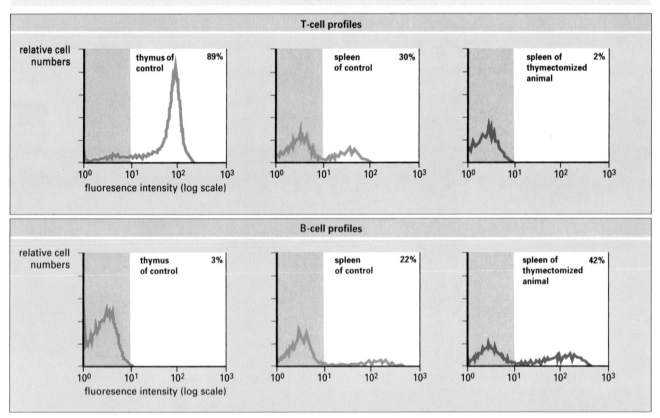

T and B cell population in *Xenopus*

Fig. 14.37 Cells from the thymus and spleen of a control (4-month-old) *Xenopus*, and from the spleen of a 7-day thymectomized sibling, were stained first with either mouse anti-T-cell (XT–1) monoclonal antibody (mAb) or with mouse anti-B-cell (anti-IgM) mAb. FITC-labelled anti-mouse-Ig was used as secondary antibody. T and B cells were then identified using a fluorescence-activated cell sorter. Early larval thymectomy deletes XT-1$^+$ positive T cells from the spleen, which now shows a proportional increase in B cell numbers. The percentage shown on each graph represents the proportion of positive cells, i.e. those to the right of the marker (grey) set to exclude 98% background fluorescence.

Sequential emergence of T cell subsets

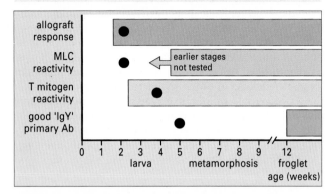

Fig. 14.38 Ontogeny of immune reactivity, and the effect of thymectomy at different ages in *Xenopus*. The allograft response, mixed lymphocyte reactivity and T-mitogen reactivity all appear early. They are followed much later by TH cells, particularly those TH cells which permit the 'IgY' primary antibody response. • Indicates the age after which thymectomy will no longer impair this particular function.

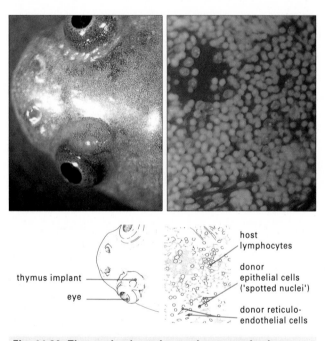

Fig. 14.39 Thymus implantation to thymectomized *Xenopus*. Left: The toad (*X. laevis*) was thymectomized at 7 days of age. A thymus from a larval *X. borealis* donor was then implanted subcutaneously in late larval life. This thymus implant grew well, lying adjacent to the left eye following metamorphosis. Right: A section of the implanted thymus was examined by fluorescence microscopy. Donor-derived cells can be distinguished from host cells, because *X. borealis* nuclei display brightly fluorescent spots, whereas *X. laevis* cells stain homogeneously dull green. The thymus is now repopulated with host lymphocytes, whereas many stromal cell types remain 'spotted' (i.e. they are of donor origin). Quinacrine stain, × 300.

THYMIC EDUCATION

Foreign thymus, grafted into early-thymectomized *Xenopus*, can promote the differentiation of host precursor cells along a T-cell pathway (Fig 14.39). The *in vivo* construction of thymuses, with epithelial and lymphoid compartments having different MHC markers, can readily be achieved by a different surgical approach. This involves joining the anterior part of one 24-hour embryo, containing the thymic epithelial buds, to the posterior portion of an MHC-incompatible embryo, from which the haemopoietic stem cells, including lymphocytes, arise (Fig. 14.40).

These two experimental systems have been used to explore the role played by thymic stromal cells in thymic education. This involves negative selection (establishing tolerance of T cells to self antigens) and positive selection (restricting the MHC-antigen specificities with which helper and effector T-cell populations preferentially interact). These experiments on *Xenopus* have indicated involvement of the foreign thymus epithelium in inducing tolerance towards skin grafts of thymus MHC type, although interestingly this tolerance does not appear to prevent a mixed lymphocyte reaction towards cells of this MHC type. Recently, similar findings have been made with bird and mammal embryos. However, in mammals the view persists that thymic interdigitating (dendritic) cells, which are a stromal population of extrinsic origin, rather than thymic epithelial cells, play a crucial role in inducing thymocyte tolerance by clonal deletion of T cells with high

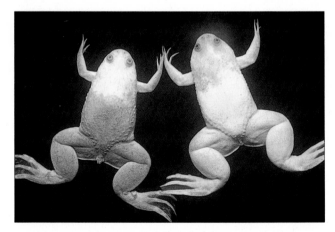

Fig. 14.40 Chimeric toads. Chimeric *Xenopus* were made by exchanging the anterior and posterior regions of two embryos 24 hours after fertilization. At this stage, the thymic anlage (e.g. thymic epithelium) is in the anterior region, whereas all the lymphocyte precursors are in the posterior region. One embryo was from an albino variant with white skin and red eyes, the other embryo was from a normal *Xenopus*. These chimeras are proving useful for studying thymic education. (Courtesy of Dr Martin Flajnik and Dr Louis DuPasquier.)

affinity for self MHC. A role of the amphibian thymus in positive selection has been suggested from *in vivo* experiments with chimeric *Xenopus*.

ONTOGENY OF ALLOIMMUNITY AND ALLOTOLERANCE

Onset of alloimmunity (to MHC antigens) in tadpoles correlates with the lymphoid maturation of the thymus and, presumably, the appearance of the necessary T-cell populations in the periphery (Fig. 14.41). Later in development, a more vigorous alloimmune response is seen, concomitant with a rapid phase of lymphoid organ differentiation. Immunocompetent larvae (but not adults) can, nevertheless, be rendered tolerant of allogeneic skin; allotolerance induction is particularly easy at metamorphosis (Fig. 14.42). The size of grafts applied and the degree of histoincompatibility appear to be critical. Those that are only slightly incompatible are always tolerated by larval and peri-metamorphic

Xenopus. These alloimmune 'deficiencies' of tadpoles may well relate to the finding that MHC class I molecules are not expressed prior to metamorphosis (see earlier section).

IMMUNOLOGY OF METAMORPHOSIS

Immunologists are intrigued to know how amphibians escape the risk of dying from an autoimmune disease at metamorphosis, since adult-specific cell markers are first expressed at this time. The involvement of suppressor cell populations seems likely. On the other hand, high plasma corticosteroid levels and increased expression of corticosteroid receptors on lymphocytes are found during the metamorphic climax. Such hormonal alterations may directly impair cell-mediated immunity, possibly by inhibiting IL-2 production. The significance of MHC class I first being expressed at metamorphosis remains to be elucidated. Amphibian metamorphosis is a fascinating period for probing the interplay between endocrine and immune systems, which will undoubtedly have significance outside purely phylogenetic considerations.

MODELS FOR THE STUDY OF LYMPHOID CELL ORIGINS

Embryonic transplantation of gill buds in *Rana pipiens*, *Xenopus laevis* and the newt *Pleurodeles waltlii* have revealed that thymic lymphocytes develop from extrinsic precursor cells which colonize the thymus. In *Xenopus*, lymphoid precursor cells destined for the thymus have now been shown to arise from both ventro-lateral plate mesoderm (ventral blood islands) and dorso-lateral plate mesoderm of the embryo.

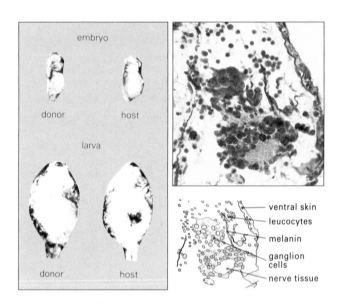

Fig. 14.41 Transplantation of embryonic tissue in *Rana* – ontogeny of alloimmunity. Left: A piece of neural fold removed from one embryo (tail-bud stage) is transplanted to the mid-ventral surface of another embryo (host). Intimately associated with the neural folds are the neural crest elements which are precursors of diverse cell types, including pigment cells. The pigment cells that differentiate provide an externally visible means of following the progress of the embryonic transplant. The host larva has developed a distinctive mass of graft-derived pigment cells. Right: The section shows differentiated graft elements (large ganglion cells with prominent nucleoli, other nervous tissue and melanin), 15 days after transplantation. Despite the earliness of the transplantation, lymphocytes and granulocytes are invading the graft. H&E stain, × 100. (Courtesy of Dr E. P. Volpe.)

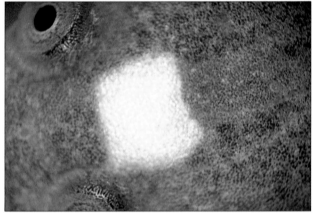

Fig. 14.42 Skin graft tolerance in *Xenopus*. Allogeneic skin, even from an MHC-disparate donor, may be tolerated by a larval or metamorphosing recipient. Subsequent skin grafts (here a piece of white belly skin) from the same donor are similarly retained by the adult frog. However, skin from a different donor is rejected within 3 weeks at 25°C.

These transplantation experiments use cytogenetically distinct lines, which can be identified by the number of chromosomes per cell (triploid/diploid). Similar studies with ventral mesoderm cells have revealed that thymocyte- and B-cell-specific precursors differentiate in this embryonic layer by 20 hours of development. Such experiments illustrate the usefulness of amphibian embryos for exploring the embryonic origins of T and B cells.

 SUMMARY OF IMMUNOEVOLUTION

Salient features of immunologic phylogeny in vertebrates and invertebrates are summarized in Fig. 14.43.

It should be additionally noted that molecular and genetic characterization of immunoglobulins, MHC proteins, T-cell receptors, complement and cytokines of lower vertebrates is in progress.

Immune responses in invertebrate and vertebrate phyla

invertebrates
phagocytosis/encapsulation important in eliminating non-self material
cell-mediated immunity evident early in evolution
different classes and subclasses of immunocyte plus haemopoietic tissue present in coelomates
inducible, broad spectrum, humoral immunity in some coelomates, but immunoglobulins absent from all phyla
lectins and prophenoloxidase involved in recognition of self/non-self in at least some phyla

vertebrates
all display cell-mediated and humoral immunity
all possess a range of lymphoid tissues, which become more complex in 'higher' forms
all possess B lymphocytes; T-equivalent cells identified in bony fishes and all terrestrial vertebrates
all have IgM; jawed vertebrates possess additional, non-μ, heavy chains

Fig. 14.43 Summary of the immune responses found in invertebrate and vertebrate phyla.

FURTHER READING

Beck G, Habicht GS. Primitive cytokines: harbingers of vertebrate defence. *Immunol Today* 1991;**12**:180.

Brehelin M, ed. *Immunity in Invertebrates*. Heidelberg: Springer-Verlag, 1986.

Cohen N, Sigel MM, eds. *The Reticuloendothelial System. Ontogeny and Phylogeny*. New York: Plenum, 1982.

Cohen N, ed. First international symposium on the immunology of ectothermic vertebrates. *Devel Comp Immunol* 1987;**11**:435.

Cooper EL, ed. *Developmental and Comparative Immunology*. New York: Pergamon Press, 1992.

Cooper EL, Langlet C, Bierne J, eds. *Developmental and Comparative Immunology*. New York: AR Liss, 1987.

Du Pasquier L. Evolution of the immune system. In: Paul WE. *Fundamental Immunology*. 2nd ed. New York: Raven Press, 1989.

Du Pasquier L, Schwager J, Flajnik MF. The immune system of *Xenopus*. *Annu Rev Immunol* 1989;**7**:251.

Ellis AE, Tatner MF, eds. *Fish and Shellfish Immunology*. London: Academic Press, 1992.

Flajnik M, Hsu E, Kaufman JF, DuPasquier L. Changes in the immune system during metamorphosis of *Xenopus*. *Immunol Today* 1987;**8**:58.

Horton JD. Immune system of *Xenopus*: T cell biology. In:Tinsley RC, Kubel HR, eds. *The Biology of* Xenopus. Oxford: Oxford University Press, 1993.

Lackie AM, ed. *Immune mechanisms in invertebrate vectors. Zoological Society of London Symposia, 56*. Oxford: Oxford University Press, 1986.

Litman GW, Hinds K, Kobubu F. The structure and organisation of immunoglobulin genes in lower vertebrates. In: *Immunoglobulin Genes*. London: Academic Press, 1988.

Manning MJ, Tatner MF, eds. *Fish Immunology*. London: Academic Press, 1985.

Manning MJ, Turner RJ. *Comparative Immunobiology*. Glasgow: Blackie, 1976.

Manning MJ, Tatner MF, Secombes CJ, eds. Immunology and disease control mechanisms of fish. *J Fish Biol* 1987;**31 (A)**.

Ratcliffe NA, Rowley AF, eds. *Invertebrate Blood Cells*. Vols 1 & 2. London: Academic Press, 1981.

Ratcliffe NA, Rowley AF, Fitzgerald SW, Rhodes CP. Invertebrate immunity: basic concepts and recent advances. *Int Rev Cytol* 1985;**97**:183.

Rowley AF, Ratcliffe NA, eds. *Vertebrate Blood Cells*. Cambridge: Cambridge University Press, 1988.

Smith LC, Davidson EH. The echinoid immune system and the phylogenetic occurrence of immune mechanisms in deuterostomes. *Immunol Today* 1992;**13**:356.

Solomon JB. Invertebrate receptors and recognition molecules involved in immunity and determination of self and non-self. In: *Receptors in Cellular Recognition and Developmental Processes*. London: Academic Press, 1986.

Tournefier A, Charlemagne J, eds. *Evolution of the Vertebrate Immune System*. Telford Press, 1992.

Warr G, Cohen N, eds. *Phylogenesis of Immune Functions*. Oxford: CRC Press, 1991.

Zapata AG, Varas A, Torroba M. Seasonal variations in the immune system of lower vertebrates. *Immunol Today* 1992;**13**:142.

chapter 15

Immunity to Viruses, Bacteria and Fungi

 IMMUNITY TO VIRUSES

The viruses are a group of organisms which must enter a host cell to proliferate, since they lack the necessary biochemical machinery to manufacture proteins and metabolize sugars. Some viruses also lack the enzymes required for nucleic acid replication, and are dependent on the host cell for these functions as well. The number of genes carried by different viruses may be as few as 3 or as many as 250, but this is still much less than even the smallest bacteria. The course of a generalized virus infection is illustrated in Fig. 15.1.

The prions are a poorly characterized group of pathogens, originally described as 'slow viruses'. These include the causative agents of scrapie, a neurological disorder of sheep, and two similar human diseases, Kuru and Creutzfeld–Jakob disease. Prions are small proteinaceous infectious particles, with no nucleic acids. They are associated with a protein (PrP 27–30) which can polymerize into amyloid-like filaments; plaques of amyloid are found in infected brains. Interestingly, genes coding for a protein with the same primary sequence are found in the normal genome and are expressed in the brain. Thus the relationship of prions to true viruses remains unclear.

The illnesses produced by viruses and prions are as varied as the organisms themselves. Illness may be acute, recurrent, latent (dormant infection where the virus is not readily detectable but may recur), or subclinical (acute or chronic symptomless infection where the virus is demonstrable). The immune response evoked by these pathogens is equally varied. Infections with prions evoke no fever or inflammatory infiltrate. This is true for both natural hosts and experimental hosts, so prions are presumably not recognized by the immune system. This may be due to the existence of normal homologues of the prion protein. In contrast, many of the true viral diseases induce strong immune responses with lifelong immunity or chronic immunopathology (Fig. 15.2).

A generalized viral life cycle

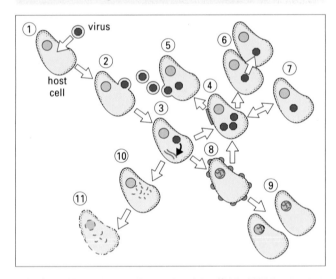

Fig. 15.1 The virion (viral particle) binds, by its receptors, to a host cell (1). It then penetrates the cell and becomes uncoated (2 and 3). Some viruses replicate their components, which then assemble in the host cell (4) and are released by budding from the cell membrane (5). The virus can also spread by cell-to-cell contact (6) without being released. It can also remain dormant within cells, to be reactivated at a later date (7). Some viruses can insert their genetic material into the host cell genome, where they remain latent (8). Their proteins may be expressed on the surface of the cell. Subsequently the cell may become productive (4) or undergo neoplastic transformation (9). Some viral infections may be abortive (10), either because the host cell is non-permissive for infection or because the virus is defective. Abortive infections (like productive infections) can lead to cell death (11).

Illness and virus infection

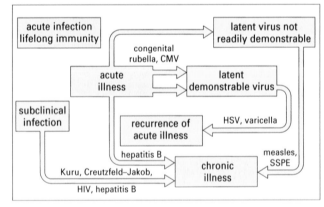

Fig. 15.2 The varied pathology of different viral infections is indicated in the red boxes. While many viruses produce an acute illness followed by sterile lifelong immunity, some are followed by later recurrence, due to virus remaining latent within cells. Examples of different types are given. (CMV = cytomegalovirus; HSV = herpes simplex virus; SSPE = subacute sclerosing panencephalitis.)

The following discussion will concentrate on those acute viral infections which usually evoke obvious immunity, since these are the only ones for which there are reliable immunological data. It must therefore be remembered that we have little understanding of the immunological mechanisms underlying the recurrent, latent, or lifelong subclinical virus infections. Even the data which relate to the acute infections must be interpreted with caution. A number of mechanisms can be shown to destroy viruses, or virus-infected cells *in vitro*, but it is more difficult to be sure which ones are important *in vivo*. This problem is crucial to vaccine design. If we do not know which effector functions normally protect us against particular viral infections, the design of vaccines is a matter of trial and error. There is, therefore, the constant danger of priming inappropriate effector functions. This could lead to disease of enhanced severity, or immunopathology in later life. Moreover, even when we do know which effector functions to prime, we still know far too little about vaccine design (discussed at the end of this chapter) to preferentially prime the chosen mechanism.

In conclusion, this first section describes a number of immune effector mechanisms, the relative importance of which, in any one human infection, remains uncertain.

VIRAL INFECTION

A typical viral infection starts with local invasion of an epithelial surface and then, after one or more viraemic phases (viruses in the blood), results in infection of the target organ, for example the skin, or nervous system. Different viruses infect different cell types, and this is partly dependent on how the virus receptors are distributed on cells. For example, the Epstein–Barr virus primarily infects B cells because it attaches via the complement receptor CR2, and Human Immunodeficiency Virus (HIV) enters cells expressing CD4 (Fig. 15.3).

Since different immunological mechanisms are effective against different forms of antigen (for example, free antigen on host cell surfaces), the relevance of any particular mechanism will depend on the way the viral antigens and virion are encountered. This in turn depends on the species of virus and phase of the infection (Fig. 15.4).

Interferon, (discussed below), has a non-specific action against all viruses, and is therefore part of the innate (non-adaptive) immune system. It acts in a protective capacity before the virus penetrates a cell, by inducing a state of resistance in host cells to viral multiplication.

Mechanisms that may combat a generalized viral infection

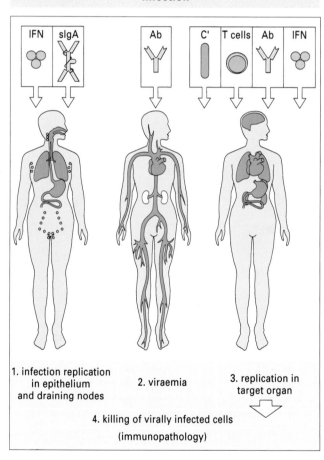

1. infection replication in epithelium and draining nodes

2. viraemia

3. replication in target organ

4. killing of virally infected cells (immunopathology)

Fig. 15.4 The first line of defence is interferon (IFN) and secretory IgA of epithelial surfaces (1). Some viruses which replicate entirely on these surfaces may be checked at this stage. Other viruses have one or two viraemic phases (viruses in blood), susceptible to serum antibody (2). Virus in cells is attacked by a variety of cellular and humoral mechanisms (3). Generally, killing of virally infected cells is beneficial, but sometimes the immune reactions cause more damage than the original infection (4).

Virus receptors

virus	receptor	cell type infected
human immunodeficiency virus (HIV)	CD4 receptor	TH cells
rabies virus	acetylcholine receptor	neurons
vaccinia (cowpox) virus	epidermal growth factor receptor	epidermal cells
Epstein–Barr virus	complement receptor type 2 (CR2)	B cells
influenza A virus	glycophorin A receptor	many cell types

Fig. 15.3 Viruses attach to cells via specific receptors and this partly determines which cell types become infected.

The adaptive immune response depends on antibodies and T-cell receptors which recognize specific antigens on the virus and on virally-infected cells.

Antibody is only capable of directly binding to extracellular viruses, not to those that have become intracellular. IgG and IgM antibodies are limited in their actions to plasma and tissue fluids, whereas secretory IgA (sIgA) may protect epithelial surfaces. sIgA is therefore particularly important in protecting against viruses which lack a viraemic phase. Antibody in association with complement (C1–C9) can lyse host cells carrying viral antigens, or directly damage enveloped viruses.

The cell-mediated immune reactions (Tc cells, antibody-dependent cytotoxic cells) are potentially effective against intracellular viruses, which are recognized by the presence of viral antigens in the membrane of the infected cell.

It is important to differentiate between viral antigens, encoded, at least in part, by the viral genome, and host antigens, induced in the cell by the virus (Fig. 15.5).

Although these 'host-coded' antigens are potentially useful as markers of virus infection, they are of little use in producing protective immunity.

Viral antigens are largely proteins or glycoproteins. The glycoproteins are often glycosylated by the host cell during the budding process. A virion's internal antigens are not usually relevant to antibody-mediated immunity (Fig. 15.6), though they can be important for T-cell responses.

T-CELL RECOGNITION OF VIRAL ANTIGENS

The response to viral antigens is almost entirely T-cell dependent. Even the antibody response requires T-cell help. Thus susceptibility to virus infections is particularly associated with T-cell dysfunction, though this tells us little about the effector mechanisms involved, since T cells are required both for antibody production and for some cytotoxic reactions.

Recognition of influenza antigens by class II-restricted Tc cells appears to require processing of the antigens within the endosomes of APCs. Thus it resembles the processing required for recognition by class II-restricted TH cells, and can be blocked by agents which disrupt lysosomes. These Tc cells can 'recognize' non-infected cells if viral antigens are added, suggesting that intact antigen is processed in endosomes before associating with the class II molecules.

Viral antigens associated with infected cells

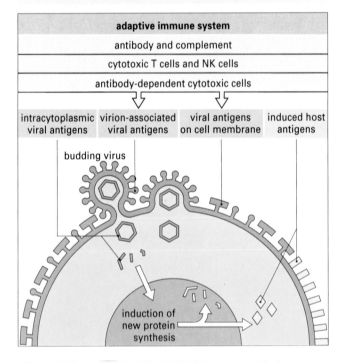

Fig. 15.5 An infected cell is shown diagrammatically with its virally-encoded antigens (dark blue). These antigens may be either inside the cell, on the cell membrane or associated with assembling virions or virus metabolism. Viruses also induce new host proteins (light blue) which are expressed in the nucleus and cytoplasm or on the plasma membrane. The actions of the adaptive immune system are only effective against antigens that are expressed on the cell surface.

Internal and external viral antigens

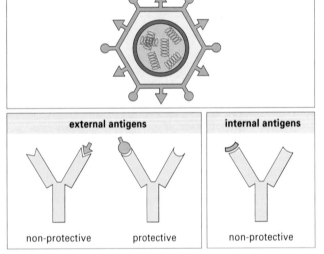

Fig. 15.6 Diagram of a virion showing internal and external antigens surrounding the viral genetic material. Antibody is only capable of binding to external antigens, although it may be produced to all antigens. IgG and IgM act as plasma and tissue fluid, whereas secretory IgA is important in protecting epithelial surfaces. Antibodies to internal antigens are not protective, although T-cell responses to these antigens may be.

In contrast, recognition of virus-infected cells by class I-restricted Tc cells is not affected by disruption of lysosomes, but does require protein synthesis. These Tc cells do not recognize uninfected cells in the presence of purified exogenous antigen. On the other hand they do recognize L cells (a murine cell line of fibroblast origin), if these cells are transfected with both the viral antigen gene and the appropriate class I gene. This implies that the antigen associates with the class I molecule during or following its synthesis, but does not require processing in endosomes.

Antigenic shift and drift in influenza virus

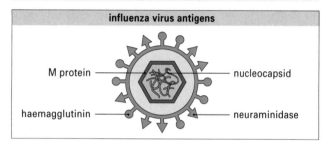

influenza virus antigens

M protein — nucleocapsid

haemagglutinin — neuraminidase

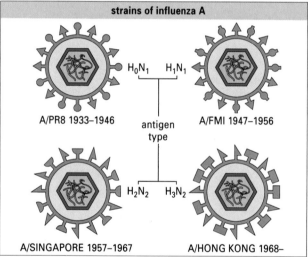

strains of influenza A

H_0N_1 H_1N_1

A/PR8 1933–1946   antigen type   A/FMI 1947–1956

H_2N_2 H_3N_2

A/SINGAPORE 1957–1967   A/HONG KONG 1968–

Fig. 15.7 The major surface antigens of influenza virus are haemagglutinin and neuraminidase. The haemagglutinin is involved in attachment to cells, and antibodies to haemagglutinin are protective (critical site). Antibodies to neuraminidase are much less effective, and those to the internal components are ineffective (non-critical sites). The influenza virus can change its surface slightly (antigenic drift) or radically (antigenic shift). Alterations in the structure of the haemagglutinin antigen render earlier antibodies ineffective and thus new virus epidemics break out. The diagram indicates new strains which have emerged by antigenic shift since 1933.
 The official influenza antigen nomenclature is based on the type of haemagglutinin (H_0, H_1 etc.) and neuraminidase (N_1, N_2 etc.) molecules expressed on the surface of the virion. New strains replace old strains but the internal antigens remain unchanged.

EFFECTS OF ANTIBODY

Antibody may upset the interactions between virus and host cell which lead to binding, penetration, uncoating, or replication. For instance, some viruses have envelopes which, following entry into the phagocytic vacuole, interact with the vacuolar membrane and cause its dissolution, liberating the viral nucleic acid into the cytoplasm. However, the essential interaction with the vacuolar membrane can be blocked if the virion is coated with antibody.

Antibody to critical sites on the virus surface (for example, haemagglutinin of the influenza virus) neutralizes more effectively than antibody to other, non-critical components (for example, neuraminidase) (Fig. 15.7). Complement assists neutralization, by coating the virus or by lysing those with lipid membranes. Antibody plus complement can lyse a variety of human cell lines infected with the virus responsible for measles, influenza or mumps. The alternative complement pathway is required to amplify the triggering of the lytic sequence by the classical pathway, which is not by itself sufficient to cause damage.

Antibody may also produce effects which are not beneficial to the host (Fig. 15.8). For example, it may strip viral antigens from the cell surface, so that the infected cell avoids destruction by cytotoxic cells. It may also increase the rate of infection of cells bearing Fc receptors, by stimulating those cells to take up the virus. This is seen with HIV. Coinfection with viruses such as cytomegalovirus (CMV), which induces Fc-receptor expression, can also theoretically potentiate HIV infection.

The relative importance of the different mechanisms remains unclear. Thus in the intensively studied influenza model, passive transfer of antibody to nude mice does not result in clearing of the virus, though it suppresses shedding, and hence the spread of infection to other mice. Furthermore, mice made artificially agammaglobulinaemic, so that they produce no detectable antibody to haemagglutinin, recover and are subsequently immune. Thus cell-mediated responses appear to be important.

However, there is no doubt that passively administered antibody can protect humans against measles, hepatitis A and B, varicella, and possibly mumps and rubella, if given before, or soon after exposure.

ANTIBODY-DEPENDENT CELL-MEDIATED CYTOTOXICITY

Cells with cytotoxic potential which also express membrane Fc receptors (K cells), may be involved in combating some virus infections. They can lyse virus-infected cells after binding to specific antibody on the cell surface (see Chapter 8).

Immunity to vaccinia virus is mediated by K cells rather than Tc cells. This is because cells carrying Fc receptors are essential to the process, and most Tc cells do not have Fc receptors (Fig. 15.9). The clinical importance of this mechanism is unknown, but it may be more significant in humans than in mice.

NATURAL KILLER (NK) CELLS IN VIRAL IMMUNITY

There is good evidence that NK cells play a role in immunity to murine cytomegalovirus (CMV). If mice are depleted of NK cells by treatment with antibody to asialo–GM1 they show an increased susceptibility to the virus. In a similar way, the transfer of NK-enriched normal spleen cells, or cloned NK cells, to suckling mice protects them from the infection. It is not clear whether the same is true in man *in vivo*, but there are reports of preferential lysis *in vitro*, by human NK cells, of CMV-infected target cells.

Tc CELLS AND MHC RESTRICTION

There is evidence for Tc cells being involved in the response to some virus infections. Vaccination of human subjects with killed whole influenza A virus results in an increased ability to mount an *in vitro* MHC-restricted Tc cell response against host cells infected with viruses of the same or different strains (Fig. 15.10). The lack of strain-specificity agrees with several reports that, in mice, Tc cells generated by one variant can protect against serologically distinct variants (see Fig. 15.11). This may prove important in devising effective vaccines – influenza A virus avoids the antibody response because its surface haemagglutinin and neuraminidase glycoproteins change every few years.

The antiviral effects of antibody

effector	advantages		disadvantages
antibody only	blockage of critical sites ⇨	neutralization	persistent fraction
antibody + complement	lysis of virus with lipid membranes ⇨	neutralization	
antibody + complement	coating ⇨	removal by phagocyte via C3 receptors	may infect the phagocyte
antibody + alternative complement pathway	lysis of infected cell		may 'strip' virus and protect cell from other mechanisms

Fig. 15.8 Note that antibody is not always entirely beneficial.

Immunity to vaccinia virus infection

effector cells	fibroblast target cells	effect on target
1. leucocytes	infected	killed
2. leucocytes	non-infected	no effect
3. non-T cells	infected	killed
4. leucocytes	allogeneic infected	killed
5. cells lacking Fc receptors	infected	no effect
6. leucocytes with blocked Fc receptors	infected	no effect

Fig. 15.9 Human volunteers who had been vaccinated in childhood were revaccinated with vaccinia virus. Peripheral blood leucocytes (effector cells), taken 7 days after vaccination, killed virus-infected HLA-matched target cells (1) but not uninfected cells (2). This was not apparently due to Tc cells, since the effect is mediated by non-T cells (3) and the killing was not restricted to HLA matched targets (4). (In this and the next figure, HLA difference between target and effector cells is indicated in red.) The immunity was apparently due to K cells, since removal of cells with Fc receptors removed the effect (5), and blocking of antibody binding to Fc receptors (with F[ab']₂ anti-IgG Fc) also blocked killing (6).

Tc-cell activity to influenza A in humans

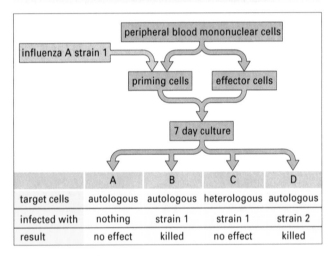

target cells	autologous	autologous	heterologous	autologous
	A	B	C	D
infected with	nothing	strain 1	strain 1	strain 2
result	no effect	killed	no effect	killed

Fig. 15.10 Peripheral blood lymphocytes from a person vaccinated 28 days previously with killed influenza A virus (strain 1) were harvested and divided into two aliquots. One aliquot (10% of the total) was incubated with influenza A strain 1 for 90 minutes, giving a preparation of priming cells. These were then mixed with uninfected (effector) cells and cultured for 7 days. The aim is to keep the effector cell population free from infection. Tc cells generated in the culture were tested on either autologous MHC-identical cells or heterologous MHC- mismatched cells infected with strain 1 or strain 2 virus. The effector cells killed MHC-matched infected targets (B) but not uninfected (A) or mismatched infected targets (C). The Tc cells are not virus-strain specific (D). Tc cells are implicated in these experiments since the cytotoxicity is restricted to infected autologous cells.

Antibodies to these proteins are less useful because they are type-specific and so do not block infection with different strains. Note that MHC restriction implies that Tc cells are involved, unlike the K-cell activity described above.

Immunity in man appears to be virus strain-specific but this does not rule out a role for cross-reactive Tc cells in the recovery phase of influenza infection. Rapid boosting of Tc cell memory during an established infection may be essential for rapid recovery, but this boosted response is short-lived and may not be able to block reinfection with another strain.

Other evidence for T-cell activity is provided by studies involving human volunteers, in which it is found that high Tc-cell activity before challenge with live influenza virus correlates with little or no subsequent shedding of virus particles, which in time correlates with protection.

DELAYED HYPERSENSITIVITY TO VIRAL ANTIGENS

In the mice, delayed type hypersensitivity (DTH) responsiveness – a measure of T-cell sensitization – can be transferred to syngeneic recipients by either class II-restricted CD4$^+$ T cells, or by class I-restricted CD8$^+$ T cells. However, only the CD8$^+$ cells are protective against influenza infection. Indeed the CD4$^+$ cell type results in accelerated death following challenge with live virus (Fig. 15.11). This result illustrates the heterogeneity of the phenomena covered by the term 'delayed hypersensitivity'.

INTERFERON

The term interferon (IFN) is used for several unrelated classes of proteins, which have antiviral effects. Some of them are glycosylated. The classification of these molecules is constantly changing as new classes and sub-types are described.

IFN$_\alpha$ exists as at least 15 subtypes, the genes for which show 85% homology. These, together with IFN$_\beta$, formed the original Type 1 IFN. IFN$_\gamma$ is the original Type II or 'immune' IFN, and shows no homology with any of the other types. IFN$_\gamma$ is a lymphokine as well as an IFN. There are two main types of IFN receptors: one for IFN$_\gamma$, the other for IFN$_\alpha$ and IFN$_\beta$.

IFNs are released from many cell types in response to viral infection, double-stranded RNA, endotoxin (lipopolysaccharide, or LPS), and mitogenic and antigenic stimuli. In general, IFN$_\gamma$ differs from the others as it is only released as a lymphokine from activated T cells.

The antiviral effects of IFNs are exerted via many complex pathways. Among the best studied and understood (Fig. 15.12) are the following:

1. Increased expression of Class I and Class II MHC glycoproteins facilitating recognition of viral antigens by the immune system
2. Activation of cells with the ability to destroy virus infected targets; these include NK cells and macrophages
3. Direct inhibition of viral replication.

Lack of correlation between delayed hypersensitivity and protection in murine influenza

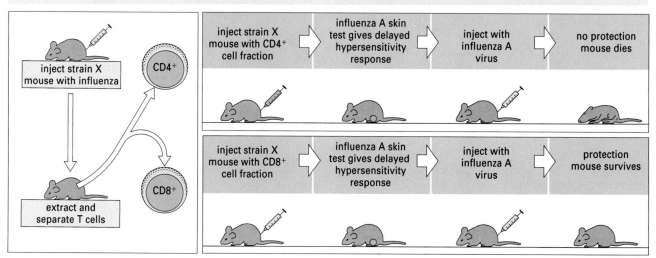

Fig. 15.11 A strain X mouse is infected with influenza A virus. T cells are later removed and divided into those carrying CD4 markers, and those carrying CD8. These two cell populations are injected into other strain X mice. Both are skin-tested with influenza A and give a delayed hypersensitivity response. Subsequent infection of the mice with virus results in the accelerated death (compared with controls) of the mouse which received CD4$^+$ T cells. The mouse which received CD8$^+$ cells is protected from the virus. Thus the ability to produce a delayed hypersensitivity response to a virus does not necessarily imply protective immunity.

Several mechanisms contribute to the third pathway. Released IFN binds to receptors on neighbouring cells and induces synthesis of antiviral proteins. These include a protein kinase and a 2',5'-adenyl synthetase, both of which are activated by double-stranded RNA which is produced during virus-induced metabolism, so that they only become activated if virus enters the cell. The kinase inactivates an enzyme needed for ribosome assembly, and the synthetase catalyses a cascade of enzymes resulting in cleavage of mRNA. These and other mechanisms result in inhibition of protein synthesis, with some selectivity for the viral proteins. However this selectivity is not absolute, which may account for the ability of IFN to inhibit cell growth (including some anti-tumour activity). It may also contribute to the decrease in cell-mediated responses seen early in virus infections.

There are also reports that IFNs can inhibit other viral processes such as penetration of cells, uncoating of the viral nucleic acid, and budding from infected cells.

The clearest evidence for the antiviral efficacy of IFNs *in vivo* came from experiments in which mice were treated with antibody to murine IFNs. They were killed by several hundred times less virus than that needed to kill control animals.

The action of interferon

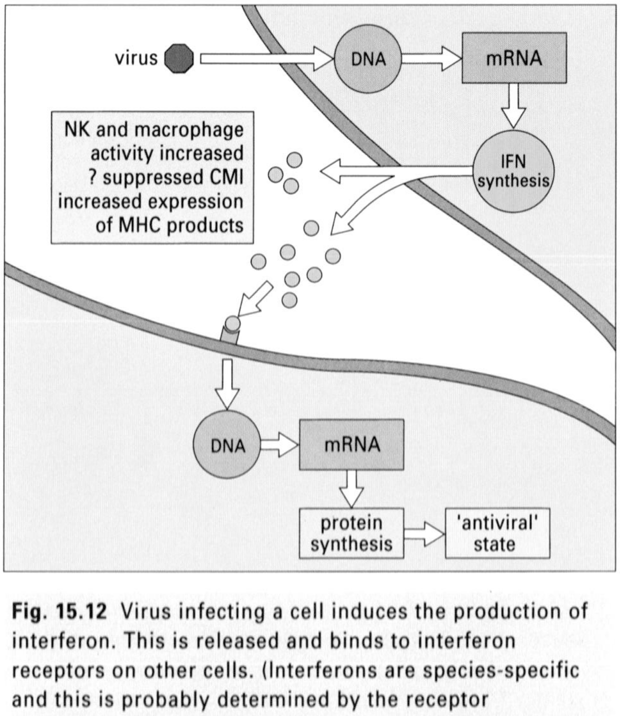

Fig. 15.12 Virus infecting a cell induces the production of interferon. This is released and binds to interferon receptors on other cells. (Interferons are species-specific and this is probably determined by the receptor specificity.) The interferon induces production of antiviral proteins which are activated if virus enters the second cell. Interferon also has many other actions, some of which are still poorly defined.

ANTIVIRAL EFFECTS OF TUMOUR NECROSIS FACTOR (TNF)

TNF exerts several antiviral activities which are similar to those of IFN$_\gamma$, but which apparently work through a separate pathway. Thus, treatment of cultured cells with TNF for 24 hours before addition of vesicular stomatitis virus (VSV) profoundly inhibits virus yield, whereas IFN$_\gamma$ has no effect. In contrast, IFN$_\gamma$ is more effective than TNF when encephalomyocarditis virus (EMCV) is used. However, when added together, TNF and IFN$_\gamma$ show synergistic inhibition of both these RNA viruses. The same effect is seen with DNA viruses such as herpes simplex virus (HSV). If TNF is added to cells after virus infection, it can selectively kill them, even when the cell line is normally TNF-resistant. This effect is also synergistic with that of IFN$_\gamma$.

HUMAN IMMUNODEFICIENCY VIRUS (HIV)

Many of the points raised in previous sections are illustrated by the retrovirus responsible for Acquired Immunodeficiency Syndrome (AIDS). Infection with HIV is characterized by prolonged clinical latency, ineffective immunity, continuous virus mutation, neuropathology, and a tendency to infect bone marrow-derived cells and lymphocytes (see Chapter 18).

HIV is taken up by T cells following binding of a viral glycoprotein (gp120) to CD4 (see Fig. 15.13). It also enters macrophages and other antigen-presenting cells (APCs) by this route. However, entry into cells bearing Fc receptors can be enhanced by antibody, suggesting that this provides an alternative route into phagocytic cells, or enhances entry when CD4 is scarce. There is then a long, but variable period of clinical latency. In about 50% of patients, progression to AIDS does not occur for 10 years. During this latent period, HIV can exist as a provirus, integrated within the host's genomic DNA, without any transcription occurring. Numerous factors can lead to the activation of transcription. *In vitro* both TNF and IL-6 cause increased production of infectious virus from latently infected T cell lines. This may be important *in vivo* because monocytes from individuals carrying HIV tend to release abnormally large quantities of these cytokines. So it is possible that *in vivo* there is a cycle of TNF and IL-6 release, leading to enhanced virus transcription (see Fig. 15.13). This could lead to infection of further cells, and release of more cytokine. Other factors which increase virus production include infection with herpes virus and adenovirus. Production is increased *in vitro* by other cytokines and lymphokines and by mitogens and phorbol esters. Elimination of the virus does not occur for a variety of reasons, including latency, viral mutation (giving rapid antigenic drift), and progressive immunodeficiency.

IMMUNOPATHOLOGY

The immune response to viruses can cause damage to the host via the formation of immune complexes, or by direct damage to infected cells. Complexes can form in body fluids or on cell surfaces, or following capping and stripping of expressed virus. Chronic immune-complex glomerulonephritis can occur in mice infected neonatally with lymphocytic choriomeningitis (LCM) virus (Fig. 15.14). Direct damage to infected cells by a T-cell-dependent mechanism is responsible for most of the tissue damage in infection of adult mice. A similar mechanism has been postulated for chronic active hepatitis in man. Thus, *in vitro* correlates of cell-mediated immunity are present in a proportion of patients with chronic active hepatitis, but absent in asymptomatic carriers. In human HIV infection, some of the neuropathology may be due to inappropriate cytokine release from infected brain macrophages.

VIRUSES AND AUTOIMMUNITY

Viruses may also evoke autoimmunity, possibly by release of antigens normally concealed from the immune system, or by inducing expression of developmental antigens, or by directly stimulating autoreactive cells. Retroviruses, when they are integrated into the host genomic DNA, can lead to the expression of novel histocompatibility antigens.

 IMMUNITY TO BACTERIA

The defence mechanisms appropriate for a bacterial infection can be related to the structure of the invading bacteria (and hence the immunological mechanisms to which they are susceptible), and to the mechanism of their pathogenicity. These two points are considered in more detail below.

THE STRUCTURE OF BACTERIA

There are four main types of bacterial cell wall (Fig. 15.15), belonging to the following groups:
1. Gram-positive bacteria
2. Gram-negative bacteria
3. mycobacteria
4. spirochaetes.
The outer lipid bilayer of Gram-negative organisms is of particular importance because it is often susceptible to mechanisms which can lyse membranes such as complement and certain cytotoxic cells. Killing of the other types usually requires uptake by phagocytes.

The outer surface of the bacterium may also contain fimbriae or flagellae, or be covered by a protective capsule. These can impede the functions of phagocytes or complement, but also act as targets for the antibody response, the role of which is discussed later.

THE MECHANISMS OF PATHOGENICITY OF BACTERIA

There are two extreme patterns of pathogenicity:
1. toxicity without invasiveness
2. invasiveness without toxicity (Fig. 15.16).

Infection of lymphocytes and macrophages by HIV

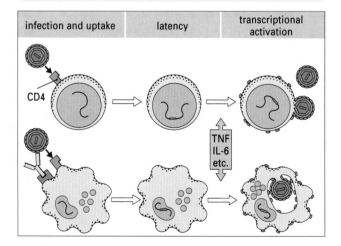

Fig. 15.13 The gp120 on the surface of HIV virions binds to CD4 on the lymphocyte membrane, and this triggers uptake. The virus also enters macrophages which express much less CD4, but this may be assisted by binding through antibody to Fc receptors. The virus remains latent, integrated in the host cell's genomic DNA, until some stimulus (e.g. cytokines) causes transcriptional activation. Then virus buds from the outer membrane of T cells, or into intracytoplasmic vacuoles of macrophages, where a large reservoir of potentially infectious particles can build up.

Lymphocytic choriomeningitis virus (LCM) in mice

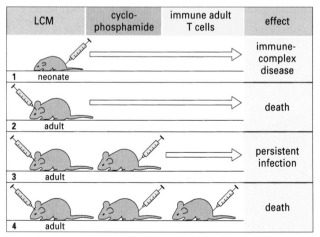

Fig. 15.14 The different effects of LCM are related to differences in immune status. Infection of neonatal mice (1) produces chronic virus shedding and immune-complex disease, manifesting itself as glomerulonephritis and vasculitis. Intracerebral infection of adult mice (2) results in death. This is due to a T-cell reaction, since suppression of immunity with cyclophosphamide (3) leads to persistent infection, but prevents death. This 'protective' effect produced by cyclophosphamide can be reversed by T cells from an immune animal (4).

However, most bacteria are intermediate between these extremes, with some invasiveness assisted by some locally acting toxins and spreading factors (tissue-degrading enzymes).

Corynebacterium diphtheriae and *Vibrio cholerae* are examples of organisms which are toxic but not invasive. Since their pathogenicity depends almost entirely on toxin production, neutralizing antibody to the toxin

Bacterial cell walls

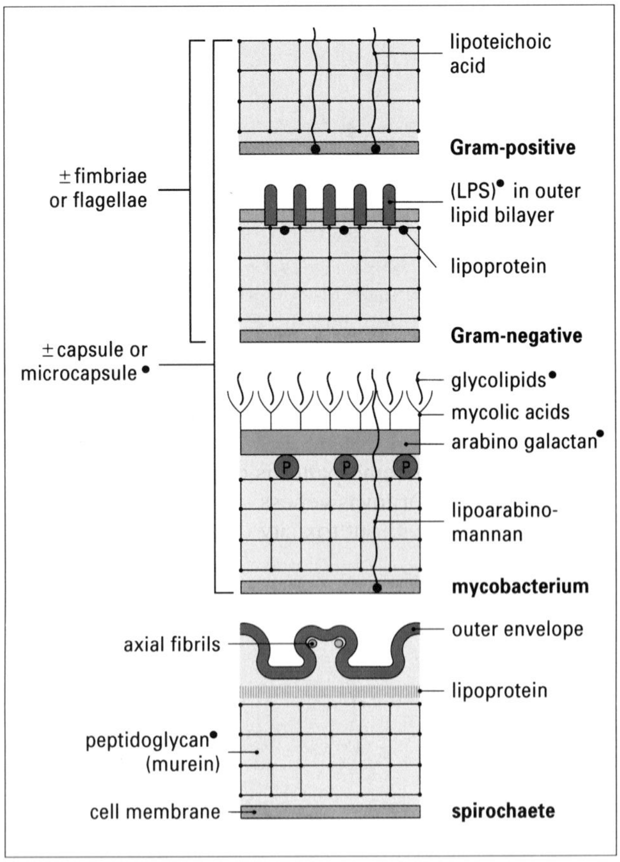

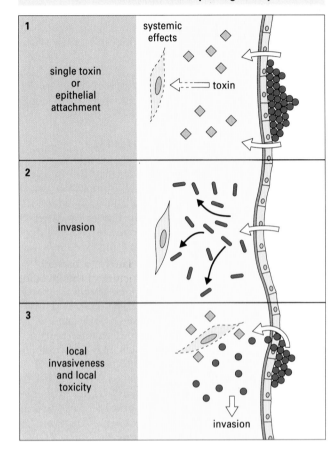

Mechanisms of immunopathogenicity

Fig. 15.15 Different immunological mechanisms have evolved to destroy the cell wall structure of the different groups of bacteria. All types have an inner cell membrane and a peptidoglycan wall. Gram-negative bacteria also have an outer lipid bilayer in which lipopolysaccharide (LPS) is embedded. Lysosomal enzymes and lysozyme are active against the peptidoglycan layer, while cationic proteins and complement are effective against the outer lipid bilayer of the Gram-negative bacteria. The compound cell wall of the mycobacteria is extremely resistant to breakdown, and it is likely that this can only be achieved with the assistance of the bacterial enzymes working from within. Some bacteria also have fimbriae or flagellae, which can provide targets for the antibody response. Others have an outer capsule which renders the organisms more resistant to phagocytosis, or to complement. The components indicated with a black spot (•) all have adjuvant properties, that is, they are recognized by the immune system as a non-specific signal that boosts immune activity.

Fig. 15.16 Mechanisms of pathogenicity, and their relationship to protective immunity.
1. Some bacteria cause disease only because of a single toxin (e.g. *Corynebacterium diphtheriae, Clostridium tetani*) or because of an ability to attach to epithelial surfaces, without invading the host's tissues (e.g. in group A streptococcal sore throat). Immunity to such organisms may require only antibody to neutralize this critical function.
2. At the other extreme there are organisms which are not toxic, and cause disease by invasion, where damage results mostly from the bulk of organisms, or from immunopathology (e.g. *lepromatous leprosy*). These organisms must be destroyed and degraded by the cell-mediated immune response.
3. Most organisms fall between the two extremes, with some local invasiveness assisted by local toxicity and enzymes which degrade extracellular matrix (e.g. *Staphylococcus aureus, Clostridium perfringens*). Antibody and cell-mediated responses are both involved in resistance.

is probably sufficient for immunity, though antibody, binding to the bacteria themselves and so blocking adhesion to the epithelium, may also be important.

In contrast, the pathogenicity of most invasive organisms does not rely so heavily on a single toxin, so immunity requires killing of the organisms themselves.

ANTIBACTERIAL MECHANISMS WHICH DO NOT DEPEND ON ANTIGEN RECOGNITION BY T CELLS OR ANTIBODY

The body's first line of defence against pathogenic bacteria consists of simple barriers to the entry or establishment of the infection. Thus the skin and exposed epithelial surfaces have protective systems which limit the entry of potentially invasive organisms (Fig. 15.17). Only a minute proportion of the potentially pathogenic organisms around us ever gain access to the tissues.

RECOGNITION OF COMMON BACTERIAL COMPONENTS

If the organisms do enter the tissues, they can be combated initially by the innate immune system. Numerous bacterial components are recognized in ways which do not rely on the antigen-specific receptors of either B cells or T cells. These types of recognition are phylogenetically ancient 'broad spectrum' mechanisms that evolved before antigen-specific T cells and immunoglobulins, allowing protective responses to be triggered by common microbial components. Many organisms, such as non-pathogenic cocci, are probably removed from the tissues as a consequence of these pathways, without the need for a specific adaptive immune reaction. Fig. 15.18 shows some of the microbial components involved, and the host responses which are triggered. It is interesting to note that the 'Limulus assay', used to detect contaminating lipopolysaccharide (LPS) in preparations for use in man is based on one such recognition pathway found in an invertebrate species. In *Limulus polyphemus* (the horseshoe crab) tiny quantities of LPS trigger formation of fibrin which walls off the LPS-bearing infectious agent.

There are several consequences of these lymphocyte-independent bacterial recognition pathways.

Activation of complement via the alternative pathway

This may result in the killing of some bacteria, particularly those with an outer lipid bilayer susceptible to the lytic complex (C5–9). It also releases the chemotactic products, C3a and C5a. These cause smooth muscle contraction and mast cell degranulation, as well as attracting and activating neutrophils. The consequent release of histamine and leukotriene contributes to further increases in vascular permeability. Attachment to the bacteria of derivatives of C3 is important in subsequent interactions with phagocytes.

Chemotaxis

This may be due both to complement activation, and to direct chemotactic effects of bacterial products. It attracts more phagocytes to the site of infection.

Cytokine release

The rapid release from macrophages of cytokines such as TNF and IL-1 leads to systemic activation of phagocytic cells, and their increased adhesion to endothelium, facilitating passage into inflamed tissue.

Release of lymphokines from NK cells

When murine NK cells are stimulated by both microbial components and TNF, they can release IFN$_\gamma$. This in turn can activate macrophages. This T-cell-independent pathway helps to explain the unexpected resistance of mice with SCID (Severe Combined Immunodeficiency, a defect in T-cell maturation) to infections such as *Listeria monocytogenes*.

Adjuvant effects

'Adjuvant' is derived from the Latin (*adjuvare*, to help). It refers to the fact that, when given experimentally, soluble antigens evoke stronger T- and B-cell-mediated responses if they are mixed with bacterial components. Components with this property are indicated in Fig. 15.15. The best known adjuvant in laboratory use, known as Complete

Non-specific barriers to infection

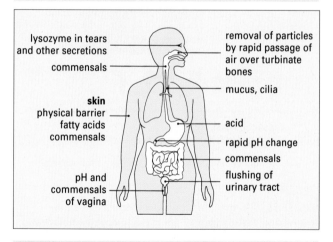

lysozyme in tears and other secretions
commensals

skin
physical barrier
fatty acids
commensals

pH and commensals of vagina

removal of particles by rapid passage of air over turbinate bones

mucus, cilia

acid

rapid pH change

commensals

flushing of urinary tract

Fig. 15.17 Invasion by potentially pathogenic organisms is limited by a variety of non-specific mechanisms.
1. Intact skin is impenetrable to most bacteria. Additionally, fatty acids produced by the skin are toxic to many organisms. The pathogenicity of some strains correlates with their ability to survive on the skin.
2. Epithelial surfaces are cleansed, for example, by ciliary action in the trachea, or by flushing of the urinary tract.
3. Many bacteria are destroyed by pH changes in the stomach and vagina – both are acidic. In the vagina, the epithelium secretes glycogen which is metabolized by particular species of commensal bacteria, producing lactic acid. This also limits pathogen invasion.
4. Commensals occupy a particular ecological niche, and so stop pathogens gaining access to it. Thus infections by *Candida* or *Clostridium difficile* can occur when the normal flora is disturbed by antibiotics.

Freund's adjuvant, consists of killed *Mycobacterium tuberculosis* suspended in oil, which is then emulsified with the aqueous antigen solution. This effect probably reflects the fact that, when the antigen-specific immune response evolved, it did so in a tissue environment already containing these pharmacologically active bacterial components. The response to a pure bacterial antigen, injected without adjuvant-active bacterial components can be regarded as an artificial situation that does not occur in nature.

Selection of the appropriate lymphocyte-mediated response Different bacteria exert optimal adjuvant effects on different parameters of the immune system. This may reflect the need for the immune response to perform some elementary 'taxonomy' on the infecting organism, so that it can activate the appropriate effector functions. Cytokine release by bacteria may also assist in this decision-making step, which is described in greater detail in Chapter 8.

Selection of inappropriate lymphocyte responses Adjuvanticity is clearly an adaptation of the host. However, some organisms may exploit it to disturb immunoregulation, and so activate an inappropriate subset of helper T (TH) cells. This has been most clearly demonstrated in a model of infection of mice with the protozoan parasite *Leishmania major*. In this model, activation of TH2 cells leads to fatal disease, whereas activation of TH1 cells is fully protective.

Shock syndromes If cytokine release is sudden and massive, several acute tissue-damaging syndromes can result and these are potentially fatal. They are described in a later section dealing with immunopathology.

THE ROLE OF ANTIBODY AND COMPLEMENT
Interactions of bacteria with antibody
Antibody clearly plays a crucial role in dealing with bacterial toxins. It neutralizes diphtheria toxin by blocking the attachment of the binding portion of the molecule to its target cells. Similarly it may block locally-acting toxins or extracellular matrix-degrading enzymes which act as spreading factors, and it can interfere with motility by binding to flagellae. An important function on external surfaces, often performed by sIgA, is to stop bacteria binding to epithelial cells. For instance, antibody to the M proteins of Group A streptococci

Protective mechanisms not involving antigen-specific B or T cells

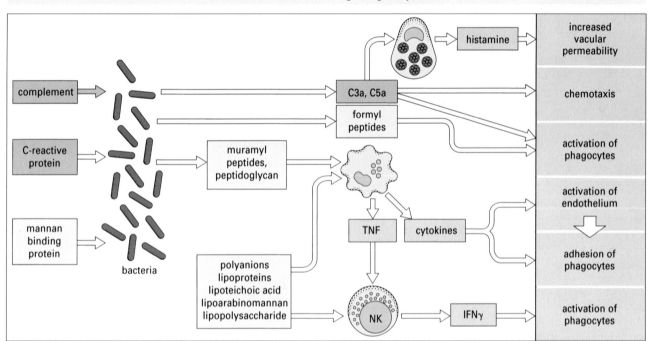

Fig. 15.18 Several common bacterial components are recognized by molecules present in serum, and by receptors on cells. These recognition pathways result in: activation of the alternative complement pathway (Factors C3, B, D, P, C5), with consequent release of C3a and C5a; activation of neutrophils and macrophages; triggering of cytokine release; mast cell degranulation leading to increased blood flow in the local capillary network; increased adhesion of cells and fibrin to endothelial cells. These mechanisms, plus tissue injury caused by the bacteria, may activate the clotting system and fibrin formation, which limit bacterial spread.

gives type-specific immunity to streptococcal sore throats. It is also likely that some antibodies to the bacterial surface can block functional requirements of the organism such as the binding of iron-chelating compounds or the intake of nutrients (Fig. 15.19). However, the most important role of antibody in immunity to non-toxigenic bacteria is the more efficient targeting of complement. With the aid of antibodies, even organisms which resist the alternative pathway (see below) are damaged by complement, or become coated with C3 products, which then enhance the binding and uptake by phagocytes (Figs 15.20 and 15.21). The most efficient complement-fixing antibodies in man are IgG1, IgG3 and IgM. IgG1 and IgG3 are also the subclasses with the highest affinity for Fc receptors.

Avoidance of complement by pathogenic bacteria

Many organisms have devised strategies to resist the detrimental effects of complement (Fig. 15.22). Some bacterial capsules are very poor activators of the alternative pathway. Alternatively long side-chains (O antigens) on lipopolysaccharide may fix C3b at a distance from the vulnerable lipid bilayer. Similarly, smooth Gram-negative organisms (*Escherichia coli, Salmonella* spp., *Pseudomonas* spp.) may fix but then rapidly shed the C5b–C9 membrane complex. Other organisms exploit the physiological mechanisms which block destruction of host cells by complement. When C3b has

The antibacterial roles of antibody

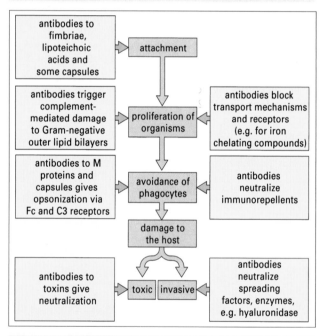

Fig 15.19 This diagram lists the stages of bacterial invasion (blue) and indicates the antibacterial effects of antibody that operate at different points (yellow). Antibodies to fimbriae, lipoteichoic acid and some capsules block attachment of the bacterium to the host cell membrane. Bacteria trigger complement-mediated damage to Gram-negative outer lipid bilayers. Antibody directly blocks bacterial surface proteins which pick up useful molecules from the environment and transport them across the membrane. Antibody to M proteins and capsules opsonizes the bacteria via Fc and C3 receptors for phagocytosis. Immunorepellents – factors which interfere with normal phagocytosis and may be toxic for leucocytes – are neutralized. Following host-cell damage, the bacterial toxins may be neutralized by antibody, as may bacterial spreading factors, which facilitate invasion for example by the destruction of connective tissue or fibrin.

Effect of antibody and complement on rate of clearance of virulent bacteria from the blood

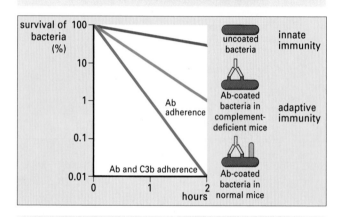

Fig. 15.20 The uncoated bacteria are phagocytosed rather slowly; on coating with antibody, adherence to phagocytes is increased many-fold. The adherence is somewhat less effective in animals temporarily depleted of complement.

The interaction between bacteria and phagocytic cells

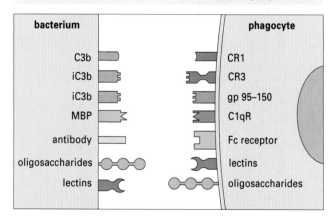

Fig 15.21 A variety of molecules facilitate the binding of the organisms to the phagocyte membrane. The precise nature of the interaction may determine whether uptake occurs, and whether appropriate killing mechanisms are triggered.

attached to a surface it can either interact with factor B leading to further amplification, or it can become inactivated by factors H and I. Capsules rich in sialic acid (as host cell membranes are) seem to promote the interaction with H and I. *Neisseria meningitidis, E. coli* K1, and Group B streptococci all resist complement attachment in this way. The M protein of Group A streptococci acts as an acceptor for factor H, thus potentiating C3bB dissociation. Also these bacteria house a gene for a C5a protease.

Avoidance of complement-mediated damage

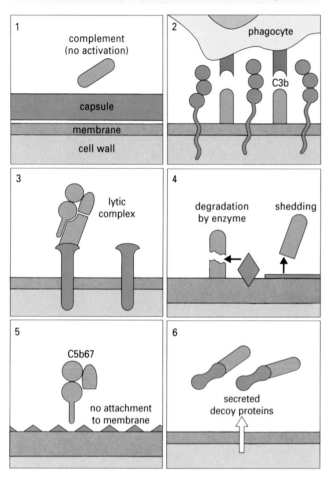

Fig. 15.22 Bacteria avoid complement-mediated damage by a variety of strategies. (1) An outer capsule or coat prevent complement activation. (2) An outer surface can be configured so that complement receptors on phagocytes cannot obtain access to fixed C3b. (3) Surface structures can be expressed which divert attachment of the lytic complex (MAC) from the cell membrane. (4) Membrane-bound enzyme can degrade fixed complement, or cause it to be shed. (5) The outer membrane can resist the insertion of the lytic complex. (6) Secreted decoy proteins can cause complement to be deposited on them and not on the bacterium itself.

INTERACTION WITH PHAGOCYTES

Ultimately most bacteria are killed by phagocytes. This process involves several steps (Fig. 15.23).

Chemotaxis in which bacterial components, such as f-Met.Leu.Phe, and complement products, such as C5a, attract the phagocytes.

Attachment of the phagocyte to the organism   This is an important interaction which may determine whether uptake subsequently occurs, and whether killing mechanisms are triggered during uptake. The binding can be mediated by the following entities.

1. Lectins on the organism, for example the mannose-binding lectin on the fimbriae of *E. coli*.
2. Lectins on the phagocyte. Of particular interest in this respect are the complement receptors CR3 and p150,95 and the related molecule LFA-1, which have multiple binding sites specific for different carbohydrate moieties. They can bind to β-glucans and to the lipopolysaccharide endotoxin of Gram-negative bacteria.
3. Complement deposited via the alternative or classical pathways. It has recently been discovered that complement can also be fixed by mannose-binding lectin present in serum, which can itself bind to C1q receptors.
4. Fc receptors, which link to antibody bound to the bacteria (see Fig. 15.20).

Bacterial killing by phagocytes

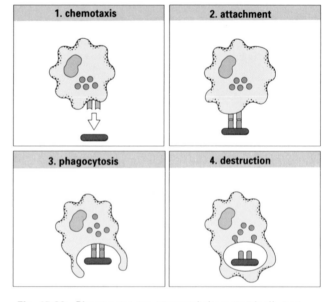

Fig. 15.23 Phagocytes are attracted chemotactically to a bacterial infection. The phagocytes attach to the bacterium via numerous receptors, as indicated in Fig. 15.21. The organism is then phagocytosed. Finally the organism is exposed to a sequence of killing mechanisms, some of which involve fusion of lysosomes with the phagosome.

Triggering of uptake The binding of an organism to a receptor on the macrophage membrane does not always lead to its uptake. For example, zymosan particles (derived from yeast) bind via the glucan-recognizing lectin-like site on CR3 and are taken up, whereas erythrocytes coated with C3bi are not, although the C3bi also binds to CR3.

Triggering of microbicidal activity Just as binding of an organism to membrane receptors does not guarantee uptake, so uptake does not guarantee the triggering of killing mechanisms. It seems that interaction with CR3 is particularly likely to trigger killing.

THE KILLING MECHANISMS OF PHAGOCYTIC CELLS
Once the organism has been internalized it is exposed to an array of killing mechanisms.

Oxygen–dependent killing mechanisms
Reactive oxygen intermediates (ROIs) This pathway involves an enzyme in the phagocyte membrane which reduces oxygen (O_2) to superoxide anion (O_2^-), a reactive oxygen intermediate (ROI). This in turn generates other ROIs (Fig. 15.24). Cells from patients with chronic granulomatous disease (CGD) lack this pathway, and are unable to kill some microorganisms. The disease is characterized by chronic inflammatory lesions involving pyogenic organisms, for example staphylococci. The monocytes of individuals with congenital myeloperoxidase deficiency may show defective microbicidal activity. However, it remains unclear whether sufficient halide is available in phagosomes *in vivo*. Moreover, tissue macrophages do not contain peroxidase and thus do not carry out the peroxidase-dependant reactions.

Reactive nitrogen intermediates (RNI) This recently discovered pathway (Fig. 15.25) may be particularly important. It results in the formation of NO (nitric oxide) which is toxic for bacteria and tumour cells. For optimal expression of this mechanism, macrophages need both activation by IFN$_\gamma$, and triggering by TNF. This is the mechanism which enables murine macrophages to kill mycobacteria.

Oxygen-independent killing mechanisms
These mechanisms may be more important than was previously thought. Many organisms can be killed by cells from patients with chronic granulomatous disease, who cannot produce reactive oxygen intermediates, or from patients with myeloperoxidase deficiency, who cannot produce hypohalous acids. Some of this killing may be due to NO, but many organisms can be killed anaerobically, so other mechanisms must exist.

Cationic proteins with antibiotic-like properties The defensins are cysteine- and arginine-rich cationic peptides of 30–33 amino acids, found in rabbit macrophages and human neutrophil polymorphs, where they comprise 30–50% of the granule proteins. They form ion-permeable channels in lipid bilayers. They are most effective at pH 7.0 so they probably act early after phagolysosome formation before acidification takes place. Defensins can kill organisms as diverse as *Staphylococcus aureus*, *Pseudomonas aeruginosa*, *Escherichia coli*, *Cryptococcus neoformans* and the enveloped virus *Herpes simplex*. There are several other cationic proteins with different pH optima, including cathepsin G and azurocidin, both of which are related to elastase but which have activity against Gram-negative bacteria; this is unrelated to their enzyme activity.

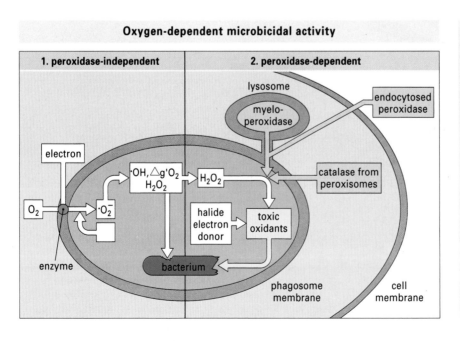

Oxygen-dependent microbicidal activity

1. peroxidase-independent	2. peroxidase-dependent

lysosome
myelo-peroxidase
endocytosed peroxidase
electron
'OH, $\triangle$g'O_2, H_2O_2
H_2O_2
catalase from peroxisomes
O_2
$\cdot O_2^-$
halide electron donor
toxic oxidants
enzyme
bacterium
phagosome membrane
cell membrane

Fig. 15.24 1. An enzyme in the phagosome membrane reduces oxygen to superoxide anion ($\cdot O_2^-$). This can give rise to hydroxyl radicals ($\cdot OH$), singlet oxygen, ($\Delta g^1 O_2$) and hydrogen peroxide (H_2O_2), all of which are potentially toxic. Lysosome fusion is not required for these parts of the pathway, and the reaction takes place spontaneously following internalization of the phagosome. 2. If lysosome fusion occurs, myeloperoxidase may enter the phagosome. Myeloperoxidase (or under some circumstances, catalase from peroxisomes) acts on peroxides in the presence of halides (preferably iodide), additional toxic oxidants, such as hypohalite (HIO, HCIO), are generated.

Other antimicrobial mechanisms Following lysosome fusion there is a transient rise in pH before acidification (a fall in pH) of the phagolysosome takes place. This occurs within 10–15 minutes. Some organisms may be killed by the acidification itself, although this is more likely to be related to the low pH optima of lysosomal enzymes. Certain Gram-positive organisms with readily exposed peptidoglycan may be killed by lysozyme. A variety of other substances, such as lactoferrin (produced by neutrophil polymorphs), have also been implicated in killing. Lactoferrin can bind iron and render it unavailable to bacteria even at an acid pH; thus the ability of polymorphs to kill some bacteria is lost if they are loaded with iron. These mechanisms may all require phagolysosome fusion (Figs 15.26 and 15.27).

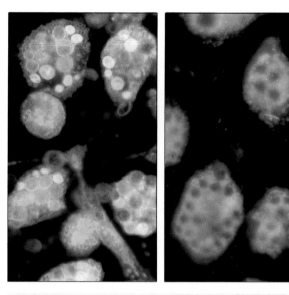

Fig. 15.26 Inhibition of fusion of secondary lysosomes with yeast-containing phagosomes by the addition of ammonium chloride. Mouse peritoneal macrophages were incubated in acridine orange, which concentrates in secondary lysosomes. Live baker's yeast was then added – these assume the appearance of 'holes' in the cell. Normally, the secondary lysosomes fuse with the phagosomes, and the acridine orange enters them, fluorescing green, yellow or orange depending on the concentration (left). However, in the presence of ammonium chloride, fusion does not occur and the 'holes' remain dark (right). Such blocking of lysosomal fusion may be employed by *Mycobacterium tuberculosis* and some leishmania, which secrete ammonia. Some polyanions, such as polyglutamic acid or suramin, can also do this. (Courtesy of Mr R. Young and Dr P. D. Hart.)

The nitric oxide pathway

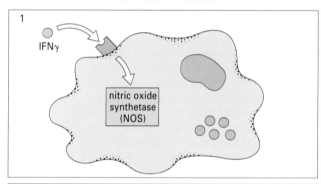

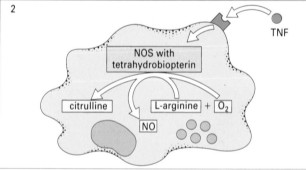

Fig. 15.25 Nitric oxide synthetase combines oxygen with the guanidino nitrogen of L-arginine to give nitric oxide, which is toxic for bacteria and tumour cells. Tetrahydrobiopterin is needed as a cofactor. IFN$_\gamma$ activates the pathway (1), which is then optimally triggered by TNF (2). Paradoxically, it is doubtful whether human macrophages can make tetrahydrobiopterin, but neutrophils and other human cell types can do so. This pathway may therefore be important for the self-defence of non-immunological tissue cells.

Mechanism involved in bacterial killing

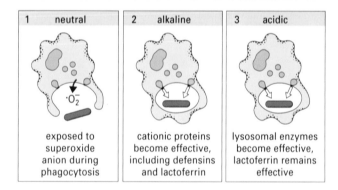

Fig. 15.27 During phagocytosis there is immediate exposure to superoxide anion (1). This leads to a transient increase in pH when cationic proteins may be effective (2). Subsequently the pH falls, as H$^+$ ions are pumped into the phagolysosome and lysosomal enzymes with low pH optima become effective (3). Lactoferrin acts by chelating free iron, and can do so at alkaline or acidic pH.

ACTIVATION OF MACROPHAGES

Although macrophages and monocytes possess killing mechanisms in the resting state, these mechanisms can be enhanced, and new mechanisms can be expressed when they are activated. Activation occurs through exposure to microbial products, and to lymphokines derived from T cells. Similarly, the decline which normally occurs if the cells are kept in culture for a week can be reversed by treatment with suitable activating stimuli (Fig. 15.28).

Activation by Microbial Products

A number of microbial products cause direct activation of monocytes and macrophages, or indirect activation by triggering cytokine release from them. The cytokines then activate the phagocytes – an autocrine effect. This was discussed earlier in relation to the non-lymphocyte-dependent recognition of bacteria.

Lymphokine-Mediated Activation

In vivo, lymphokines released during T-cell-mediated responses are often required for phagocytes to become fully activated. The lymphokine most often implicated is IFN$_\gamma$, which enhances both oxygen-dependent and oxygen-independent killing mechanisms. There are also reports implicating IL-2, GM–CSF, TNF, and other lymphokines. As discussed in greater detail in Chapter 8, activation of some functions requires combinations of cytokines.

Lymphokines *in vivo* have two effects on phagocytes – attracting them and activating them – and the relative importance of these two components differs for different organisms. Thus for immunity to *Listeria monocytogenes*, which can be killed by the baseline levels oxygen-dependent mechanisms in both monocytes and neutrophils, it is the attraction of the cells to the lesion which is most important. In contrast, for *Mycobacterium tuberculosis*, which thrives inside neutrophils and monocytes, it is the activation of the cells which is critical.

The contrast between human and murine macrophages

Mycobacteria illustrate the complexity of this topic. IFN$_\gamma$ can activate murine macrophages to destroy mycobacteria completely. This appears to be due to the nitric oxide pathway. However, the same lymphokine acting on human macrophages causes, at best, feeble inhibition of *M. tuberculosis* or, at worst, significantly increased growth. This may be because human macrophages, unlike murine ones, seem unable to make tetrahydrobiopterin, an essential cofactor for nitric oxide production (see Fig. 15.25). On the other hand, human cells do something which the murine cells cannot – IFN$_\gamma$ causes human (but not murine) macrophages to express a 1-hydroxylase enzyme which converts the circulating inactive form of 25-hydroxy-cholecalciferol (vitamin D$_3$) into an active metabolite, 1,25-dihydroxycholecalciferol. This metabolite activates antimycobacterial mechanisms in the macrophages rather more efficiently than IFN$_\gamma$ itself.

Bacterial mechanisms for the avoidance of phagocyte-mediated killing

Since most organisms are ultimately killed by phagocytes, it is not surprising that successful pathogens have evolved an array of mechanisms to counteract this risk (Fig. 15.29).

ANTI-BACTERIAL ACTIVITY OF NON-PHAGOCYTIC CELLS
Direct contact

There are reports that some organisms, particularly Gram-negative bacteria, can be killed by contact with NK cells, or even Tc cells. This probably involves the

Antibacterial function of human monocytes and macrophages

bacteria	cells at day 0 untreated	cultured for 7 days	
		untreated	treated with IFN$_\gamma$
Escherichia coli	killed	killed	n/a
Salmonella typhimurium *Listeria monocytogenes*	killed	not killed	killed (this effect not blocked by glucocorticoids)
Legionella pneumophila	not killed	not killed	
Nocardia asteroides	killed	?	killed (this effect blocked by corticosteroids)
Mycobacterium tuberculosis	not killed	not killed	variable (some stasis, but no killing by cells from some donors; 1,25-dihydroxycholecalciferol is more active than IFN$_\gamma$ in this system)
Chlamydia psittaci	killed	not killed	killed
Chlamydia trachomatis	killed	killed	n/a
C. trachomatis biovar *lymphogranuloma venereum*	killed	not killed	killed

Fig. 15.28 Table indicating the ability of various monocyte or macrophage preparations to kill the indicated organisms. These cells have an intrinsic ability to kill many bacteria. This may be partly lost after 7 days in culture, but can often be restored by treatment with IFN$_\gamma$. Other organisms are killed only after lymphokine-mediated activation, while a few may not be killed at all. This emphasizes the complexity of the killing pathways.

membrane-lysing mechanism of these cells (see Chapter 8), acting on the outer lipid bilayer which is characteristic of Gram-negative organisms.

Killing of infected cells by Tc cells
There is speculation that some organisms, such as mycobacteria, which thrive inside host phagocytes, may need to be released from the parasitized host cell and exposed to other killing mechanisms. Tc cells may perform this function.

γδ T cells
A large proportion of T cells bearing γδ receptors seem to proliferate in response to bacterial antigens. Some subsets of these cells home to epithelial surfaces. Thus it seems likely that they have a role in infection, but this is not yet understood. In general they are cytotoxic, so they may destroy parasitized cells.

Activation of protective mechanisms in tissue cells
It is usually forgotten that tissue cells which are not components of the immune system can also harbour bacteria such as *M. leprae,* invasive *Shigella* and *Salmonella* species, or *Rickettsia* and *Chlamydia.* Activation of fibroblasts by IFN$_\gamma$ can inhibit growth of such internal organisms, probably via the nitric oxide pathway, which is not confined to phagocytic cells.

MECHANISMS OF BACTERIAL IMMUNOPATHOLOGY
Endotoxic shock
This occurs when there is massive production of cytokines, usually caused by bacterial products, particularly endotoxin (LPS), released during septicaemic episodes. There can be life-threatening fever, circulatory collapse, diffuse intravascular coagulation, and haemorrhagic necrosis, leading eventually to multiple organ failure (see Fig. 15.30).

The Shwartzman reaction
Shwartzman observed that if Gram-negative organisms were injected into the skin of rabbits, and then a second dose was given intravenously 24 hours later, haemorrhagic necrosis occurred at the prepared skin site. This is known as Shwartzman reaction (see Fig. 15.31). He also noted that two intravenous injections 24 hours apart caused a systemic reaction, commonly involving circulatory collapse and bilateral necrosis of the renal cortex. Sanarelli had made similar observations and this is now known as the Systemic Shwartzman or Sanarelli–Shwartzman reaction. These reactions can also be accompanied by necrosis in the pancreas, pituitary, adrenals and gut. There is marked diffuse intravascular coagulation and thrombosis. Many other organisms are now known to 'prepare' the skin in the same way, including streptococci, mycobacteria, *Haemophilus* spp., corynebacteria and vaccinia virus. Endotoxin (LPS) is the active component of the intravenous 'triggering' injection. Early work implicated endothelial changes and neutrophil accumulation and degranulation as mediating the damage. However, it now seems probable that TNF and IL-1 induce these reactions (see Chapter 8). Direct injection of TNF into sites of inflammation (evoked by a previous injection of bacteria) causes a similar type of necrosis; the injected TNF may be doing the same work as TNF arriving via the circulation, following an intravenous dose of LPS.

This phenomenon explains the characteristic haemorrhagic rash seen in children with meningococcal

Evasion mechanisms of bacteria

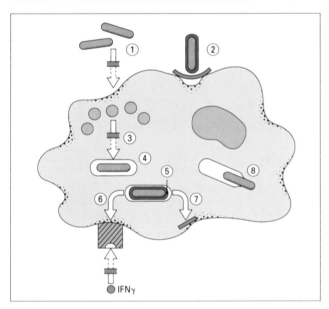

Fig. 15.29 Bacteria, particularly those which are successful intracellular parasites, have evolved the ability to evade different aspects of phagocyte-mediated killing. Some can secrete repellents or toxins which inhibit chemotaxis (1). Others have capsules or outer coats which inhibit attachment by the phagocyte (2). Once ingested some, such as *Mycobacterium tuberculosis*, secrete molecules which inhibit lysosome fusion with the phagosome (3). They may also secrete catalase which breaks down hydrogen peroxide (4). Organisms such as *M. leprae* have highly resistant outer coats. *M. leprae* surrounds itself with a phenolic glycolipid which scavenges free radicals (5). Mycobacteria also release a lipoarabinomannan which blocks the ability of macrophages to respond to the activating effects of IFN$_\gamma$ (6). Infected cells may also lose their efficacy as antigen-presenting cells (7). Several organisms (e.g. *M. leprae*), can escape from the phagosome to multiply in the cytoplasm (8). Finally the organism (e.g. *M. tuberculosis)* may kill the phagocyte.

meningitis. A first episode of septicaemia results in widespread inflammatory sites which are small and subclinical at the time, but which remain cytokine-sensitive. A second, larger septicaemic episode triggers enough cytokine release to cause necrosis in those sites.

The Koch phenomenon

This is a necrotic skin-test response to antigens of *M. tuberculosis*, originally demonstrated by Robert Koch in tuberculous guinea pigs (Fig. 15.32). It may be related to the necrosis which also occurs in the lesions in this disease. It is at least partly due to the release of cytokines into a T-cell mediated inflammatory site (delayed hypersensitivity site). Such sites are exquisitely sensitive to the tissue-damaging effects of cytokines.

Fig. 15.33 uses examples to illustrate the relationship between the nature of the organism, the disease and immunopathology caused, and the mechanism of immune response which leads to protection.

NEW TOPICS IN BACTERIAL IMMUNOLOGY
Superantigens

These recently recognized bacterial components are so named because they bind directly to the variable regions of β-chains on certain subsets of T cells, and cross-link them to the MHC of APCs. As a result, all T cells bearing the relevant V_β gene product are activated, without any requirement for the processing and presentation of the superantigen as peptides in the cleft of the MHC. Such superantigens have been found in staphylococci, mycoplasmas, and probably mycobacteria. The full biological significance of this bacterial adaptation is not yet clear, but one obvious effect can be the toxicity of the massive cytokine/lymphokine release resulting from the simultaneous stimulation of a large subset of T cells. The staphylococcal toxins responsible for the Toxic Shock Syndrome (TSST-1 etc.) appear to operate in this way.

Heat shock proteins (stress proteins)

These proteins are found in all eukaryotic and prokaryotic cells, where they have essential roles in the assembly, folding and transport of other molecules. Cells exposed to abnormally elevated temperatures express higher levels of these proteins, which reflects their role in the stabilization of protein structure. Their amino acid sequences are very highly conserved and there is currently much speculation that, because bacterial heat shock proteins are so similar to human ones, they may be involved in the initiation of autoimmunity.

Septicaemic shock

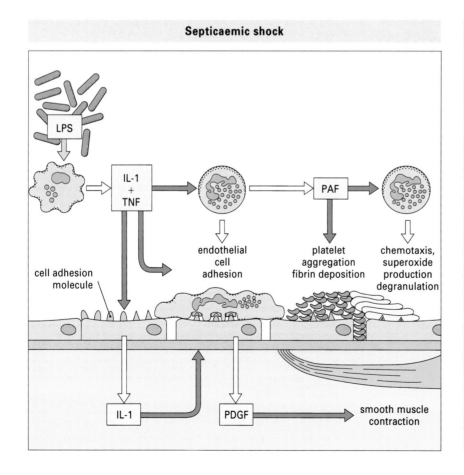

Fig. 15.30 Excessive release of cytokines, often triggered by the endotoxin (LPS) of Gram-negative bacteria, can lead to diffuse intra-vascular coagulation (DIC) with consequent defective clotting, changes in vascular permeability, loss of fluid into the tissues, a fall in blood pressure, circulatory collapse, and haemorrhagic necrosis, particularly in the gut. This figure illustrates some important parts of this pathway at the cellular level. The cytokines TNF and IL-1 cause endothelial cells to express cell adhesion molecules and tissue thromboplastin. These promote adhesion of circulating cells and deposition of fibrin respectively. Platelet activating factor (PAF) enhances these effects. In experimental models, shock can be blocked by neutralizing antibodies to TNF, and greatly diminished by antibodies to tissue thromboplastin, or by inhibitors of platelet activating factor (PAF). Gram-positive bacteria can induce shock. (PDGF = platelet-derived growth factor, produced by both platelets and endothelium.)

Paradoxically, in spite of their similarity to host proteins, they seem to be target antigens in the protective response against many infectious organisms.

IMMUNITY TO FUNGI

Little is known about the precise mechanisms involved in immunity to fungal infections, but it is thought that they are essentially similar to those involved in resistance to bacterial infections. The fungal infections of man fall into four major categories.
1. Superficial mycoses. These are caused by fungi known as dermatophytes, and are usually restricted to the non-living keratinized components of skin, hair and nails.
2. Subcutaneous mycoses. Saprophytic fungi can cause chronic nodules or ulcers in subcutaneous tissues following trauma, for example chromomycosis, sporotrichosis and mycetoma.
3. Respiratory mycoses. Soil saprophytes produce subclinical or acute lung infections (rarely disseminated), or granulomatous lesions, for example histoplasmosis and coccidiomycosis.
4. Candidiasis. *Candida albicans* (a ubiquitous commensal) causes superficial (rarely systemic) infections of skin and mucous membranes.

Cutaneous fungal infections are usually self-limiting and recovery is associated with a certain limited resistance to reinfection. Resistance is apparently based on cell-mediated immunity since patients develop delayed type hypersensitivity reactions to fungal antigens, and the occurrence of chronic infections is associated with a lack of these reactions. T-cell immunity is also implicated in resistance to other fungal infections, since resistance can sometimes be transferred with immune T cells. It is presumed that TH cells release cytokines which activate macrophages to destroy the fungi (Fig. 15.34). In respiratory mycoses, spectra of disease activity somewhat similar to the spectrum of activity in leprosy can be seen (see Chapter 22). Disturbance of normal physiology by immunosuppressive drugs, or of normal flora by antibiotics, can predispose to invasion by *Candida*. *Candida* infections are also common in immunodeficiency diseases (severe combined immunodeficiency, thymic aplasia, AIDS etc.) implying that the immune system is involved in confining the fungus to its normal commensal sites.

There is also evidence for neutrophil polymorph involvement in immunity to some respiratory mycoses such as mucormycosis (Fig. 15.35). It is possible that the cationic proteins (defensins) are important for protection from fungi, since phagocytes from patients with defective oxygen reduction pathways usually kill yeast and hyphae with near normal efficiency (Fig. 15.36). However, the nitric oxide pathway is effective against *Cryptococcus,* and this mechanism may turn out to be important for many fungi.

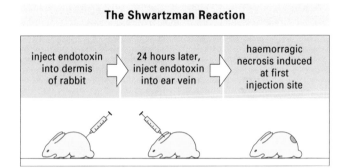

Fig. 15.31 Shwartzman observed that if Gram-negative bacteria are injected into the skin of rabbits, a subsequent intravenous injection of more bacteria 24 hours later will induce haemorrhagic necrosis at the original skin site (LPS has the same effect). More recent studies have revealed that the inflammatory skin site is exquisitely sensitive to the systemically released cytokines resulting from the later intravenous injection. At the local cellular level this phenomenon probably has much in common with that shown in Fig. 15.30. The complement system and neutrophils are also involved.

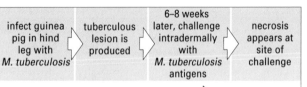

Fig. 15.32 Robert Koch observed that injection of *M. tuberculosis,* or soluble antigens from *M. tuberculosis,* into the skin of tuberculous guinea-pigs resulted in a necrotizing reaction both at the challenge site, and in the original tuberculous lesion. This is at least partly due to the fact that the delayed hypersensitivity reaction to mycobacterial antigens can, like the LPS-injected site in the Shwartzman reaction, be very sensitive to the toxicity of cytokines. These may be released locally in the skin-test site. A similar reaction is seen in humans who have, or have had, tuberculosis. Responses to the same antigen in individuals who are skin-test positive as a result of BCG vaccination, do not usually show necrosis.

VACCINE DESIGN

In order to design a vaccine, it is necessary to answer the following questions:

1. Which microbial antigens are likely to produce a useful, protective response?
2. At what anatomical site is the immune response required?
3. Which immunological mechanism(s) is(are) required?
4. What adjuvant and immunization schedule is both safe to use, and likely to evoke the relevant response (Fig. 15.37)?

When dealing with organisms which owe their pathogenicity to a single identified immunogenic toxin, all four questions are easily answered. Toxins such as those of *Corynebacterium diphtheriae* and *Clostridium tetani* lose their toxicity when heated, but retain their immunogenicity. Such a toxoid will evoke a systemic antibody response when injected with a simple adjuvant such as Al(OH)$_3$ or killed *Bordetella pertussis*. Thus, adjuvants for systemic antibody responses are not a problem. However, vaccine design is usually more difficult, as the following paragraphs illustrate.

MICROBIAL ANTIGENS

Organisms such as *Streptococcus pyogenes* and *S. pneumoniae* have large numbers of serotypes, so that an effective vaccine becomes a complex mixture which is expensive to make and incomplete in its coverage. Problems are still greater when there are numerous toxic products, with little definitive information as to which antigens provoke a protective response, or even the mechanism of protection. *B. pertussis* is an example of this, where the efficacy of a crude killed vaccine in protecting against whooping cough is due to luck rather than science. Neither its action nor its occasional association with brain damage are understood, so a truly rational and safe vaccine cannot yet be designed. For many bacteria, such as *Mycobacterium leprae* or *M. tuberculosis*, the antigens that induce protection have not been identified. It is not even clear whether protection is associated with just one, or with several antigens of these complex organisms.

LOCALIZATION OF EFFECT

With some infections, there is a need to achieve expression of immunity in certain sites, such as the genitourinary tract or gut. Experimentally direct intravaginal immunization with antigens of *Neisseria gonorrhoeae* is much more effective than systemic immunization in evoking a response in this site. Similarly, the conventional *Vibrio cholerae* vaccine injected intramuscularly has a very limited protective effect, while experiments suggest that oral vaccines can

Immunity in some important bacterial infections

infection	pathogenesis	major defence mechanisms
Corynebacterium diphtheriae	non-invasive pharyngitis–toxin	neutralizing antibody
Vibrio cholerae	non-invasive enteritis–toxin	neutralizing and adhesion-blocking antibodies
Neisseria meningitidis (Gram-negative)	nasopharynx →bacteraemia →meningitis →endotoxaemia	killed by antibody and lytic complement; opsonized and phagocytosed
Staphylococcus aureus (Gram-positive)	locally invasive and toxic in skin etc.	osponized by antibody and complement, killed by phagocytes
Mycobacterium tuberculosis	invasive, evokes immunopathology, ? toxic	? macrophage activation by cytokines from T cells
Mycobacterium leprae	invasive, space-occupying and/or immunopathology	

Fig. 15.33 This table provides examples of how a knowledge of the organism, and the mechanism of disease, can lead to a prediction of the relevant protective mechanism.

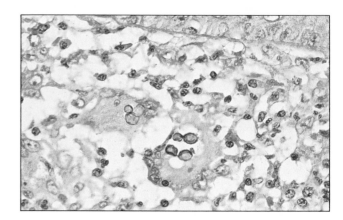

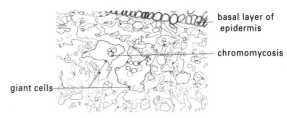

Fig. 15.34 Evidence for T-cell immunity in chromomycosis. The pigmented fungal cells of chromomycosis (a subcutaneous mycosis) are visible inside giant cells in the dermis of a patient. The area is surrounded by a predominantly mononuclear cell infiltrate.
H&E stain, × 400. (Courtesy of Dr R. J. Hay.)

be more effective. Developing a safe oral vaccine is difficult. The answer probably lies in the development of stable mutants of pathogenic organisms which, when swallowed, initiate an infection and invade the local epithelium or lymphoid tissue, but die after a limited number of replication cycles. Thus, derivatives of *Salmonella typhimurium* have been constructed which carry stable mutations determining the period of survival in the gut-associated lymphoid tissue and spleen. Such mutations can be transferred into other species. Alternatively, the genes for relevant antigenic determinants from other pathogens can be inserted into the mutant, in the hope that they will be expressed in a way which will evoke appropriate responses.

IMMUNOLOGICAL MECHANISMS

When the required response is cell-mediated, there are serious problems for the designer of vaccines. An adjuvant is required which is acceptable for use in man and which can activate the appropriate subset of TH cells. Activation of an inappropriate subset (e.g. TH2 cells before challenge with *Leishmania*) can increase rather

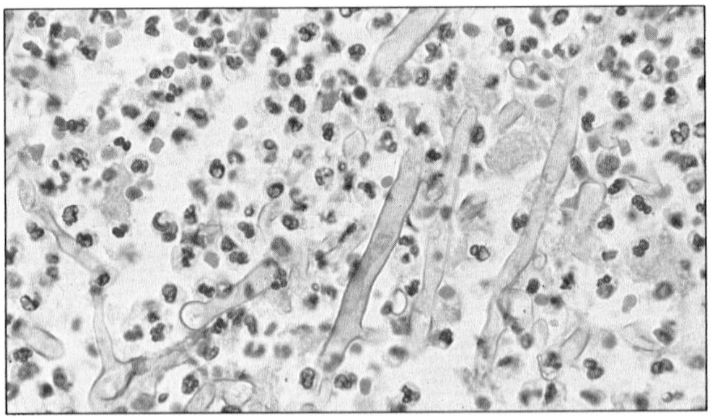

Fig. 15.35 Evidence for neutrophil-mediated immunity to mucormycosis. Section through a lung of a patient suffering from mucormycosis – an opportunistic infection in an immunosuppressed subject. The inflammatory reaction consists almost entirely of neutrophil polymorphs around the fungal hyphae. The disease is particularly associated with neutropenia (lack of neutrophils). Silver stain, × 400. (Courtesy of Dr R. J. Hay.)

Monocyte/macrophage killing of fungi

organism	source of monocytes/macrophages		
	normal	chronic granulomatous disease	myeloperoxidase deficiency
Candida albicans	killed	sometimes killed	sometimes killed
Candida parapsilosis	killed	not killed	unknown
Cryptococcus neoformans	killed	unknown	killed
Aspergillus fumigatus conidia	killed	killed	unknown
Aspergillus fumigatus hyphae	killed	killed	unknown

Fig. 15.36 Many fungi are killed by monocytes or macrophages. Since cells from patients with chronic granulomatous disease and individuals with myeloperoxidase deficiency can also effect killing, this shows the importance of non-oxygen dependent mechanisms.

Requirements for vaccine design

organism	antigen	mechanism	adjuvant	site
Corynebacterium diphtheriae *Clostridium tetani*	toxin	neutralizing antibody	Al(OH)$_3$ or pertussis	systemic
Streptococcus pneumoniae	capsular polysaccharide but many serotypes	antibody	not known	systemic
Bordetella pertussis	not certain: various toxins	? antibody	not known	systemic and secretory
Neisseria gonorrhoeae	pili, LPS	antibody	? recombinant commensal	GU tract
Vibrio cholerae	toxin, LPS		? recombinant organism	gut
Mycobacterium tuberculosis	not known	? T-cell-dependent macrophage activation	BCG – but often fails, and is a live vaccine	systemic

Fig. 15.37 Different organisms require different strategies for vaccine design. In general those further down this list present greater problems.

than decrease susceptibility. Unfortunately we understand very little about the way the 'decision' to activate a particular TH cell subset is made. Moreover live vaccines usually seem to be needed.

Various strategies are under investigation by trial and error in different contexts. These include the expression of specific microbial antigens in existing vaccine carriers such as live BCG (Bacille Calmette–Guerin, an attenuated strain of *Mycobacterium bovis*), or in orally ingested *Salmonella* mutants, or in vaccinia virus.

ADJUVANTS

Attempts are being made to develop safe adjuvants derived from the concept of Complete Freund's Adjuvant (a water-in-oil emulsion containing killed mycobacteria in the oil phase – see p. 15.11). This is effective, but has severe adverse effects in humans. Isolated or synthetic adjuvant-active components of bacteria, such as derivatives of muramyl dipeptide, suspended in a metabolizable oil such as squalene, might prove acceptable in man.

FURTHER READING

General
Roitt IM, Delves PJ, eds. *Encyclopedia of Immunology*. London: Academic press, 1992. (See numerous entries under names of individual fungi and bacteria and viruses.)

Viruses
Bean B. Antiviral therapy: current concepts and practices. *Clin Microbiol Rev* 1992;**5**:146-82.

Borden EG, Rosenzweig IB, Byrne GI. Interferons: from virus inhibitor to modulator of amino acid and lipid metabolism. *J Interferon Res* 1987;**7**:591.

Doherty PC, Allan W, Eichelberger M, Carding SR. Roles of α/β and γ/δ T cell subsets in viral immunity. *Annu Rev Immunol* 1992;**10**:123–51.

Mims CA, White DW. *Viral Pathogenesis and Immunology*. Oxford: Blackwell Scientific Publications, 1984.

Moore JB, Smith GL. Steroid hormone synthesis by a vaccinia enzyme: a new type of virulence factor. *EMBO J* 1992;**11**:1973–80.

Murray K. Application of recombinant DNA techniques in the development of viral vaccines. *Vaccine* 1988;**6**:164.

Nash AA, Jayasuriya A, Phelan J, Cobbold SP, Waldman H, Prospero T. Different roles for L3T4[+] and Lyt2[+] T cell subsets in the control of an acute herpes simplex virus infection of the skin and nervous system. *J Gen Virol* 1987;**68**:825.

Ray CA, Black RA, Kronheim SK, *et al*. Viral inhibition of inflammation: cowpox virus encodes an inhibitor of the interleukin-1β converting enzyme. *Cell* 1992;**69**:597–604.

Sissons JG, Oldstone MBA. Antibody-mediated destruction of virus-infected cells. *Adv Immunol* 1980;**31**:1.

Stroop WG, Baringer JR. Persistent slow and latent viral infections. *Prog Med Virol* 1982;**28**:1.

Wiley DC, Wilson IA, Skehel JJ. Structural identification of the antibody binding sites of Hong Kong influenza haemagglutinin and their involvement in antigenic variation. *Nature* 1981;**289**:373.

Wraith DC. The recognition of influenza A virus-infected cells by cytotoxic T lymphocytes. *Immunol Today* 1987;**8**:239.

Zinkernagel RM, Doherty PC. MHC-restricted cytotoxic T cells. Studies on the biological role of polymorphic major transplantation antigens determining T cell restriction, specificity, function and responsiveness. *Adv Immunol* 1979;**27**:51.

Bacteria
Catterall JR, Black CM, Leventhal JP, Rizk NW, Wachtel JS, Remington JS. Nonoxidative microbicidal activity in normal human alveolar and peritoneal macrophages. *Infect Immun* 1987;**55**:635.

Chan J, Xing Y, Magliozzo RS, Bloom BR. Killing of virulent *Mycobacterium tuberculosis* by reactive nitrogen intermediates produced by activated murine macrophages. *J Exp Med* 1992;**175**:1111–22.

De Libero G, Kaufmann SHE. Antigen-specific Lyt2[+] cytolytic T lymphocytes from mice infected with the intracellular bacterium *Listeria monocytogenes*. *J Immunol* 1986;**137**:2688.

Ganz T, Selsted ME, Szklarek D, *et al*. Defensins: natural peptide antibiotics of human neutrophils. *J Clin Invest* 1985;76:1427.

Joiner KA, Brown EF, Frank MM. Complement and bacteria: chemistry and biology in host defence. *Annu Rev Immunol* 1984;**2**:461.

Lynn WA, Golenbock DT. Lipopolysaccharide antagonists. *Immunol Today* 1992;**13(7)**:271–76.

Mims CA. *The Pathogenesis of Infectious Disease*. 3rd ed. London: Academic Press, 1987.

Mitchell GF. The way ahead for vaccines and vaccination: symposium summary. *Vaccine* 1988;**6**:200.

Ofek I, Sharon N. Lectinophagocytosis: a molecular mechanism of recognition between cell surfaces sugars and lectins in the phagocytosis of bacteria. *Infect Immun* 1988;**56**:539.

Rook GAW, Al Attiyah R. Cytokines and the Koch phenomenon. *Tubercle* 1991;**72**:13-20.

Rothstein JL, Schreiber H. Synergy between tumour necrosis factor and bacterial products causes haemorrhagic necrosis and lethal shock in normal mice. *Proc Natl Acad Sci U S A* 1988;**85**:607.

Sibley LD, Krahenbuhl JL. *Mycobacterium leprae*-burdened macrophages are refractory to activation by gamma-interferon. *Infect Immunity* 1987;**55**:446.

Yamamura M, Uyemura K, Deans RJ, *et al*. Defining protective responses to pathogens: cytokine profiles in leprosy lesions. *Science* 1991;**254**:277–79.

Fungi
Bullock WE, Wright SD. Role of the adherence-promoting receptors CR3 LFA-1 and p150,95 in binding of *Histoplasma capsulatum* by human macrophages. *J Exp Med* 1987;**165**:195.

Calderon RA, Hay RJ. Cell-mediated immunity in experimental murine dermatophytosis. Adoptive transfer of immunity to dermatophyte infection by lymphoid cells from donors with acute or chronic infections. *Immunol* 1984;**53**:4.

Cox RA. Immunologic studies of patients with histoplasmosis. *Am Rev Respir Dis* 1979;**120**:143.

Murphy JW. Mechanisms of natural resistance to human pathogenic fungi. *Annu Rev Microbiol* 1991;**45**:509–38.

Rogers TG, Balish E. Immunity to *Candida albicans*. *Microbiol Rev* 1980;**44**:660.

chapter 16

Immunity to Protozoa and Worms

Parasite infections typically stimulate a number of immunological defence mechanisms, both antibody- and cell-mediated, and the responses that are most effective depend upon the particular parasite and the stage of infection. The general principles of immunity to parasitic diseases are considered here, illustrated by some of the more important infections of man.

Parasitic protozoa may live in the gut (e.g. amoebae), in the blood (e.g. African trypanosomes), within erythrocytes (*Plasmodium* spp.), in macrophages (e.g. *Leishmania* spp., *Toxoplasma gondii*), including those of the liver and spleen (e.g. *Trypanosoma cruzi* and *Leishmania* spp.), or in muscle (e.g. *Trypanosoma cruzi*).

Parasitic worms which infect man include some trematodes or flukes (e.g. Schistosomes), some cestodes (e.g. tapeworms) and some nematodes or roundworms (e.g. *Trichinella spiralis*, hookworms, *Ascaris* and the filarial worms). Tapeworms and hookworms inhabit the gut while adult schistosomes live in blood vessels, while other worms, for example the filarial worms, live in the lymphatics. Many parasitic worms pass through complicated life cycles, including migration through various parts of the host's body and development of different stages in different organs, before they reach the site where they finally mature and spend the rest of their lives.

Parasites infect very large numbers of people (Fig. 16.1) and present a major medical problem, especially in tropical countries: malaria, for example, kills 1–2 million people a year. The diseases caused are diverse and the immune responses which are effective against the different parasites vary considerably. Parasitic infections do, however, share a number of common features.

GENERAL FEATURES OF PARASITIC INFECTIONS

Protozoan parasites and worms are considerably larger than bacteria and viruses (Fig. 16.2), although some protozoa are still small enough to live inside human cells. For this they have evolved a special mode of entry: for example, the merozoite, the invasive form of the blood stage of the malarial parasite, binds to certain receptors on the surface of the erythrocyte and uses a specialized organ, the rhoptry, to enter the cell. *Leishmania* parasites, which inhabit macrophages, simply allow the cell to engulf them, but then need a special strategy to survive in this unfavourable milieu. Larger size means that these parasites carry more antigens, both in number and kind. Many parasites can also change their surface antigens, a process known as antigenic variation. In the case of parasites which have more complicated life histories, some antigens may be specific to a particular stage of development, so that host immunity is stage-specific. For example, the protein coat of the sporozoite, the infective stage of the malarial parasite transmitted by the mosquito, is not recognised by antibodies which react with the erythrocytic stage.

Over millions of years of evolution parasites have become well adapted to their host and show marked

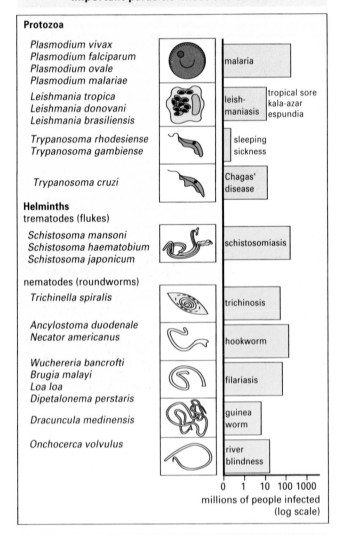

Important parasitic infections of man

Protozoa

Plasmodium vivax
Plasmodium falciparum
Plasmodium ovale
Plasmodium malariae — malaria

Leishmania tropica
Leishmania donovani
Leishmania brasiliensis — leish-maniasis — tropical sore / kala-azar / espundia

Trypanosoma rhodesiense
Trypanosoma gambiense — sleeping sickness

Trypanosoma cruzi — Chagas' disease

Helminths
trematodes (flukes)

Schistosoma mansoni
Schistosoma haematobium
Schistosoma japonicum — schistosomiasis

nematodes (roundworms)

Trichinella spiralis — trichinosis

Ancylostoma duodenale
Necator americanus — hookworm

Wuchereria bancrofti
Brugia malayi
Loa loa
Dipetalonema perstaris — filariasis

Dracuncula medinensis — guinea worm

Onchocerca volvulus — river blindness

0 1 10 100 1000
millions of people infected
(log scale)

Fig. 16.1 Data from the World Health Organization (1990).

host specificity. For example, the malarial parasites of birds, rodents or man can each multiply only in its own particular kind of host. There are some exceptions to this general rule, for example, the tapeworm of the pig is also able to infect man, but frequently a parasite cannot complete its life cycle in the incorrect host. Within a species, hosts vary in their resistance, which depends upon a variety of immune response genes. Strains of mice carrying some MHC genes – and some people – do not make antibody to one of the peptides of the malarial sporozoite coat because their T cells do not become sensitized. Non-MHC genes can also be important here. For example, innate resistances of mice to infection by *Leishmania donovani,* and to several other parasites, is determined by a single dominant gene controlling macrophage activation (see Chapter 9).

There are always several immunological effector mechanisms involved in host defence against particular parasites, and the parasites have many different ways of evading them. Some even exploit cells and molecules of the immune system to their own advantage: thus *Leishmania* spp. live in macrophages and use complement receptors to effect their entry, so avoiding destruction by toxic products of the oxidative burst.

It is not in the interests of the parasite to kill its host, and parasitic infections are usually chronic. Among the consequences of chronic infection are the presence of circulating antigens, persistent antigenic stimulation and the formation of immune complexes (Fig. 16.3). Characteristically, levels of immunoglobulins are raised: IgM in trypanosomiasis and malaria; IgG in malaria and visceral leishmaniasis, and IgE in worm infections. Splenomegaly occurs in most parasitic infections, and some parasite antigens can act directly as polyclonal mitogens for lymphocytes. Immunosuppression and immunopathological effects often occur.

In general terms, cell-mediated responses are more effective against intracellular protozoa, while antibody is more effective against extracellular parasites in blood and tissue fluids, but the type of response conferring most protection depends upon the parasite. Antibody alone, or with complement, can damage some extracellular parasites, but it is more effective acting in combination with certain effector cells, for instance by opsonizing for phagocytosis, or by promoting antibody-dependent cell-mediated cytotoxicity (ADCC). The effects are local and many cell types secreting many different mediators may be present at sites of immune rejection.

Within a single infection different immune responses may act against different developmental stages of the parasite. Thus in malaria, while antibody against extracellular forms blocks their capacity to invade new cells, cell-mediated immunity prevents the development of the liver stage within the hepatocytes. Protective immunity to malaria does not correlate with antibody levels and even occurs in the absence of antibody. This was shown in mice immunized with genetically engineered *Salmonella typhimurium* carrying a gene coding for the malaria sporozoite surface antigen and later challenged with sporozoites: although the mice did not make specific antibody, they developed immunity to the parasite.

Comparative size of various infective agents

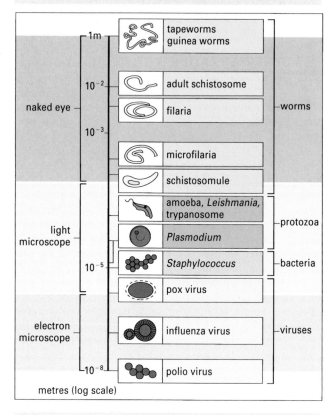

Fig. 16.2   Comparative size of various infective agents, whose sizes range over 8 orders of magnitude.

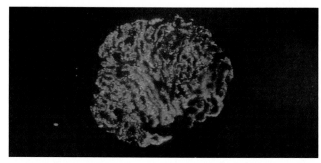

Fig. 16.3 Immune complex deposition in quartan malaria nephrotic syndrome. Low power fluorescence micrograph of a renal glomerulus in a biopsy specimen from a Nigerian child with the syndrome. People infected with *Plasmodium malariae* may develop glomerulonephritis as a result of the deposition of immune complexes. The section was stained with FITC conjugated anti-human IgG and shows granular deposition of immunoglobulin throughout the capillary loops of the glomerulus. (Courtesy of Dr V. Houba.)

EFFECTOR MECHANISMS

Various kinds of effector cells such as macrophages, neutrophils, eosinophils and platelets, help defend the host against parasites and act to control the multiplication and spread of parasites already in residence. The anatomical location of these effector cells is obviously important: for example, the cercariae of *Schistosoma mansoni* enter through the skin and experimental depletion of macrophages, neutrophils and eosinophils from the skin of mice immune to this parasite increases their susceptibility to infection.

Most of the anti-parasitic activities of effector cells are enhanced by the action of cytokines produced in response to infection; cytokines may also affect cell migration. Principally, cytokines are secreted by T lymphocytes and by macrophages, but some may be derived from B lymphocytes, or from fibroblasts or the endothelial cells of blood vessels. Endothelial cells can act as part of the immune system, themselves secreting cytokines and responding to them, for example, by increased expression of MHC antigens or secretion of reactive O_2 metabolites. These are toxic to parasites, but may also damage the host's own tissues.

Parasite infections in T-deprived mice

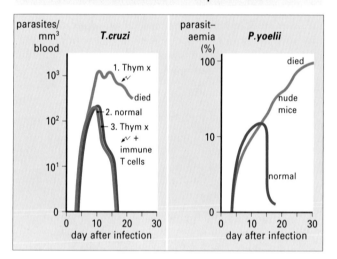

Fig. 16.4 These graphs plot the increase in number of blood-borne parasites (parasitaemia) following infection. *Trypanosoma cruzi* multiplies faster (and gives fatal parasitaemia) in mice that have been thymectomized (Thym x) and irradiated (⚡) to destroy T cells (1). In normal mice, parasites are cleared from the blood by 16 days (2). Reconstitution of T-deprived mice with T cells from immune mice (immune-T) restores their ability to control the parasitaemia (3). In these experiments both experimental groups (1 and 3) were given fetal liver cells to restore vital haematopoietic function. *Plasmodium yoelii* causes a self-limiting infection in normal mice and the parasites are cleared from the blood by day 20. In nude mice the parasites continue to multiply, killing the mice after about 30 days.

T CELLS

T cells are fundamental to the control of parasite multiplication. In most parasite infections, protection can be conferred experimentally on normal animals by the transfer of spleen cells, especially T cells, from immune animals. However, transfer of T cells from acutely infected animals can in some cases (for example, susceptible mouse strains infected with *Leishmania tropica*) suppress the protective response and cause the death of the recipients.

The T cell requirement is demonstrable by the way in which nude (athymic) or T-deprived mice fail to clear otherwise non-lethal infections, for example of *Trypanosoma cruzi* and *Plasmodium yoelii,* the latter being a malarial parasite of rodents (Fig. 16.4).

The type of T cell responsible for controlling infections varies, and how it acts depends on both the parasite and the stage of infection. For example, CD4$^+$ T cells transfer protective immunity against *Leishmania major* and *L. tropica* from immune mice of a genetically resistant strain to mice of a susceptible strain. Antibodies against the CD4 molecule enhance the size of skin lesions in resistant mouse strains and cause an increase in the number of parasites present. CD4$^+$ cells are also necessary for the mouse to eliminate *Giardia muris* which inhabits the gut lumen.

In malaria, both CD4$^+$ and CD8$^+$ cells are necessary, to protect against different phases of infection. For example, CD4$^+$ T cells mediate immunity against blood stage *P. yoelii* while CD8$^+$ cells protect against the liver stage of *P. berghei*, as demonstrated by depleting the host of the respective cell type. The CD8$^+$ Tc cells destroy infected hepatocytes and they also secrete IFN$_\gamma$ which inhibits the multiplication of the parasites within the hepatocytes. Since hepatocytes are MHC Class II negative, CD4$^+$ T cells do not recognise them and are not stimulated to secrete IFN$_\gamma$. Cytotoxic T cells, acting in an antigen-specific class I-restricted manner, are also known to destroy cells infected with *Theileria parva*, a parasite which lives in the lymphocytes of cattle.

CYTOKINE SECRETION BY T CELLS

The role of cytokines in parasitic infections has been elucidated by administering the cytokine to infected animals, or eliminating it with monoclonal antibodies. Many cytokines act on effector cells to enhance their cytotoxic or cytostatic capabilities and to increase cell numbers. The monocytosis of malaria and the characteristic enlargement of the spleen, caused by an enormous increase in cell numbers, are T cell-dependent. So too is the accumulation of macrophages in the granulomata that develop in the liver in schistosomiasis, and the eosinophilia characteristic of worm infections. Activated T cells secrete colony-stimulating factors, such as IL-3 and GM-CSF, which act on cells of the myeloid lineage inducing an increase in their number and then their differentiation and activation. For example eosinophils activated by colony-stimulating factors, including IL-3 and GM-CSF, have an enhanced ability to kill schistosome larvae.

In some circumstances, secretion of cytokines may harm the host. Administration of IL-3 to mice infected with *Leishmania major*, for instance, leads to an exacerbation of the local infection and increases dissemination of the parasites. This is probably due to proliferation of bone marrow precursors of the cells the parasites inhabit.

Some apparent paradoxes have recently been explained by the differentiation of Th1 and Th2 subsets of CD4+ T cells. Thus Th1 cells are better at dealing with intracellular parasites, and Th2 cells with extracellular parasites. Although the same clear distinctions have not been shown for human T cells, immune responses occurring during the course of many parasitic infections can be described as Th1-like or Th2-like. The balance of these may change with age.

There are also host differences in the importance of the different cytokines in different infections. In man, Th2 effects in schistosomiasis appear to be important for immunity, whereas in the mouse, Th1 cells and IFN$_\gamma$ are needed for protection, while Th2 cells may give rise to immunopathology.

One or other type of the T-helper cell subset usually predominates. In mice infected with *Leishmania*, Th1 cells are required for immunity. Thus the resistance of some strains of mice to infection by *L. major* depends upon the production of IFN$_\gamma$. In sensitive mice with progressive disease, the CD4+ cells do not secrete IFN$_\gamma$ but secrete IL-3 and IL-4 (Fig. 16.5). Transfer of CD4+ cells secreting IL-4 inhibits the beneficial effects of IFN$_\gamma$ and exacerbates the disease. IL-4 *in vitro* also inhibits the IFN$_\gamma$-induced activity of human monocytes against *L. donovani* (Fig. 16.6). Immunity to *Leishmania* is best induced by peptides which preferentially activate Th1 cells.

Cytokine production and the spread of infection

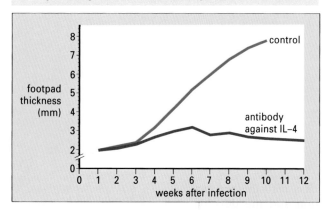

Fig. 16.5 The susceptibility of a sensitive mouse strain to infection by *Leishmania major* is due to the production of interleukin-4. Mice were infected in the footpad and the size of the lesion was measured each week. Weekly treatment with a monoclonal antibody against IL-4 prevented the multiplication of the parasite.

Action of Th1 and Th2 cells in *Leishmania* infection

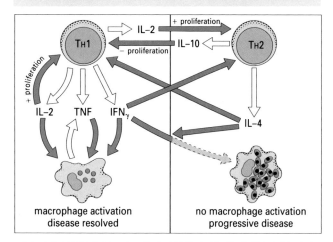

Fig. 16.6 Development of the immune response to *Leishmania* infection illustrating the cytokines secreted by the different subsets of T cells and their effect on the resolution of the disease.

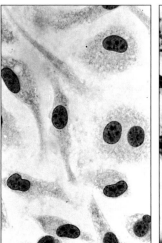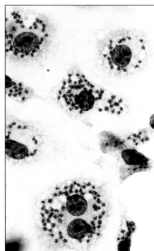

Fig. 16.7 Inhibition of parasite multiplication in macrophages treated with cytokines. Peritoneal macrophages from BALB/c mice, infected 72 hours previously with 10^7 amastigotes of *Leishmania donovani*, were treated with either a supernatant from activated T cells (containing cytokines) or a control supernatant. Cells treated with cytokines do not contain any parasites following culture (left) whereas untreated macrophages contain many parasites (right). Subsequent studies using recombinant IFN$_\gamma$ and monoclonal antibody against IFN$_\gamma$ showed that the inhibition was mediated by this cytokine. (Courtesy of Dr H. Murray, with permission from *J Immunol* 1982;**129**: 344–357, © by American Association of Immunologists.)

Both T-helper cell subsets may occur sequentially within a self-limiting infection. TH1 cells often appear at the onset of infection and secrete IFNγ. This controls parasite multiplication non-specifically by activating effector cells and increasing the expression of receptors that enhance phagocytosis. It also augments expression of MHC Class II molecules and therefore antigen presentation.

TH2 cells prevail later on, and help produce antibodies to add specificity to the immune reaction. For example in malaria, where protection against the blood stage depends upon CD4+ cells and an intact but modified spleen (reversal of immunity cannot be overcome by the transfer of normal spleen cells), parasite elimination could take place in the spleen via activated effector cells and antibody dependent cytotoxicity.

The pattern of cytokine production in a non-immune infected host may be different from that in an immune host. Thus, in mice infected with *Schistosoma mansoni*, IL-5-producing TH2 cells predominate during infection, but in mice which have become immune following vaccination with irradiated cercariae, IgE levels and eosinophil numbers are low and IFNγ-producing TH1 cells predominate. A soluble egg antigen, released later on during infection when adult worms start to produce eggs, appears to be responsible for the difference between susceptible and immune mice. This antigen reduces TH1 function and levels of IFNγ and increases TH2 production of IL-5.

Interleukin-2 IL-2, secreted by proliferating lymphocytes, is deficient in some parasitic infections, for example, malaria, African trypanosomiasis and Chagas' disease. When T cells from mice infected with *Trypanosoma brucei* are cultured and challenged with mitogen, IL-2 production and the expression of the IL-2

receptor are both abnormally low. In mice infected with *T. cruzi*, injection of IL-2 restores T-helper cell activity, leading to more parasite-specific IgM and IgG, fewer parasites in the blood and longer survival time.

Interferon-γ (IFNγ) IFNγ is involved in immune mechanisms that control the multiplication of many parasites, presumably by activating effector cells. Treatment of macrophages with IFNγ *in vitro* renders them resistant to invasion by some intracellular parasites which multiply within them (e.g. *Toxoplasma gondii* and *Leishmania* spp.) and leads to the elimination of parasites already resident. The ability of crude lymphokine preparations to stimulate macrophages to kill these parasites (Fig. 16.7) is abolished by antibodies against IFNγ. That these findings reflect events that occur *in vivo* has been shown by the therapeutic effects of IFNγ on mice infected with *Trypanosoma cruzi* (Fig. 16.8). Furthermore, mice treated with an antibody that blocks the binding of IFNγ to its receptor succumbed to infection by a normally avirulent strain of *Toxoplasma gondii*. Peritoneal macrophages taken from the treated mice were not activated and supported multiplication of the parasite, whereas those from control mice were activated and resistant.

Similarly, resistance to *Leishmania donovani* correlates with the production of IFNγ, macrophage activation and the development of granulomata; none of these events occur in nude (athymic) mice, in which the parasites multiply unchecked. Spleen cells taken from genetically resistant mice during acute phase infection, and cultured with parasite antigen, do not secrete IFNγ or IL-2, but those taken when the infection is beginning to resolve do so, and giving IFNγ during the acute phase blocks parasite multiplication. Likewise, treatment of mice with antibody against IFNγ abrogates natural resistance, allowing dissemination of the parasites. In man too, it is notable that T cells from patients fail to secrete IFNγ when cultured with parasite antigen.

Extracellular parasites, for example, *Entamoeba histolytica* and *Schistosoma mansoni*, are also susceptible to the effects of IFNγ activation of macrophages. These effects may be enhanced by the presence of antibody, through ADCC.

In malaria, administration of human IFNγ to chimpanzees infected with sporozoites of *Plasmodium vivax* diminished parasitaemia. The ability of immune mice to withstand challenge by sporozoites of *P. berghei* was overcome by treatment with an antibody against IFNγ.

MACROPHAGES
Apart from acting as antigen-presenting cells in the initiation of an immune response, macrophages affect the course of parasitic infection in two ways.
1. They act as effector cells which inhibit the multiplication of parasites or destroy them.
2. They secrete molecules which regulate the inflammatory response. Some, IL-1, TNFα and the CSFs, enhance

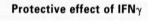

Protective effect of IFNγ

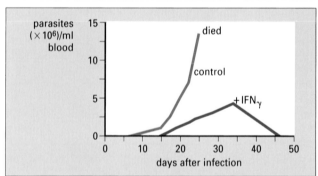

Fig. 16.8 The effect of administration of the T cell cytokine IFNγ on acute infection caused by *Trypanosoma cruzi*. In this strain of mice, the parasites multiply to kill their host in about 3 weeks. Administration of recombinant mouse IFNγ controls their multiplication and is followed ultimately by their elimination.

immunity by activating other cells or stimulating their proliferation. Others, like prostaglandins and TGF_β, may be immunosuppressive.

Activation of macrophages is a general feature of the early stages of infection and all their functions are then enhanced. The macrophages are activated mainly by cytokines secreted from T cells, (for example IFN_γ, GM-CSF, IL-3 and IL-4), but not all activation is mediated by T cells.

Some parasite products, such as the soluble antigens of malarial parasites and of *Trypanosoma brucei*, induce macrophages to secrete TNF_α, for example, which itself then activates other macrophages. NK cells can be a source of IFN_γ.

Phagocytosis Phagocytosis by macrophages is important against the smaller parasites and its effectiveness is markedly enhanced by opsonization of the parasite with antibodies and complement C3b, leading for instance to more rapid clearance of protozoan parasites from the blood. African trypanosomes such as *T. brucei* are quickly taken up by macrophages in the liver, particularly when opsonized with antibody and C3b. Comparison of strains of mice with various immunological defects for their resistance to infection by *T. rhodesiense* shows that the destruction of trypanosomes by macrophages is a major effector mechanism.

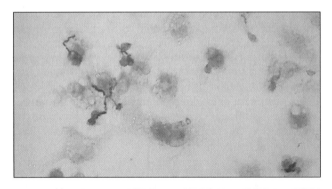

Fig. 16.9 The triggering of the respiratory burst of macrophages by *Leishmania donovani*. This picture shows a culture of resident peritoneal macrophages that have ingested promastigotes of *L. donovani* in the presence of nitroblue tetrazolium (NBT). The development of a black precipitate shows that the NBT has been reduced by products of the respiratory burst, which was triggered by contact with the parasites. More than 80% of promastigotes (the stages injected by the insect vector) are destroyed by normal macrophages but some escape from the phagolysosomes to become amastigotes. Amastigotes do not trigger the respiratory burst as effectively as promastigotes and survive well in normal macrophages. They can, however, be eradicated *in vitro* by incubation of the cells with lymphokines. Both stages are killed by H_2O_2 but not by the other oxygen metabolites.
(Courtesy of Dr J. Blackwell.)

Phagocytosis also provides a means of entry into macrophages for parasites that multiply inside those cells. The promastigotes of *Leishmania* fix complement by the alternative pathway and then bind to the CR3 complement receptors on the macrophage cell surface, triggering their uptake by phagocytosis. Binding can be blocked experimentally by antibodies against the receptor. The parasites can also gain entry by binding to the mannose-fucose receptor on the macrophage surface.

Parasite Killing Properties Macrophages secrete scores of soluble factors, many of which can be cytotoxic, so they can also kill parasites without ingesting them.

When activated, they can kill relatively small extracellular parasites, such as the erythrocytic stages of malaria and even larger parasites, such as the larval stages of the schistosome. They can also act as killer cells through antibody dependent cell-mediated cytotoxicity (ADCC); specific IgG and IgE, for instance, enhance their ability to kill schistosomules. They also secrete various cytokines (e.g. TNF_α and IL-1) that interact with other types of cell, and which can render hepatocytes resistant to malarial parasites.

Reactive oxygen intermediates (ROIs) are generated by macrophages and granulocytes following phagocytosis of many parasites, including *Trypanosoma cruzi*, *Toxoplasma gondii*, *Leishmania* spp., malarial parasites, filarial worms and schistosomes (Fig. 16.9). Macrophages activated by cytokines release more superoxide and hydrogen peroxide than normal resident macrophages and their O_2^--independent killing mechanisms are more potent.

Human macrophages, however, kill *T. gondii* by an O_2^--independent mechanism. This may explain our innate resistance to infection by this organism, which is lost in immunocompromised individuals.

Nitric oxide (NO) is one potent O_2^--independent toxin whose synthesis is greatly enhanced by cytokines such as TNF_α and IFN_γ, especially when they act together. Nitric oxide is a product of the metabolism of L-arginine, and endothelial cells are another source of this cytotoxic molecule. Nitric oxide contributes to host resistance in leishmaniasis, schistosomiasis and malaria, and may be generally important in the control of parasitic infections (Fig. 16.10).

Tumour Necrosis Factor (TNF_α) Although lymphocytes secrete TNF_α, activated macrophages are the most important source of this molecule. Protective responses to several protozoa (e.g. *Leishmania*) (Fig. 16.11) and to helminths (e.g. *Schistosoma mansoni*) are mediated by TNF_α. It may, however, have harmful as well as beneficial effects on the infected host, depending on the amount produced and whether it is free in the circulation or locally confined. Administration of TNF_α cures a susceptible strain of mice infected with the rodent malarial parasite, *Plasmodium chabaudi*, but kills a genetically resistant strain. Presumably the latter can make enough TNF_α to control parasite replication, and any more has toxic effects.

Toxic effect of NO on *Leishmania in vitro*

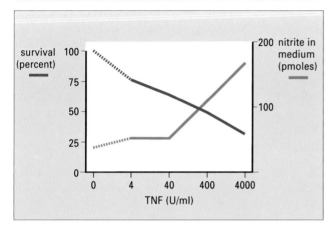

Fig. 16.10 Evidence that the killing of *Leishmania major* by activated macrophages is correlated with the release of nitric oxide. Macrophages in culture are activated by recombinant TNF in a dose-related fashion, the highest doses decreasing parasite survival to about a third of that in control cultures. At the same time, the amount of NO released, measured as nitrite present in the culture medium, increases. Interference with NO production allows parasites to survive. (Based on data from Liew, Li, Millott. *Immunol* 1990; **71**:556.)

Control of cutaneous Leishmaniasis by TNF

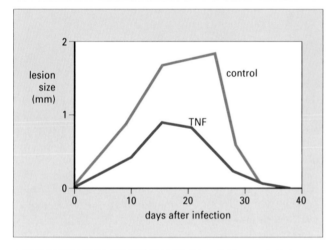

Fig. 16.11 TNF control of the size of lesions in murine cutaneous leishmaniasis. These graphs plot the mean size of the lesion induced in the footpad of groups of mice by *L. major* against time after infection. Administration of recombinant TNF caused a reduction in the thickness of the footpad.
Lymph node cells from infected mice of a resistant strain secrete TNF when cultured with specific antigen, whereas those from the sensitive strain do not. (Based on data from Titus *et al.*, *J Exp Med* 1989;**170**:2097.)

TNF_α activates macrophages, eosinophils and platelets to kill the larval form of *Schistosoma mansoni* and its effects are enhanced by IFN_γ. The cytotoxicity of activated macrophages for the schistosomules appears to be mediated through TNF_α because it is greatly diminished by the addition of antibody against TNF_α, but the fact that it is not completely abolished suggests that another factor is also involved.

Granuloma Formation in the Liver and Fibrous Encapsulation In some parasitic infections, the immune system cannot completely eliminate the parasite, and the body reduces damage by walling off the parasite behind a capsule of inflammatory cells. This reaction, which is T-dependent, is a chronic cell-mediated response to locally released antigen, and is mediated by cytokines, including IFN_γ and TNF_α. Macrophages accumulate and release fibrogenic factors which stimulate the formation of granulomatous tissue and ultimately fibrosis. In schistosomiasis, granuloma formation in response to a particular soluble egg antigen occurs around worm eggs which have become trapped in the liver. Although this reaction may benefit the host, in that it insulates the liver cells from toxins secreted by the worm eggs, it is the major source of pathology, causing irreversible changes in the liver and the loss of liver function. In the absence of T cells, there is no granuloma formation and no subsequent fibrous encapsulation (Fig. 16.12).

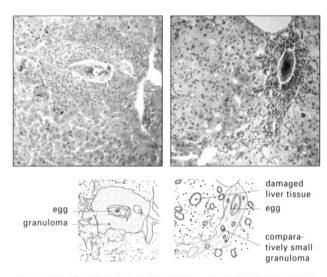

Fig. 16.12 T cell-dependence of granuloma formation around schistosome eggs in the liver. Many of the eggs of schistosome worms are carried to the liver where they become insulated behind a capsule of inflammatory cells. In normal mice, the granulomata consist predominantly of eosinophils and are the result of a T cell-dependent reaction (left). In T-cell-deficient mice, eggs of *Schistosoma mansoni* do not induce much granuloma formation and as a result toxic products of the eggs can diffuse out and cause damage to the surrounding liver tissue (right). (Courtesy of Dr M. Doenoff.)

The interaction of cells in response to a worm infection

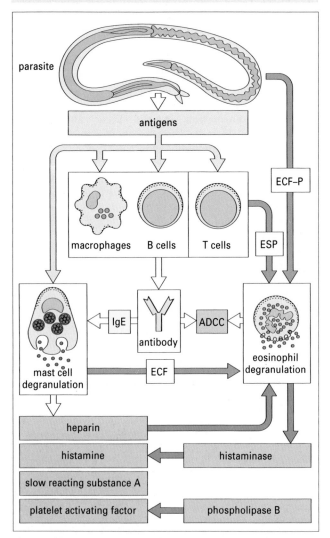

Fig. 16.13 Antigens released by the parasite stimulate T cells and macrophages to interact with B cells to produce specific antibody. Specific IgE antibody sensitizes local mast cells so that they degranulate when they come into contact with antigen, releasing a variety of effector molecules, some of which increase the permeability of blood vessels around the parasite. The mast cells also release eosinophil chemotactic factors (ECF). Eosinophils are attracted towards the worm by these and by parasite-derived chemotactic factors (ECF-P). They are stimulated to proliferate by eosinophil stimulation promoter (ESP) derived from antigen-stimulated T cells. The eosinophils act in two main ways.
1. In association with specific antibody they kill the parasite by antibody-dependent cell-mediated cytotoxicity (ADCC).
2. Enzymes released from the eosinophil granules exert a controlling effect on the substances released from the mast cells.
Heparin inhibits eosinophil degranulation. (Green arrows indicate stimulation, and red arrows inhibition.)

GRANULOCYTES
Neutrophils   Like macrophages, neutrophils are phagocytic cells that can kill a variety of parasites, large and small, and many of their effector properties are similar. They can kill by both O_2^--dependent and -independent mechanisms, including nitric oxide. They produce a more intense respiratory burst than macrophages and their secretory granules contain highly cytotoxic proteins.

Neutrophils too can be activated by cytokines, such as IFN_γ or TNF_α. When pretreated with GM-CSF they kill the parasite *Trypanosoma cruzi* more rapidly. Extracellular destruction in this case is mediated by H_2O_2, whereas granular components are involved in intracellular destruction of ingested organisms. Neutrophils are present in parasite-infected inflammatory lesions and probably act to clear parasites from bursting cells. Their membranes bear Fc receptors and receptors for complement that render them effective participants in antibody-dependent cytotoxic reactions. Thus they can kill the larvae of *Schistosoma mansoni* by mechanisms that are enhanced in the presence of antibody or complement. They may be more destructive than eosinophils against several species of nematode, including *Trichinella spiralis,* although the relative effectiveness of the two types of cell may depend upon the isotype and specificity of antibody.

Eosinophils   Eosinophilia and the production of high levels of IgE are the common consequences of infection by parasitic worms. It has been suggested that the eosinophil has evolved specially as a defence against the tissue stages of parasites that are too large to be phagocytosed, and that the IgE-dependent mast-cell reaction has evolved primarily to localize eosinophils near the parasite and then enhance their anti-parasitic functions.

The increase in the number of eosinophils in worm infections like schistosomiasis and ascariasis is T-cell dependent, and the cells show an enhancement in their state of activity. In schistosomiasis in man, TH2-like effects appear to be associated with immunity. Both IgE and eosinophilia, the hallmarks of worm infections, are controlled by cytokines secreted by TH2 cells. Experimentally, giving mice antibody against IL-4 decreases the amount of circulating IgE to background levels, while antibody against IL-5 inhibits worm-induced eosinophilia.

T cells also recruit eosinophils into the gut mucosa in worm infections of the gastrointestinal tract. The recruitment is mediated by a specific factor, eosinophil stimulation promoter (ESP) (Fig. 16.13). The importance of these effector cells *in vivo* has been shown by experiments using antiserum against eosinophils. Mice infected with *Trichinella spiralis* and treated with the antiserum developed more cysts in their muscles than controls: without protection by eosinophils the mice cannot eliminate the worms but encyst the parasites to minimise damage. Similarly, treatment of immune mice with antiserum to eosinophils abrogates their ability to resist infection by *Schistosoma mansoni.*

Eosinophils are less phagocytic than neutrophils, but like neutrophils they can kill parasites by both O_2^--dependent and -independent mechanisms; their activities are also enhanced by cytokines such as TNF_α and GM-CSF. They degranulate in response to perturbation of their surface membrane, so that binding to the larvae of worms (e.g. *S. mansoni* and *T. spiralis*), especially when the larvae are coated with IgE or IgG, releases granular contents onto the surface of the worms. Damage to schistosomes can be caused by the major basic protein (MBP) of the eosinophil crystalloid core (Figs 16.14 and 16.15). MBP is not specific for any tar-

get, but since it is confined to a small space between the eosinophil and the schistosome, there is little damage to nearby host cells. Killing of *S. mansoni* by eosinophils is enhanced by mast cell products, and when studied *in vitro*, eosinophils from patients with schistosomiasis are more effective than those from normal subjects. The antigens released cause local IgE-dependent degranulation of mast cells and the release of mediators. These selectively attract eosinophils to the site and further enhance their activity. Other products of eosinophils later block the mast cell reactions. The importance of these effector mechanisms *in vivo* has

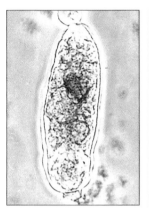
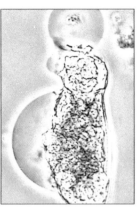
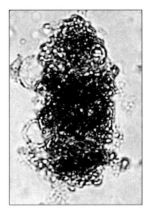

Fig. 16.14 Effect of major basic protein of eosinophils on schistosome larvae. Killing of schistosomules by eosinophils can be effected by the major basic protein of the granules. These pictures show progressive surface damage and disruption of a larva caused by incubation in this cell product: intact worm (left); initial stage of damage to the tegument and worm surface (middle); total destruction of the worm (right). (Courtesy of Dr D. McLaren.)

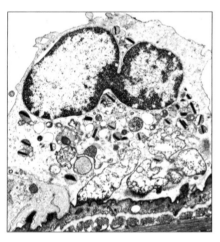
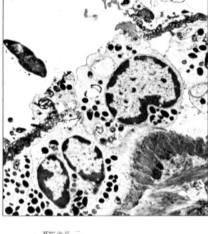
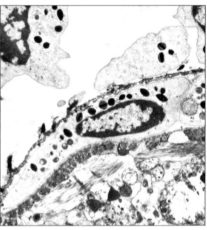

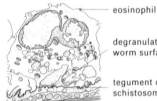
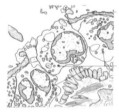

eosinophil

degranulation at worm surface

tegument of schistosomule

tegument

eosinophil

tegument

eosinophil

schistosomule

Fig. 16.15 Killing of schistosome larvae by eosinophils. Eosinophils can adhere to schistosomules and kill them. The damage is associated with degranulation of the eosinophils and the release of the contents of the granules onto the surface of the worm. This series of electron micrographs

shows adherence of the eosinophils and degranulation onto the surface of the worm larva (left), and stages in the breakup of the worm tegument and migration of eosinophils through the lesions (middle and right). (Courtesy of Dr D. McLaren.)

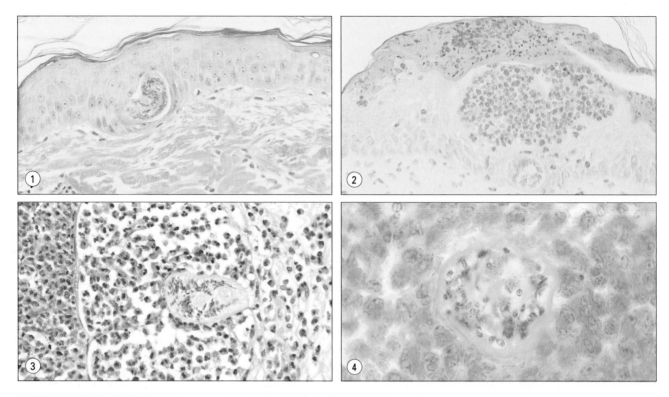

Fig. 16.16 Immunity to *Schistosoma mansoni in vivo*.
Normal or previously infected baboons were infected
percutaneously with 1000 cercariae of *S. mansoni*.
1. In control animals at 72 hours after challenge, there is no
inflammatory or immune reaction and the schistosomes lie
just above the basement membrane. H & E stain, × 160.
2. In animals infected 2 years previously, an inflammatory
infiltration surrounds the schistosome by 24 hours after the

challenge, and is predominantly eosinophilic.
Giemsa stain, × 160.
3. In the immune animal 24 hours after challenge the
schistosomule is trapped in an abscess of adherent
eosinophils. Giemsa stain, × 250.
4. The same animal as (3) showing a killed parasite in
which the eosinophils have invaded its interior. × 640.
(Courtesy of Dr B. J. Cottrell and Dr H. M. Seitz.)

Two-stage expulsion of nematodes from the gut

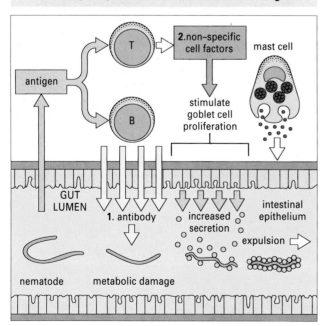

Fig. 16.17 The expulsion of some intestinal nematodes
occurs spontaneously a few weeks after primary infection.
It depends upon two sequential steps, following antigen
sensitization of specific T cells and B cells.
1. Antibody (mainly IgG1) damages the worms but is not
itself sufficient to cause their elimination.
2. T cells do not adhere directly to the worms but they
release non-specific factors which act on mucus-secreting
goblet cells in the intestinal epithelium. The mucus coats
the worms and leads to their expulsion. The numbers of
goblet cells in the jejunal epithelium and the secretion of
mucus increase in proportion to the worm burden. The
antigen-specific effector T cells are generated early in
infection and the rate-limiting step is the onset of antibody
damage.

been shown in monkeys, in which schistosome killing is associated with eosinophil accumulation (Fig. 16.16).

MAST CELLS

The cytoplasmic granules of mast cells contain a number of preformed mediators (see Chapter 19). They are also a source of many different cytokines, including IL-3, IL-4, GM-CSF and TNF$_\alpha$. Unstimulated mouse peritoneal mast cells contain about twice as much TNF$_\alpha$ as stimulated peritoneal macrophages. These stores of TNF$_\alpha$ are ready for immediate release when the cell is stimulated, in contrast to macrophages which must synthesize it.

Mucosal mast cells are induced by antigen-activated T cells in worm infections and mast cell mediators appear to enhance activity of other effector processes. They interact with eosinophils and also play an important (though not essential) role in accelerating the expulsion of nematodes from the gut (Fig. 16.17). Mast cell products, including a protease, cause changes in the permeability of the gut and shedding of the epithelium which may help eject some protozoan parasites. In intestinal infections caused by nematodes, the mucosa coats the worms in mucus just before expulsion (Fig. 16.18). In a new host, the worms may bind to the gut wall, but in an immune animal they are trapped in mucus and fail to do so. Antibody and complement appear to promote mucus trapping. By altering mucosal permeability mast-cell mediators allow complement and serum antibodies to leak into the gut lumen. The mediators can also act on intestinal smooth muscle to facilitate expulsion by peristalsis.

PLATELETS

Platelets are capable of killing various types of parasite, including the schistosomule stage of flukes, *Toxoplasma gondii* and *Trypanosoma cruzi*. Like other effector cells, their cytotoxic activity is enhanced by treatment with cytokines (e.g. IFN$_\gamma$ and TNF$_\alpha$). For example, in *Schistosoma mansoni*-infected rats, platelets become larvicidal before antibody can be detected but when acute-phase reactants appear in the serum. Incubation of normal platelets in such serum can cause their activation. Platelets also bear Fc$_\epsilon$ receptors on their surface membrane, by which they mediate antibody-dependent cytotoxicity.

ANTIBODY

In addition to the rise in specific antibodies, many parasite infections provoke a non-specific hypergammaglobulinaemia. Specific responses are mostly T cell-dependent, but much of the non-specific antibody production is probably due to substances released from the parasites acting as B-cell mitogens. Specific antibody is particularly important in the control of extracellular parasites and in preventing the invasion of cells by blood-borne intracellular parasites, but is ineffective once the parasite has entered its host cell. The importance of antibody-dependent relative to antibody-independent responses varies with the infection (Fig. 16.19). The mechanism by which specific antibody controls parasite infections and its effects are summarized in Fig. 16.20 and are as follows.

1. Antibody can act directly on protozoa to damage them, either by itself or by activating the complement system (Fig. 16.21).

2. Antibody can neutralize a parasite directly by blocking attachment to a new host cell, as with *Plasmodium* spp., whose merozoites enter red blood cells through a special receptor: their entry is inhibited by specific antibody (Fig. 16.22). Antibody may also act to prevent spread, for example in the acute phase of infection by *Trypanosoma cruzi*.

3. Antibody can enhance phagocytosis by macrophages. Phagocytosis is increased even more by the addition of complement. These effects are mediated by Fc and C3 receptors on the macrophages, which may increase in number as a result of macrophage activation. Phagocytosis plays an important role in the control of infections of *Plasmodium* spp. and *T. brucei*.

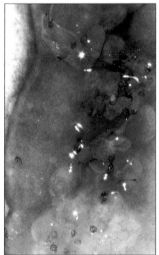
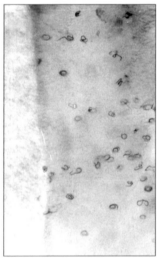

Fig. 16.18 Effect of mucus secretion on worm expulsion. Stereomicrographs of the intestine of rats challenged with 1000 intestinal worms (*Nippostrongylus brasiliensis*), 2 hours previously. Animals on the left were primed, 18 days previously, with a subcutaneous infection of the parasite; in these animals the worms become enveloped in globules of mucus. In unimmunized rats (right) there is no mucus production and the worms become attached to the wall of the intestine. (Courtesy of Dr H. R. P. Miller, with permission from *Immunology* 1981;**44**: 419–429.)

Relative importance of antibody-dependent and -independent responses in protozoal infections

parasite and habitat		antibody–dependent			antibody–independent	
		importance	mechanism	means of evasion	importance	mechanism
T. brucei free in blood	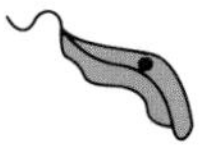	+ + + +	lysis with complement which also opsonizes for phagocytosis	antigenic variation	–	
Plasmodium inside red cell	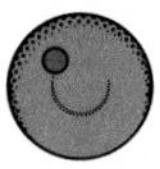	+ + +	blocks invasion, opsonizes for phagocytosis	intracellular; antigenic variation	liver stage + + + blood stage + + +	cytokines macrophage activation
T. cruzi inside macrophage	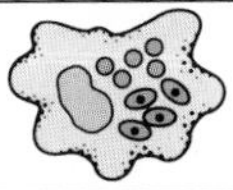	+ +	limits spread in acute infection, sensitizes for ADCC	intracellular	+ + + (chronic phase)	macrophage activation by cytokines and killing by NO and metabolites of O_2
Leishmania inside macrophage	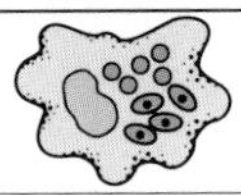	+	limits spread	intracellular	+ + + +	

Fig. 16.19 This table summarizes the relative importance of the two immune responses, the mechanisms involved and, for antibody, the means by which the protozoan can evade damage by antibody. Antibody is the most important part of the immune response against those parasites that live in the bloodstream, such as African trypanosomes and malarial parasites, whereas cell-mediated immunity is active against those like Leishmania that live in the tissues. Antibody can damage parasites directly, enhance their clearance by phagocytosis, activate complement or block their entry into their host cell and so limit the spread of infection. Once inside, the parasite is safe from its effects. Trypanosoma cruzi and Leishmania are both susceptible to the action of oxygen metabolites released by the respiratory burst of macrophages and to nitric oxide. Treating macrophages with cytokines enhances release of these products and diminishes entry and survival of the parasites. Malarial parasites within the red cell may be destroyed by some secreted products of activated macrophages, including hydrogen peroxide and other cytotoxic factors.

Control of parasite infections by specific antibody

parasite	Plasmodium sporozoite, intestinal worms, trypanosome	Plasmodium sporozoite and merozoite, Trypanosoma cruzi, Toxoplasma gondii	Plasmodium, trypanosome	schistosomes, Trichinella spiralis, filarial worms
mechanism	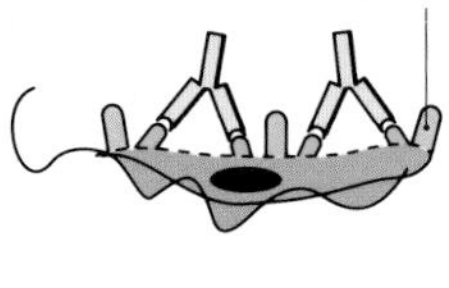	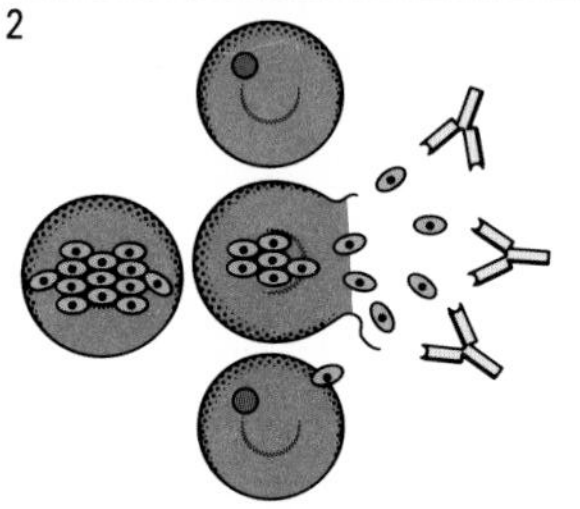	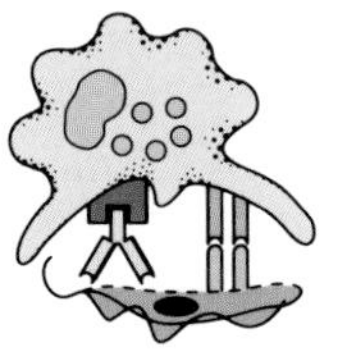	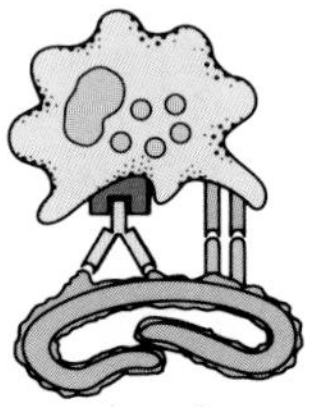
effect	direct damage or complement-mediated lysis	prevents spread by neutralizing attachment site, prevents escape from lysosomal vacuole, prevents inhibition of lysosomal fusion	enhancement of phagocytosis	antibody-dependent cell-mediated cytotoxicity (ADCC)

Fig. 16.20 1. Direct damage. Antibody activates the classical complement pathway, causing damage to the parasite membrane and increasing susceptibility to other mediators. 2. Neutralization. For example, parasites such as Plasmodium spp. spread to new cells by specific receptor attachment; blocking the merozoite binding site with antibody prevents attachment to the receptors on the erythrocyte surface and hence prevents further multiplication.

3. Enhancement of phagocytosis. Complement C3b deposited on parasite membrane opsonizes it for phagocytosis by cells with C3b receptors (e.g. macrophages). Macrophages also have Fc receptors. 4. Eosinophils, neutrophils, platelets and macrophages may be cytotoxic for some parasites when they recognize the parasite via specific antibody (ADCC). The reaction is enhanced by complement.

4. Antibody is also involved in antibody-dependent cell-mediated cytotoxicity, for example, in infections caused by *Trypanosoma cruzi, Trichinella spiralis, Schistosoma mansoni* and filarial worms. Cytotoxic cells such as macrophages, neutrophils and eosinophils adhere to antibody-coated worms by means of their Fc and C3 receptors (Fig. 16.23) and release their granular contents, ROIs etc. in apposition to the parasite.

Different kinds of antibody and cell may act at different stages in the life cycle. For example, eosinophils are more effective than other cells at killing the newly hatched larvae of *T. spiralis*, whereas macrophages are more effective against the microfilariae. In each case, the antibody mediating the reaction is stage-specific: IgG mediates killing by eosinophils, while IgE mediates killing by macrophages.

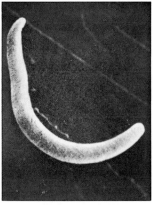
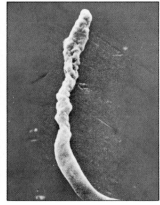

Fig. 16.21 Direct effect of specific antibody on sporozoites of malarial parasites. These scanning electron micrographs show a sporozoite of *Plasmodium berghei*, which causes malaria in rodents, before (left) and after (right) incubation in immune serum. The surface of parasite is damaged. Specific antibody protects against infection with *Plasmodium* spp. at several of the extracellular stages of the life cycle. The antibody is stage-specific in each case. Specific antibody perturbs the outer membrane of the sporozoite, causing leakage of fluid. (Courtesy of Dr R. Nussenzweig.)

Effect of antibody on malarial parasites

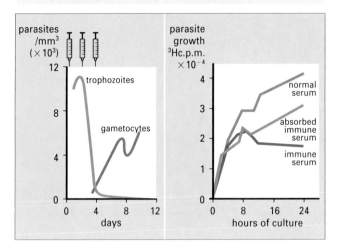

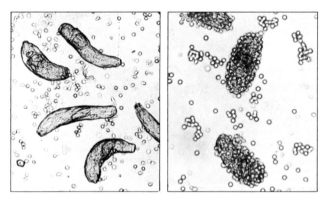

Fig. 16.22 Left: Transfer of γ-globulin from immune adults to a child infected with *Plasmodium falciparum* caused a sharp drop in parasitaemia. Specific antibody acts at the merozoite stage in the life of the parasite and prevents the initiation of of further cycles of multiplication in the blood. The development of gametocytes from existing intracellular forms is unaffected.
Right: In culture, the presence of immune serum blocks the continued increase in number of *P. knowlesi* (a malarial parasite of monkeys), as measured by incorporation of ³H-leucine. It stops multiplication at the stage after schizont rupture by preventing the released merozoites from invading fresh red blood cells. The inhibitory activity of the immune serum can be reduced by prior absorption of the specific antibody with free schizonts.

Fig. 16.23 Antibody-dependent cytotoxicity against schistosomes mediated by neutrophils. These photographs show schistosomules of *Schistosoma mansoni* incubated with neutrophils in the presence of normal rat serum (left) and in the presence of fresh immune serum containing active complement (right). The adherence of neutrophils to the surface of the larva, mediated by antibody and complement can be seen. This is the first step in the killing of the parasite. The worm is probably killed by hydrogen peroxide and other oxygen metabolites released from the neutrophil during the respiratory burst. This follows the membrane perturbation resulting from contact between parasite and neutrophil. Neutrophils from patients with chronic granulomatous disease, which are incapable of generating ROIs, are markedly impaired in their ability to kill schistosomules. However, they retain some activity, indicating the existence of an O_2^--independent cytotoxic mechanism. (Courtesy of Dr D. MacLaren.)

Different antibody isotypes may have different effects. In children in The Gambia infected with *Schistosoma haematobium,* parasite-specific IgE is associated with protection against the adult worms and there is an inverse relationship between the amount of IgE in their blood and reinfection. IgG4 appears to block its action and reinfection is more likely in children who have high levels of IgG4. The development of immunity seems to depend upon a switch from IgG4 to IgE that occurs with age, and infection rates are highest in 10- to 14-year-olds when IgG4 levels are highest.

In many infections it is difficult to distinguish between cell-mediated and antibody-mediated responses, since both act in concert against the parasite. This is illustrated in Fig. 16.24 which summarizes the immune reactions which may occur against the schistosome larva.

NON-SPECIFIC EFFECTOR MECHANISMS

Tissue macrophages, monocytes and granulocytes all have some intrinsic anti-parasite activity. However, this is greatly enhanced by antibodies and the cytokines secreted by sensitized lymphocytes.

Of the serum-soluble factors, complement has already been mentioned for its interaction with specific antibody via the classical pathway. Several types of parasite, including the adult worms and infective larvae of *Trichinella spiralis* and the schistosomules of *Schistosoma mansoni,* carry molecules in their surface coats which activate the alternative pathway.

ESCAPE MECHANISMS

It is a necessary characteristic of all successful parasite infections that they can, in different ways, evade the full effects of their host's immune responses.

An ability to resist destruction by complement often correlates with virulence. *Leishmania tropica,* which is easily killed by complement, causes a localized self-healing infection in the skin, whereas *L. donovani,* which is ten times more resistant to complement, becomes disseminated throughout the viscera, causing a disease which is often fatal. The mechanisms whereby parasites can resist the effect of complement differ. The lipophosphoglycan surface coat of *Leishmania major* activates complement, but the complex is then shed so the parasite avoids lysis. The trypomastigotes of *Trypanosoma cruzi* bear a surface glycoprotein that has activity that resembles DAF, which limits the complement reaction.

ANATOMICAL SEQUESTRATION

Parasites which live inside cells are safe from the action of some of the host's defences during their intracellular phase of existence. Other parasites are protected by cysts (for example, *Trichinella spiralis, Entamoeba histolytica)* or live in the gut (intestinal nematodes).

Those that live inside macrophages have evolved different ways of avoiding being killed by oxygen metabolites and lysosomal enzymes (Figs 16.25 and 16.26).

Coordinated response to schistosomules

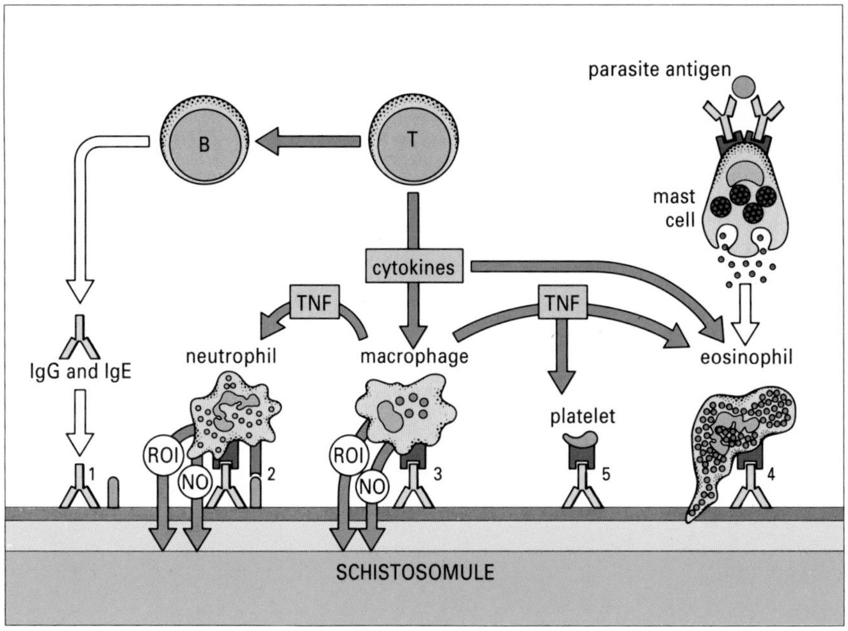

Fig. 16.24 This diagram illustrates the various effector mechanisms that have been shown to damage schistosomes *in vitro*. Antibody and complement at high levels damage worms (1), and at lower levels antibody sensitizes neutrophils (2), macrophages (3), eosinophils (4) and platelets (5) for antibody-dependent cell-mediated cytotoxicity. Neutrophils and macrophages probably act by releasing toxic oxygen and nitrogen metabolites, whereas eosinophils damage the worm tegument by release of major basic protein. The response is potentiated by cytokines (e.g. TNF$_\alpha$). IgE antibody is important both in sensitizing eosinophils and in sensitizing local mast cells, which release a variety of mediators, including mediators which activate the eosinophils.

Toxoplasma gondii penetrates the macrophage by a non-phagocytic pathway and so avoids triggering the oxidative burst; *Leishmania* organisms can enter by binding to complement receptors, another way of avoiding stimulating the respiratory burst. In addition, they possess enzymes that inhibit the progression of the burst, superoxide dismutase which protects them against the action of superoxides, and a lipophosphoglycan surface coat (LPG) that acts as a scavenger of oxygen metabolites and affords protection against

The different means by which protozoa that multiply within macrophages escape digestion by lysosomal enzymes

Fig. 16.25 *Toxoplasma gondii*. Live parasites coated with host laminin enter the cell actively, into a membrane-bound vacuole, by binding to a member of the integrin family of receptors on the surface of the macrophage. They are not attacked by enzymes because lysosomes do not fuse with this vacuole. Dead parasites, however, are taken up by normal phagocytosis into a phagosome (by interaction with the Fc receptors on the macrophage if they are coated with antibody) and they are then destroyed by the enzymes of the lysosomes which fuse with it.
Trypanosoma cruzi. Survival of these parasites depends upon their stage of development; trypomastigotes escape from the phagosome and divide in the cytoplasm whereas epimastigotes do not escape and are killed. The proportion of parasites found in the

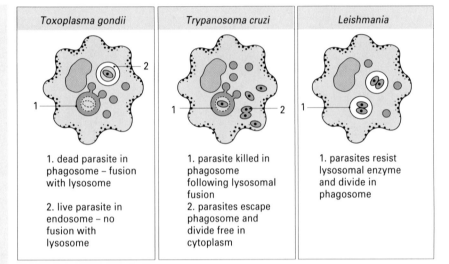

Toxoplasma gondii	*Trypanosoma cruzi*	*Leishmania*
1. dead parasite in phagosome – fusion with lysosome 2. live parasite in endosome – no fusion with lysosome	1. parasite killed in phagosome following lysosomal fusion 2. parasites escape phagosome and divide free in cytoplasm	1. parasites resist lysosomal enzyme and divide in phagosome

cytoplasm is decreased if the macrophages are activated.
Leishmania spp. These parasites multiply within the phagosome and the presence of a surface protease helps them resist digestion. If the macrophages are first activated by cytokines the number of parasites entering the cell and the number that replicate diminish.

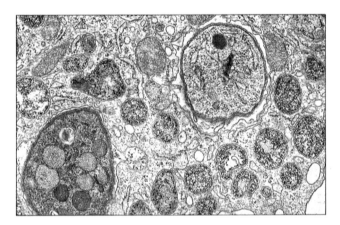

Fig. 16.26 Electron micrograph showing part of a macrophage infected with *Toxoplasma gondii*. Following infection, the macrophages were treated with thorotrast to make the contents of the secondary lysosomes electron dense. The live parasite has inhibited fusion of secondary

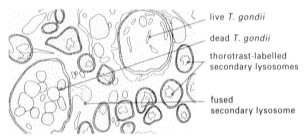

live *T. gondii*

dead *T. gondii*

thorotrast-labelled secondary lysosomes

fused secondary lysosome

lysosomes with its phagosome. Several dead parasites lie in a phagosome that contains thorotrast; it can be seen that a phagosome has just fused with the vacuole and emptied its contents into it. × 14 000. (Courtesy of Prof. T. C. Jones.)

Two surface antigens of *Leishmania*

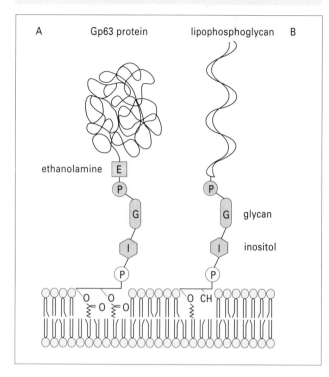

enzymatic attack. A glycoprotein, Gp63 (Fig. 16.27), inhibits the action of the macrophage's lysosomal enzymes. *Leishmania* spp. can also down-regulate the expression of MHC Class II on the macrophages they inhabit, thus reducing their capacity to stimulate Tн cells. These escape mechanisms, however, are of more limited efficiency in the immune host.

Fig. 16.27 Schematic representation of two surface antigens of *Leishmania* that are anchored to the membrane by phosphatidylinositol tails.
A This protein antigen, Gp63, has protease activity. That of *L. mexicana,* together with LPG, binds complement. This enables the promastigote to enter the macrophage through the C3 complement receptor.
B This glycolipid antigen, a lipophosphoglycan (LPG), imparts resistance to complement-mediated lysis. That of *L. major* binds C3b, the third component of complement, enabling the promastigote to enter through the CR1 complement receptor. Antibodies to both antigens confer protection against murine cutaneous leishmaniasis.

Antigenic variation in African trypanosomes

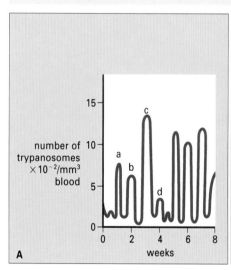

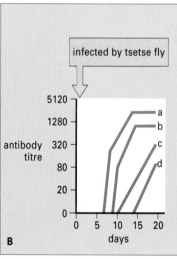

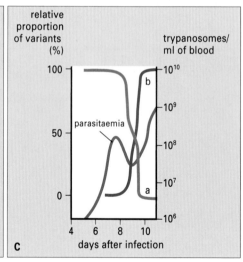

Fig. 16.28 Trypanosome infections may run for several months giving rise to successive waves of parasitaemia. Graph A shows a chart of the fluctuation in parasitaemia in a patient with sleeping sickness. Although infection was initiated by a single parasite, each wave is caused by an immunologically distinct population of parasites (a,b,c,d); protection is not afforded by antibody against preceding variants. There is a strong tendency for new variants to appear in the same order in different hosts. Variation does not occur in immunologically compromised animals (that is, animals treated to deprive them of some aspect of immune function). Graph B shows the time-course of production of antibody against four variants in a rabbit bitten by a tsetse fly carrying *Trypanosoma brucei*. Antibody to successive variants appears shortly after the appearance of each variant and rises to a plateau. The appearance of antibody drives the parasite towards another variant type. Graph C shows the kinetics of one cycle of antigenic variation. A rat was infected with a homogeneous population of one variant (a) of *T. brucei*. The second wave of parasitaemia develops as the new variant (b) emerges and predominates.

AVOIDANCE OF RECOGNITION

Parasites that are vulnerable to specific antibody have evolved different methods of evading its effects. The African trypanosome undergoes antigenic variation: it can change the molecule that forms its surface coat, the VSG (variable surface glycoprotein) which protects the underlying surface membrane from the host's defence mechanisms. New populations of parasites are antigenically distinct from previous ones (Fig. 16.28) which can be shown by immunofluorescence or radioimmunoassay. Several antigens of malarial parasites also undergo antigenic variation.

Other parasites, such as schistosomes, acquire a surface layer of host antigens, so that the host does not distinguish them from 'self' (Fig. 16.29). Schistosomules cultured in medium containing human serum and red blood cells can acquire surface molecules containing A,B and H blood-group determinants. They can also acquire MHC molecules. However, schistosomules maintained in medium devoid of host molecules also become resistant to attack by antibody and complement, indicating that protective changes in the parasite tegument occur that are independent of the adsorption of host antigens.

SUPPRESSION OF THE HOST'S IMMUNE RESPONSES

Immunosuppression is an evasion mechanism practiced universally by parasites. Some can cause disruption of lymphoid cells or tissue directly, e.g newly hatched larvae of *Trichinella spiralis* which release a soluble lymphocytotoxic factor. Similarly, schistosomes can cleave a peptide from IgG that inhibits many cellular immune responses. Older worms can acquire host DAF. This molecule has a GPI anchor, and it is thought that after being shed from host cells it can become inserted into the lipid layer of the worm's tegument through its phospholipid tail. Its presence may explain why, in contrast to cercariae and young schistosomules, older worms do not fix complement by the alternative pathway.

Soluble parasite antigens, which are released in enormous quantities, may impair the host's response by a process termed immune distraction. Thus the soluble antigens (the S- or heat-stable antigens) of *Plasmodium falciparum* are thought to mop up circulating antibody, providing a smokescreen and diverting it from the body of the parasite. Many of the surface antigens that are shed are soluble forms of molecules inserted into the

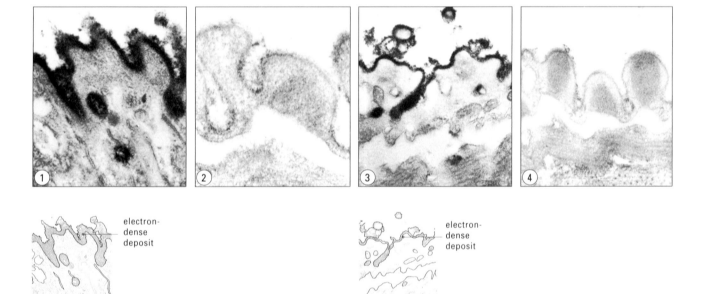

Fig. 16.29 Acquisition of host antigens by schistosomes. These electron micrographs show sections of the surface of schistosomes that have been incubated with labelled antibody against schistosome antigens or against mouse red blood cells. Presence of each antigen is shown by the layer of electron-dense deposit of labelled antibody. Young 3-hour schistosomules bind parasite-specific antibody *in vitro* (1) but not after 4 days in a mouse host (2). Antibody against mouse antigens binds to the 4-day-old lung-stage parasite (3) but not to the newly transformed schistosomules (4). Thus, older worms express the species-specific antigens of their host but not their own antigens. Lung-stage worms are immune to attack by complement and antibody-mediated effectors *in vitro*. Worms transferred from one species to another die within 24 hours. They are only susceptible to attack by specific antibody *in vitro* if they are not coated with host protective antigens.(Courtesy of Dr D. McLaren.)

parasite membrane by a GPI anchor, including the VSG of *Trypanosoma brucei*, the LPG or 'excreted factor' of *Leishmania* (see Fig. 16.27) and several surface antigens of schistosomules. These are released by endogenous phosphatidylinositol-specific phospholipases.

Non-specific immunosuppression is a universal feature of parasite infection (Fig. 16.30) and has been demonstrated for both antibody (Figs 16.31 and 16.32) and cell-mediated responses. Much of the suppression may be due to macrophages becoming overloaded with free antigen. In mice infected with African trypanosomes, antigen presentation by macrophages is diminished and IL-1 secretion is reduced. Macrophages also release prostaglandins and other suppressive molecules which subdue inflammatory reactions.

Antigen-specific suppression may also occur, as has been demonstrated in leishmaniasis (Fig. 16.33). T cells from patients infected with *L. donovani* when cultured with specific antigen do not secrete IL-2 or IFN$_\gamma$. Their production of IL-1 and expression of MHC Class II is also decreased, while their secretion of prostaglandins is enhanced. Such patients benefit from treatment with IFN$_\gamma$ combined with pentavalent antimony.

However, immunosuppression may benefit both the host and parasite, as is seen in schistosomiasis. Many immune responses, particularly those of T$_H$ cells, are depressed in this infection. A factor produced by the worm inhibits lymphocyte proliferation directly, as do suppressive molecules secreted by T cells and macrophages. Liver granulomata surrounding schistosome

Interference with host's immune response by free antigens released from the parasite

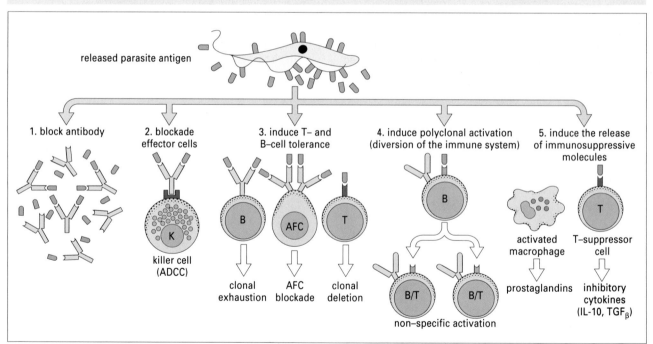

Fig. 16.30 Free antigens can:
1. Combine with antibody and divert it from the parasite. The variant surface glycoprotein of *Trypanosoma brucei* and the soluble antigens of *Plasmodium falciparum* , which are also polymorphic and contain repetitive sequences of amino acids, are thought to act in this way as a smokescreen or decoy.
2. Blockade effector cells, either directly or as immune complexes. Circulating complexes, for example, are able to inhibit the action of cytotoxic cells active against *Schistosoma mansoni*.
3. Induce T- or B-cell tolerance, presumably by blockage of

antibody-forming cells (AFC) or by depletion of the mature antigen-specific lymphocytes (i.e. clonal exhaustion).
4. Cause polyclonal activation. Many parasite products are mitogenic to B or T cells, and the high serum concentrations of non-specific IgM (and IgG) commonly found in parasitic infections probably result from this polyclonal stimulation. Its continuation is believed to lead to impairment of B cell function, the progressive depletion of antigen-reactive B lymphocytes and thus immunosuppression.
5. Activate T cells, or macrophages, or both, to release suppressive molecules.

Polyclonal activation by African trypanosomes

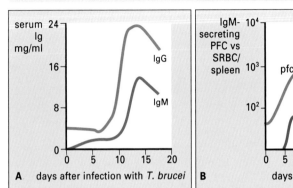
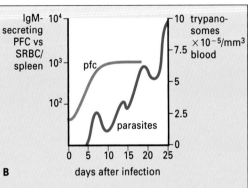
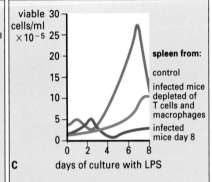

Fig. 16.31 Graph A shows increasing concentrations of serum immunoglobulins observed in mice infected with *Trypanosoma brucei*. These levels are only consistent with polyclonal activation and not specific antibody alone. Graph B shows the increase in number of IgM-secreting cells forming plaques with sheep red blood cells (SRBC) that occurs spontaneously during infection, that is, without injection of SRBC. The number increases with the parasitaemia to reach a plateau of 20–30 times normal. Cells secreting antibody against other antigens increase similarly. Soluble fractions derived from parasites have been shown to be mitogenic, their activity being enhanced by macrophages. Trypanosomes (and other parasites) thus cause proliferation of B lymphocytes and this may lead to the progressive depletion of antigen-reactive B cells. Graph C shows the failure of spleen lymphocytes taken from infected mice (at day 8) to proliferate in response to stimulation by lipopolysaccharide (LPS) *in vitro*. Removal of T cells and macrophages from spleens taken soon after infection partly restores the response, but not later on when the B cell potential appears to become exhausted. Macrophages collected early in infection can also depress the ability of normal spleen cells to respond to LPS.

Depression of non-specific antibody production in mice with malaria

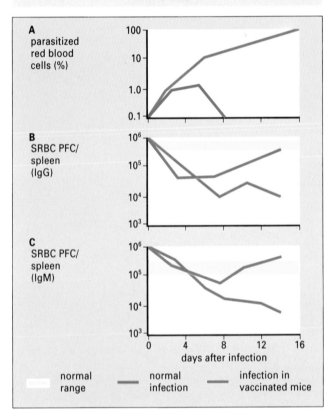

Fig. 16.32 Graph A shows the course of parasitaemia in unvaccinated and vaccinated mice infected with a lethal variant of *Plasmodium yoelii;* unvaccinated mice die about 16 days later, vaccinated mice survive and all parasites disappear from the blood by 8 days. As graphs B and C show, the time-course of parasitaemia correlates with the generalized, non-specific immunosuppression. The numbers of IgM- and IgG-producing plaque-forming cells (PFC)/spleen obtained 5 days after infection in response to sheep red blood cells (SRBC) was measured in two groups of mice. Antibody-producing cells decreased during infection, but in vaccinated mice they returned to normal as the mice recovered. The depression of PFC appears to reflect parasite load. Its mechanism is unknown.

eggs diminish in size with time, probably as a result of changes in local production of cytokines. This immuno-suppression benefits both host and parasite, because although extensive granulomata damage the host's liver, some macrophage accumulation is helpful in protecting the tissue against the toxic secretions of the egg.

Some of the escape mechanisms discussed above are summarized in Fig. 16.34.

IMMUNOPATHOLOGICAL CONSEQUENCES OF PARASITE INFECTIONS

Apart from the directly destructive effects of some parasites and their products on host tissues, many immune responses themselves have pathological effects. In malaria, sleeping sickness and visceral leishmaniasis, the increased number and heightened activity of macrophages and lymphocytes in the liver and spleen lead to enlargement of those organs.

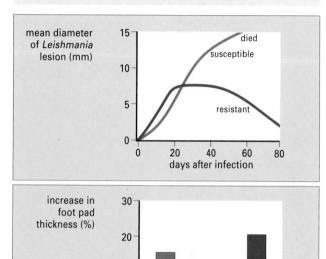

Depression of specific delayed hypersensitivity in mice infected with Leishmania

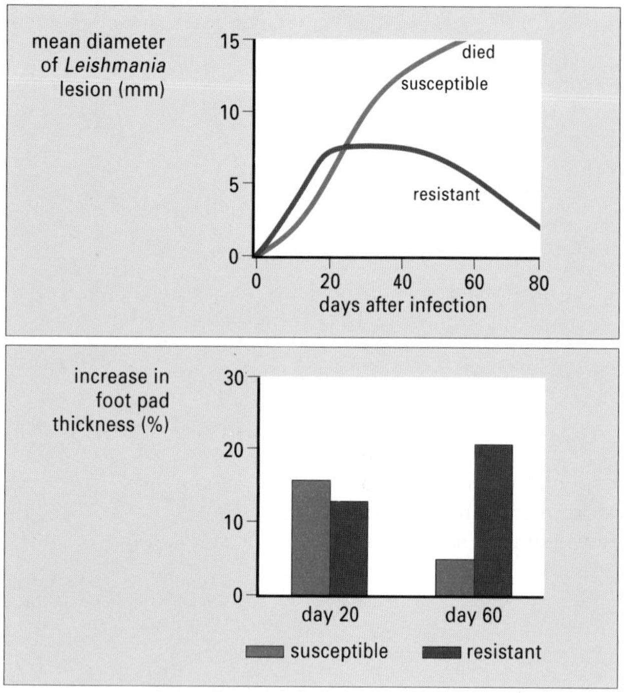

Fig. 16.33 Upper left: The course of infection of *L. tropica*, as determined by the size of lesion, is plotted for a susceptible stain and a resistant strain of mouse. Mice of the susceptible stain die about 70 days after infection. Left: Delayed hypersensitivity to specific antigen injected into the footpad is illustrated as the percentage increase in footpad thickness. In resistant mice the response increases as the mice recover, whereas it is significantly depressed in the susceptible mice. The depression is antigen-specific and is mediated by cells which inhibit delayed hypersensitivity, but not antibody production. Recovery from this infection is mediated by T cells.

Mechanisms by which parasites avoid host defences

parasite	habitat	main host effector mechanism	method of avoidance
Trypanosoma brucei	bloodstream	antibody + complement	antigenic variation
Plasmodium spp.	liver (hepatocyte) blood cell	cytokines, antibody	unknown, antigenic variation
Toxoplasma gondii	macrophage	O_2 metabolites lysosomal enzymes	failure to trigger, inhibits fusion of lysosomes
Trypanosoma cruzi	macrophage	O_2 metabolites lysosomal enzymes	unknown, escapes into cytoplasm, so avoiding digestion
Leishmania	macrophage	O_2 metabolites lysosomal enzymes	O_2 burst impaired and products scavenged, avoids digestion
Trichinella spiralis	gut, blood, muscle	myeloid cells, antibody + complement	encystment in muscle
Schistosoma mansoni	skin, blood, lungs, portal vein	myeloid cells, antibody + complement	acquisition of host antigens, blockade by soluble antigen and immune complexes

Fig. 16.34 A summary of the various methods which parasites have evolved to avoid host defence mechanisms in the host

The formation of immune complexes is common; they may be deposited in the kidney, as in the nephrotic syndrome of quartan malaria, and may give rise to many other pathological changes. For example, tissue-bound immunoglobulins have been found in the muscles of mice infected with African trypanosomes and in the choroid plexus of mice with malaria.

The IgE of worm infections can have severe effects on the host through the release of mast-cell mediators: Anaphylactic shock may occur when a hydatid cyst ruptures. Asthma-like reactions occur in *Toxocara canis* infections, and in tropical eosinophilia when filarial worms migrate through the lungs.

Autoantibodies, which probably arise as a result of polyclonal activation, have been detected against red blood cells, lymphocytes and DNA (e.g. in trypanosomiasis and in malaria). Antibodies against the parasite may cross-react with host tissues. For example, the chronic cardiomyopathy, enlarged oesophagus and megacolon that occur in Chagas' disease are thought to result from the autoimmune effects on nerve ganglia of antibody and of cytotoxic T cells that cross-react with *Trypanosoma cruzi.*

Excessive production of some cytokines may contribute to some of the manifestations of disease. Thus the fever, anaemia, diarrhoea and pulmonary changes of acute malaria closely resemble the symptoms of endo-toxaemia and are probably caused by TNF. The severe wasting of cattle with trypanosomiasis may also be mediated by TNF_α. Several immunological mechanisms may combine in producing pathological effects, as is likely in the anaemia of malaria (Fig. 16.35).

Lastly, the non-specific immunosuppression that is so widespread probably explains why people with parasite infections are especially susceptible to bacterial and viral infections (e.g. measles). It may also account for the association of Burkitt's lymphoma with malaria.

VACCINES

Some vaccines composed of attenuated living parasites have proved successful in veterinary practice but now, as a result of recent exciting advances in the field of molecular biology, much effort is being directed towards the development of subunit vaccines against the important parasitic diseases of man. One of the biggest difficulties, however, is the polymorphic and rapidly changing nature of many parasite antigens, especially of trypanosoma and malarial parasites. Moreover, immunization could lead to the selection of new parasite antigens and induce the appearance of a new variant.

To be effective, a vaccine must induce a long-lived response (i.e. memory) from the right kind of T cells: those that produce a strong cell-mediated immunity and do not induce suppression. Since antigens that are recognised by T cells often show marked genetic restriction the antigen used as a vaccine must be presented by most MHC haplotypes. Antigens that may induce the wrong kind of immune response or autoimmunity must be avoided. In some circumstances, parasite antigens can induce antibodies that cause dissemination of the parasites, and some cell-mediated responses may cause pathology.

Possible causes of development of anaemia in malaria

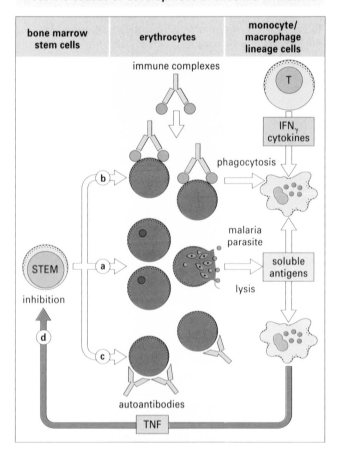

Fig. 16.35 There is more destruction of erythrocytes in malaria than can be accounted for by the number infected by parasites. In addition to those lost by lysis when the schizont ruptures (a), immunopathological mechanisms probably contribute to the anaemia. Parasite antigens, or immune complexes containing parasite antigens, may bind to unparasitized erythrocytes and accelerate their clearance by cells of the macrophage/monocyte lineage in the spleen and liver (b). There is also some autoantibody produced against erythrocytes which again accelerates their breakdown (c). TNF released in response to infection inhibits red blood cell development from bone marrow stem cells (d).

STRATEGIES IN VACCINE DESIGN

The usual strategy has been to identify protective antigens and then the key immunogenic portion of the molecule, which is likely to be distinct from the portion causing suppression. Although antigens are more easily identified by reactions with antibody, antigens that are useful in vaccination have to be identified by their reactions with T cells, since protection usually depends upon development of good cell-mediated immunity. Humoral responses are likely to be stronger against the parasite's surface antigens, but the parasite may be able to evade such antibodies. Cell-mediated immunity is often independent of surface antigens. Better protection may be obtained using antigens from within the parasite, such as the paramyosin of schistosomes. Internal antigens appear to be able to stimulate T cells to release cytokines and activate macrophages. Even if complete protection cannot be achieved, it may still be worth developing a vaccine that reduces parasite load.

Another possible approach is the development of vaccines which do not block initial infection but prevent the clinical manifestations of disease. In malaria, the aim would be to vaccinate against the antigens which induce cytokines like TNF_α, which is thought to be responsible for many of the symptoms of the disease.

Preparation of Antigens Once promising antigens have been identified there are several courses of action.
1. If they are proteins or peptides, the genes coding for them may be cloned and transferred to microbial or insect cells, which will secrete the recombinant antigens. However, recombinant molecules may differ from natural ones: recombinant glycoproteins, for instance, remain unglycosylated.
2. Molecules whose sequence has been determined, can be synthesized chemically in the laboratory.
3. Antigens can be used to produce idiotypic vaccines which mimic the immunogenic structures. Idiotypic vaccines have the advantage that they can be made to mimic carbohydrate moieties of antigens and they avoid the need to use the antigen itself.

Enzyme Antigens Parasite enzymes which differ from those of the host may be useful targets for immunological attack, since their specific disablement would impair the parasites' development. One good candidate is the protease (Gp63) on the surface of the promastigotes of *Leishmania*. Antibody against the purified enzyme is not protective, but when the enzyme is used to vaccinate mice it induces strong cell-mediated responses and protection. Similarly, an aldolase from blood-stage malarial parasites has been cloned and used to vaccinate monkeys. Despite some homology with mammalian aldolase, it gives partial protection.

Leishmaniasis Two surface antigens of promastigotes containing phospholipids are known to be protective and are giving promising results as vaccines when incorporated into liposomes.

Malaria A number of antigens of *Plasmodium falciparum,* which are possible vaccine candidates, have been cloned. The circumsporozoite protein, which coats the surface of the sporozoite, has been sequenced and a small section synthesized. It is composed of a repeating sequence of 4 amino acid residues, which may be repeated up to 40 times in the whole molecule, depending upon the strain of parasite from which it is derived. Both cloned antigens and synthetic peptides induce the development of neutralizing antibodies against sporozoites, but protection appears to require more than that. Unfortunately these responses show a clear genetic restriction, a feature of highly repetitive epitopes; in mice, response to such sequences is related to their MHC haplotype.

Several antigens from blood-stage parasites of *Plasmodium falciparum* have also been cloned and sequenced, and synthetic peptides prepared that are similar to selected regions of the molecules. Again, these molecules contain many repeated sequences that are immunodominant and induce antibody production. It is possible, however, that epitopes inducing the necessary cell-mediated immunity lie outside these regions of repeats, within variable regions of the molecules. Vaccine trials of a mixture of synthetic peptides from both the sporozoite and merozoite are in progress.

Ultimately, it seems likely that combinations of antigens will be the most successful, given with a carrier, an adjuvant and possibly a cytokine. The route of administration is also important since it affects antigen presentation. Living carriers have a great advantage, as they multiply. BCG bacilli are already widely used as a vaccine and themselves act as an adjuvant. Similarly, *Salmonella* spp. which have been rendered avirulent by genetic engineering, and can be given by mouth, are already undergoing clinical trials.

FURTHER READING

Brophy PM, Pritchard DI. Immunity to helminths: ready to tip the biochemical balance. *Parasitol Today* 1992;**8**:419.

Capron AR. Immunity to schistosomes. *Curr Opin Immunol* 1992;**4**:419.

Colley DG, Nix NA. Do schistosomes exploit the host pro-inflammatory cytokine TNF-α for their own survival? *Parasitol Today* 1992;**8**:355.

Cox FEG, Liew EY. T-cell subsets and cytokines in parasitic infections. *Parasitol Today* 1992;**8**:371.

Cox FEG. Vaccination against parasites. In: Behnke JM. *Parasites: Immunity and Pathology. The consequences of parasitic infection in mammals.* London: Taylor & Francis, 1990:396–416.

James SL. The effector functions of nitrogen oxides in host defense against parasites. *Exp Parasitol* 1991;**73**:223.

Kwiatkowski D. Malaria: becoming more specific about non-specific immunity. *Curr Opin Immunol* 1992;**4**:425.

Locksley RM, Louis JA. Immunology of leishmaniasis. *Curr Opin Immunol* 1992;**4**:413.

chapter 17

Tumour Immunology

The idea that there might be immune responses to tumours is an old one. At the turn of the century, Paul Erhlich suggested that in humans there was a high frequency of 'aberrant germs' (tumours), which if not kept in check by the immune system, would overwhelm us. Thus tumours came to be regarded as similar to grafted tissue recognizable by the immune system. This, in turn, led to attempts to stimulate the immune system to reject them. Occasional regressions following treatment with bacterial vaccines (Coley's toxin), or occurring spontaneously, were taken as evidence of an effective immune response.

Early in the century, experimentalists began to investigate tumour immunity and noted that transplanted tumours usually regressed. However, much of the early work fell into disrepute when it was realized that this was simply a consequence of the genetic disparity of host and tumour, and did not reveal immune responses to tumours. It was only in the post-war years, when genetically homogeneous inbred rodents became available, that it was possible to investigate the immune responses of tumour-bearing animals. An added impetus to these studies was provided by Burnett and Thomas, who developed Ehrlich's idea of immune responses to 'aberrant germs', elaborating it into the theory of Immune Surveillance.

Tumour viruses and immunodeficiency

cause of immunodeficiency	common tumour types	viruses involved
inherited immunodeficiency	lymphoma	EBV
immunosuppression for organ transplants or AIDS	lymphoma	EBV
	cervical cancer	papilloma virus
	Kaposi's sarcoma	not known
malaria	Burkitt's lymphoma	EBV
autoimmunity	lymphoma	EBV

Fig. 17.1 In all forms of immunodeficiency, the greatest increase is in tumours of the lymphoid system. Epstein–Barr virus (EBV) is involved in many of these. Most normal adults carry EBV throughout life with no ill effects. Most epithelial cancers, which show no viral association, are not increased in patients who are immunosuppressed or immunodeficient.

IMMUNE SURVEILLANCE

Burnett and Thomas' idea was that the immune system continually surveyed the body for the presence of abnormal cells, which were destroyed when recognized. The immune response to a tumour was therefore thought to be an early event, leading to the destruction of the majority of tumours before they became clinically apparent. It was also proposed that the immune system played an important role in delaying the growth, or causing regression of established tumours. A variety of evidence was adduced to support these ideas:

1. postmortem data suggest that there may be more tumours than become clinically apparent
2. many tumours contain lymphoid infiltrates and in some tumours this may be a favourable sign
3. spontaneous regression of tumours occurs
4. tumours occur more frequently in the neonatal period and in old age, when the immune system functions less effectively.

Although at first sight this appears impressive evidence in favour of the theory, on closer examination the strongest point, the association between immunosuppression and increased tumour incidence, is less conclusive. In all instances of immunodeficiency or immunosuppression in man, the spectrum of tumours which arise is limited and there is evidence that viruses are involved in causing many of them (Fig. 17.1). This suggests that the immune response may be important in preventing the spread of potentially oncogenic viruses, rather than surveillance against all tumours. Normal humans who become infected with EBV carry the virus for life and show a strong cytotoxic T-cell response to the virus. Increased virus replication, and shedding of viral particles in secretions, has been demonstrated in immunodeficient individuals, so it is clear that the immune response limits virus replication under normal circumstances (Fig. 17.2).

Animal experimental data supports the view that immune surveillance is largely directed towards viruses rather than tumours. A large study of athymic nude mice did not show a general increase in tumour frequency. However, a high proportion of the mice developed tumours caused by the small DNA polyoma virus, which seldom causes tumours in normal animals. The same result was seen in a study of the effects of long term treatment with anti-lymphocyte serum on immune responses.

None of this evidence necessarily implies that there is no immune response to the majority of tumours. It does suggest that, for the majority of tumours, the immune response may be relatively late and ineffective.

TUMOUR ANTIGENS

In man few tumours are known to be caused by viruses (Fig. 17.3), but there is abundant evidence of genetic alterations (mutation, gene amplification, chromosomal deletion or translocation) in most, if not all, tumours. It is known that at least some of these lead to the expression of altered proteins in tumour cells. These altered proteins might be expected to provide antigenic targets for host immune responses. Experimentally, they are detectable by immunizing other species with tumour material.

TUMOUR ASSOCIATED TRANSPLANTATION ANTIGENS (TATAs)

TATAs are of two types. The first are antigens which are shared by many tumours, even though these may not even be of the same tissue of origin. The second are antigens which are specific to an individual tumour. Tumours may express both specific and shared antigens.

SHARED TUMOUR ANTIGENS

These antigens are found on tumours induced by viruses such as the small DNA polyomaviruses and the SV40 viruses, which can cause tumours in experimental animals, and the papillomaviruses, which are implicated in human cervical cancer. These viruses code for T (tumour) antigens which are shared by other viruses of the same group. T antigens are nuclear proteins which play a role in the maintenance of the transformed (cancerous) state.

In animals there are many infectious RNA oncogenic viruses which cause leukaemias and sarcomas, and at least one human leukaemia virus has been discovered (see Fig. 17.3). These viruses bud from the cell membrane of infected cells, and the viral envelope's glycoprotein can be detected at the host cell membrane. There are strong humoral and cell-mediated responses to both DNA- and RNA-tumour viruses, which can protect against tumour challenge (Fig 17.4).

In some strains of mice, activation of endogenous RNA tumour viruses occurs regularly, leading to leukaemia. In others, when carcinogenic chemicals are given, the resulting tumours may express viral antigens and produce infectious mouse leukaemia virus (MuLV). Such tumours express common tumour-associated antigens as well as the tumour specific transplantation antigens (TSTAs) discussed below. Host immune responses to endogenous RNA viruses are weak, perhaps because of immunological tolerance (see Chapter 10).

Role of EBV in tumorigenesis

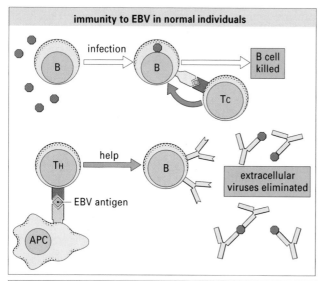

immunity to EBV in normal individuals

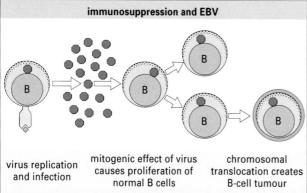

immunosuppression and EBV

virus replication and infection

mitogenic effect of virus causes proliferation of normal B cells

chromosomal translocation creates B-cell tumour

Fig. 17.2 In normal individuals EBV infects B lymphocytes but spread of infection is prevented by Tc cells and antibody, which eliminate infected cells and virus. In immunosuppressed individuals, and in some patients receiving cyclosporin, the virus replicates and infects more B cells. The virus is also mitogenic for B cells so in an immunosuppressed individual, infected B cells tend to proliferate more rapidly. A chromosomal translocation in an infected B cell can lead to malignant transformation.

Viruses and human tumours

tumour	virus
liver cancer	hepatitis B
cervical cancer	human papillomaviruses (HPV 16 and 18)
Burkitt's lymphoma and other lymphomas in immunosuppression	EBV
nasopharyngeal cancer	EBV
adult T cell leukaemia	human T leukaemia virus I (HTLV I)

Fig. 17.3 EBV is associated with Burkitt's lymphoma in Africa and nasopharyngeal cancer in China, suggesting that co-factors, either genetic or environmental, are required to cause the tumours. Adult T-cell leukaemia is found mainly in Japan and the Caribbean.

TUMOUR SPECIFIC TRANSPLANTATION ANTIGENS (TSTAs)

TSTAs are antigens which can provoke an immune response to injected tumour cells, but only if the animal has been previously immunized with the same tumour (Fig. 17.5). These antigens were first detected using tumours from inbred mice that had been induced by chemical carcinogens. For many years the nature of these antigens remained obscure, but they have now been elucidated.

A transplantable (therefore poorly immunogenic) tumour of DBA2 strain mice was exposed *in vitro* to a powerful mutagen. This produced mutant subclones some of which would no longer grow *in vivo*, unless very large numbers of tumour cells were implanted.

The mutants had clearly become more immunogenic than the parent tumour. One of these tumour- (tum-) variant clones was used to immunize syngeneic mice. This generated Tc cells, which would kill only the immunizing tumour and not the parental tumour line or other tum- variants (Fig. 17.6). The Tc cells were then used as probes to identify the presence of the mutated tumour antigen during molecular cloning of the tumour antigen gene. Ultimately the mutant gene coding for the tumour antigen (the tum- gene) was identified and sequenced. Comparison of this gene with the homologous gene from the parental tumour showed a single amino acid difference. Formal proof that this mutation could generate the immunogenic antigen recognized by the Tc cells was then obtained: parental tumour cells

Immunization to tumour antigens

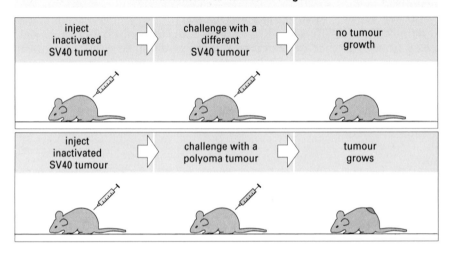

Fig.17.4 Demonstration of common tumour associated transplantation antigens (TATAs). Inbred mice were immunized with an SV40 virus-induced tumour by repeated injection of tumour cells inactivated by irradiation. Half the mice were challenged with a different SV40 tumour and half with a tumour induced by polyomavirus. The mice could reject the SV40 but not the polyomavirus tumour, showing that they were immune to T antigens of SV40.

Demonstration of tumour specific antigens of chemically-induced tumours

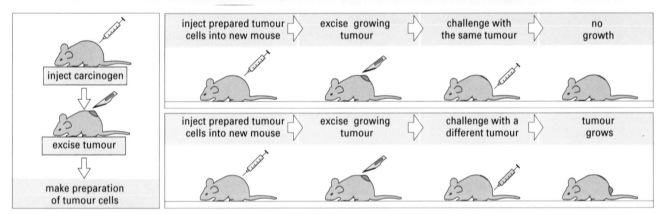

Fig. 17.5 Mice were induced to produce tumours by the injection of a chemical carcinogen (methyl cholanthrene). Tumour cells from these mice were then injected subcutaneously into genetically identical mice. Later, the growing tumours were removed surgically. Mice challenged with the same tumour were able to reject it, but those challenged with a different tumour (induced with the same carcinogen) were not.

incubated with a ten-amino acid peptide having the tum- sequence could be killed, while if they were incubated with the homologous peptide from parental cells they were not (Fig. 17.7). (Tc cells are MHC class I restricted, so it seems likely that the tumour-specific protein is processed within the cell to generate a peptide which then becomes associated with MHC class I and is transported to the cell surface.)

There is good evidence that there are class II restricted responses to human tumours, but much less is known about tumour antigens recognized in association with MHC class II. These are discussed in more detail below.

TUMOUR ASSOCIATED ANTIGENS

There have been many attempts to detect antigens unique to tumours, using either serum from the tumour-bearing host (autologous typing) or sera derived from animals deliberately immunized with tumour material (heterologous typing). Recent work has relied on monoclonal antibodies, derived from either autologous or heterologous B cells. Although there is very little evidence for molecules uniquely expressed in tumours, several types of antigen (some neo-antigens and some differentiation antigens) associated with tumours in some way have been identified.

WIDELY DIFFERENTIATED ANTIGENS

These are widely distributed on, or more commonly in, tumour and normal cells. These are the types of antigen most often detected with sera from tumour-bearing patients, or monoclonal antibodies derived from them. The antibodies are often IgM and of low affinity. Similar monoclonal antibodies can be derived by immortalizing B lymphocytes from normal individuals. These antibodies detect autoantigens and their importance in the host response to tumours (if any) is unclear.

NORMAL DIFFERENTIATION ANTIGENS WITH RESTRICTED DISTRIBUTION

Most tumour cells represent the clonal progeny of a single cell, and cells of that type may be relatively rare. The tumour cells may therefore express antigens present on only a few normal cells. The Common Acute Lymphoblastic Leukaemia Antigen (CALLA or CD10) is an example (Fig. 17.8).

ONCOFETAL ANTIGENS

Tumours may express antigens normally not expressed, or expressed at very low levels, in adult life but present during fetal development. Examples of this are α-fetoprotein, which is produced by liver cancer cells, and carcinoembryonic antigen (CEA) produced by colon cancer cells and other epithelial tumours.

Specificity of tumour immunity

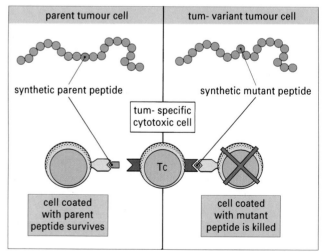

Specificity of Tc cells for a tumour antigen peptide

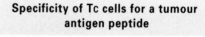

Fig. 17.6 The production of a highly immunogenic (tum-) variant tumour and Tc cells specific for it. After inducing mutations in the parent tumour cells, subclones were obtained, some of which would no longer grow in DBA2 mice. Spleen Tc cells from mice injected with these tum- cells could kill tum-, but not the parent tumour, *in vitro*.

Fig. 17.7 Tc cells were taken from a mouse immunized with a tum- variant tumour. *In vitro*, they killed tumour cells coated with a peptide from the tum- gene sequence, but not cells coated with the cumulated homologous peptide from the parental tumour. The two peptides differ by a single amino acid.

ALTERED ANTIGENS

Glycosylation is altered in many tumours. This may give rise to the expression of new carbohydrate epitopes, such as the Thomsen–Friedenreich antigen, a disaccharide which is usually hidden on normal cells. Aberrant blood groups can also be created in this way. Alterations in glycosylation may also reveal epitopes on the protein backbone which are rarely detected in normal cells. For example, polymorphic epithelial mucins are produced by many normal epithelial cells. They are high molecular weight glycoproteins with a repeating core peptide carrying the carbohydrate side chains. In epithelial tumours, a new protein epitope can be detected in the repeating core structure.

 ## IMMUNE RESPONSES TO HUMAN TUMOURS

THE IMMUNE RESPONSE TO TUMOURS *IN SITU*

Histological studies of human tumours have shown that the majority contain a marked infiltrate of inflammatory cells (Fig. 17.9). Lymphocytes and macrophages usually predominate but other cells can be detected including dendritic cells, granulocytes and mast cells. The use of monoclonal antibodies to detect lymphoid cell subtypes has allowed a more refined analysis of cell types within tumours (Fig. 17.10), and has shown that most major lymphocyte subtypes can be found in tumours.

Expression of CALLA in normal cells and lymphomas

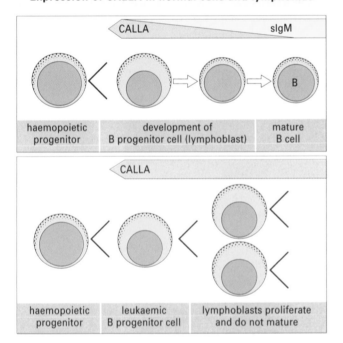

Fig. 17.8 CALLA is normally expressed only on B cell progenitors or lymphoblasts, which make up <1% of normal bone marrow cells. CALLA becomes much more abundant in the commonest form of childhood leukaemia.

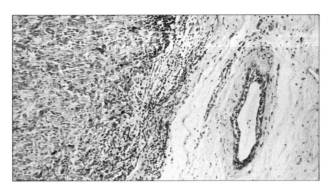

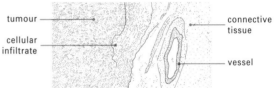

Fig. 17.9 Immunological reaction to a mammary carcinoma. The section shows a mammary tumour heavily infiltrated with mononuclear cells. Such inflammation suggests that tumours may be recognized by cells of the immune system which are potentially active in limiting or eliminating the tumour cells. H&E stain, ×50.

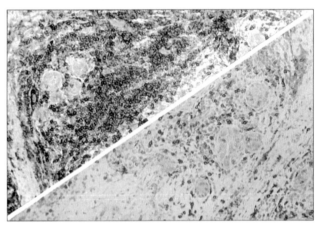

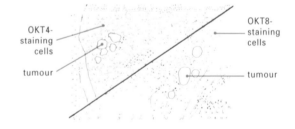

Fig. 17.10 CD4$^+$ and CD8$^+$ T cells in carcinoma of the breast. CD4$^+$ and CD8$^+$cells were detected by the immunoperoxidase technique (dark stain) using OKT4 or OKT8 antibodies respectively. The sections are counterstained with haematoxylin. With OKT4 (upper) CD4 cells were seen throughout the tumour, whereas OKT8 (lower) showed that there were fewer CD8 cells, and these were around the edge of the tumour.

The state of activation of the cells can also be analysed using monoclonal antibodies (mAbs) specific for the IL-2 receptor, MHC class II molecules and other activation markers. However no very clear associations have yet emerged between the presence of particular subtypes of lymphoid cells and the cancer patient's prognosis. This may be because only a small fraction of the infiltrating cells observed are actually recruited specifically to the the tumour site. This difficulty in interpretation has led to attempts to analyse the function of tumour infiltrating lymphocytes *in vitro*. These studies are discussed in the next section.

DETECTION OF IMMUNE RESPONSES *IN VITRO*
Early attempts to detect cell-mediated responses to human tumours used colony inhibition assays. The tumour target cells were incubated with peripheral blood lymphocytes, and after a period of time surviving tumour cells grew into colonies which could be counted. These early data showed that lymphocytes from tumour patients would kill their own tumour cells, but would also kill tumour cells from other patients, if these were of the same cytological tumour type. The cytotoxicity therefore appeared to be tumour-type specific but not genetically restricted. Later it was realized that lymphocytes of normal individuals were also cytotoxic to tumour cells. It became clear that most of this cytotoxicity was due to natural killer (NK) cells and that tumour patients and controls differed little in the target specificity of their NK cells.

MIXED LYMPHOCYTE–TUMOUR INTERACTIONS
The discovery of NK activity and the later realization that Tc cells generally require an *in vitro* boost with antigen before their cytotoxicity is revealed, led to many experiments in which lymphocytes from patients were stimulated by inactivated tumour cells in mixed lymphocyte–tumour interaction (MLTI) (Fig. 17.11) to see whether the patient's immune system could react to the tumour. The lymphocytes might be taken from peripheral blood, from tumour-draining lymph nodes or from the tumour itself (the latter are known as tumour-infiltrating lymphocytes or TILs).

The MLTI assay is designed to measure the ability of the patient's T cells to respond to their tumour, but in these assays Tc cells are generated and it is possible to measure their cytotoxic activity by ^{51}Cr-release assay (see Chapter 25). Tc cells can also be stimulated by culturing them in IL-2 to expand any effector cells generated *in vivo*. One should distinguish the activity of Tc cells from that of NK cells, which can be done by assaying the expanded lymphocyte population on appropriate target cells.

The mixed lymphocyte–tumour interaction

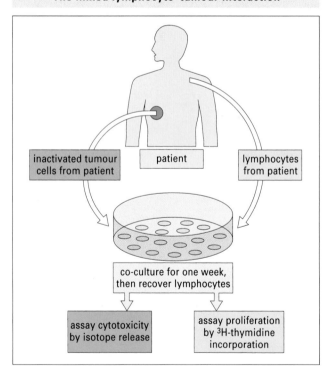

Fig. 17.11 Lymphocytes taken from blood, from draining lymph nodes or directly from tumour tissue, are co-cultured with autologous tumour cells, which have been inactivated by x-irradiation or treatment with mitomycin-C. After a suitable period of culture, the lymphocytes are assayed for proliferation by incorporation of ^{3}H–thymidine (included in the culture medium). They can be assayed for their ability to lyse target cells in isotope release assays.

Patterns of response generated in MLTI

target cell	responder lymphocytes			
	tumour specific Tc	autoreative Tc	tumour specific MHC-restricted cytotoxic cells	NK cells ± Tc cells
NK target	–	–	–	+
allogeneic tumour	–	–	+	+
autologous normal cell	–	+	–	+
autologous tumour	+	+	+	+

Fig 17.12 Lymphocytes harvested from MLTI are assayed in a ^{51}Cr release assay on several different tumour or normal cells. Killing is detected by release of isotope into the supernatant of the cultures. Several patterns of specificity can be detected in the lymphocytes from different patients, varying from lysis of the autologous tumour only, to non-specific lysis of all target cells. The latter may be due to either activated NK cells or T cells. Among the T cells, CD4 and CD8 cells behave in a similar way, both showing the same variety of responses.

SPECIFICITY OF HUMAN ANTI-TUMOUR LYMPHOCYTES

The specificities of both CD4 and CD8 cells are similar and show a variety of patterns of reactivity against different targets in different patients (Fig. 17.12).

1. In both cases a minority of cloned T cells are specific for autologous tumour.

2. Some clones react to autologous tumour and all, or a proportion, of autologous tissues tested.

3. Some clones show reactivity to autologous and some allogeneic tumours.

4. The remaining cells show broad reactivity to many tumour targets.

The third pattern is reminiscent of the tumour type specificity described for the early colony inhibition experiments (see p. 17.6). Recent data suggest that this type of clone may respond in a specific but unrestricted fashion to the repeating core peptide of mucin. It is not yet clear whether the peptide is presented by MHC molecules or in some other fashion (for example acting as a superantigen). Mucin-responsive cells may be of CD4 or CD8 type.

The *in vivo* significance of the cytotoxic responses detected *in vitro* remains uncertain, but in animal model experiments, cloned anti-tumour cytolytic cells can cause tumour regression.

IMMUNE ESCAPE MECHANISMS

Since spontaneous tumours grow and kill the host, many tumours must escape the host immune response. A variety of mechanisms have been proposed. The most obvious is that the tumour is non-immunogenic. If a tumour is immunogenic, several mechanisms may protect it. First it might 'sneak through', meaning that when the tumour is small it is not recognized by the immune system, and by the time it stimulates a response the tumour is too large to be contained. This phenomenon has been demonstrated experimentally (Fig 17.13). Alternatively, blocking or suppressive mechanisms might operate on the immune system. Although the role of blocking antibodies and Ts cells is uncertain, some tumours produce cytokines (e.g. TGFβ) that can inhibit immune responses.

Tumour cells may also evade immune responses by loss of molecules important for immune recognition. Loss of an MHC class I allele, or even all class I molecules, is well recognized in tumours (Fig 17.14). Alternatively tumours may lack molecules required for adhesion of lymphocytes, such as LFA-1 and LFA-3, or acquire molecules which alter their metastatic capability, such as CD44. For example, Burkitt's lymphoma cells are resistant to Tc-mediated lysis, because of low expression of LFA-1. Another example is the expression of an alternatively spliced form of CD44 in metastatic tumour cells of rat. Another protective mechanism may occur on cells which increase their levels of surface ICAM-1 expression – this occurs in disease progression in melanoma. ICAM-1 has some homology with complement-binding proteins and may protect against complement-mediated lysis.

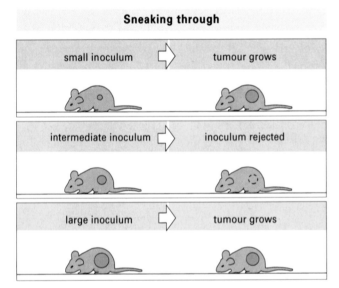

Sneaking through

small inoculum ⇨ tumour grows

intermediate inoculum ⇨ inoculum rejected

large inoculum ⇨ tumour grows

Fig. 17.13 Graded doses of tumour cells are injected into non-immune mice. Small doses grow progressively, because they do not stimulate an immune response until the tumour is established, intermediate doses are rejected, while large doses overwhelm the response and once more grow progressively.

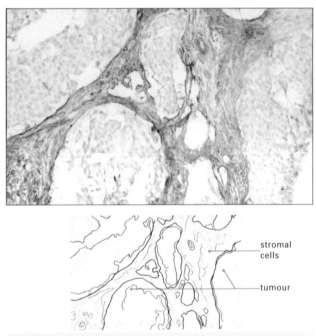

stromal cells

tumour

Fig. 17.14 Breast cancer tissue reactive with monoclonal antibody (2A1) to the monomorphic determinant of HLA class I antigens. Only stromal cells are stained, as malignant epithelial cells fail to express normal MHC class I antigens. Some 50% of primary human breast cancers fall into this category. Aberrant class II expression may also occur on some tumours. (Indirect immunoperoxidase technique, counterstained with haematoxylin.)

IMMUNODIAGNOSIS

Although there are few molecules which are exclusive to tumour cells, antibodies to tumour-associated molecules can be very useful in tumour diagnosis, by either detecting increased amounts of an antigen or the presence of an antigen in an abnormal site.

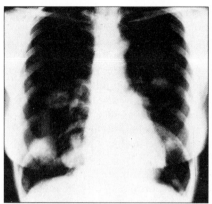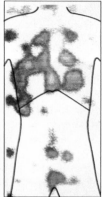

Fig. 17.15 Chest radiograph and immunoscintigraphy scan of a patient with carcinoma of the colon who has lung and liver metastases. The monoclonal antibody YPC2/12.1, raised against human colorectal cancer, binds to carcino-embryonic antigen. (It reacts with a glycoprotein of 180 kD.) The antibody was radiolabelled with ^{131}I and administered intravenously. Scintigrams were obtained after 48 hours. The image is that obtained after a subtraction procedure to eliminate background blood-borne antibody. (Courtesy of Professor K. Sikora.)

IN VIVO

Radiolabelled antibodies against tumour-associated molecules have been used for detection of tumours (Fig. 17.15) but the method is seldom more sensitive than modern methods of computerized tomography or nuclear magnetic resonance imaging. In addition immunoscintigraphy has the disadvantage that antibodies need to be freshly labelled for each patient, and different antibodies are optimal for different tumour types.

IN VITRO

Antibodies are useful for identifying the cell of origin of undifferentiated tumours (Fig. 17.16) and for the detection of micrometastases in bone marrow, cerebrospinal fluid, lymphoid organs or elsewhere (Fig. 17.17). There are also immunoassays available for several tumour-associated molecules which can be detected in the serum. These include CEA and AFP. Raised levels of either of these molecules may be useful in diagnosis, but neither is associated with only one tumour type, so they are generally more useful in following the course of treatment (Fig. 17.18).

IMMUNOTHERAPY

Immunotherapy has a long history but it is rarely the treatment of first choice. Intervention may be active or passive, specific or non-specific. Figure 17.19 summarizes the possibilities.

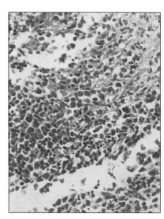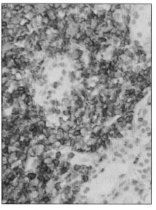

Fig.17.16 Identification of the cell of origin of an undifferentiated tumour. Conventional histology of a biopsy of this tumour showed a sheet of undifferentiated tumour cells which could not be identified. When the tumour was stained by the indirect immunoperoxidase method with an antibody against CD45 (the leucocyte common antigen), it was found to be strongly positive, identifying it as a lymphoma.

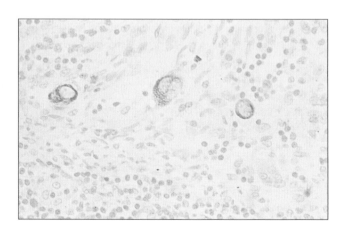

Fig 17.17 Detection of micrometastases using a monoclonal antibody. The figure shows a section of tumour draining lymph node taken from a patient with cancer of the breast. The section is stained by the indirect immunoperoxidase method with an antibody against a cytokeratin. Carcinoma cells express cytokeratins and are clearly stained brown. Scattered single tumour cells, such as are present in this lymph node, are easily missed by conventional histological examination.

ACTIVE IMMUNIZATION

Specific active immunization with inactivated tumour cells has shown some success in animal models where immunization occurred before tumour challenge.

Attempts to induce regression of established tumours have been much less successful. While much effort has been expended in designing means of making tumour cells more immunogenic (Fig 17.20), most of these antedate present day understanding of the way in

Monitoring serum CEA level in colon carcinoma

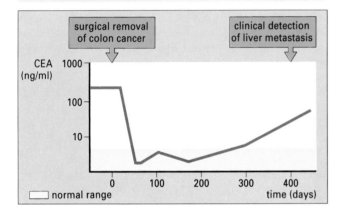

Fig. 17.18 Relationship of serum carcinoembryonic antigen (CEA) level to clinical course in a patient with carcinoma of the colon. At presentation there is a high CEA level, which falls following surgery. A rise is found well before the clinical detection of metastatic tumour.

Immunotherapy of tumours

active	non-specific	BCG, *Corynebacterium parvum*, levamisole
	specific	preventive vaccines of tumour cells, cell extracts, purified or recombinant antigens, or idiotypes
passive	non-specific	LAK cells, cytokines
	specific	antibodies alone or coupled to drugs, pro-drugs, toxins or radioisotopes bi-specific antibodies T cells
	combined	LAK cells and bi-specific antibody

Fig. 17.19 Non-specific mechanisms boost general immune functions or specific killer cells, often in conjunction with cytokines. Specific antibody-mediated cytotoxicity may also be effective.

Augmentation of host response

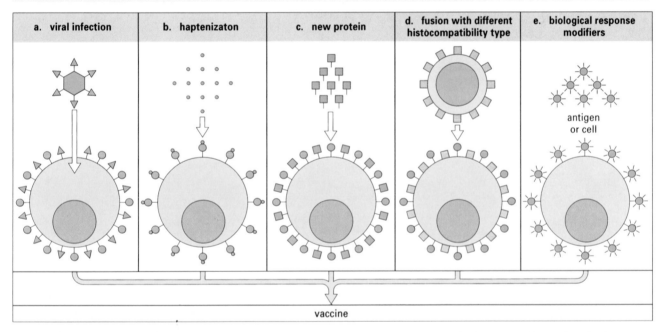

Fig. 17.20 Vaccination against tumours is aimed at increasing the host response to tumour by: a. infecting the tumour with virus, b. coupling haptens to the tumour surface antigens, c. coupling protein antigens to the tumour surface, d. fusing the tumour with cells of a different histocompatibility type, e. increasing the immune response with adjuvants and other biological response modifiers. These procedures have been tried in experimental animals, before or after challenge with tumours, and some (e.g. e) have also been tried in humans.

which antigenic epitopes are presented to T cells in association with MHC molecules. Where these strategies work, they probably act mainly by inducing an inflammatory response, which promotes expansion of antigen-specific T cells and might help to overcome any inhibitory effects of the tumour. There is little evidence however that specific active immunization has been effective so far in man.

A variety of agents have been used to stimulate the immune response non-specifically (Fig. 17.21). Most attempts at systemic therapy in man have not been conspicuously successful, but intralesional BCG can cause regression of melanoma, and non-specific local immunization with BCG is effective against bladder tumours.

Since there is increasing evidence for a role of viruses in some human cancers, the most promising avenue for active immunization may be in preventing infection with potentially oncogenic agents. Successful mass immunization against hepatitis B virus will certainly decrease the incidence of primary hepatoma. It may be possible eventually to vaccinate at-risk populations against papillomaviruses, HTLV-1 or EBV.

 ## PASSIVE IMMUNOTHERAPY

THERAPY WITH ANTIBODIES

Early attempts at passive immunotherapy with polyclonal antisera were limited because of the difficulty of achieving high titre and specificity. The advent of monoclonal antibodies promised to overcome these difficulties, but so far progress has been slow. This is because,

with the exception of B-cell and T-cell idiotypes on lymphomas, no antigens unique to tumours have yet been discovered. Nevertheless some antigens show increased expression on certain tumour cells, which may open the way to antibody treatment. In other cases, damage to normal body cells carrying the same antigen may be unimportant or tolerable. Monoclonal antibodies may be used either alone, or coupled to drugs, pro-drugs, toxins, cytokines or isotopes (Fig. 17.22). There are however a number of limitations to antibody therapy.

1. Antibody penetration into large tumour masses is often poor. In principle this might be overcome by smaller molecules that retain specific antigen binding, e.g. F(ab') fragments, or by engineered single-domain antibodies. Alternatively, it may be possible to target therapy to the endothelium of tumour blood vessels.

2. Antibodies are bound by any normal cells expressing the target antigen, and non-specifically by cells bearing Fc receptors or receptors for immunoglobulin carbohydrates. Chemical modification or genetic engineering of the antibody molecules may partially overcome these difficulties. Better discrimination between tumour and normal cells might be obtained with bi-specific antibodies against two different antigens which are both present on the tumour cells but only found separately on normal cells.

3. Antibodies are immunogenic and may therefore be attacked by the immune system. Even chimeric or humanized antibodies may induce an immune response to their idiotype. The use of different MAbs for successive courses of therapy might solve this problem.

Examples of biological response modifiers

type of BRM	examples	major effect
bacterial products	BCG, *C. parvum*, muramyl dipeptide, trehalase dimycolate	activate macrophages and NK cells
synthetic molecules	pyran copolymer, MVE, poly I:C, pyrimidines	induce interferon production
cytokines	IFN$_\alpha$, IFN$_\beta$, IFN$_\gamma$, IL-2, TNF	activate macrophages and NK cells
hormones	thymosin, thymulin, thymopoietin	modulate T cell function

Fig. 17.21 Biological response modifiers (BRMs) are used to enhance immune responses to tumours and fall into four major groups. Broadly speaking, bacterial products have adjuvant effects on macrophages; a variety of synthetic polymers, nucleotides and polynucleotides induce interferon production and release; the cytokines administered directly act on macrophages and NK cells, and a variety of hormones including the thymic hormones, can be used to enhance T cell function. (MVE = maleic anhydride divinyl ether.)

Therapeutic modification of monoclonal antibodies

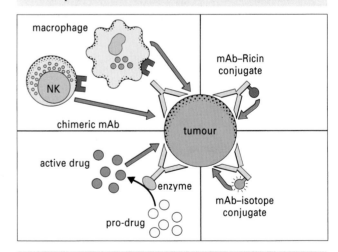

Fig. 17.22 Genetically engineered chimeric antibodies with a human Fc portion reduce the risk of an immune response to the mAb. Human Fc will also recruit human effector mechanisms. Alternatively, various molecules can be coupled to mAbs for targeting to tumour cells. These include toxins, radioactive isotopes, cytotoxic drugs or enzymes capable of activating pro-drugs.

Because of these difficulties (which may eventually be overcome) antibody therapy has been most effective when penetration to the tumour can be ensured, for example for blood-borne tumours (leukaemias) or those in the peritoneal cavity. MAbs may also be used *in vitro* to purge bone marrow of tumour cells before bone marrow transplantation (Fig. 17.23).

In vitro purging of tumour-infiltrated bone marrow

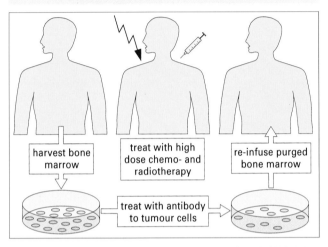

Fig. 17.23 Bone marrow containing tumour cells can be purged using monoclonal antibodies and complement, antibody–toxin conjugates or antibodies coupled to magnetic beads. The purged marrow is stored while the patient is given high dose chemo- and radiotherapy. The purged marrow is then returned to the patient. This therapy has given encouraging results in some leukaemia and lymphoma patients who were not helped by conventional therapy.

Antibody-targeted cellular therapy

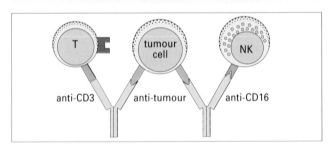

Fig 17.24 Bi-specific antibodies can be constructed either by chemical coupling of two mAbs or by making quadromas by fusion of two different monoclonal antibody-secreting hybridomas. A bi-specific antibody can be used to target effector cells to a tumour surface antigen. Antibodies to some leucocyte cell surface molecules (e.g. CD3 on T cells) have the additional advantage that they activate T cells. *In vitro* this method of targeting can significantly increase specific killing of tumour cells.

LYMPHOKINE ACTIVATED KILLER (LAK) CELLS

When human peripheral blood mononuclear cells are cultured *in vitro* with IL-2, they become highly cytotoxic to a wide variety of tumour targets, many of which are resistant to freshly isolated NK cells. Initial animal and human experiments, in which LAK cells were re-infused, gave some good results, especially when IL-2 was given at the same time. However, controlled trials have given less encouraging results and the therapy, involving high-dose IL-2, has significant toxicity. It seems likely that few LAK cells localize in tumours, and this may contribute to the poor results. To overcome this, bi-specific mAbs have been used. In these, one antibody is directed against a tumour molecule and the other against lymphocyte surface markers. In theory these antibodies should help to localize the LAK cells on the tumour (Fig 17.24). While such strategies certainly work *in vitro*, their effectiveness *in vivo* is less clear.

TUMOUR INFILTRATING LYMPHOCYTES (TILs)

T cells extracted from tumour sites can be grown *in vitro* using IL-2 and eventually re-infused. In a proportion of cases the cultured T cells show relative specificity for the tumour from which they were derived. In animal model systems there is no doubt that tumour-specific cytotoxic T cells can cause dramatic regression of tumour. The tumour toxicity of such TILs may be increased by transfecting into them genes coding for cytokine production. However, the real efficacy of such strategies in humans remains to be tested.

Cytokine therapy for tumours

cytokine	tumour type and results	cytokine effects and possible anti-tumour mechanisms
IFN$_\alpha$	prolonged remissions of hairy-cell leukaemia	possible cytostatic effect on tumour
	weak effects on some carcinomas	increased expression of MHC class I, cytostasis
IFN$_\gamma$	ineffective systemically, remissions of peritoneal carcinoma of the ovary	increased MHC class I and II macrophage activation, Tc activation, cytostasis
IL-2	remissions in renal cancer and melanoma	T cell activation and proliferation, NK cell activation
TNF$_\alpha$	can reduce malignant ascites	?increased tumour cell adhesion, macropage and lymphocyte activation

Fig 17.25 Most cytokines have been given systemically in high doses. The mechanism of the anti-tumour effect is uncertain in most cases. *In vitro*, IFNs and TNF$_\alpha$ are cytostatic for some tumour cells, but *in vivo* any effects seen may be indirect, since many cytokines induce production of other cytokines (the cytokine cascade). The fact that some patients treated with IL-2 suffer transient autoimmune thyroiditis provides some evidence that cytokine administration does potentiate immune responses.

CYTOKINES

Many cytokines have been cloned, expressed and used for tumour therapy. (Fig. 17.25 gives information on those which have been most thoroughly investigated so far.) Successes have so far been few and far between, though IFN_α can induce prolonged remission of the rare hairy-cell leukaemia and IL-2 is effective in a proportion of melanomas and renal carcinomas. There are also encouraging results in treatment of intra-peritoneal ovarian tumours with IFN_γ and TNF_α. However, it is possible that cytokines have so far been used in an inappropriate way. Generally they have been used in a similar fashion to cytotoxic drugs, that is in the highest tolerable dose. Recent data in head and neck cancer suggests that lower doses may be equally, if not more, effective. Used in this way, cytokines also have far fewer adverse effects.

Some cytokines are finding a useful role in supportive therapy. Colony stimulating factors can shorten the period of aplasia after bone marrow transplantation or cytotoxic therapy, and erythropoietin can relieve the anaemia.

FURTHER READING

Balkwill FR. *Cytokines in Cancer Therapy*. Oxford: Oxford University Press, 1989.

Cancer immunotherapy update. *Immunol Today* 1990;**11**:190–200.

De Plaen E, Lurquin C, Van Pel A, *et al*. Tum- variants of mouse mastocytoma P815. Cloning of the gene of tum- antigen O91A and identification of the tum- mutation. *Proc Nat Acad Sci* 1988;**85**:2274–78.

Fanger MW, Segal DM, Romet-Lemonne J-L. Bispecific antibodies and targeted cellular cytotoxicity. *Immunol Today* 1991;**12**:51–54.

Franks LM, Teich N. *Introduction to the cellular and molecular biology of cancer*. Oxford: Oxford University Press, 1991.

Herlyn M, Menrad A, Koprowski H. Structure, function and clinical significance of human tumour antigens. *J Nat Cancer Inst* 1990;**82**:1883–89.

Koprowski H, Rovera G. Cancer. *Curr Opin Cancer* 1990; **2**:681–82.

Perussia B. Lymphokine-activated killer cells, natural killer cells and cytokines. *Curr Opin Immunol* 1991;**3**:49–55.

Topalian SL, Solomon D, Rosenberg SA. Tumour-specific cytolysis by lymphocytes infiltrating human melanomas. *J Immunol* 1989;**142**:3714–25.

chapter 18

Immunodeficiency

Immunodeficiency disease results from the absence, or failure of normal function, of one or more elements of the immune system. Specific immunodeficiency diseases involve abnormalities of T or B cells, the cells of the adaptive immune system. Non-specific immunodeficiency diseases involve abnormalities of elements such as complement or phagocytes, which act non-specifically in immunity. Primary immunodeficiency diseases are due to intrinsic defects in cells of the immune system and are for the most part genetically determined. Secondary immunodeficiency diseases result from extrinsic factors, such as drugs, irradiation, malnutrition or infection. Thus AIDS is a secondary immunodeficiency resulting from a virus infection.

Immunodeficiency diseases cause increased susceptibility to infection in patients. The infections encountered in immunodeficient patients fall, broadly speaking, into two categories. Patients with defects in immunoglobulins or complement proteins or phagocytes are very susceptible to recurrent infections with encapsulated bacteria, such as *Haemophilus influenzae*, *Streptococcus pneumoniae*, *Staphylococcus aureus*, etc. They are called pyogenic infections because these bacteria give rise to pus formation. On the other hand, patients with defects in cell-mediated immunity, i.e. in T cells, are susceptible to overwhelming, even lethal, infections with microorganisms that are ubiquitous in the environment and to which normal people rapidly develop resistance. For this reason, they are called opportunistic infections; opportunistic microorganisms include yeast and common viruses such as chickenpox.

B-CELL DEFICIENCIES

Common defects in B-cell function are listed in Fig. 18.1. Patients with these defects have recurrent pyogenic infection such as pneumonia, otitis media and sinusitis. If untreated, they develop severe obstructive lung disease (bronchiectasis) from recurrent pneumonia, which destroys the elasticity of the airways.

X-LINKED AGAMMAGLOBULINEMIA (X-LA)

The model B-cell deficiency is X-linked agammaglobulinaemia. It was the first immunodeficiency disease to be understood in detail, the underlying deficiency being discovered in 1952. Affected males have no B cells in their blood or lymphoid tissue; consequently their lymph nodes are very small and their tonsils are absent. Their serum contains no IgA, IgM, IgD or IgE and only small amounts of IgG (less than 100 mg/dl). For the first 6–12 months of life, they are protected from infection by maternal IgG that crossed the placenta into the fetus. As this supply of IgG is exhausted, affected males develop recurrent pyogenic infections. If they are infused intravenously with large doses of gammaglobulin they remain healthy.

The X-LA gene is on the long arm of the X-chromosome (Fig. 18.2). This is the site of many other immuno-

Primary B-cell deficiencies

X-linked agammaglobulinaemia
IgA deficiency
IgG subclass deficiency
immunodeficiency with increased IgM
common variable immunodeficiency
transient hypogammaglobulinaemia of infancy

Fig. 18.1 The range of B-cell deficiencies varies from a delayed maturation of normal immunoglobulin production, through single isotype deficiencies to X-linked agammaglobulinaemia, where affected male children have no B cells and no serum immunoglobulins.

The X-linked immunodeficiencies

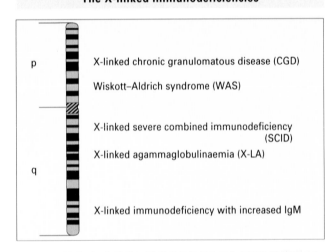

Fig. 18.2 The genes for many immunodeficiency diseases are located on the long arm of the X-chromosome. Except for CGD, it is not yet known what these various loci encode or what leads to the immunodeficiency. (Adapted from Schwaber J, Rosen FS. *Immunodeficiency Rev* 1990:2;235.)

deficiency diseases; the localization of these genes facilitates prenatal diagnosis. Except for chronic granulomatous disease (see below), it is not known what these various loci encode or what leads to the immunodeficiency, but rapid progress is being made in isolating these genes. Bone marrow of males with X-LA contains normal numbers of pre-B cells which, for unknown reasons, cannot mature into B cells (Fig. 18.3).

IgA DEFICIENCY AND IgG SUBCLASS DEFICIENCY

IgA deficiency is the most common immunodeficiency. One in 700 Caucasians have the defect, but it is not found, or is found only rarely, in other ethnic groups. People with IgA deficiency tend to develop immune-complex disease (Type II hypersensitivity). About 20% of IgA-deficient individuals also lack IgG2 and IgG4, and are very susceptible to pyogenic infections. In humans, most antibodies to the capsular polysacchar-

ides of pyogenic bacteria are in the IgG2 subclass. A deficiency in IgG2 alone therefore results in recurrent pyogenic infections as well. For reasons that are unclear, individuals with deficiency of IgG3 only are also susceptible to recurrent infections. These class and subclass deficiencies result from failures in terminal differentiation of B cells (see Fig. 18.3).

IMMUNODEFICIENCY WITH INCREASED IgM

A peculiar immunodeficiency results in patients who are IgG- and IgA-deficient but synthesize large amounts (more than 200 mg/dl) of polyclonal IgM. They are susceptible to pyogenic infections and should be treated with intravenous gamma-globulin. They tend to form IgM autoantibodies to neutrophils, platelets and other elements of the blood, as well as to tissue antigens, thereby adding the complexities of autoimmune disease to the immunodeficiency. The tissues, particularly of

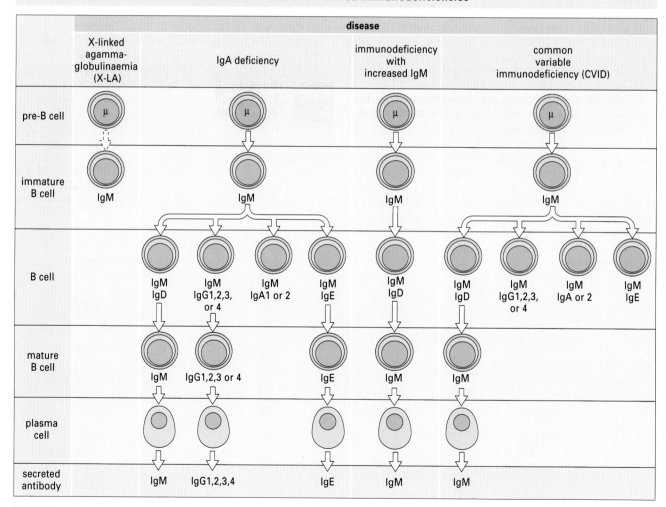

B-cell maturation in X-linked immunodeficiencies

Fig. 18.3 **X-LA**-affected male infants have no B cells and no serum immunoglobulins, except for small amounts of maternal IgG. In **IgA deficiency**, IgA-bearing B cells and in some cases IgG2- and IgG4-bearing B cells, are unable to differentiate into plasma cells. People with **immunodeficiency with increased IgM** lack IgG and IgA. **CVID** B cells of most isotypes are unable to differentiate into plasma cells.

the gastrointestinal tract, become infiltrated with IgM-producing cells (Fig. 18.4).

COMMON VARIABLE IMMUNODEFICIENCY (CVID)

Individuals with CVID have acquired agammaglobulinaemia in the second or third decade of life, or later. Both males and females are equally affected and the cause of the acquisition of agammaglobulinaemia is generally not known, but may follow infection with viruses such as Epstein–Barr virus (EBV), which causes infectious mononucleosis. Patients with CVID, like males with X-LA, are very susceptible to pyogenic organisms and to the intestinal protozoan, *Giardia lamblia*, which causes severe diarrhoea (Fig. 18.5). Most patients (80%) with CVID have B cells that do not function properly. The B-cell defects are very variable, however, and some patients also have decreased T cell function. CVID should be treated with intravenous gamma-globulin as it provides protection against recurrent pyogenic infections. Many patients with CVID develop autoimmune diseases, most prominently pernicious anaemia, and the reason for this is not known. CVID is not hereditary, but is commonly associated with the MHC haplotypes HLA-B8 and HLA-DR3.

TRANSIENT HYPOGAMMAGLOBULINAEMIA OF INFANCY

As mentioned above, infants are protected initially by their mother's IgG. The maternal IgG is catabolized, with a half-life of approximately 30 days. By three months of age, normal infants begin to synthesize antibodies, although antibody formation to bacterial capsular polysaccharides does not commence in earnest until the second year of life. In some infants, the onset of normal IgG synthesis is retarded for as long as 36 months and, until then, such infants are susceptible to pyogenic infections. The B cells of these infants are normal but they appear to lack help from CD4$^+$ T cells to synthesize antibodies.

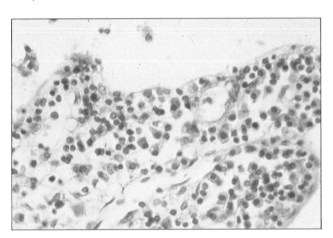

Fig. 18.4 Gall bladder from a patient with immuno-deficiency with increased IgM. The submucosa is filled with cells with pink-staining cytoplasm and eccentric nuclei. The cells are synthesizing and secreting IgM.

T-CELL DEFICIENCIES

The major T-cell deficiencies are shown in Fig. 18.6. Patients with no T cells, or poor T-cell function, are susceptible to opportunistic infections. Since B-cell function in humans is T-cell dependent, T-cell deficiency also results in humoral immunodeficiency; in other words T-cell deficiency leads to a combined deficiency of both humoral and cell-mediated immunity.

SEVERE COMBINED IMMUNODEFICIENCY (SCID)

The most profound hereditary deficiency of cell-mediated immunity occurs in infants with severe combined immunodeficiency. Infants with SCID develop recurrent infections early in life (in contrast to X-LA). They have prolonged diarrhoea due to rotavirus or bacterial infection of the gastrointestinal tract. They develop pneumonia, usually due to the protozoan, *Pneumocystis carinii*.

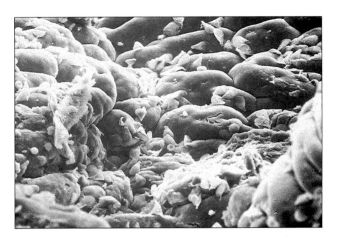

Fig. 18.5 *Giardia lamblia*. Innumerable giardia parasites can be seen swarming over the mucosa of the jejunum of a patient with common variable immunodeficiency.

Primary-T cell deficiencies

severe combined immunodeficiency
adenosine deaminase deficiency
purine nucleoside phosphorylase deficiency
MHC class II deficiency
DiGeorge anomaly
hereditary ataxia telangiectasia
Wiskott–Aldrich syndrome

Fig. 18.6 There is a wide range of causes for T-cell deficiencies, ranging from absence of lymphocytes, to enzyme deficiency, through to MHC deficiency. All affect the ability of T cells to function properly which in turn leads to humoral deficiency, i.e. combined T- and B-cell deficiency.

The common yeast organism *Candida albicans* grows luxuriantly in their mouth or on their skin (Fig. 18.7). If they are vaccinated with live organisms, such as vaccinia virus (used for immunization against smallpox) or Bacille Calmette–Guerin (used for immunization against tuberculosis) they die of progressive infection from these ordinarily benign organisms. SCID is incompatible with life and affected infants usually die within the first two years unless they are rescued with transplants of bone marrow. In this case they are rendered into lymphocyte chimeras and can survive and live normally.

Infants with SCID have very few lymphocytes in their blood (fewer than 3000/µl). Their lymphoid tissue also contains no or few lymphocytes. The thymus gland has a fetal appearance (Fig. 18.8) containing the endodermal stromal cells derived embryonically from the third and fourth pharyngeal pouch. Lymphoid stem cells, which normally populate the thymus by six weeks of human gestation, have failed to appear and the thymus does not become a lymphoid organ.

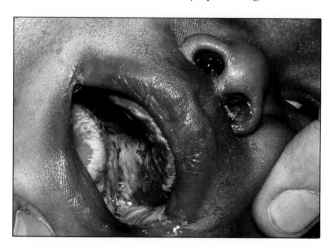

Fig. 18.7 *Candida albicans* **in the mouth, in a patient with severe combined immunodeficiency.** This organism grows luxuriantly in the mouth and on the skin of SCID patients.

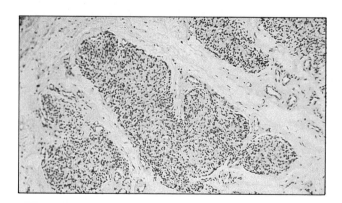

Fig. 18.8 Thymus of severe combined immunodeficiency. Note that the thymic stroma has not been invaded by lymphoid cells and no Hassall's corpuscles are seen. The gland has a fetal appearance.

SCID is more common in male than female infants (3:1). This is because over 50% of SCID cases are caused by a gene on the X-chromosome. The remaining cases of SCID are due to recessive genes on other chromosomes; of these, half have a genetic deficiency of adenosine deaminase (ADA) or purine nucleoside phosphorylase (PNP). Deficiency of these purine degradation enzymes results in the accumulation of metabolites that are toxic to lymphoid stem cells, namely dATP and dGTP (Fig. 18.9). These metabolites inhibit the enzyme ribonucleotide reductase, which is required for DNA synthesis and, therefore, for cell replication. Since ADA and PNP are found in all mammalian cells, why should these defects only affect lymphocytes? The explanation appears to lie in the relative deficiency of 5'-nucleotidase in lymphoid cells; this enzyme normally compensates for defective ADA or PNP by preventing dAMP and dGMP accumulation.

The optimal treatment for SCID is a bone marrow transplant from a histo-identical donor, usually a normal sibling. About 40% of patients do not have a histo-identical sibling, in which case haplo-identical parental marrow has sometimes been transplanted successfully. Recently a retroviral vector, into which the ADA gene had been inserted, has been used to transfect the lymphocytes of children who are ADA deficient. This was the first example of successful 'gene therapy'.

Possible role of ADA and PNP deficiency in SCID

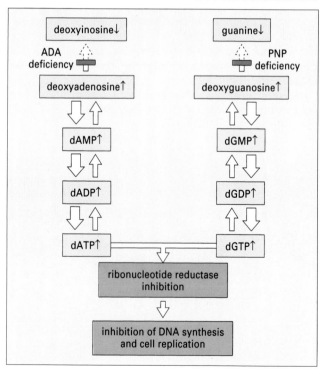

Fig. 18.9 It is thought that deficiencies of ADA and PNP lead to accumulations of dATP and dGTP respectively. Both of these metabolites are powerful inhibitors of ribonucleotide reductase, an essential enzyme for DNA synthesis.

MHC CLASS II DEFICIENCY

The failure to express class II major histocompatibility molecules on antigen-presenting cells (macrophages and B cells) is inherited as an autosomal recessive characteristic, which is not linked to the major histocompatibility locus on the short arm of chromosome 6. Affected infants have recurrent infections, particularly of the gastrointestinal tract. Because the development of CD4$^+$ T cells depends on positive selection by MHC class II molecules in the thymus, MHC class II deficient infants have a deficiency of CD4$^+$ T cells. This lack of TH cells leads to a deficiency in antibodies as well.

MHC class II deficiency results from a defect in promoter proteins that bind to the 5' untranslated region of the class II genes.

THE DiGEORGE ANOMALY

As previously mentioned the thymic epithelium is derived from the third and fourth pharyngeal pouches by the sixth week of human gestation. Subsequently the endodermal anlage is invaded by lymphoid stem cells that undergo development into T cells. The parathyroid glands are also derived from the same embryonic origin. A congenital defect in the organs derived from the third and fourth pharyngeal pouches results in the DiGeorge anomaly. Affected infants have distinctive facial features (Fig. 18.10) in that their eyes are widely separated (hypertelorism), the ears are low set, and the philtrum of the upper lip is shortened. These infants also have congenital malformations of the heart or aortic arch. They have neonatal tetany from the hypoplasia or aplasia of the parathyroid glands. The T-cell deficiency is variable, depending on how badly the thymus gland is affected.

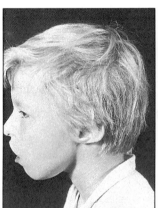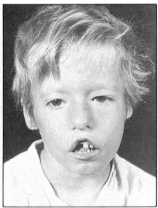

Fig. 18.10 DiGeorge anomaly. Note the wide-set eyes, low-set ears and shortened filtrum of upper lip.

HEREDITARY ATAXIA–TELANGIECTASIA (AT)

AT is inherited as an autosomal recessive trait. Affected infants develop a wobbly gait (ataxia) at about 18 months of age. Telangiectasia (dilated capillaries) appear in the eyes and on the skin by six years of age. AT is accompanied by a variable T-cell deficiency. About 70% of AT patients are IgA deficient and some also have IgG2 and IgG4 deficiency. They develop severe sinus and lung infections. Their cells exhibit chromosomal breaks, usually in chromosome 7 and chromosome 14, at the sites of the T-cell receptor genes and the genes encoding the heavy chains of immunoglobulins. AT patients, as well as the cells from AT patients *in vitro*, are very susceptible to ionizing irradiation; they appear to have a defect in DNA repair but the reason for this is not known.

WISKOTT–ALDRICH SYNDROME (WAS)

WAS is an X-linked immunodeficiency disease. Affected males have small and profoundly abnormal platelets; they are also few in number (thrombocytopenia). Boys with WAS develop severe eczema as well as pyogenic

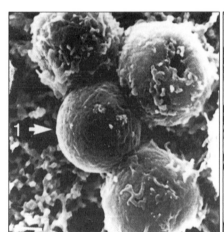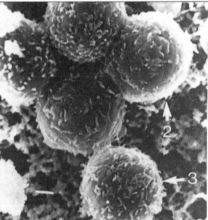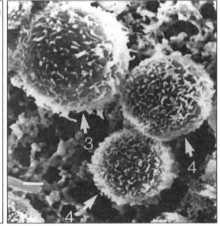

Fig. 18.11 Scanning electron micrographs of lymphocytes in Wiskott–Aldrich syndrome. WAS blood lymphocytes (1 and 2) have fewer surface microvilli than normal blood lymphocytes (3 and 4). (Courtesy of Dr D. Kenney, from Remold-O'Donnel E, Rosen FS. *Immunodeficiency Rev*:2;167, with permission.)

Schematic diagram of HIV

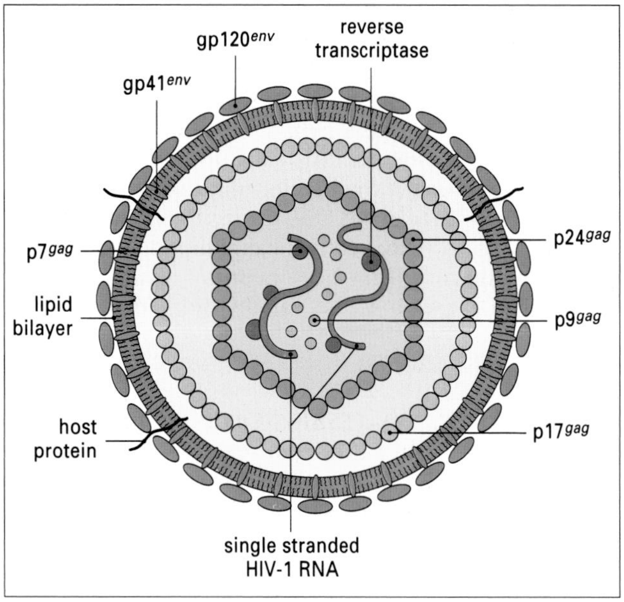

gp120*env*

gp41*env*

reverse transcriptase

p7*gag*

lipid bilayer

host protein

p24*gag*

p9*gag*

p17*gag*

single stranded HIV-1 RNA

and opportunistic infections. Their serum contains increased amounts of IgA and IgE, normal levels of IgG and decreased amounts of IgM. Their T cells are defective in function and this malfunction of cell-mediated immunity gets progressively worse. Their T cells have a uniquely abnormal appearance as shown by scanning electron microscopy (see Fig. 18.11). They have fewer microvilli on the cell surface than normal T cells. The sialoglycoproteins in the membranes of both platelets and T cells are abnormal but the cause of this is at present unknown.

Fig. 18.12 There are two proteins contained in the membranous envelope (*env*), two making up the capsid (*gag*) and two in the nuclear region (*gag*) with the diploid RNA genome. Also in the nuclear region is reverse transcriptase, a DNA polymerase that uses RNA as a template. (Adapted from Greene WC. *New Engl J Med* 1990:**324**;309.)

Life cycle of HIV-1

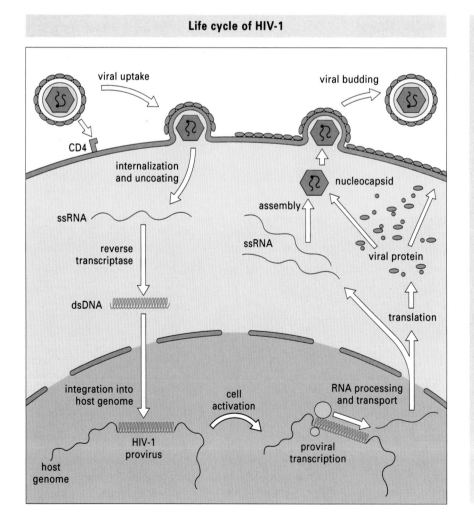

viral uptake

viral budding

CD4

internalization and uncoating

ssRNA

reverse transcriptase

dsDNA

integration into host genome

HIV-1 provirus

host genome

cell activation

proviral transcription

RNA processing and transport

translation

viral protein

assembly

nucleocapsid

ssRNA

Fig. 18.13 After the interaction of gp120^env with the CD4 membrane receptor, gp41-mediated membrane fusion occurs, leading to the entry of HIV-1 into the cell. After uncoating, reverse transcription of viral RNA begins, and this results in the production of the double-stranded DNA form of the viral genome. In turn, the HIV-1 integrase promotes the insertion of this viral DNA duplex into the host genome, giving rise to the HIV-1 provirus. The expression of the HIV-1 gene is stimulated initially by the action of particular inducible and constitutive host transcription factors with binding sites in the long terminal repeat. Stimulation leads to the sequential production of various viral mRNAs. The first mRNAs produced are the multiply spliced species of approximately 2.0 kb encoding the Tat, Rev, and Nef regulatory proteins. The structural proteins of the virus are then produced, allowing the assembly of virions. The free HIV-1 virions produced by viral budding from the host cell can then reinitiate the retroviral life cycle by infecting other CD4⁺ target cells. (Adapted from Greene WC. *New Engl J Med* 1990:**324**;309.)

SECONDARY IMMUNODEFICIENCY DISEASES

Secondary immunodeficiencies are those that result from extrinsic or environmental causes. For example, most drugs used in cancer chemotherapy are cytotoxic for T cells. Worldwide, protein malnutrition is probably the leading cause of immunodeficiency in children; it leads to a profound T-cell deficiency and susceptibility to opportunistic infections. Loss of immunoglobulin into the bowel, in inflammatory bowel disease, may lead to a humoral immunodeficiency. Burns can also lead to a severe loss of immunoglobulins through damaged skin. Infections may cause immunodeficiency by parasitizing cells of the immune system, as in AIDS.

ACQUIRED IMMUNODEFICIENCY SYNDROME (AIDS)

AIDS is caused by infection with the human immunodeficiency virus (HIV). HIV can be transmitted by sexual contact, or from mother to child through the placenta, or by transfer of whole blood or blood products. There are no other well-established modes of transmission of HIV. Exposure to HIV by one of these routes may or may not result in infection.

When an individual is first infected with HIV he or she may develop a transient illness characterized by fever, swollen lymph nodes, a rash and inflammation of the meninges. This occurs in about 15% of infected individuals. The remainder are asymptomatic at the time of initial infection. As time passes, an individual with HIV infection may develop swollen lymph nodes; this is called progressive generalized lymphadenopathy (PGL). Patients with PGL may revert to an asymptomatic state. Patients with PGL, as well as asymptomatic individuals, may have progression to what is called the AIDS-related Complex (ARC). ARC is characterized by fever, night sweats, weight loss and perhaps minor infections such as yeast organisms in the mouth (thrush). Patients with ARC do not revert to an asymptomatic state, unlike patients with PGL. In time, ARC progresses into full-blown AIDS, the patient has develops a major opportunistic infection, or one of the bizarre malignancies associated with AIDS.

The most prominent malignancies observed in patients with AIDS are Kaposi's sarcoma, a tumour of endothelial cells that gives rise to prominent purplish spots on the skin, and Burkitt's lymphoma, which involves B cells. At any time in the course of HIV infection, patients may develop thrombocytopenia (low platelet count), or diseases of the nervous system leading to dementia and paralysis.

The structure of HIV is shown schematically in Fig. 18.12. Its membrane envelope contains two linked glycoproteins, gp120 and gp41, cleaved from a common precursor, gp160. The gp120 protein binds to CD4 and the virus enters cells carrying this marker. These include CD4$^+$ T cells (T$_H$ cells), and cells of the monocyte/ macrophage lineage, such as the dendritic cells of lymphoid tissue and skin (Langerhans' cells), and the microglia of the central nervous system.

The nucleocapsid of HIV contains four proteins, p24, p17, p9 and p7. These four proteins are cleaved from the 53 kDa molecule (p53) encoded by the *gag* gene of the virus. Individuals infected with HIV make antibodies to gp120, gp41 and, most prominently of the gag proteins, to p24. Because of difficulties in detecting the virus itself, infection is defined by the appearance, in the serum, of antibodies to any or all of these proteins. The appearance of antibodies (called seroconversion) can take up to three months from the initial infection.

The life cycle of the virus is depicted in Fig. 18.13. Having entered a cell, HIV loses its coat, and a single stranded DNA copy of the viral RNA is made. This is mediated by the viral enzyme HIV reverse transcriptase. Ultimately, a complementary strand of DNA is made to give a double-stranded DNA replica of the viral genome. This is incorporated into the host genome. A DNA copy of the virus RNA may remain dormant within the cell for months or years. Infectious viral particles are subsequently made, particularly when an infected T cell is activated. Shortly after the primary infection, as many as 1 in 100 T cells may contain HIV. Host defence mechanisms decrease the viral burden at first, but ultimately the virus overcomes them and progressively infects more and more T cells. Enumeration of CD4$^+$ cells in the patient's blood is the best indicator of the progress of the infection. When the absolute number of CD4$^+$ T cells falls below 600/µl the patient begins to lose cell-mediated immunity and opportunistic infections ensue (Fig. 18.14). During the early phases of the infection there is polyclonal expansion of B cells and the serum contains large amounts of IgG, IgM and IgA. In the late stages of AIDS, the amount of immunoglobulin in the serum falls dramatically and the antibody titres to gp120 and p24 decrease concomitantly.

The only successful therapy for HIV infection thus far has been the use of dideoxynucleosides, principally azidothymidine or zidovudine. These compounds inhibit the reverse transcriptase of HIV, so impairing the production of DNA replicas of the virus.

Common opportunistic infections

Pneumocystis carinii
Candida albicans
Mycobacterium avium–intracellulare
Toxoplasma gondii
Cryptosporidium spp.
genital and anal *herpes simplex*

Fig. 18.14 Some of the many organisms that can affect the immunocompromised host, especially patients with AIDS. The lower the blood levels of CD4$^+$ T cells, the greater the likelihood of opportunistic infection.

DEFECTS IN THE COMPLEMENT PROTEINS

The proteins of the complement system and their interactions are discussed in Chapter 12. Genetic deficiencies of almost all the complement proteins have been found in human beings (Fig. 18.15) and these deficiencies reveal much about the normal function of the complement system. Deficiencies of the classical pathway components, C1q, C1r and C1s, C4 or C2, result in a propensity to develop immune-complex diseases such as systemic lupus erythematosus. This correlates with the known function of the classical pathway in the dissolution of immune complexes. Deficiencies of C3, Factor H or Factor I result in increased susceptibility to pyogenic infections; this correlates with the important role of C3 in opsonization of pyogenic bacteria. Deficiencies of the terminal components, C5, C6, C7, C8 , and of the alternative pathway components, Factor D and properdin, result in remarkable susceptibility to infection with the two pathogenic species of the *Neisseria* genus: *N. gonorrhoeae* and *N. meningitidis*. This clearly demonstrates the importance of the alternative pathway and the macromolecular attack complex in the bacteriolysis of this genus of bacteria. All these complement component deficiencies are inherited as autosomal recessive traits, except for properdin deficiency, which is inherited as an X-linked recessive, and C1 inhibitor deficiency, which is inherited as an autosomal dominant.

Genetic deficiencies of human complement

group	type	deficiency	heredity		
			AR	AD	XL
I	immune-complex deficiency	C1q	•		
		C1 or C1r and C1s	•		
		C2	•		
		C4	•		
II	angioedema	C1 inhibitor		•	
III	recurrent pyogenic infections	C3	•		
		Factor H	•		
		Factor I	•		
IV	recurrent Neisserial infections	C5	•		
		C6	•		
		C7	•		
		C8	•		
		properdin			•
		Factor D	?	?	?
V	asymptomatic	C9	•		

Fig. 18.15 Genetic deficiencies of human complement. (AR = phenotypically autosomal recessive; AD = autosomal dominant; XL = X-linked recessive.)

Hereditary Angioneurotic Oedema (HAE)

Clinically, the most important deficiency of the complement system is that of the C1 inhibitor. This molecule is responsible for dissociation of activated C1, by binding $C1r_2C1s_2$. The deficiency results in the well known disease, hereditary angioneurotic oedema (Fig. 18.16). This disease is inherited as an autosomal dominant trait. Patients with HAE have recurrent episodes of circumscribed swelling of various parts of the body (angioedema). When the oedema involves the intestine, excruciating abdominal pains and cramps result, with severe vomiting. When the oedema involves the upper airway, the patients may choke to death from respiratory obstruction. Angioedema of the upper airway therefore presents a medical emergency, which requires rapid action to restore normal breathing.

C1 inhibitor not only inhibits the classical pathway of complement but also joint elements of the kinin, plasmin and clotting systems. The oedema is mediated by two peptides generated by uninhibited activation of the complement and contact systems: a peptide derived from the activation of C2, called C2 kinin, and bradykinin derived from the activation of the contact system (Fig. 18.17). The effect of these peptides is on the post-capillary venule, where endothelial cells contract, forming gaps that allow leakage of plasma (Fig. 18.18).

There are two genetically determined forms of HAE. In type I, the C1 inhibitor gene is defective and no transcripts are formed. In type II, there are point mutations in the C1 inhibitor gene so that defective molecules are synthesized. This distinction is important because the diagnosis of type II disease cannot be made by quantitative measurement of serum C1 inhibitor alone. Simultaneous measurements of C4 must also be done. C4 is always decreased in the serum of hereditary angioneurotic oedema patients, because of its destruction by uninhibited, activated C1.

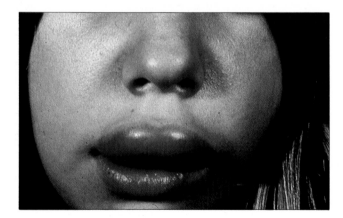

Fig. 18.16 Hereditary angioneurotic oedema. This clinical photograph shows the transient localized swelling which occurs in this condition.

Pathogenesis of hereditary angioneurotic oedema

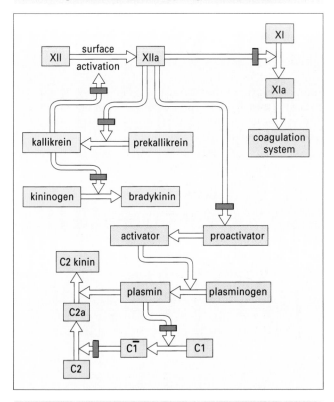

Fig. 18.17 C1 inhibitor is involved in inactivation of elements of the clotting, kinin, plasmin and complement systems, which may be activated following the surface dependent activation of Factor XII (Hageman factor). The points at which C1 inhibitor acts are shown in red. Uncontrolled activation of these pathways results in the formation of bradykinin and C2 kinin, which induce oedema formation.

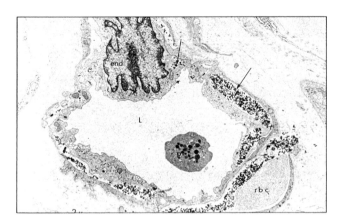

Fig. 18.18 Postcapillary venule of guinea pig. The guinea pig was injected intravenously with India ink (carbon particles). Subsequently the skin was injected with C1s. Gaps formed between the endothelial cells and the carbon particles can be seen leaking from the blood vessel. (Courtesy of Professor Kaethe Willms.)

C1 inhibitor deficiency may be acquired later in life. In some cases an autoantibody to C1 inhibitor is found. In others, there is a monoclonal B-cell proliferation such as occurs in chronic lymphocytic leukemia, multiple myeloma or B cell lymphoma. Such patients make an anti-idiotype to their over-produced immunoglobulin; the idiotype–anti-idiotype interaction, for unknown reasons, causes consumption of C1, C4, C2 and C1 inhibitor without formation of an effective C3 convertase (which would cause C3 deposition and removal of the complex).

DEFECTS IN PHAGOCYTOSIS

Phagocytic cells – polymorphonuclear leucocytes and cells of the monocyte/macrophage lineage – are important in host defence against pyogenic bacteria and other intracellular microorganisms. A severe deficiency of polymorphonuclear leucocytes (neutropenia) can result in overwhelming bacterial infection. Two genetic defects of phagocytes are clinically important in that they result in susceptibility to severe infections and are often fatal: chronic granulomatous disease (CGD) and the leucocyte adhesion deficiency (LAD).

CHRONIC GRANULOMATOUS DISEASE (CGD)

Reduction of O_2 to O_2^-, by the reaction

$$NADPH + 2O_2 \rightarrow NADP^+ + 2O_2^- + H^+$$

is important in intracellular killing of ingested bacteria.

Patients with CGD are incapable of forming oxygen radicals (O_2^-) and hydrogen peroxide in their phagocytes, following ingestion of microorganisms by the phagocytes. Thus they cannot kill ingested bacteria or fungi, particularly catalase-producing organisms.

As a result, microorganisms remain alive in phagocytes of patients with CGD. This gives rise to a cell-mediated response to persistent intracellular microbial antigens, and granulomas form. Children with CGD develop pneumonia, infections in the lymph nodes (lymphadenitis) and abscesses in the skin, liver and other viscera.

The diagnosis of CGD is made by the inability of their phagocytes to reduce nitroblue tetrazolium (NBT) dye after a phagocytic stimulus. NBT, a pale, clear, yellow dye, is taken up by phagocytes when they are ingesting a particle. When NBT accepts H^+ and is reduced, as a result of NADPH oxidation, it forms a deep purple precipitate inside the phagocytes. The reduction of NBT does not occur in the phagocytes of CGD patients (Fig. 18.19).

The NADPH oxidase reaction is complicated and the enzyme complex has many subunits. In resting phagocytes the membrane contains a phagocyte-specific cytochrome, cytochrome b_{558}. This cytochrome is composed of two chains, one of 91 kDa, encoded by a gene on the short arm of the X-chromosome, and one of 22 kDa, encoded by a gene on chromosome 16.

When phagocytosis occurs, several proteins from the cytosol become phosphorylated, move to the membrane and bind to cytochrome b_{558}. The complex that is formed acts as an enzyme, catalysing the NADPH oxidation reaction and thereby activating oxygen radical production (Fig. 18.20). The most common form of CGD is X-linked and involves a defect in the 91 kDa chain of cytochrome b_{558}. Three types of CGD are autosomal recessive and result from defects in the 22 kDa chain of the cytochrome b_{558}, or from defects in one or other of two proteins, called p47^{phox} or p67^{phox} (*phox* is an abbreviation for phagocytic oxidase).

LEUCOCYTE ADHESION DEFICIENCY (LAD)

The receptor in the phagocyte membrane, that binds to C3bi on opsonized microorganisms, is critical for the ingestion of bacteria by phagocytes. This receptor, called complement receptor 3 or CR3, is deficient in patients with LAD and consequently they develop severe bacterial infections, particularly of the mouth and gastrointestinal tract.

CR3 is composed of two polypeptide chains: an α chain of 165 kDa (CD11b), and a β chain of 95 kDa (CD18). In LAD, there is a genetic defect of the β chain, encoded by a gene on chromosome 21. Two other proteins share the same β chain, namely lymphocyte function associated antigen (LFA-1) and p150,95 (see Chapter 12). Although they have unique α chains (CD11a and CD11c respectively), these proteins are also defective in LAD. LFA-1 is important in cell adhesion and interacts with intercellular adhesion molecule 1 (ICAM-1) on endothelial cell surfaces and other cell membranes. Because of the defect in LFA-1, phagocytes from patients with LAD cannot adhere to vascular endothelium and thus cannot migrate out of blood vessels into areas of infection. Thus patients with LAD cannot form pus efficiently; this allows the rapid spread of bacterial invaders.

NADPH oxidase and the forms of CGD

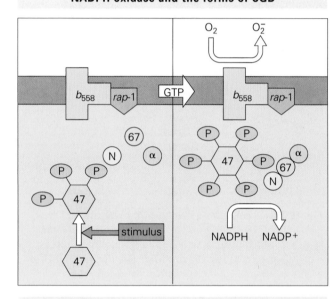

Fig. 18.20 Prevailing knowledge of the NADPH oxidase suggests that, in its dormant state, some of its component parts are in the membrane (cytochrome b_{558} and possibly *rap*-1) while others are in the cytosol (p47^{phox}, p67^{phox}, the NADPH-binding component, N, and a putative fourth component, α). After phagocytosis, the cytosolic components associate and move to the membrane, an event possibly mediated by phosphorylation of p47^{phox}. Once the cytosol components are associated with the membrane components, the oxidase becomes catalytically active and p47^{phox} is phosphorylated further. (Adapted from Curnutte JT. *Blood* 1991:**77**;673, with permission.)

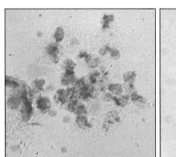
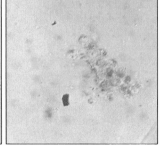

Fig. 18.19 Nitroblue tetrazolium (NBT) test. Left: In normal polymorphs and monocytes, reactive oxygen intermediates (ROIs) are activated by phagocytosis, and yellow NBT is converted to blue formazan. Right: Patients with CGD cannot form ROIs and so the dye stays yellow. (Courtesy of Professor A. R. Hayward.)

FURTHER READING

Rosen FS, Seligman M. *Immunodeficiency Reviews*. Vols 1–3. London: Gordon Breech, 1988–1992.

chapter 19

Hypersensitivity – Type I

 TYPES OF HYPERSENSITIVITY

When an adaptive immune response occurs in an exaggerated or inappropriate form causing tissue damage, the term hypersensitivity is applied. Hypersensitivity is a characteristic of the individual concerned. It cannot be manifested on first contact with the particular antigen evoking the hypersensitivity reaction, but usually appears on subsequent contact. Coombs and Gell described four types of hypersensitivity reaction (Types I, II, III and IV), but in practice these types do not necessarily occur in isolation from each other. These reactions are no more than beneficial immune responses acting inappropriately, and sometimes causing inflammatory reactions and tissue damage. The first three types are antibody-mediated; the fourth is mediated primarily by T cells and macrophages.

Type I, or immediate hypersensitivity, occurs when an immunoglobulin E (IgE) response is directed against innocuous environmental antigens, such as pollen, house-dust mites or animal dander. The resulting release of pharmacological mediators by IgE-sensitized mast cells produces an acute inflammatory reaction with symptoms such as asthma or rhinitis. Type II, or antibody-dependent cytotoxic hypersensitivity, occurs when antibody binds to either self antigen or foreign antigen on cells, and leads to phagocytosis, killer cell activity or complement-mediated lysis. Type III hypersensitivity develops when immune-complexes are formed in large quantities, or cannot be cleared adequately by the reticulo-endothelial system, leading to serum-sickness type reactions. Type IV or delayed type hypersensitivity (DTH), is most seriously manifested when antigens (for example those on tubercle bacilli) are trapped in a macrophage and cannot be cleared. T cells are then stimulated to elaborate lymphokines which mediate a range of inflammatory responses. Other aspects of DTH reactions are seen in graft rejection and allergic contact dermatitis. These four types of hypersensitivity reaction are summarized in Fig. 19.1.

The four types of hypersensitivity reaction

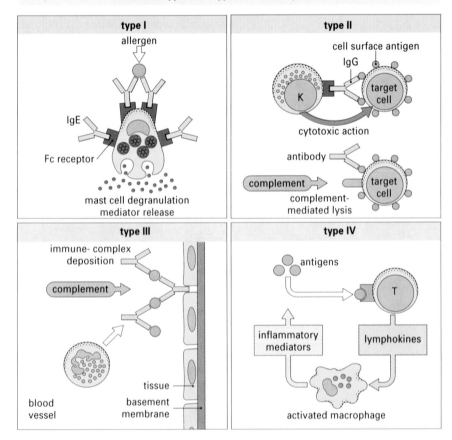

Fig. 19.1 There are four types of hypersensitivity reaction.
Type I Mast cells bind IgE via their Fc receptors. On encountering allergen the IgE becomes cross-linked, inducing degranulation and release of mediators.
Type II Antibody is directed against antigen on an individual's own cells (target cell) or foreign antigen, such as transfused red blood cells. This may lead to cytotoxic action by K cells, or by complement-mediated lysis.
Type III Immune-complexes are deposited in the tissue. Complement is activated and polymorphs are attracted to the site of deposition, causing local damage.
Type IV Antigen-sensitized T cells release lymphokines following a secondary contact with the same antigen. Lymphokines induce inflammatory reactions and activate and attract macrophages which release mediators.

19.1

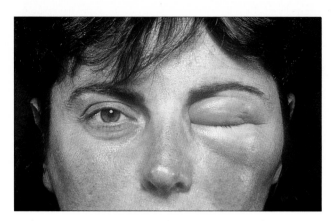

Fig. 19.2 The anaphylactic response to bee venom. The immediate reaction is a clear cut example of Type I hypersensitivity due to the release of pharmacological mediators, including histamine, from mast cells. This is a localized reaction to a facial sting. The reaction can also produce generalized anaphylaxis and even death, as the allergen is injected into the patient rather than being inhaled. The reaction can be aggravated by mellitin in the venom, which can trigger mast cells non-immunologically.

TYPE I – IMMEDIATE HYPERSENSITIVITY

DEFINITION

Type I hypersensitivity is characterized by an allergic reaction (Fig. 19.2) that occurs immediately following contact with the antigen, which is referred to as the allergen. The term 'allergy', meaning 'changed reactivity' of the host when meeting an 'agent' on a second or subsequent occasion, was originally coined in 1906 by von Pirquet. He made no strictures as to the type of immunological response made by the host. It is only in recent years that 'allergy' has become synonymous with Type I hypersensitivity. These reactions are dependent on the specific triggering of IgE-sensitized mast cells by allergen. The mast cells release pharmacological mediators which produce the inflammatory responses typical of Type I hypersensitivity reactions (Fig. 19.3).

Important new research has shown that multiple, multifunctional lymphokines and cytokines are also released as a result of IgE-mediated mast cell activation. IL-3 and IL-4 may have significant autocrine effects on the mast cell itself and these and other cytokines may facilitate IgE production by B cells. In addition, several cytokines, including products of the IL-8/IL-9 gene family,

Induction and effector mechanisms in Type I Hypersensitivity

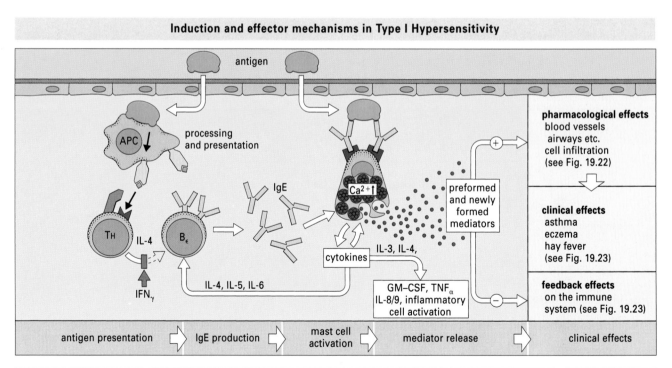

Fig. 19.3 Innocuous environmental antigens (allergens) enter via mucosal surfaces, and are taken up by local antigen-presenting cells (APCs) which process and present them to TH cells. Cognate recognition between the TH cell and B cell, and the release of soluble factors, are also required for B cell proliferation and differentiation, which leads to the production of allergen-specific IgE. The IgE binds, via Fcε receptors (FcεRI), to mast cells thus sensitizing them. When allergen subsequently reaches the sensitized mast cell it cross-links surface-bound IgE, causing an increase in intracellular Ca^{2+} which triggers the release of pre-formed mediators such as histamine and proteases and lipid-derived mediators such as leukotrienes and prostaglandins, which are newly-synthesized. These produce the clinical effects of allergy. Feedback effects of mediators on cells of the immune system may help damp down the allergic reactions.

may be important in the chemotaxis and activation of inflammatory cells at allergic reaction sites. However, it is important to note that the role of the mast-cell-derived cytokines remains to be elucidated *in vivo*.

ATOPY

Originally described by Coca and Cooke in 1923, the term atopy describes the clinical presentations of Type I hypersensitivity, which include asthma, eczema, hay fever and urticaria. These usually occur in subjects with a family history of these or similar conditions, who show immediate wheal-and-flare skin reactions to common environmental allergens.

It had already been suggested that anaphylaxis in animals, discovered by Portier and Richet in 1902, was related to hay fever or asthma in humans. But whereas 90% of animals develop precipitating antibodies to injected heterologous proteins or toxins, only 5–10% of the human population exposed to an airborne allergen become sensitized to it. Furthermore, human allergy shows strong hereditary linkages which were not then appreciated in the animal model. Thus, Coca and Cooke considered that human allergic diseases were different from animal anaphylaxis and called them 'atopic diseases'. There is still some advantage in keeping the term atopy as it is convenient umbrella term for a number of diseases which share some common features, such as asthma, eczema and hay fever.

The first description of the mechanism of the allergic reaction was by Prausnitz and Küstner (1921), who showed that serum taken from an allergic subject and injected into the skin of a normal subject, would produce the same allergic reaction at the site of injection. Küstner was allergic to fish, and injection of his serum into the skin of Prausnitz led to an immediate wheal-and-flare reaction when fish antigen was subsequently injected into the skin of a sensitized site. (This is similar to the PCA test (see below), used for the assay of IgE production in experimental animals.) Some 45 years later, Ishizaka and colleagues showed that this 'atopic reagin' was a new class of immunoglobulin – IgE.

IMMUNOGLOBULIN E

Following the initial contact of allergen with the mucosa there is a complex series of events before IgE is produced. The IgE response is a local event occurring at the site of the allergen's entry into the body, that is, at mucosal surfaces and/or at local lymph nodes. IgE production by B cells depends on allergen presentation by antigen-presenting cells (APCs) and cooperation between the B cells and T_H cells. Locally produced IgE first sensitizes local mast cells; 'spill-over' IgE then enters the circulation and binds to specific receptors on both circulating basophils and tissue-fixed mast cells throughout the body.

The structure of IgE is compared with that of IgG1 in Fig. 19.4. Like other immunoglobulins, IgE comprises two heavy and two light chains, but the IgE heavy chain has five domains.

The major characteristics of IgE include its sensitivity to heat and its ability to bind to mast cells and basophils with high affinity. It is notable that although the serum half-life of IgE is only days, mast cells may remain sensitized for weeks or months due to the high affinity of binding to the $Fc_{\epsilon}RI$, and the consequent protection from proteolysis by serum proteases. Early experiments by Stanworth demonstrated this elegantly. He sensitized twelve separate skin sites on his own arm with atopic serum and then challenged single sites at weekly intervals for three months. There was still an immediate wheal-and-flare on the last site showing that adequate amounts of IgE were still attached to local skin mast cells three months after sensitization.

The skin-sensitizing capacity of IgE resides in the Fc portion of the molecule, and by heating the immunoglobulin at 56°C for half an hour it is destroyed. However, the antigen-binding capacity which resides in the Fab portion is preserved. In passive cutaneous anaphylaxis (PCA) tests, skin sites are sensitized by specific IgE antibody before and after heating the serum and subsequently challenged by an antigen. PCA tests can distinguish IgE from other antibodies which may sensitize mast cells, for example IgG1 (in the guinea-pig), which is not heat-labile.

The structures of IgG1 and IgE

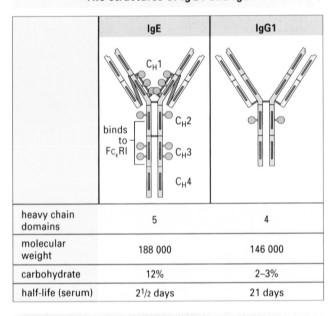

	IgE	IgG1
heavy chain domains	5	4
molecular weight	188 000	146 000
carbohydrate	12%	2–3%
half-life (serum)	2½ days	21 days

Fig. 19.4 IgE is a trace protein in serum (<0.001% of total serum immunoglobulin). It has five domains in the heavy chain and varies from the basic IgG structure as shown. A part of the Fc region of IgE (C_H3 and C_H4) is involved in binding to Fc_{ϵ} receptors ($Fc_{\epsilon}R$) on mast cells and basophils. This Fc binding is heat labile and activity is destroyed by heating at 56°C for 30 minutes. Antigen-binding to the Fab portions is not heat labile.

IgE LEVELS IN DISEASE

IgE levels are often raised in allergic disease and grossly elevated in parasitic infestations. When assessing children or adults for the presence of atopic disease, a raised level of IgE aids the diagnosis although a normal IgE level does not exclude atopy (Fig. 19.5). The determination of IgE alone will not predict an allergic state as there are also genetic and environmental factors which play an important part in the expression of clinical symptoms. However, if a patient does have a very high IgE and no evidence of a worm infection, allergy does become increasingly likely. When skin tests are performed on large numbers of subjects, many more have positive skin test reactions than complain of symptoms. A recent survey has shown that up to 30% of a random group of 5000 subjects had a positive skin test reaction to one or more common allergens. Thus, these subjects can produce specific IgE but lack some factor (factor X, see Fig. 19.35), which precipitates them into the symptoms of atopy.

CONTROL OF IgE PRODUCTION
Early Studies

Studies by Tada and colleagues in the early 1970s using rats clearly demonstrated the importance of T cells in controlling IgE production. Animals immunized with the antigen DNP–*Ascaris*, along with *Bordetella pertussis* as adjuvant, showed a rise in IgE titres which peaked after 5–10 days and returned to normal over the next 6 weeks. If these animals were thymectomized or irradiated as adults, the IgE response was enhanced and prolonged. If, during this phase of enhanced IgE production, the thymectomized animal was passively given thymocytes or spleen cells from *Ascaris*-primed animals, IgE production was suppressed (Fig. 19.6). The suppression of the IgE response was due to the

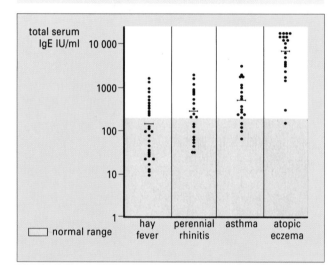

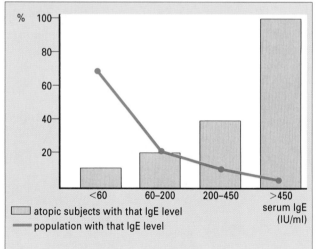

Fig. 19.5 Upper: The serum concentration of IgE (around 100 IU/ml) is 10^5 times less than that of IgG (around 10 mg/ml) and comprises less than 0.001% of the total immunoglobulin. Levels in atopic patients tend to be raised, especially so in atopic eczema. (1 IU = 2 ng). Lower: The higher the level of IgE the greater the likelihood of atopy; where the level is greater than 450 IU/ml the majority of subjects are atopic.

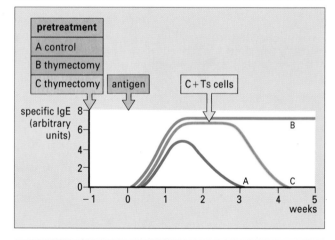

Fig. 19.6 The IgE response is under both T-helper (T_H) and T-suppressor (T_S) cell control. This experiment uses three groups of rats – a control group (A), receiving no pretreatment 1 week before antigen challenge, and two groups which are first thymectomized (B and C). Following antigen challenge the IgE response is measured regularly. On immunization with antigen there is a transient rise in antigen-specific IgE in the controls. Thymectomy (or irradiation) causes a prolonged response (B) which can be curtailed by the addition of antigen-stimulated spleen cells containing T_S cells (C). In neonatally thymectomized rats, no IgE response is seen, indicating the basic requirement for T_H cells.

activity of Ts cells in the transferred cell population suggesting that thymectomy or irradiation treatment reduces suppressor activity. The IgG and IgM levels were unchanged by the cell transfer, showing that IgE responses are particularly sensitive to the effects of Ts cells. However, neonatal thymectomy completely abolishes the capacity to produce IgE to DNP–*Ascaris*, showing the need for TH cells in the IgE response. In several clinical conditions there is an association between low Ts cell numbers and high levels of IgE, indicating that T cell control of IgE production is also important in man.

Recent Studies

It is now known that subsets of TH cells that produce particular profiles of lymphokines are responsible for the regulation of IgE production by B cells. The cellular mechanisms involved in this regulation are outlined in Fig. 19.7. Evidence from studies in both animals and man has shown that IL-4 produced by TH2 cells enhances IgE production, whereas IFN$_\gamma$ from TH1 cells is inhibitory (Fig. 19.8).

The crucial role of these lymphokines *in vivo* has been shown in mice where neutralizing antibodies to IL-4, or administration of IFN$_\gamma$, both lead to an inhibition of IgE

Molecular control of IgE – recent studies

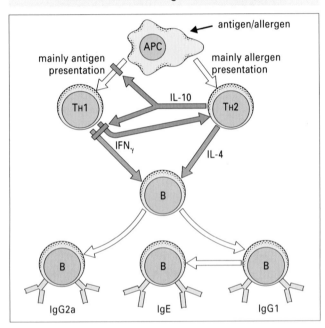

Fig. 19.7 In the mouse there are two populations of TH cells, characterized by the profile of lymphokines they produce. Thus, TH1 cells produce IFN$_\gamma$ and IL-2, while TH2 cells produce IL-4 and IL-5. In an immune response to an allergen, TH2 cells seem to be preferentially stimulated by APCs, resulting in the release of IL-4 which promotes the isotype switch of B cells to IgE production. With antigens such as tetanus toxoid, TH1 cells are preferentially activated. They release IFN$_\gamma$ which leads to the production of IgG2a by B cells and inhibition of the TH2 response to antigen.

In response to allergen, TH2 cells can equally suppress the response of TH1 cells by producing IL-10, which may act by interfering with allergen presentation to TH1 cells. It may also inhibit IFN$_\gamma$ production. In man, the roles of IL-4 and IFN$_\gamma$ are similar to those seen in the mouse, but the lymphokine profiles of TH1 and TH2 cells are not so clear cut.

The effects of IFN$_\gamma$ on induced IgE synthesis

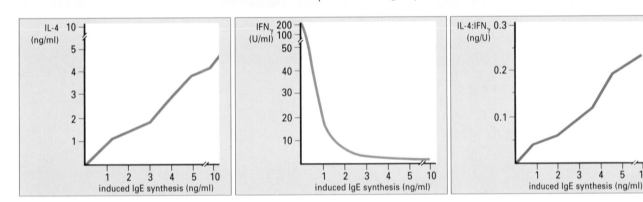

Fig. 19.8 The ability of T cell clones to induce IgE synthesis correlates with their secreted IL-4 and IFN$_\gamma$. For example, supernatant IL-4 from activated T cell clones induces the secretion of IgE by B cells (left). Interestingly, T cell supernatants devoid of IL-4 were unable to induce IgE synthesis.

Where IFN$_\gamma$ is secreted (centre) there is an inhibition of IgE secretion. If both IL-4 and IFN$_\gamma$ are present, the supernatant can induce the synthesis of IgE provided the ratio of the two is in favour of IL-4 (right). (Based on data from Del Prete G et al. *J Immunol* 1988;**140**:4193–4198.)

responses. Furthermore, mice homozygous for a mutation that inactivates the IL-4 gene cannot produce IgE after a nematode infection. In patients with hyper-IgE syndrome, giving IFN$_\alpha$ (used in preference to IFN$_\gamma$ because of the fewer adverse effects) also leads to a reduction in serum IgE levels. The molecular mecha-

nisms by which IL-4 causes B-cell switching to IgE production remain to be elucidated.

It is noteworthy that TH2 cells also produce IL-5, which promotes the synthesis and secretion of IgA from B cells and is crucial in stimulating eosinophil development and activation. The production of IL-4 and IL-5 by

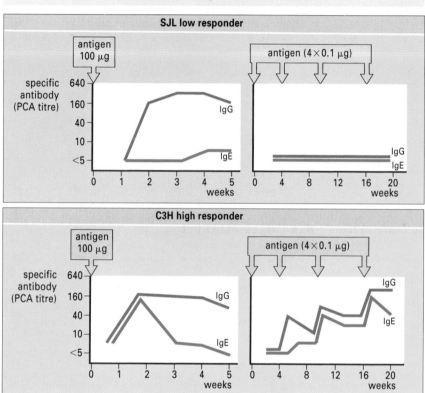

Fig. 19.9 Dependence of the IgE response on the antigen dose and the genetic constitution of the animal. The two genotypes of mouse are selected whose immune response may reflect human atopy. A 'low responder' SJL mouse makes predominantly IgG to a single large dose (100 µg) of antigen, but makes little or no specific IgG or IgE in response to repeated small doses (0.1 µg). By contrast a C3H 'high responder' mouse (bottom) makes a transient large IgE response to a single high antigen dose which decays over 3–4 weeks, whilst repeated low dose antigen stimulation which mimics natural exposure produces rising titres of both IgE and IgG with each injection.

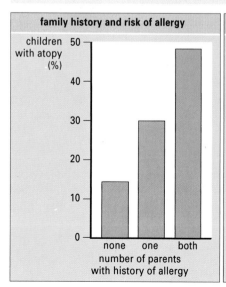

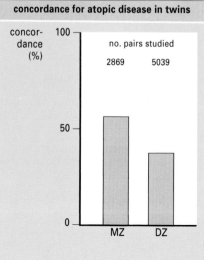

Fig. 19.10 The role of heredity and environment in atopy. Left: The greater the parental history of allergy, the greater the likelihood of the children being atopic.
Right: The concordance of atopic disease in dizygotic (DZ – non-identical) twins is slightly greater than that found in the general population, which is approximately 17%. However, the concordance in monozygotic (MZ – identical) twins is well below the 100% that might be expected if the genotype was the sole factor in determining the development of atopy. These two findings suggest that both genetic and environmental factors are important in the expression of atopic disease.

TH2 cells may explain the eosinophilia that is so frequently associated with IgE-mediated allergic reactions. Clearly, influencing the profile of lymphokine production, or the effect of lymphokines, could be useful in future treatment of IgE-mediated disorders.

Genetic Control of IgE in Mice

The finding that different strains of animals vary in their ability to make IgE responses, suggests that IgE production is under direct genetic control. Low responder strains of mice, such as SJL, do not produce high titres of IgE even when subjected to an optimum immunization schedule for its production. In these studies, both the dose of antigen and the mode of its administration is critical (Fig. 19.9). It must be emphasized that although many animal model systems are available for studying IgE production, these are not models of allergy; there are no strains of laboratory mouse that develop allergic symptoms spontaneously, although they are exposed to environmental allergens. Humans are sensitized by multiple low-dose exposures to environmental allergens, such as pollen during the summer, and the route of sensitization is usually via mucosal surfaces and not by injection, except in the case of wasp or bee stings. The production of IgE in response to allergen, which is under genetic control, is just one factor in the development of atopy (see below).

■ GENETICS OF THE ALLERGIC RESPONSE IN MAN

Early studies in the 1920s showed that allergic parents tended to have a higher proportion of allergic children than parents who were not allergic. When large numbers of families are examined the figures show that with two allergic parents there is a greater than 50% chance of the children having allergy. Even with one allergic parent the chances are still almost 30%. Thus, both genetic background and elevated serum IgE levels are risk factors (Fig. 19.10).

A variety of non-genetic factors may also play an important role, such as the quantity of the exposure, the nutritional status of the individual and the presence of chronic underlying infections or acute viral illnesses (see Fig. 19.36). As regards the quantity of exposure, the annual challenge of individuals by airborne pollens is in the order of 1μg. It is perhaps surprising that some 15% of the population respond to this exceptionally low-dose challenge.

There are three main genetic mechanisms regulating the allergic response; these mechanisms affect the total IgE levels, the allergen-specific response and general hyperresponsiveness, and are discussed in more detail below.

TOTAL IgE LEVELS

Studies of families in which at least one member has high IgE levels have confirmed the hypothesis that a low IgE level is associated with a dominant gene.

HLA-LINKED ALLERGEN-SPECIFIC RESPONSE

The association between HLA types and a specific response to allergen is most striking when ultrapure (>99.5% pure) allergen preparations are used. It is most pronounced for very low-dose allergen exposure and especially for low molecular weight minor determinants, for example the ragweed allergen, *Amb a* V (5 kDa), than for abundant high molecular mass allergens, for example Ragweed *Amb a* I (AgE, 38 kDa). With *Amb a* V, more than 90% of IgE responders are HLA-Dw2, whereas with AgE there is as yet no HLA association (Fig. 19.11).

The association is greater with IgE antibody and immediate hypersensitivity skin tests than with IgG antibody. However, following hyposensitization to ragweed it is only the HLA-Dw2, *Amb a* V⁺ subjects who make a good IgG response, showing that immune response to *Amb a* V is not restricted to IgE, but includes other immunoglobulin classes.

Lastly, there is a higher degree of HLA linkage when the subject has a low total IgE. For example, of patients who are allergic to ragweed, only 1 in 6 respond to *Amb a* III (Ra3), which is a minor determinant. Of the *Amb a* III⁺ patients with low levels of total IgE, 90% of subjects carry HLA-A2 (see Fig. 19.12). With increasing total IgE levels, the HLA association disappears.

GENERAL HYPERRESPONSIVENESS

The possibility of genetic factors in general hyperresponsiveness – revealed by positive skin tests to a broad range of antigens – has been tested in patients attending an allergy clinic (see Fig. 19.13). The results showed that HLA-B8 and HLA-Dw3, but not HLA-A1, are present at a significantly higher frequency in the allergic group. A more specific hyperresponsiveness

Allergens and HLA associations

systematic name	old name	mol.wt (daltons)	primary association	*p* value
Ambrosia (Ragweed) spp.				
Amb a I	AgE	37 800	none	–
Amb a III	Ra3	12 300	A2	0.01
Amb a VI	Ra6	11 500	DR5	$<10^{-7}$
Amb a V	Ra5	5000	DR2/Dw2	$<10^{-9}$
Amb t V	Ra5G	4400	DR2/Dw2	$<10^{-3}$
Lolium (ryegrass) spp.				
Lol p I	Rye I	27 000	DR3/Dw3	$<10^{-3}$
Lol p II	Rye II	11 000	DR3/Dw3	$<10^{-3}$
Lol p III	Rye III	11 000	DR3/Dw3	$<10^{-4}$

Fig. 19.11 HLA association of IgE responses to allergens from ragweed and ryegrass. (Courtesy of Dr D. Marsh.)

Atopy: IgE levels and tissue type

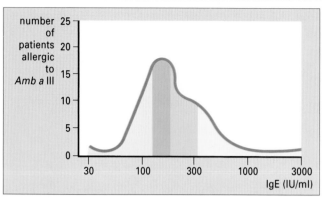

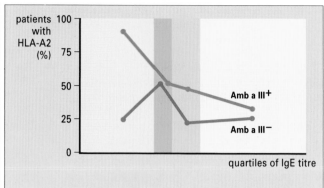

Fig. 19.12 Left: Graph showing the number of ragweed-allergic patients (*Amb a* III⁺) with given levels of total IgE; quartiles of the range are indicated in different shades. Right: Graph showing the percentage of patients in the four quartiles possessing HLA-A2. This is shown for both *Amb a* III⁺ and *Amb a* III⁻ individuals. It appears that a person is more likely to be sensitive to *Amb a* III if she or he possesses HLA-A2, and this association is most marked where the IgE level is low, where the linkage is very high. HLA-A2 is present in 47% of the population.

IgE response: genetic association

HLA	Skin test		P
	positive (%)	negative (%)	
A1	28.7	24.1	0.400
B8	22.3	11.5	0.010
Dw3	25.2	11.7	0.002

Fig. 19.13 There is a significant association between HLA-B8 and HLA-Dw3 positive skin tests to a number of common environmental allergens (e.g. pollens, house dust mite). The IgE response to allergens is clearly genetically linked, both in terms of the response to a specific allergen, and the general atopic tendency to produce IgE antibody in response to any antigen.

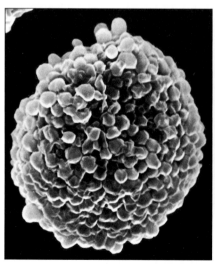

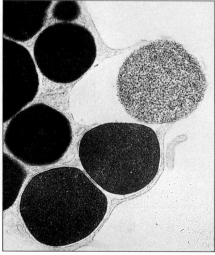

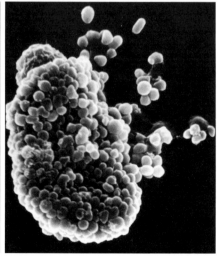

Fig. 19.14 Electron micograph study of rat mast cells – I. Left: An intact rat peritoneal mast cell with the cell membrane shrunk onto the granules. Scanning electron micrograph, × 1500. Centre: A granule during exocytosis. Transmission electron micrograph, × 15 000. Right: A rat peritoneal mast cell degranulating following incubation with anti-IgE for 30 seconds. Scanning electron micrograph, × 1500. (Courtesy of Dr T. S. C. Orr.)

can also be seen in those already making anti-ragweed IgE antibodies, where patients with HLA-B8 have higher titres of antibody and also higher levels of total IgE.

HLA-B8 is also strongly associated with other forms of immune 'hyperactivity', for example autoimmune diseases. This raises the possibility that HLA-B8 is linked to Ts cell control of immune responses, since depressed Ts cell activity is thought to be involved in the development of both autoimmune and IgE responses.

MAST CELLS

It has long been recognized that there is a species difference in mast cell morphology. These morphological differences may be seen not only in the staining properties of the cells and the outer structure of their granules, but also in the detailed mechanism of the degranulation process. This last point can be clearly demonstrated; in man, the membranes surrounding the mast cell granules fuse before exocytosis (compound exocytosis), whereas in rats the granules are expelled singly (Figs 19.14 and 19.15).

In addition to the morphological differences there are also functional differences between species and even between mast cells derived from different sites within the same animal. The functional differences are seen in response to drugs which stimulate mast cell degranulation (Ca^{2+} ionophores, compound 48/80 etc.) or sodium cromoglycate, which inhibits histamine release only from particular mast-cell populations.

It used to be thought that mast cells comprised a homogeneous population, with a morphology similar to that of the cells now recognized as connective tissue mast cells (CTMCs). The staining technique used to demonstrate CTMCs involves formalin fixation of sections and toluidine blue staining. It is now realized that these stains do not adequately show up the mucosal mast cell (MMC) which is only shown with special fixatives and stains (Figs 19.16 and 19.17).

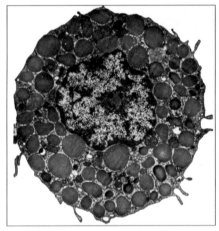 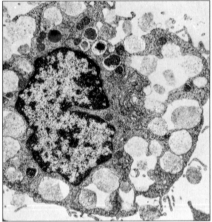

Fig. 19.15 Electron micrograph study of rat mast cells – II.
Left: Rat peritoneal mast cells showing electron-dense granules. Right: Following incubation with anti-IgE, vacuolation with exocytosis of the granule contents has occurred. Transmission electron micrographs, × 2700. (Courtesy of Dr D. Lawson.)

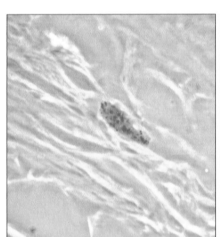 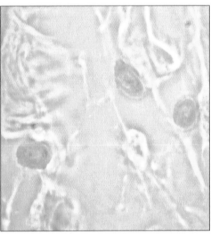

Fig 19.16 Histological appearances of rat ileum mast cells.
Left: Connective tissue mast cell showing both blue and brown granules. Right: Three mucosal mast cells with only blue granules. Fixed in formol saline, alcian blue and safranin stain, × 600. (Courtesy of Dr T. S. C. Orr.)

DISTRIBUTION OF MAST CELLS

CTMCs are found around blood vessels in most tissues. Although CTMCs from different sites have similar properties, the gross morphology of CTMCs from the peritoneum and the skin for example, may be quite different in terms of the number and size of the granules, the density of staining and their pharmacological properties (Fig. 19.18). MMCs have a different distribution from CTMCs; in man the highest concentrations are found in the mucosa of the midgut and in the lung. During parasitic infections there is a marked increase in MMCs in the gut mucosa as seen, for example in rats infected with *Nippostrongylus brasiliensis*. This increase is also seen in Crohn's disease and ulcerative colitis, and there is an increase of CTMCs in the synovium of patients with rheumatoid arthritis. The role that mast cells play in these diseases is not clear. It has been suggested that the precursors of gut MMCs arise in the mesenteric lymph nodes which drain the gut and then migrate via the thoracic duct back to the intestine. It is clear that MMC proliferation after a parasitic infection is dependent on T-cell derived lymphokines including IL-3 and IL-4. CTMC clones arise in culture from fibroblast layers, independent of T cells or T-cell factors.

Recent evidence suggests that MMCs and CTMCs are derived from the same precursor cell, with the end-cell phenotype depending on factors found in the local microenvironment.

MAST CELL NEUTRAL PROTEASES

Recently a number of mast-cell-granule proteases have been cloned and sequenced. Two of these, tryptase and chymase, have been used to define mast-cell subpopulations which have different tissue distribution in man (Fig. 19.19).

These proteases are of clinical interest in that tryptase

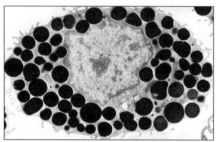 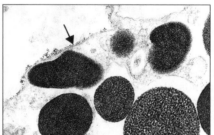 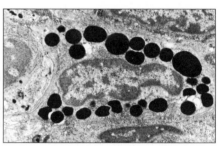

Fig. 19.17 Electron micrograph study of rat mast cells – III. Left: The connective tissue mast cell (CTMC) has electron-dense granules characteristic of the rat. Far right: The mucosal mast cell (MMC) of an ileal villus has fewer granules, with considerable diversity of size. Centre: At far higher magnification, a rat CTMC on which membrane-bound IgE has been marked with colloidal gold particles (indicated with arrows). (Courtesy of H. Coleman.)

Differences between mast cell populations – I

	mucosal mast cell	connective tissue mast cell
location *in vivo*	gut and lung	ubiquitous
life span	<40 days (?)	>40 days (?)
T-cell-dependent	+	–
number of Fc_ϵ receptors	25×10^5	3×10^4
histamine content	+	+ +
cytoplasmic IgE	+	–
major AA metabolite $LTC_4:PGD_2$ ratio	25:1	1:40
DSCG/theophylline inhibits histamine relese	–	+
major proteoglycan	chondroitin sulphate	heparin

Fig. 19.18 Much of this data comes from rodent studies and may not apply to man. There are at least two subpopulations of mast cells, the mucosal mast cells (MMCs) and the connective tissue mast cells (CTMCs). The differences in their morphology and pharmacology suggest different functional roles *in vivo*. MMCs are associated with parasitic worm infections and possibly allergic reactions. In contrast to the CTMC, the MMC is smaller, shorter lived, T-cell dependent, has more Fc_ϵ receptors and contains intracytoplasmic IgE. Both cells contain histamine and serotonin in their granules; the higher histamine content of the CTMC may be accounted for by the greater number of granules. Major arachidonic acid metabolites (prostaglandins and leukotrienes), are produced by both mast cell types, but in different amounts. For example, the ratios of production of the leukotriene LTC_4 to the prostaglandin PGD_2 are 25:1 in the MMC and 1:40 in the CTMC. The effect of drugs on degranulation is different between the two cell types. Sodium cromoglycate (DSCG) and theophylline both inhibit histamine release from the CTMC but not from the MMC. (This may have important implications in the treatment of asthma.)

can cause bronchial hyperresponsiveness and chymase stimulates bronchial mucus secretion – both of which are hallmarks of asthma (see Fig. 19.34). Both proteases can also degrade vasoactive intestinal peptide (VIP), a mediator of bronchial relaxation.

CLINICAL STUDIES

A number of recent clinical studies have demonstrated that MMCs infiltrate the nasal epithelium in patients with hay fever during, but not before, the pollen season. Similarly, increased numbers of mast cells (the exact identity of which is not clear) are found in the bronchoalveolar lavage fluid of asthmatics. Since the mucosal surface is the first site of contact for inhaled allergen, the interaction of superficial mast cells and allergen will lead to the release of mediators and result in increased permeability of the mucosa to allergen. This leads to further mediator release by submucosal mast cells, thereby amplifying the clinical symptoms.

A better understanding of the nature of these superficial, bronchoalveolar mast cells and their responsiveness to anti-allergic drugs could have important therapeutic implications. For instance, in rats infected with the nematode parasite *Nippostrongylus brasiliensis*, the accumulation of MMCs in the gut is rapidly and dramatically suppressed by treatment with corticosteroids. Interestingly, locally applied corticosteroids also suppress the increase in nasal mast cell numbers seen in hay-fever patients during the pollen season. The mechanism of this suppression is not clear, but it is known that corticosteroids inhibit lymphokine production by TH cells, including IL-3 and IL-4. Both of these have mast-cell growth factor activity.

Differences between mast cell populations – II

cell type	location	amount per cell (pg)	
		tryptase	chymase
MC$_T$ (MMC)	lung and nasal cavity, intestinal mucosa	10	<0.04
MC$_{TC}$ (CTMC)	skin, blood vessels, intestinal submucosa	35	4.5
Basophil	circulation	0.04	<0.04

Fig. 19.19 Tryptase is a tetramer of 134 kDa which may comprise as much as 25% of the mast cell protein. Chymase is a monomer of 30 kDa. The relative proportions of these proteases in mast cells defines MC$_T$ and MC$_{TC}$ population, which have different distributions in human tissues. Basophils have very low amounts of both proteases. (The suffixes T and TC represent the content of tryptase and chymase in the respective cells.)

EFFECT OF DRUGS

The effect of drugs on mast cell degranulation is crucial, both functionally and clinically. In the rat, sodium cromoglycate and theophylline both inhibit histamine release from CTMCs but not from MMCs. Because of mast cell heterogeneity and species differences, it is unsafe to extrapolate these results to man. The development of 'pure' human mast cell lines could be of great use in developing drugs for the management of the allergic patient.

THE STRUCTURE AND FUNCTION OF Fc RECEPTORS

Two different receptors for IgE on cells are now known (Fig. 19.20). The high affinity receptor (Fc$_\epsilon$RI) is found on mast cells and basophils and is the 'classical' IgE receptor. This receptor is part of the immunoglobulin supergene family and quite distinct from the low affinity Fc receptor for IgE (Fc$_\epsilon$RII) found on leucocytes and lymphocytes. The low affinity receptor has not evolved from the immunoglobulin supergene family but has substantial homology with several animal lectins.

THE HIGH AFFINITY RECEPTOR – Fc$_\epsilon$RI

Analysis of the Fc$_\epsilon$RI receptor was initiated in the mid-1970s. It is now known to have the tetrameric structure shown in Fig. 19.20.

The α-chain (45 kDa) is glycosylated and exposed on the surface. Antibodies against the α-chain can block IgE binding to the receptor and trigger histamine release from rat basophil leukaemia cells. The carbohydrate probably protects the α-chain from serum protease activity, as with many cell-surface proteins. It is unlikely that the carbohydrate chain plays a role in IgE-binding and IgE-mediated histamine release *per se*. However, carbohydrate-binding lectins can trigger histamine release, probably by this route. This reaction may not be of importance under physiological conditions.

The single β-chain (33 kDa) and the two disulphide-linked γ-chains (9 kDa) are essential components of the αβγ$_2$ receptor unit, being required for receptor expression on the cell surface and perhaps playing a role in signal transduction.

The receptor interacts with the distal portion of the IgE heavy chain, that is, regions of the C$_H$2 and/or C$_H$3 domains. The interaction is highly specific and the binding constant for IgE is also very high (approximately 10^{10} M^{-1}). Neither the interaction of monovalent IgE with the receptor complex, nor the binding of substrate to a single IgE, appear to activate mast cells or basophils, since no histamine release occurs. It is the cross-linking of several surface-bound IgEs, by antigen or by other molecules, which stimulates degranulation.

The carbohydrate associated with IgE itself does not seem to be of importance in its interaction with Fc$_\epsilon$RI. Its role seems to be in the secretion of IgE from B cells. The high-affinity receptor was thought to be limited to mast cells and basophils, but some recent data suggest that receptors may also be found on Langerhans' cells.

THE LOW AFFINITY RECEPTOR – FC$_\epsilon$RII

The human lymphocyte Fc$_\epsilon$RII or CD23 antigen (45 kDa) shows the characteristics of a membrane-bound molecule, i.e. a transmembrane domain, but it is unusual in that it lies 'upside down' in the cell membrane, the C-terminus being extracellular (see Fig. 19.20). Unlike other Fc receptors, Fc$_\epsilon$RII is not a member of the immunoglobulin supergene family but belongs to a primitive superfamily of animal lectins.

Two forms of the human Fc$_\epsilon$RII have now been identified, cloned and sequenced. They differ only in the N-terminal cytoplasmic region, the extracellular domains being identical. The Fc$_\epsilon$RIIa is normally expressed on B cells, whereas expression of Fc$_\epsilon$RIIb on T cells, B cells, monocytes and eosinophils requires induction by IL-4 (Fig. 19.21). This may explain the observed difference in Fc$_\epsilon$RII subtype function on B cells during normal B cell activity on the one hand, and the effector phase of IgE-mediated immunity on the other. Thus, it it notable that Fc$_\epsilon$RIIb+ lymphocytes and monocytes are increased in the circulation of some atopics, particularly those with atopic eczema. In patients with hay fever, the rise in expression on lymphocytes occurs at the same time as increased IgE levels seen during the pollen season. Normal alveolar macrophages which express Fc$_\epsilon$RIIb, when sensitized with allergen-specific IgE and then challenged with the allergen, release enzymes. This suggests that these cells may be involved in the pathogenesis of allergen-induced lung disease, whether asthma or alveolitis.

While the role of Fc$_\epsilon$RIIa in B cell differentiation and adhesion has been demonstrated, the function of the various soluble CD23 molecules (so-called IgE binding factors), is not yet clear. They can be viewed as another form of cytokine, being an autocrine growth factor for B cells and essential for isotype switching to IgE.

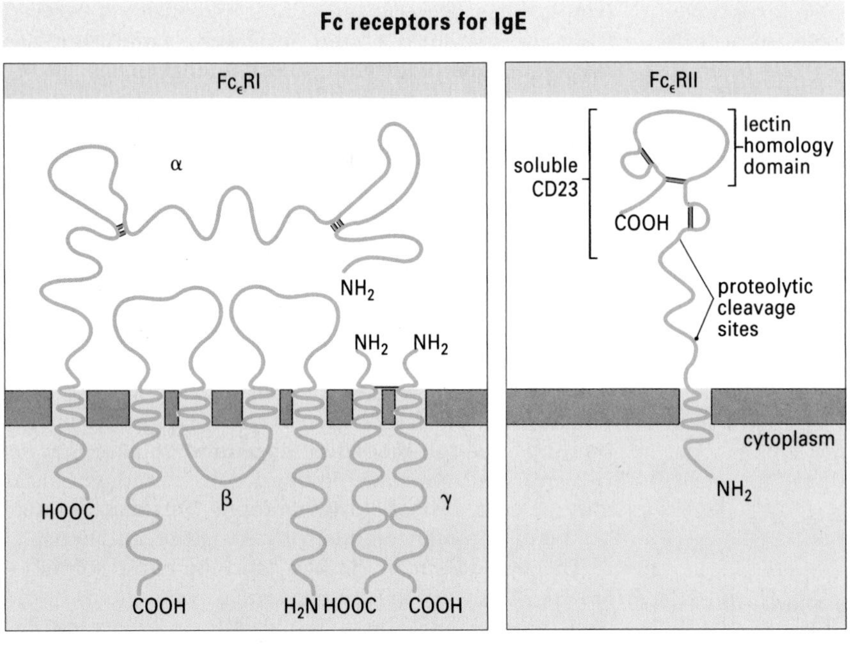

Fc receptors for IgE

Fig. 19.20 The model for Fc$_\epsilon$RI proposes a tetramer consisting of one α-chain with two disulphide-linked immunoglobulin-like loops. The β-chain has two extracellular portions near two γ-chains which are linked by a disulphide bonds (yellow). The α-chain is crucial for IgE binding. The hypothetical model for the Fc$_\epsilon$RII is based on sequence data and the homology with animal lectins. Proteolytic cleavage can release several IgE-BF species including the 25 kDa soluble CD23 molecule, which contains the lectin binding domain. This cleavage is inhibited by IgE, accounting for the apparent increase of Fc$_\epsilon$RII expression on lymphocytes cultured in the presence of IgE.

IgE binding on cells other than mast cells

receptors	cells	comment
Fc$_\epsilon$RIIa	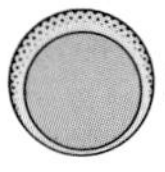 B cells	expressed in normal B cells functions as cell growth and adhesion molecule
Fc$_\epsilon$RIIb	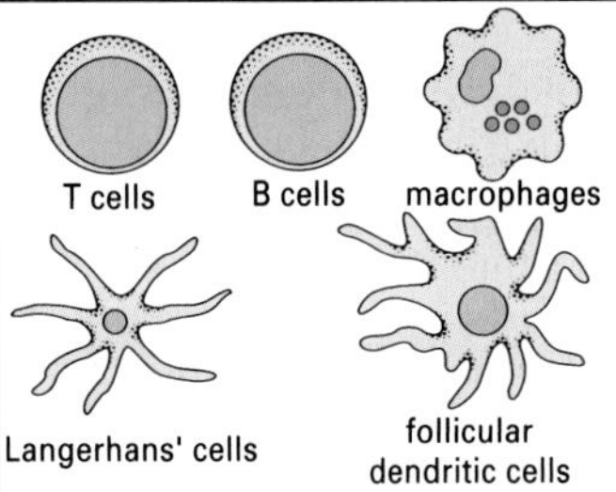 T cells, B cells, macrophages, Langerhans' cells, follicular dendritic cells	induced by IL-4 on normal cells expressed routinely by some T and B cells, monocytes and eosinophils, Langerhans' cells and follicular dendritic cells

Fig. 19.21 IgE binding on cells other than mast cells. Compared to those on mast cells and basophils, receptors on other cells (Fc$_\epsilon$RII) have a much lower affinity for IgE. Fc$_\epsilon$RIIa is constitutively expressed on normal B cells whereas Fc$_\epsilon$RIIb expression is induced on various cell types by IL-4. T cells, B cells, monocytes and macrophages express Fc$_\epsilon$RIIb as do Langerhans' cells when in skin. This latter cell may also express the high affinity receptor Fc$_\epsilon$RI.

OTHER CELLS THAT CAN BIND IgE

Normal eosinophils and platelets, when sensitized with IgE, have enhanced cytotoxicity against some parasites, including schistosomes. In addition, these cells may become sensitized by circulating immune complexes containing IgE in allergic patients. They could contribute to the allergic response, since they both contain a variety of mediators and inflammatory proteins capable of exacerbating allergic reactions. However, recent evidence suggests that IgE binds to these cells, not through an Fc receptor for IgE, but by another type of receptor not yet identified.

Langerhans' cells in the skin of patients with atopic eczema have surface-bound IgE through CD23 which may be important in antigen presentation and inflammation. Such IgE-binding Langerhans' cells are not seen in normal skin or in atopic subjects without eczema.

MAST-CELL TRIGGERING

Once IgE has bound to $Fc_\epsilon RI$ on mast cells and basophils, degranulation can be triggered by IgE cross-linking. This is achieved by allergen or other molecules, and leads to aggregation of the Fc_ϵ receptors. Degranulation is also effected by manoeuvres which directly cross-link the receptors (Fig. 19.22). Lectins, such as PHA and ConA, can cross-link IgE by binding to carbohydrate residues on the Fc region, thus causing degranulation. This might explain the urticaria induced in some individuals by strawberries, which contain large amounts of lectin.

Other compounds are extremely active in degranulating mast cells. Probably the most important of these *in vivo* are the breakdown products of complement activation, that is, C3a and C5a. The anaphylatoxins

Mast cell activation and physiological effects of mast-cell derived mediators

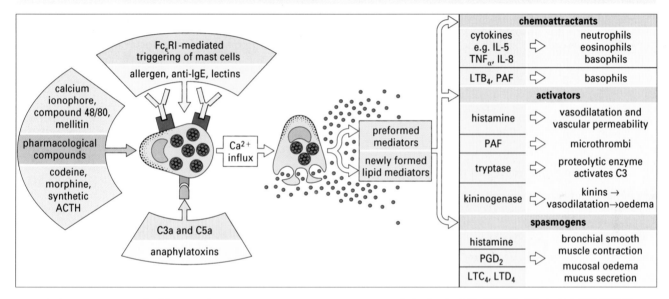

Fig. 19.22 Mast cell activation can be produced by immunological stimuli which cross-link Fc_ϵ receptors, and by other agents such as anaphylatoxins and secretagogues (e.g. compound 48/80, mellitin, calcium ionophore, a23187). Some other drugs such as codeine, morphine and synthetic ACTH have also been found to act on mast cells directly. The common feature in each case is the influx of Ca^{2+} ions into the mast cell, which is crucial for degranulation.
Microtubule formation, and movement of the granules to the cell membrane, lead to fusion of the granule and plasma membrane, and the release of preformed granule-associated mediators. Changes in the plasma membrane, associated with activation of phospholipase A_2, release arachidonic acid; this can then be metabolized by lipoxygenase or cyclooxygenase enzymes, depending on the mast-cell type. These newly-formed lipid metabolites include prostaglandins (PGD_2), thromboxanes, produced by the cyclooxygenase pathway, and leukotrienes (LTC_4, LTD_4 and chemotactic LTB_4), produced by the lipoxygenase pathway.

Both the preformed, granule-associated lipid mediators and the newly-formed lipid mediators have three main areas of action.
Chemotactic agents. A variety of cells are attracted to the site of mast cell activation, in particular eosinophils, neutrophils and mononuclear cells including lymphocytes. In addition, recent evidence suggests that certain of the preformed cytokines released from degranulating mast cells are also chemotactic for inflammatory cells.
Inflammatory activators can cause vasodilatation, oedema and, via platelet activating factor (PAF), microthrombi, leading to local tissue damage. Tryptase, the major neutral protease of human lung mast cells can activate C3 directly, this function being inhibited by heparin. Kininogenases are also released and these affect small blood vessels by generating kinins from kininogens, again leading to inflammation.
Spasmogens have a direct effect on bronchial smooth muscle, but could also increase mucus secretion leading to bronchial plugging.

also affect many other cells, including neutrophils, platelets and macrophages. There are also a number of compounds that can directly activate mast cells, for example calcium ionophore, mellitin and compound 48/80, as well as some drugs, such as synthetic ACTH, codeine and morphine. All of these compounds lead to the activation of mast cells by causing an influx of calcium ions. The anaphylactic response induced by these agents is identical to that seen in IgE-mediated reactions although, of course, they act by IgE-independent mechanisms.

T CELLS AND MAST CELL TRIGGERING

The mucosal mast cell needs T cell factors (IL-3, IL-4) for maturation, but there also seems to be a more direct interaction with T cells in the induction of mediator release. Antigen-specific T cell factors can arm mast cells to release mediators following contact with antigen. These factors, produced by TDTH cells, sensitize mast cells for a few hours only, whereas IgE sensitizes them for months. The non-specific mediator, histamine-releasing factor (HRF), is produced by all stimulated human lymphocytes and can trigger the release of histamine from basophils. This release is additional to that

due to IgE and antigen. HRF may be involved in the non-specific amplification of delayed hypersensitivity, and in modulation of Type I hypersensitivity reactions.

MEDIATOR RELEASE

The antigen-induced calcium ion influx into mast cells has two main results. Firstly, there is an exocytosis of granule contents with the release of preformed mediators, the major one in man being histamine. Secondly, there is the induction of synthesis of newly formed mediators from arachidonic acid leading to the production of prostaglandins and leukotrienes, which have a direct effect on the local tissues. In the lung they cause immediate bronchoconstriction, mucosal oedema and hypersecretion leading to asthma (see Fig. 19.22).

It is becoming clear that different profiles of newly formed mediators are produced by different populations of mast cells, which may explain the different clinical effects in different organs.

Drugs may block the release of mediators either by increasing the intracellular levels of cAMP (e.g. isoprenaline, which stimulates via β-adrenergic receptors) or by preventing the breakdown of cAMP by phosphodiesterase (which is the mechanism of action of theophylline). The mode of action of sodium cromoglycate in preventing histamine release is not clear, but it may involve inhibition of the initial allergen-induced calcium influx. There are also inhibitory feedback effects of mediators such as histamine (Fig. 19.23) and prostaglandins on cells of the immune system.

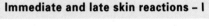

Histamine receptors and their effects

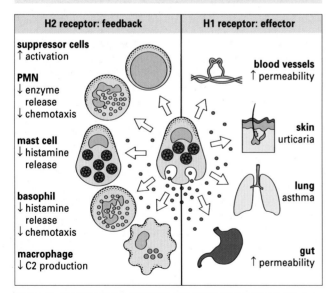

Fig. 19.23 Histamine has functions mediated by H1 and H2 receptors. The inflammatory effect of histamine is due to its pharmacological effects on blood vessels, smooth muscle and mucosal surfaces, all mediated by H1 receptors. The anti-inflammatory feedback effects are mediated by H2 receptors, via the secondary messenger cAMP.

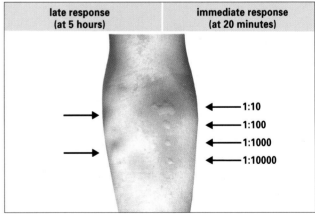

Fig. 19.24 Skin tests were performed 5 hours (left) and 20 minutes (right) before the photograph was taken. The tests on the right show the typical end-point result of a Type 1 immediate wheal-and-flare reaction. The late phase skin reaction (left) can be clearly seen at 5 hours, especially where a large immediate response has preceded it. Figures for dilution of the allergen extract are given.

BASIS OF IMMUNOPATHOLOGY OF ALLERGIC DISORDERS

CUTANEOUS REACTIONS
Skin Prick Test

It is remarkable that the skin prick test, the most simple diagnostic test for allergy, tells us so much about the immunopathology of allergic reactions. The classical skin test in atopy is the Type I wheal-and-flare reaction in which allergen introduced into the skin leads to the release of preformed mediators; these cause increased vascular permeability, local oedema and itching (Figs 19.24 and 19.25). A positive skin test usually correlates with a positive radioallergosorbent test (RAST, a laboratory test for allergen-specific IgE in serum) and a positive relevant provocation test, for example, nasal or bronchial provocation with the allergen.

The late response following skin testing is not often seen because it is rarely looked for. When it does occur it has the appearance of a lump in the skin which is painful rather than itchy.

Immediate and late skin reactions – II

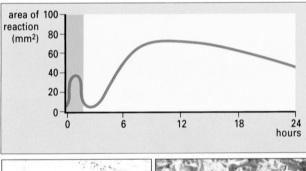

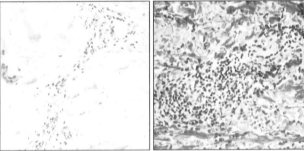

Fig. 19.25 Upper: Using skin prick or intradermal methods of skin testing, an immediate wheal-and-flare reaction is often followed by a late phase reaction, which may last 24 hours and is larger and more oedematous than the immediate response. Left: Immediate type reaction showing a sparse cellular infiltrate around the dermal vessels, consisting primarily of neutrophils. (Courtesy of Dr A. K. Black.) Right: The late reaction has a dense infiltrate, with many basophils. It can be seen after challenge of the skin, nasal mucosa and bronchi and may be particularly important in chronic asthma. (Courtesy of Dr G. Gleich.)

The fact that patients with a variety of atopic disorders show the classical immediate wheal-and-flare response following skin prick tests demonstrates that IgE is bound to skin mast cells, even though their allergic symptoms may be in the nose or bronchi. However, there is a small group of patients who give a clear-cut history of, for example, allergic rhinitis, but in whom skin tests and RAST are negative. Despite the absence of IgE in both skin and serum, these patients do make a local mucosal IgE response. This can be shown by a nasal provocation test, using the allergen, and by the presence of the relevant specific IgE in the nasal secretion, as detected by RAST.

If the lymphocytes of these patients are stimulated with allergen, lymphocyte transformation and lymphokine production result, indicating that their T cells respond to the allergen. However, this does not necessarily imply that delayed hypersensitivity is contributing directly to the disease process. It does indicate that allergen-specific T cells are present in these patients and may be providing 'help' in the IgE response.

Skin Patch Test

In patients with atopic eczema (Fig. 19.26) who have IgE antibodies to the house dust mite, it has been shown that when mite allergen is applied to lightly abraded non-affected skin, a positive patch test results (see Fig. 19.27). It is interesting that a proportion of patients with allergic rhinitis due to house dust mite (see Fig. 19.28), also show house dust mite-positive patch tests with basophil infiltration, suggesting that the infiltration is not specific to atopic eczema.

When the late-phase skin reaction was originally described, it was thought that the mechanism might have been a Type III hypersensitivity reaction (immune-complex-mediated) due to a precipitating IgG antibody, as occurs in bronchopulmonary aspergillosis. However, precipitating antibodies have not generally been found with this late reaction and further research has confirmed that the late-phase response is IgE-dependent.

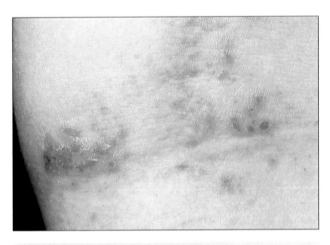

Fig. 19.26 The appearance of atopic eczema on the back of a knee in a child allergic to rice and eggs.

BRONCHIAL REACTIONS

Bronchial reactions to allergens also show an immediate and late-phase response (Fig. 19.29). Sodium cromoglycate is a very effective treatment in allergic asthma and prevents both the immediate and late phase responses which follow bronchial provocation with allergen. This implies that the development of a late reaction in the lung depends on an initial allergen–IgE–mast cell interaction; preventing degranulation with sodium cromoglycate prevents all subsequent events. If patients are pretreated with corticosteroids or prostaglandin synthetase inhibitors, late reactions alone are abolished leaving the immediate response unchanged. This indicates a role for mast cell-derived arachidonic acid metabolites, such as prostaglandins and leukotrienes, in the late response (see Fig. 19.22).

Most asthmatics with reversible airway obstruction benefit from treatment with inhaled corticosteroids. Although these drugs have little or no effect on the immediate IgE-mediated reaction, they do abolish the late reaction. This suggests that the late reaction is of

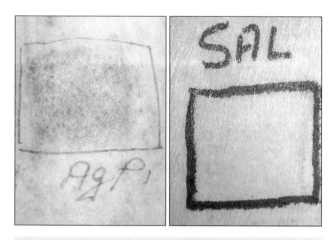

Fig. 19.27 Skin patch tests in a patient with atopic eczema using purified house dust mite (Dermatophagoides pteronyssinus) antigen. Left: The surface keratin of an unaffected area is removed by gentle abrasion and the extract is placed on the skin and occluded for 48 hours, at which time the site is examined. The lesions are macroscopically eczematous and microscopically contain infiltrates of eosinophils and basophils. Right: A saline control. (Courtesy of Dr E. B. Mitchell.)

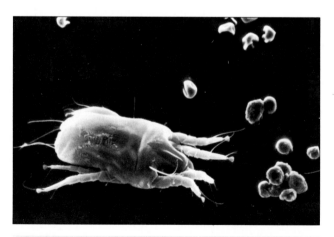

Fig. 19.28 House dust mite – a major allergen. Electron-micrograph showing a house dust mite, *Dermatophagoides pteronyssinus*, and faecal pellets (bottom right) which represent the major source of allergen. Biconcave pollen grains (top right) are shown for comparison of size, showing that the faecal pellet and not the mite itself can become airborne and reach the lungs. (Courtesy of Dr R. Tovey.)

Immediate and late-phase bronchial reactions

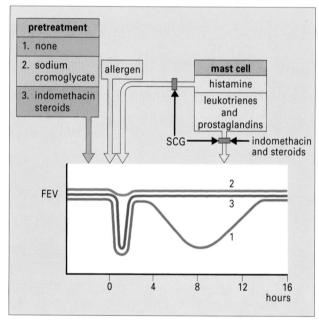

Fig. 19.29 This graph plots the forced expiratory volume (FEV), a measure of lung function, in three groups of individuals prior to and several hours after bronchial provocation with their allergen. In the control (group 1) there is a biphasic (initial and late) bronchial constriction. The initial reaction lasts for 1 hour and is followed by a late-phase reaction lasting several hours. Histamine released from degranulating mast cells is thought to be the major mediator of the immediate reaction in man. The other two groups are pretreated differently. Pretreatment with sodium cromoglycate (group 2) inhibits mast cell degranulation thus preventing both early and late-phase reactions. Pretreatment with indomethacin or corticosteroids, which block arachidonic acid metabolic pathways, inhibits the late-phase reaction but not the immediate reaction (group 3). This implicates leukotrienes and prostaglandins in the development of the late-phase reaction.

major clinical importance in chronic asthma. The beneficial effect of corticosteroids may be related to the reduction of inflammatory cell infiltration in the bronchi (Fig. 19.30).

BRONCHOALVEOLAR LAVAGE

Asthmatics have increased numbers of mast cells within the lumen of the bronchi. These cells are therefore uniquely situated to react with inhaled allergen and initiate IgE-mediated reactions in the lung. Studies on these cells, isolated by bronchoalveolar lavage (BAL), show that they have a high level of 'releasability' as indicated by high levels of mediators in the BAL fluid. These cells are likely to be the major therapeutic target for sodium cromoglycate (SCG) and perhaps other drugs. The BAL mast cells are easily inhibited by SCG compared to those obtained from the lung parenchyma (see Fig. 19.29).

Much evidence suggests a central role for inflammatory cell infiltration during the late-phase reaction. In particular, eosinophils are found in increased numbers in BAL and in the bronchial mucosa during the late phase, but not during the early phase of asthmatic reactions. Eosinophils cause damage to the respiratory epithelium through the release of eosinophil cationic protein (ECP) and major basic protein (MBP) (Fig. 19.31). This in turn may facilitate allergen entry and the access of inflammatory mediators to afferent nerve endings, causing bronchoconstriction through axon reflex pathways.

Associated with asthma is hyperreactivity of the bronchi to histamine, and to non-specific stimuli such as cold air and water vapour. Normal subjects become asthmatic following inhalation of 10 ng of histamine whereas asthmatics respond to 0.5 ng or less.

The fact that this hyperreactivity is a response to chronic allergen challenge is strongly supported by the data of Platts-Mills, who removed asthmatics from their allergenic environment (house dust mite) for up to 3 months. At the end of that time their sensitivity to histamine was greatly reduced and in some cases had returned to normal.

The inflammatory response in asthmatic bronchi

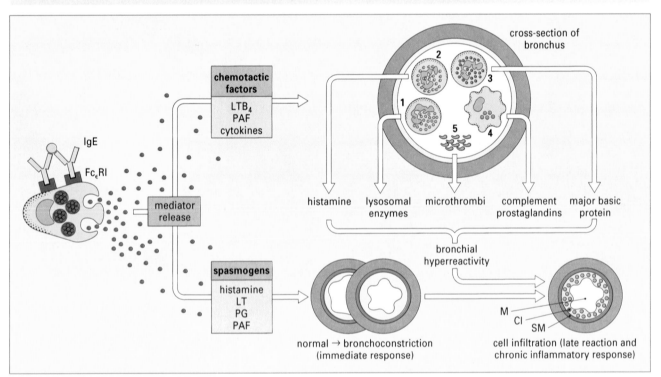

Fig. 19.30 Mast cell mediators include chemotactic and spasmogenic factors. Spasmogens produce the immediate response of bronchoconstriction and lead to increased small-vessel permeability, oedema and cell emigration. Chemotactic factors, including cytokines such as GM–CSF, IL-5 and TNF_α, lead to active accumulation of granulocytes (1), basophils (2), eosinophils (3), macrophages (4) and platelets (5). Production of a further set of inflammatory molecules by these infiltrating cells leads to the late-phase response and a chronic inflammatory response typical of asthma. Many different factors, including hypersecretion of mucus (M), smooth muscle (SM) hypertrophy and cellular infiltration (CI), with associated bronchial hyperreactivity, combine to produce subacute or chronic asthma.

FACTORS INVOLVED IN THE DEVELOPMENT OF ALLERGY

As well as the known genetic predisposition for developing allergy, it is now appreciated that other factors may also be important, and these are discussed below.

T-CELL DEFICIENCY

There is substantial evidence for a role for T cells in both the development and suppression of IgE responses (see Figs 19.6 and 19.7). This has led to the suggestion that a defect in T cells, and in particular Ts cells, may be involved in the aetiology of atopy. There are reduced numbers of CD3+ T cells and CD8+ Ts cells in patients with severe atopic eczema, but this is not seen so clearly in patients with rhinitis or asthma (Fig. 19.32). In addition, T-cell mitogen responses are reduced in severe atopics (those with eczema). These reduced T-cell responses *in vitro* correlate with reduced cell-mediated immunity, which may be reflected *in vivo* as depressed delayed hypersensitivity skin responses.

Until recently it was not clear whether this T-cell deficiency is a cause or a consequence of atopic disease. Interestingly, recent studies have provided some evidence for a causal relationship between T cell deficiency and atopy, but only in bottle-fed babies. Soothill and colleagues have shown that the incidence of eczema in children is reduced if they are breast fed,

and work by other groups has shown a relationship between bottle feeding with cows' milk in infancy, IgE levels and T cell numbers (Fig. 19.33). The implication is that bottle feeding in infancy is associated with both reduced numbers of some subsets of regulatory T cells and increased IgE levels, although it is not certain whether the bottle feeding itself affects T cell numbers. Clearly, other environmental factors are also important in the expression of allergic disorders.

MEDIATOR FEEDBACK

Mast cell mediators such as histamine, prostaglandins and leukotrienes are generally thought to be pro-inflammatory. However, recent evidence suggests an anti-inflammatory role for these compounds on a variety of cells. Histamine, a major mast cell mediator, has been particularly well studied in this respect; the major feedback effects have been outlined in Fig. 19.22.

In contrast to the inflammatory effects of histamine mediated by H1 receptors, the anti-inflammatory effects are mediated by H2 receptors and cAMP. The original hypothesis of Szentivanyi, that a defect of cAMP-mediated signalling is the basis of atopy, is now not generally accepted. However, it has been shown that the inhibition of PMN lysosomal enzyme release and activation of Ts cells by histamine, is defective in atopic subjects. Thus, the role of mediator feedback in atopy is a subject of current interest.

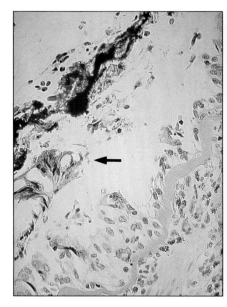
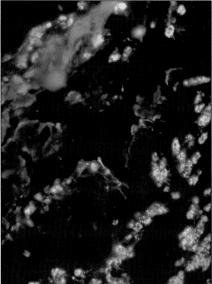
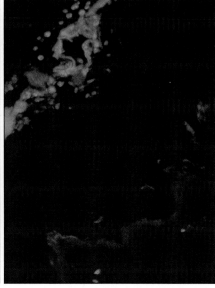

Fig. 19.31 Localization of MBP in the lung of a severe asthmatic. Left: Respiratory epithelium showing striking submucosal eosinophil infiltration and a cluster of desquamated epithelial cells in the bronchial lumen (arrowed) next to a 'stringy' deposit of soot. H&E stain. Center: The same section stained for major basic protein (MBP) showing fluorescent localization in infiltrating eosinophils. MBP deposits are also seen on desquamated epithelial cells on the luminal surface. Right: A control section stained with normal rabbit serum does not stain eosinophils or bronchial tissue but does show some non-specific staining of the sooty deposit. (Courtesy of Dr G. Gleich, from *J Allergy Clin Immunol* 1982;**70**:160–69, with permission.)

Ts cells in atopy

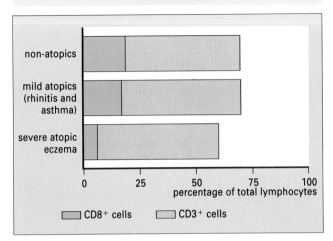

Fig. 19.32 Ts cells in atopy. Patients with severe atopic eczema, but not patients with rhinitis or asthma, have a reduced number of $CD3^+$ T cells, which is almost wholly accounted for by fewer $CD8^+$-staining Ts cells. Decreased numbers of circulating Ts cells are associated with the often grossly elevated serum IgE levels seen in atopic eczema.

ENVIRONMENTAL FACTORS

Environmental pollutants such as sulphur dioxide, nitrogen oxides, diesel exhaust particulates and fly ash may increase mucosal permeability and enhance allergen entry and IgE responsiveness. The effect of smoking seems to be biphasic; an enhancement of IgE levels with low-level cigarette consumption, and suppression at high levels. Smoking also leads to a substantial reduction in the immune response to inhaled antigens, but passive smoking may also increase the risk of asthma in children. Diesel exhaust particulates (DEP) can act as a powerful adjuvant for IgE production (Fig. 19.34). They are less than 1 μm in diameter, are buoyant in the atmosphere of polluted districts and are inhaled. The concentration in urban air is approximately 2μg/m³ of air, but on main roads can reach 30 μg/m³ and during times of peak traffic, levels of 500 μg/m³ have been recorded. DEP given intranasally with antigen produces a marked increase in antigen-specific IgE. This adjuvant effect can be seen with low-dose antigen exposure, of the order that might be experienced in the environment. The increase in allergic rhinitis and asthma in the last 3 decades parallels an increase in air pollution and diesel exhaust. Thus, environmental pollutants may be facilitating IgE responses, thereby contributing to the increase in allergic disease.

Effect of early bottle feeding and T-cell deficiency on serum IgE levels

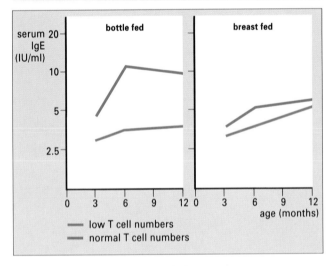

Fig. 19.33 In a survey of infants with low numbers of circulating T cells, those who had been bottle fed with cows' milk showed higher serum IgE levels than those who had been breast fed. The latter children had similar IgE levels to those infants with normal levels of T cells who were breast or bottle fed. These data show that the type of feeding and T cell number affect IgE levels, and suggest that a T-cell defect in association with an environmental factor (feeding) may influence the development of the atopic state.

Effect of pollutants on IgE responses

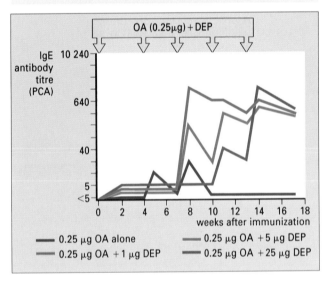

Fig. 19.34 The effects of pollutants, namely diesel exhaust particulates (DEP), on IgE anti-ovalbumin responses in mice. When mice are immunized intranasally with ovalbumin (OA), a small peak of IgE antibody is seen at week 5 and 8, and none thereafter. If DEPs are added to the OA, there is a dose-related increase in IgE persisting after immunization ceases. Thus, DEPs are good adjuvants for IgE production and may partially explain the increase in allergy in recent years. (Courtesy of Dr S. Takafuji, from *J Allergy Clin Immunol* 1987:**79**;639–45, with permission.)

THE CONCEPT OF ALLERGIC BREAKTHROUGH

It is evident that a number of factors must contribute to allergy and this has led to the hypothesis of allergic breakthrough, where clinical symptoms of allergy are only seen when an arbitrary level of immunological activity (allergic breakthrough) is exceeded (Fig. 19.35). This will depend on a number of conditions, including exposure to allergen, genetic predisposition, the tendency to make IgE, and other factors, such as the presence of upper respiratory tract viral infections, decreased Ts cell activity and transient IgA deficiency. The increasing prevalence of allergy is associated with environmental pollution, a further factor that must be taken into account in allergic breakthrough.

Viral infections can exacerbate allergic symptoms and this may be due to the fact that some viruses, for example *Herpes simplex*, enhance basophil histamine release (Fig. 19.36). Both live and ultraviolet light (UVL)-inactivated viruses can enhance histamine release, and interferon has been shown to be the mediator of this effect. Additionally, viruses can damage epithelial surfaces thereby enhancing allergen entry and increasing the responsiveness of target organs to histamine.

Allergic breakthrough in man: hypothesis

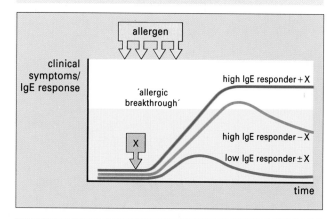

Fig. 19.35 On exposure to allergen an IgE response may develop transiently in low IgE responders before being controlled by normal Ts cell activity. In high responders, the IgE response to allergen is much greater than in low responders, but the overt expression of clinical symptoms is only seen when allergic breakthrough is exceeded. This may depend on the presence of concomitant factors (X) such as viral infections of the upper respiratory tract, transient IgA deficiency or decreased Ts cell activity, which allows unrestrained IgE responses and clinical symptoms to develop. In the absence of factors X, the high responder subject may not show clinical symptoms after a short period of allergen exposure alone, but may be induced to express clinical symptoms of allergy by further exposure to allergen and factors X.

HYPOSENSITIZATION

Hyposensitization therapy involves the injection of increasing doses of allergen. Although clinical benefit is often obtained, the exact mechanism(s) by which it occurs is unknown. Following treatment there is an increase in serum levels of allergen-specific IgG and Ts

Virus enhancement of IgE-mediated histamine release

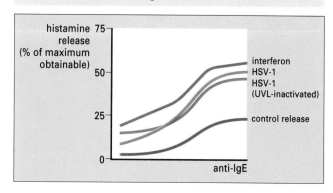

Fig. 19.36 Basophils can be induced to release histamine by anti-IgE which cross-links the IgE bound to Fc_ϵ receptors (control). Histamine release is enhanced in the presence of live *Herpes simplex* virus (HSV-1) or ultraviolet light (UVL)-inactivated HSV. Interferon is thought to be responsible for this enhancement because it mimics the virus effect. This might explain the exacerbation of asthma seen in atopics following upper respiratory tract virus infections.

Effects of hyposensitization therapy

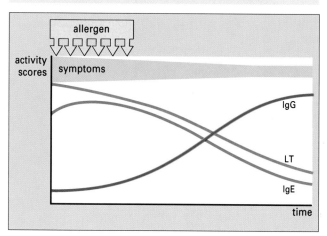

Fig. 19.37 Hyposensitization treatment involves repeated injection of increasing doses of allergen. There is an increase in antigen-specific IgG accompanied by a fall in antigen-specific IgE. This fall is thought to be due to an increase in activity of Ts cells, which is reflected in reduced antigen-induced lymphocyte transformation (LT) *in vitro*.

cell activity, while specific IgE levels tend to fall (Fig. 19.37), although in most cases there is no clear-cut correlation between any of these findings and clinical improvement in the patient. However, it has been shown that allergen-specific Ts cells develop in successfully hyposensitized ragweed allergic patients; this may have a number of effects, such as suppression of the IgE response and of T cell-dependent mast cell recruitment. In the case of people allergic to bee venom where IgG is produced by hyposensitization therapy, there is a good correlation between circulating levels of venom-specific IgG blocking antibodies and clinical protection from anaphylaxis.

There is now good evidence in experimental animals for very long-lived Ts cells and radiation-resistant (non-dividing) IgE memory B cells. In normal rats and mice, repeated inhalation of antigen (ovalbumin) results in tolerance, with suppression of IgE responses. However, using high-IgE-responder animals, Holt's group have shown that their IgE memory and IgE plasma cells are very resistant to the effects of ovalbumin-specific Ts cells and their IgE responses to ovalbumin are unaffected. However, administration of such Ts cells to unimmunized high-responder animals prevents them mounting IgE responses to ovalbumin. These results are clearly relevant, since allergic humans are clinically diagnosed after sensitization and this may explain the relative lack of success of hyposensitization therapy in many subjects. A better understanding of the mechanism(s) by which these long-lived B_ϵ cells are maintained, for example by continued presentation of allergen on dendritic cells or by the idiotypic network system, will undoubtedly be important in the future for therapy.

Interestingly, Holt's group has also shown that inhalation of noxious substances (nitrous oxides or histamine) before inhalation of antigen can induce significant IgE responses in low responder animals, supporting a role for environmental factors in promoting IgE responses, as discussed above.

The beneficial role of IgE in parasitic worm infections

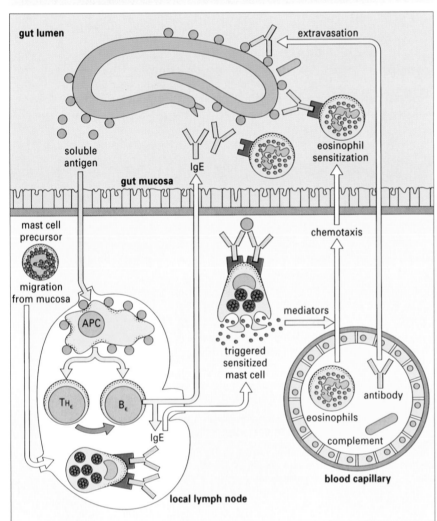

Fig. 19.38 IgE has a beneficial role in parasitic worm infections. During such an infection, soluble worm antigens diffuse across the gut mucosa into the body and are transported to the local lymph nodes, where an IgE response occurs. Mast cell precursors migrate from the gut mucosa to the same local lymph nodes where they mature, acquire worm-specific IgE on their surface and then migrate back to the gut mucosa via the thoracic duct and bloodstream. These mast cells degranulate following contact with worm antigen, releasing mediators which increase vascular permeability and attract inflammatory cells, including eosinophils, to the area. IgE from the lymph node also sensitizes the worm to attack by eosinophils which bear Fc receptors for IgE. Complement and worm-specific IgG also enter the site, due to increased vascular permeability caused by mediators such as histamine. There is also an associated increase in mucus production by goblet cells in the mucosa. All of these mechanisms lead to worm damage and expulsion.

THE BENEFICIAL ROLE OF IgE

With so many disadvantages inherent in being able to make an IgE response to innocuous environmental allergens, the question arises as to why IgE antibody has evolved. It has long been considered that IgE has evolved to play a major role in the defence against parasitic worms; the mechanisms involved are illustrated in Fig. 19.38. Parasitic worms that reside in the gut release soluble allergens that stimulate phenomenal IgE (and IgG) responses in gut-associated lymphoid tissues (GALT). Mast cells maturing in the GALT are sensitized with IgE and migrate to the gut mucosa where they are triggered to release mediators which recruit serum factors (IgG and complement), and chemotactic factors that attract eosinophils and neutrophils. These can kill IgE- or IgG-coated worms by a variety of mechanisms. Since approximately one-third of the world's population has parasitic worm infections this may have represented the evolutionary pressure which initiated development of the IgE class, allergies being an unfortunate by-product of this evolutionary step.

FURTHER READING

Brostoff J, Challacombe SJ, eds. *Food Allergy and Intolerance.* London: Ballière Tindall, 1987.

Bruynzeel-Koomen C, Wichen D, Toonstra J, Berren SL, Bruynzeel PLB. The presence of IgE molecules on epidermal Langerhans' cells in patients with atopic dermatitis. *Arch Dermatol Res* 1986;**278**:199–205.

Coca AF, Cooke RA. On the classification of the phenomenon of hypersensitiveness. *J Immunol* 1923;**8**:163.

Cooke RA, Vander-Veer A. Human sensitization. *J Immunol* 1916;**1**:201.

Finkelman FD, Holmes J, Katona IM, *et al.* Lymphokine control of *in vivo* immunoglobulin isotype selection. *Annu Rev Immunol* 1990;**8**:303–33.

Galli SJ. New insights into 'The Riddle of the Mast Cells': environmental regulation of mast cell development and phenotypic heterogeneity. *Lab Invest* 1990;**62**:5–33.

Gleich GJ, Flanahan NA, Fujisawa T, Vanhoutte PM. The eosinophil as a mediator of damage to respiratory epithelium: a model for bronchial hyperreactivity. *J Allergy Clin Immunol* 1988;**81**:776–81.

Gordon JR, Burd PR, Galli SJ. Mast cells as a source of multifunctional cytokines. *Immunol Today* 1990;**11**:458–64.

Juto P. Elevated serum immunoglobulin E in T cell deficient infants fed cow's milk. *J Allergy Clin Immunol* 1980;**66**:402.

Kaliner MA. The late-phase reaction and its clinical implications. *Hosp Prac* 1987;**15**(Oct):73–83.

Metzger H, IgE, Mast cells and the allergic response. In: *Ciba Foundation Symposium 147*. Chichester: John Wiley and Sons, 1989.

Metzger H, Alcaraz G, Hoffman R, Kinet JP, Pribluda V, Quarto R. The receptor with high affinity for immunoglobulin E. *Annu Rev Immunol* 1986;**4**:419–70.

Miller JS, Schwartz LB. Human mast cell proteases and mast cell heterogeneity. *Curr Opin Immunol* 1989;**1**:637–42.

Prausnitz C, Küstner H. In: Gell PGH, Coombes RRA, eds. *Clinical Aspects of Immunology*. Oxford: Blackwell Scientific Publications, 1962:808–16 (Appendix).

Sedgwick JD, Holt PG. Induction of IgE-secreting cells in the lymphatic drainage of the lungs of rats following passive antigen inhalation. *Int Arch Allergy Appl Immunol* 1986;**79**:329–31.

Stanworth DR. *Immediate Hypersensitivity* Amsterdam: North Holland Publications, 1973.

Takafuji S, Suzuki S, Kolzumi K, *et al.* Diesel-exhaust particulates inoculated by the intranasal route have adjuvant activity for IgE production in mice. *J Allergy Clin Immunol* 1987;**79**:639–45.

Vide L, Bennich H, Johansson SGO. Diagnosis of allergy by an *in vitro* test for allergen antibodies. *Lancet* 1967;**ii**:1105.

Yakota A, Kikutani H, Tanaka T, *et al.* Two species of human Fc$_\epsilon$ receptor (Fc$_\epsilon$RII/CD23): tissue-specific and IL-4-specific regulation of gene expression. *Cell* 1988;**55**:611–18.

chapter 20

Hypersensitivity – Type II

The different forms of hypersensitivity were originally described in terms of the mechanisms involved in damage to tissues. Both type II and type III hypersensitivity are caused by IgG and IgM antibodies. The main distinction is that type II reactions involve antibodies directed to antigens on the surface of specific cells or tissues, whereas type III reactions involve antibodies against widely distributed soluble antigens in the serum. Thus, damage caused by type II reactions is localized to a particular tissue or cell type, whereas damage caused by type III reactions affects those organs where antigen–antibody complexes are deposited (see Chapter 21).

These hypersensitivity reactions are related to normal immune responses seen against microorganisms and larger multicellular parasites. Indeed, in mounting a reaction to a pathogen, exaggerated immune reactions may sometimes be as damaging to the host as the effects of the pathogen itself. In such cases the borderline between a normal, useful immune response and hypersensitivity is blurred. Hypersensitivity reactions may also occur in many other conditions involving immune reactions, particularly autoimmunity and transplantation. The mechanisms of tissue damage which underlie autoimmune immunopathology and graft rejection are described in the chapters covering types II, III and IV hypersensitivity.

■ MECHANISMS OF DAMAGE

In type II hypersensitivity, antibody directed against cell surface or tissue antigens interacts with complement and a variety of effector cells to bring about damage to the target cells (Fig. 20.1). Antibodies can link the target cells to effector cells, such as macrophages, neutrophils, eosinophils and K cells, by means of Fc receptors on these effector cells. Alternatively, the antibodies can interact with complement by activating C1 of the classical pathway. The complement system can also act in two ways in these reactions (Fig. 20.2).

1. Antibody-sensitized target cells can be lysed by activation of the classical and lytic pathways. This results in the deposition of the C5b–9 membrane attack complex on the target cells.

2. C3b can be deposited onto target tissues by activation of the classical pathway and amplification loops. C3b binds to targets by a covalent bond, formed after the breaking of an internal thioester linkage during C3 activation by C3 convertases. After inactivation of C3b by factor I and other serum enzymes, a fragment known as C3d remains covalently bound to the target. Both C3b and C3d can act as recognition structures for effector cells carrying complement receptors, as detailed in Chapter 12.

The different antibody subclasses vary in their ability to interact with different effector cells and with the complement system. This is related to the binding characteristics of the different kinds of Fc receptor.

Both the complement fragments and IgG can act as opsonins bound to host tissues or to microorganisms, and phagocytes take up the opsonized particles. By enhancing the lysosomal activity of phagocytes, and potentiating their capacity to produce reactive oxygen

Antibody-dependent cytotoxicity

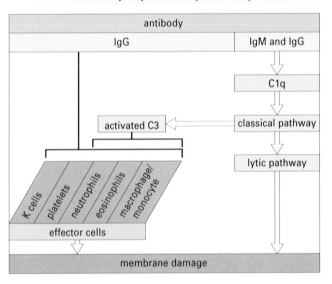

Fig. 20.1 The action of antibody occurs via Fc receptors. K cells, platelets, neutrophils, eosinophils and cells of the mononuclear phagocyte series all have receptors for Fc, by which they can engage target tissues. Activation of complement C3 can generate complement-mediated lytic damage to target cells directly, and also allows phagocytic cells with receptors for activated C3 to bind to the target.

intermediates, the opsonins increase the phagocytes' capacity to destroy pathogens, but also increase their ability to produce immunopathological damage in hypersensitivity reactions (Fig. 20.3). For example, neutrophils from the synovial fluid of patients with rheumatoid arthritis produce more superoxide when stimulated than neutrophils from the blood. This is thought to be related to their activation, in the rheumatoid joint, by mediators which include immune complexes and complement fragments.

Additionally, antibody binding to Fc receptors on phagocytes stimulates them to release arachidonic acid, the precursor for production of prostaglandins and leukotrienes, which are involved in the development of inflammation. Before they can participate in the reactions already described, phagocytes must be attracted to the site of the hypersensitivity reaction. Other complement fragments, for example C5a, act as attractants. Fibrin peptides, leukotrienes (LTB$_4$) and other chemotactic peptides from mast cells and lymphocytes are also active in signalling to incoming effector cells. This again reflects their normal functions in the development of inflammatory reactions (Fig. 20.4.)

The mechanisms by which phagocytes and other effector cells damage their targets also reflect their nor-

mal method of dealing with infectious pathogens (Fig. 20.5). Most pathogens, unless they are resistant to phagocyte-mediated attack, are killed inside the phagolysosome by a combination of oxygen metabolites, radicals, ions, enzymes, altered pH and other factors which interfere with their metabolism. Phagocytes cannot accurately ingest and kill large targets, so granule and lysosome contents are released in apposition to the sensitized target, thereby damaging it (Fig. 20.6); the process of releasing cellular contents is referred to as exocytosis. In some situations, such as the eosinophil reaction to schistosomes, exocytosis of granule contents is beneficial, but if the target is host tissue, which has been sensitized by antibody, damage, rather than benefit, will occur.

Antibodies also mediate hypersensitivity by crosslinking K cells to target tissues. K cells are mainly found in the population of large granular lymphocytes, and bind antibody via their high-affinity Fc receptors. Cytotoxicity then appears to follow the same mechanisms as used by cytotoxic T cells.

Although K-cell activity may be demonstrated against a number of different cell types *in vitro*, it is difficult to assess their impact in hypersensitivity reactions. One problem is the varying susceptibility of different target

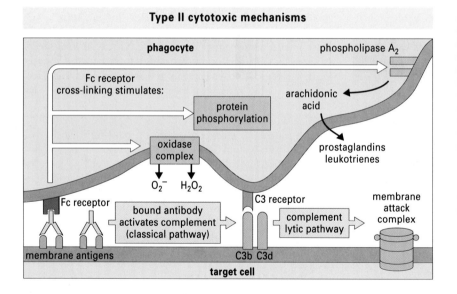

Type II cytotoxic mechanisms

Fig. 20.2 Antibody bound to membrane antigens on effector cells opsonizes them for phagocytes. Cross-linking of the Fc receptors activates a membrane oxidase complex to secrete oxygen radicals; it causes increased protein phosphorylation and hence cellular activation; it also causes increased arachidonic acid release from membrane phospholipids effected by phospholipase A. Immune complexes induce complement C3b deposition which can also interact with opsonic adherence receptors on phagocytes. Activation of the lytic pathway causes the assembly of the membrane attack complex (MAC) by components C5–C9.

Neutrophil activation

neutrophil function	activator					
	IgG	C3	IgG+C3	C5a	C5b67	IgA
adherence	+	+	+++	+	−	+
oxygen metabolism	+	±	++++	+++	++	+
lysosomal enzyme release	+	+	++++	+++	++	+
chemotaxis	+	−	+	+++	++	?
phagocytosis	+	±	++++	−	−	?

Fig. 20.3 Neutrophils are activated by complexed antibodies (IgG or IgA) and activated complement components. Each mediator has a particular spectrum of activity. Note how activated C3 (including C3b, C3bi and C3d, depending on the maturity of the cells involved) and activation via IgG potentiate each other. They present a particularly powerful signal to the cells when both are present.

cells to the actions of the various effector cells. This, in turn, depends on the amounts of particular antigens expressed on the target cell's surface and on the inher-ent ability of different target cells to sustain damage. For example, a red cell may be lysed by a single active C5 convertase site, whereas it takes many such sites to destroy most nucleated cells.

The remainder of this chapter examines some of the instances where type II hypersensitivity reactions are thought to be of prime importance in causing target cell destruction or immunopathological damage.

Chemotactic factors in hypersensitivity reactions

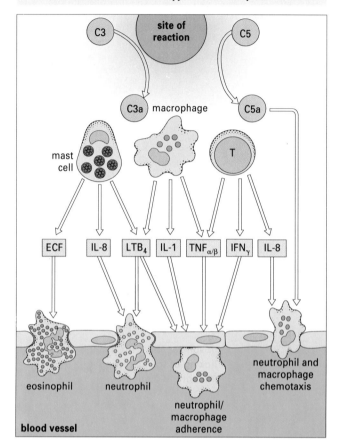

Fig. 20.4 Activated mast cells release eosinophil chemotactic factors (ECF), IL-8 and leukotriene B₄ (LTB₄). LTB₄ is also produced by macrophages and is chemotactic for neutrophils and macrophages. LTB₄, IL-I and IFN_γ act on endothelium to increase neutrophil and monocyte adherence. C5a is a major chemoattractant for both neutrophils and macrophages. Activated T cells release TNF_β and IL-8, which appear to be important in macrophage infiltration of delayed hypersensitivity reactions.

Damage mechanisms

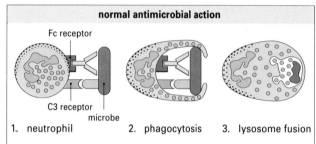

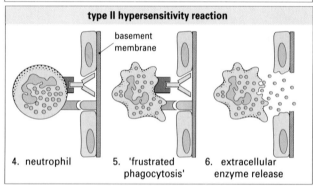

Fig. 20.5 Neutrophil-mediated damage is a reflection of normal antibacterial action. Neutrophils engage microbes with their Fc and C3 receptors (1). The microbe is then phagocytosed (2) and destroyed as lysosomes fuse to form the phagolysosome (3). In type II hypersensitivity reactions, individual host cells coated with antibody may be similarly phagocytosed, but where the target is large, for example a basement membrane (4), the neutrophils are frustrated in their attempt at phagocytosis (5). These release their lysosomal contents to the outside, causing damage to cells in the vicinity.

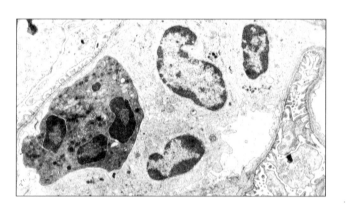

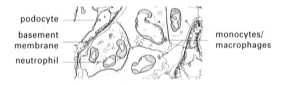

Fig. 20.6 Phagocytes attacking a basement membrane. This electronmicrograph shows a neutrophil and three monocytes binding to the capillary basement membrane in the kidney of a rabbit containing anti-basement membrane antibody. × 3500. (Courtesy of Professor G. A. Andres.)

REACTIONS AGAINST BLOOD CELLS AND PLATELETS

Some of the most clear-cut examples of type II reactions are seen in the responses to red blood cells (erythrocytes). These may occur following incompatible blood transfusions, where the recipient becomes sensitized to antigens on the surface of the donor's erythrocytes. Other important examples include autoimmune haemolytic anaemias and thrombocytopenias, where the patient becomes sensitized to his own erythrocytes or platelets, respectively.

TRANSFUSION REACTIONS

More than 200 genetic variants of erythrocyte antigens have been recognized in man. These variants are produced by at least 20 blood group systems. Each system consists of a gene locus specifying antigens on the erythrocyte surface and, in some cases, on the surface of other cells too. Within each system there may be two or more phenotypes. In the ABO system, for example, there are four phenotypes (A, B, AB and O), and these given rise to four blood groups for this system. An individual with a particular blood group can recognize red cells carrying allogeneic blood group antigens and produce antibodies to them. The antibodies may be produced naturally, without prior immunization with foreign red cells, or may only be produced in quantity after contact with foreign red cells. Some blood group systems are characterized by antigens that are stronger immunogens than others and are more likely to induce antibodies. It is important that donors and recipients are cross-matched for major blood groups before transfusion, otherwise transfusion reactions will occur. Some major human blood groups are listed in Fig. 20.7.

The ABO system is of primary importance. The epitopes concerned are located on the carbohydrate units of glycoproteins. These same epitopes occur in many

Five major blood group systems involved in transfusion reactions

system	gene loci	antigens	phenotype frequencies	
ABO	1	A, B or O	A B AB O	42% 8% 3% 47%
Rhesus	3 closely linked loci: major antigen=RhD	C or c D or d E or e	RhD⁺ RhD⁻	85% 15%
Kell	1	K or k	K k	9% 91%
Duffy	1	Fyᵃ, Fyᵇ or Fy	FyᵃFyᵇ Fyᵃ Fyᵇ Fy	46% 20% 34% 0.1%
MN	1	M or N	MM MN NN	28% 50% 22%

Fig. 20.7 Not all are equally antigenic in transfusion reactions: thus, RhD evokes a stronger reaction in an incompatible recipient than the other Rhesus antigens; and Fyᵃ is stronger then Fyᵇ. Frequencies stated are for Caucasian populations – other races have different gene frequencies.

ABO blood group reactivities

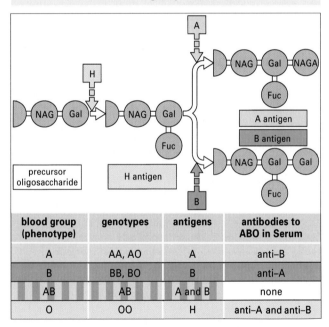

blood group (phenotype)	genotypes	antigens	antibodies to ABO in Serum
A	AA, AO	A	anti-B
B	BB, BO	B	anti-A
AB	AB	A and B	none
O	OO	H	anti-A and anti-B

Fig. 20.8 The diagram presents a simple account of the way the ABO blood groups are constructed. The enzyme produced by the H gene attaches a fucose residue (Fuc) to the terminal galactose (Gal) of the precursor oligosaccharide. Individuals possessing the A gene now attach *N*-acetylgalactosamine (NAGA) to this galactose residue, while those with the B gene attach another galactose, producing A and B antigens, respectively. People with both genes make some of each. The table indicates the genotypes and antigens of the ABO system. Most people naturally make antibodies to the antigens they lack. (NAG = *N*-acetylglucosamine.)

cell types in addition to erythrocytes. The structure of these carbohydrates, and of those determining the related Lewis blood group system, is determined by genes which code for enzymes that transfer terminal sugars to a carbohydrate backbone (Fig. 20.8). In the case of the ABO system, individuals develop antibodies to allogenic specificities without prior sensitization by foreign red cells. Identical epitopes are coincidentally expressed on a variety of microorganisms. Since antibodies to the ABO system antigens occur so widely, it is particularly important to match donor blood to the recipient for this system.

The Rhesus system is also of great importance, since it is a major cause of haemolytic disease of the newborn. Rhesus antigens are lipid-dependent proteins which are sparsely distributed on the cell surface, and are generated by three closely linked genes, of which the Rhesus D locus is most important due to its high immunogenicity.

MN system epitopes are expressed on the N-terminal glycosylated region of glycophorin A, a glycoprotein present on the erythrocyte surface. Antigenicity is determined by polymorphisms at amino acids 1 and 5. The related Ss system antigens are carried on glycophorin B. The relationship of the blood groups to erythrocyte surface proteins is listed in Fig. 20.9. Transfusion reactions caused by the minor blood groups are less common, except where repeated transfusions are given, but the risks are greatly reduced by accurately cross-matching the donor blood to the recipient.

The principle of cross-matching is to ensure that the recipient does not have antibodies which react with the donor red cells. Antibodies to ABO system antigens cause incompatible cells to agglutinate, but weaker reactions may only be detectable by an indirect Coombs' test (see below). If the individual is transfused with whole blood, it is also necessary to check that the donor's serum does not contain antibodies against the recipient's erythrocytes. Transfusion of whole blood is unusual, however; most blood donations are separated into cellular and serum fractions, to be used individually.

Transfusion of red blood cells into a recipient who has antibodies to those cells produces an immediate transfusion reaction (Fig. 20.10). The severity of the reaction depends on the class and the amounts of the antibodies involved. Antibodies to ABO system antigens are usually IgM. They cause agglutination, complement activation and intravascular haemolysis. Other blood groups induce IgG antibodies, and these agglutinate the cells less well than IgM. Severe reactions may cause red cell destruction by complement activation, but more often the IgG-sensitized cells are taken up by phagocytes in the liver and spleen. Red cell destruction may cause circulatory shock, and the released contents of the red cells can produce acute tubular necrosis of the kidneys. Transfusion reactions to incompatible blood may also develop over days or weeks in previously unsensitized individuals, as antibodies to the foreign cells are produced. This can result in anaemia or jaundice.

Transfusion reactions to other components of blood, including leucocytes and platelets, may also occur, though their consequences are not usually as severe as reactions to erythrocytes.

Erythrocyte blood group antigens

erythrocyte surface glyoprotein	blood groups expressed	number of sites per cell
anion transport protein	ABO, Ii	10^6
glycophorin A	MN	10^6
glucose transporter	ABO, Ii	5×10^5
Mr 45 000–100 000	ABO } Rh	$1 \cdot 2 \times 10^5$
Mr 30 000	ABO	
glycophorin B	N, Ss	$2 \cdot 5 \times 10^5$
glycophorins C & D	Gerbich (Ge)	10^5
DAF (delay accelerating factor)	Cromer	$< 10^4$
CD44 (80 kD)	Ina/Inb	$3 \times 10^3 – 6 \times 10^3$
Kell (93 kD)	Kell	$3 \times 10^3 – 6 \times 10^3$
Fg (40 kD)	Fg	12×10^3
lutheran (78 & 85 kD)	lutheran	$1 \cdot 5 \times 10^3 – 4 \times 10^3$

Fig. 20.9 Note that, for those blood groups which depend on carbohydrate antigens, such as ABO and Ii (expressed on the precursor of the ABO polysaccharide), the antigen may be present on different proteins, whereas antigens such as Cromer are proteins and the epitope only appears on one type of molecule.

Clinical symptoms of transfusion reactions

fever
hypotension
lower back pain
feeling of chest compression
nausea and vomiting

Fig. 20.10 A transfusion reaction takes immediate effect in a sensitized individual. The clinical symptoms of a transfusion reaction are given above.

HAEMOLYTIC DISEASE OF THE NEWBORN

Haemolytic disease of the newborn (HDNB) appears in newborn infants where the mother has been sensitized to antigens on the infant's erythrocytes and makes IgG antibodies to these antigens. These antibodies cross the placenta and react with the fetal red cells, causing their destruction (Figs 20.11 and 20.12). Rhesus D (RhD) is the most commonly involved antigen and a risk arises when a Rh$^-$ mother carries a second Rh$^+$ infant. Sensitization of the Rh$^-$ mother to the Rh$^+$ red cells usually occurs during birth of the first Rh$^+$ infant, when some fetal red cells leak back across the placenta into the maternal circulation to be recognized by the maternal immune system. For this reason the first incompatible child is usually unaffected, but the second and later children have an increasing risk of being affected as the mother is repeatedly immunized with successive pregnancies. Reactions to other blood groups may cause HDNB, the second most common being the Kell system K antigen. This is much less frequent than reactions due to RhD because of the relative infrequency of the K antigen (9%) and its weaker antigenicity.

Where haemolytic disease of the newborn due to Rhesus incompatibility is expected, there is a lower incidence of the condition if the father is of a different ABO group to the mother. This observation led to the idea that Rh$^+$ fetal cells would be rapidly destroyed in a Rh$^-$ mother by the preformed antibodies if mother and child were also ABO-incompatible. Consequently they would not be available to sensitize the maternal immune system to RhD antigen. This observation forms the basis of Rhesus prophylaxis, in which anti-RhD

Haemolytic disease of the newborn – I

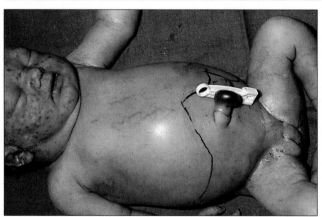

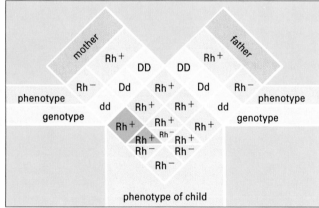

Fig. 20.11 Erythrocytes from a Rhesus$^+$ (RhD$^+$) fetus leak into the maternal circulation usually during birth. This stimulates the production of anti-Rh antibody of the IgG class postpartum. During subsequent pregnancies, antibodies are transferred across the placenta into the fetal circulation (IgM antibodies cannot cross the placenta). If the fetus is again incompatible the antibodies cause red cell destruction.

Haemolytic disease of the newborn – II

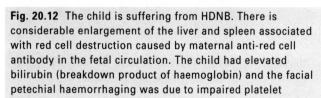

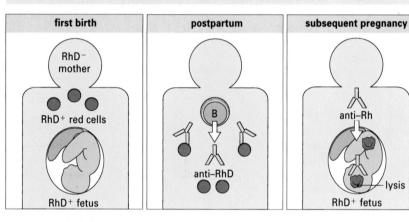

Fig. 20.12 The child is suffering from HDNB. There is considerable enlargement of the liver and spleen associated with red cell destruction caused by maternal anti-red cell antibody in the fetal circulation. The child had elevated bilirubin (breakdown product of haemoglobin) and the facial petechial haemorrhaging was due to impaired platelet function. (Courtesy of Dr K. Sloper.) The most commonly involved antigen is RhD. The table indicates the phenotypes of children from parents with different RhD phenotypes. The Rh$^+$ individuals may be homozygous (DD) or heterozygous (Dd). Rh$^-$ individuals are always homozygous (dd). The changes of HDND arises in Rh$^-$ mothers carrying Rh$^+$ children (red).

antibodies were given to Rh⁻ mothers immediately after delivery of Rh⁻ infants. This has led to a fall in the incidence of HDNB due to Rhesus incompatibility (Fig. 20.13). Although it is not certain, it is assumed that the prevention of sensitization is due to the prompt destruction of fetal red cells.

AUTOIMMUNE HAEMOLYTIC ANAEMIAS

Reactions to blood group antigens also occur spontaneously in the autoimmune haemolytic anaemias, in which patients produce antibodies to their own red cells. Autoimmune haemolytic anaemia would be suspected if a patient gave a positive result on an indirect Coombs' test (Fig. 20.14) which identifies antibodies present on the patient's red cells. These are usually antibodies directed towards erythrocyte antigens, or immune complexes absorbed onto the red cells' surface. The Coombs' test is also used to detect antibodies on

red cells caused by mismatched transfusions, and in haemolytic disease of the newborn. Autoimmune haemolytic anaemias can be divided into three types, depending upon whether they are due to:

1. warm-reactive autoantibodies which react with the antigen at 37°C
2. cold-reactive autoantibodies which only react with antigen below 37°C
3. antibodies provoked by allergic reactions to drugs.

Warm-reactive autoantibodies

Warm-reactive autoantibodies are frequently found against Rhesus system antigens, including determinants of the RhC and RhE loci as well as RhD. The type of reactivity displayed by these autoantibodies is, however, not typical of the antibodies which develop in transfusion reactions to these antigens: they appear to react with different epitopes on the Rh antigens.

Rhesus prophylaxis

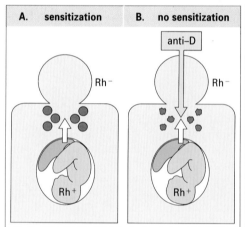

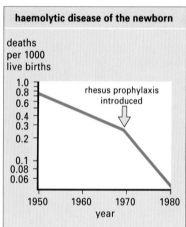

Fig. 20.13 Without prophylaxis Rh⁺ red cells leak into the circulation of a Rh⁻ mother and sensitize her to the Rh antigen(s) (A). If anti-Rh antibody (anti-D) is injected immediately postpartum it eliminates the Rh⁺ red cells and prevents sensitization (B). The incidence of deaths due to HDNB fell during the period 1950–1966 with improved patient care. The decline in the disease was accelerated by the general advent of Rhesus prophylaxis in 1969.

Indirect Coombs' test

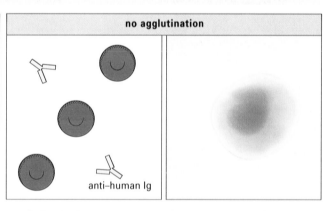

Fig. 20.14 This test, also called the direct antiglobulin test, is used to detect antibody on a patient's erythrocytes. If antibody is present the erythrocytes can be agglutinated by anti-human immunoglobulin. If no antibody is present on the red cells, they are not agglutinated by anti-human immunoglobulin.

Autoantibodies to other blood group antigens are occasionally found. The cause of the majority of warm antibody haemolytic anaemias is unknown but some are associated with other autoimmune diseases. The anaemia seen in these patients appears to be a result of accelerated clearance of the sensitized red cells by spleen macrophages more often than by complement-mediated lysis.

Cold-reactive autoantibodies

Cold-reactive autoantibodies are often present in higher titres than the warm-reactive autoantibodies. The antibodies are primarily IgM and they fix complement strongly. In most cases they are specific for the Ii blood group system. These epitopes are expressed on the precursor polysaccharides which also produce the ABO system epitopes. Incomplete glycosylation of the core polysaccharide produces increased expression of the I and i epitopes.

The reaction of the antibody with the red cells takes place in the peripheral circulation (particularly in winter) where the temperature in the capillary loops of exposed skin may fall below 30°C. This can cause peripheral necrosis, due to aggregation and microthrombosis of small vessels, in severe cases. Anaemia also occurs, but since organs such as the spleen and liver are at 37°C, and the antibodies do not bind at this temperature, this anaemia is apparently caused not by Fc-mediated removal of sensitized red cells in the centre of the body. It must therefore be due to complement-mediated destruction in the periphery. The severity of the anaemia is related to the complement-fixing ability of the patient's serum.

Most cold-reactive autoimmune haemolytic anaemias occur in older people. Their cause is unknown, but it is notable that the autoantibodies produced are usually of very limited clonality, indicating that a limited number of autoreactive clones are present. However, some cases may follow infection with *Mycoplasma pneumoniae*, and these are acute onset diseases of short duration with polyclonal autoantibodies. Such cases are thought to be due to cross-reacting antigens on the bacteria and the red cells, producing bypass of normal tolerance mechanisms, as described in Chapter 23.

DRUG-INDUCED REACTIONS TO BLOOD COMPONENTS

Drugs can provoke hypersensitivity reactions against blood cells, including erythrocytes and platelets. This can occur in three different ways (Fig. 20.15). Usually autoantibodies are produced to the drug or its metabolites, which may be bound to the erythrocytes. In this case it is necessary for both the drug and the antibody to be present to produce the reaction. The first observation of this type was made by Ackroyd, who observed thrombocytopenic purpura (destruction of platelets leading to purpuric rash) following administration of the drug Sedormid. Haemolytic anaemias have been reported following administration of a wide variety of drugs, including penicillin, quinine and sulphonamides. All these conditions are rare.

Occasionally drugs may induce allergic reactions where autoantibodies directed against the red cell antigens are produced, as is the case with 0.3% of patients given α-methyldopa. The antibodies produced are similar to those in patients with warm-reactive antibody but, unlike those diseases, the condition remits shortly after the cessation of drug treatment.

Drug-induced reactions to blood cells: ways in which drug treatment may induce damage

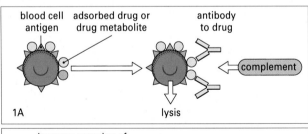

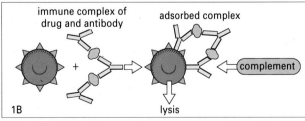

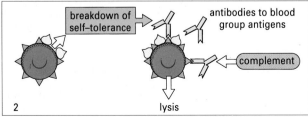

Fig. 20.15 1A. Drugs (or metabolites) adsorb to cell membranes. If the patient makes antibodies to them they will bind to the cell and complement-mediated lysis will occur.
1B. Immune complexes of drugs and antibody become adsorbed to the red cell. This appears to be mediated by the immune adherence receptor (CR1) and/or the immunoglobulin Fc region. It is uncertain whether Fc-dependent binding is specific (i.e. via an Fc receptor). Damage occurs by complement-mediated lysis.
2. Drugs, presumably adsorbed onto cell membranes, induce a breakdown of self-tolerance, possibly by stimulating T-helper (TH) cells. This leads to formation of antibodies to other blood group antigens on the cell surface. Note that in 1A and 1B the antibody is to the drug, or to a complex with the drug attached, while in 2 it is to normal cell surface antigens, therefore in 2 the antibody can destroy cells whether they carry adsorbed drug or not.

REACTIONS TO LEUCOCYTES AND PLATELETS

Autoantibodies to neutrophils (Fig. 20.16), and lymphocytes are sometimes reported. The autoantibodies to neutrophils are true tissue-specific antibodies, unlike antibodies to ABO system antigens. (ABO antigens are found on many tissues, for example, red cells, kidney, salivary gland; the neutrophil-specific antigens are found only on neutrophils.) Antibodies to both neutrophils and lymphocytes are observed in systemic lupus erythematosus (SLE), but their contribution to the pathogenesis of the disease appears to be relatively small, possibly because these cells remove bound antibodies from their surface quite rapidly.

Autoantibodies to platelets are seen in up to 70% of cases of idiopathic thrombocytopenic purpura, a disorder in which there is accelerated removal of platelets from the circulation, mediated primarily by splenic macrophages. The mechanism of removal is via the immune adherence receptors on these cells. The condition most often develops after bacterial or viral infections, but may also be associated with autoimmune diseases including SLE. In SLE, antibodies to cardiolipin, which is present on platelets, can sometimes be detected. Autoantibodies to cardiolipin and other phospholipids can inhibit one aspect of blood clotting (lupus anticoagulant) and can be associated, in some cases, with venous thrombosis and recurrent abortions. Thrombocytopenia may also be induced by drugs, by similar mechanisms to those outlined in Fig. 20.15.

HYPERACUTE GRAFT REJECTION

Hyperacute graft rejection occurs when a transplant recipient has preformed antibodies directed against the graft. The reaction occurs between a few minutes and 48 hours after completion of the transplantation; the recipient's antibodies react immediately against antigens exposed on the grafted cells. The most serious reactions of this type are due to ABO group antigens which are expressed on kidney, but since donors and recipients are now always cross-matched for these antigens, this is very rare. Preformed antibodies to other tissue antigens, including MHC class I molecules, may also cause this type of rejection. Such antibodies might arise after previous blood transfusions or failed engraftments. Hyperacute rejection is further minimized by cross-matching donor T cells with recipient sera, to ensure that the recipient lacks such antibodies.

The reaction is only seen in grafts which are revascularized directly after transplantation, such as kidney grafts. Within one hour of revascularization there is an extensive infiltration of neutrophils and this is followed by major damage to the glomerular capillaries and haemorrhage. Thrombi deposit in the arterioles and the graft is irreversibly destroyed (Fig. 20.17). The major effectors are the neutrophils and platelets, interacting with the sensitized cells via Fc, C3b and C3d receptors. These cells release reactive oxygen intermediates, enzymes, eicosanoids and vasoactive amines in the vicinity of the vessel wall. This produces increased capillary permeability and local damage to tissue cells.

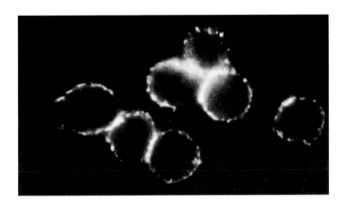

Fig. 20.16 Immunofluorescence of normal neutrophils incubated with SLE serum and goat anti-human F(ab')$_2$ FITC. Antibodies to neutrophils occur in SLE, as demonstrated by the immunofluorescence of these normal neutrophils. Acute transfusion reactions to neutrophils may cause pyrexia, presumably due to pyrogens released from the damaged neutrophils. This indicates that anti-neutrophil antibodies can damage neutrophils, although their role in the pathogenesis of SLE is uncertain. (Reproduced with permission from *Journal of Clinical Investigation* (1979) **64**;902–12.)

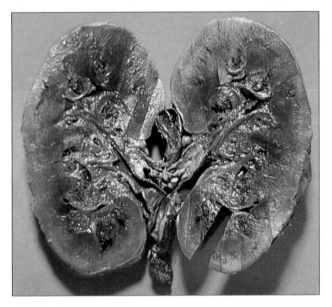

Fig. 20.17 Hyperacute graft rejection. This human kidney, removed 18 hours after transplantation, is thrombosed and haemorrhagic. The whole tissue is dark and necrotic. (Courtesy of Dr K. Welsh.)

REACTIONS TO TISSUE ANTIGENS

A number of autoimmune conditions occur in which antibodies to tissue antigens cause immunopathological damage by activation of type II hypersensitivity mechanisms. The antigens may be expressed on extracellular structural proteins, or on the surface of cells. Examples of such diseases include Goodpasture's syndrome and myasthenia gravis. There are many other examples in which it is possible to demonstrate autoantibodies to particular cell types, but in these cases the importance of the type II mechanisms is less well established.

REACTIONS TO BASEMENT MEMBRANES

A number of patients with nephritis are found to have antibodies to a glycoprotein of the glomerular basement membrane (Fig. 20.18). The antibody is usually IgG and in at least 50% of patients it appears to fix complement.

The condition usually results in severe necrosis of the glomerulus, with fibrin deposition. The association of this type of nephritis with lung haemorrhage was originally noticed by Goodpasture (hence Goodpasture's syndrome). Although the lung symptoms do not occur in all patients, the association of lung and kidney damage is due to cross-reactive autoantigens in the two tissues.

One animal model for Goodpasture's syndrome is nephrotoxic serum nephritis (Masugi glomerulonephritis). In this model heterologous antibodies to glomerular basement membrane are injected into rats or rabbits, resulting in acute nephritis. Antibody deposition occurs on the basement membranes, and there is further deposition of antibodies formed in the host animal to the injected antibody. Development of nephritis and proteinuria depends on the accumulation of neutrophils, which bind via complement-dependent and complement-independent mechanisms. Similar lesions can be

Fig. 20.18 Autoantibody to glomerular basement membrane in Goodpasture's syndrome. Antibody to a basement membrane antigen forms an evenly bound layer on the basement membrane. This is visualized with fluorescent anti-IgG. (Courtesy of Dr F. Hay.)

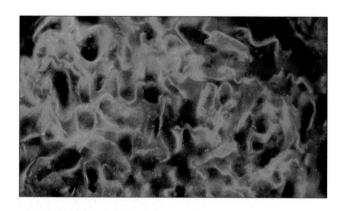

Myasthenia gravis

Fig. 20.19 Normally a nerve impulse passing down a neurone arrives at a motor endplate and causes release of the acetylcholine (ACh). This diffuses across the neuromuscular junction and combines with ACh receptors on the muscle, causing opening of ion channels in the muscle membrane which in turn triggers muscular contraction. In myasthenia gravis antibodies to the receptor block binding of the ACh transmitter, so the effect of the released vesicle is reduced and the muscle can become very weak. This is probably only one of the factors operating in the disease.

induced by immunization with heterologous basement membrane (Stablay model). Another animal model (Heyman nephritis), caused by raising autoantibodies to a protein present in the brush border of glomerular epithelial cells, resembles human membranous glomerulonephritis. Interestingly the damage in this model is mostly complement-mediated: complement depletion of the animals alleviates the condition.

MYASTHENIA GRAVIS AND LAMBERT–EATON SYNDROME

Myasthenia gravis, a condition in which there is extreme muscular weakness, is associated with antibodies to the acetylcholine receptors present on the surface of muscle membranes. The acetylcholine receptors are located at the motor endplate where the neuron contacts the muscle. Transmission of impulses from the nerve to the muscle takes place by the release of acetylcholine from the nerve terminal and its diffusion across the gap to the muscle fibre.

It was noticed that immunization of experimental animals with purified acetylcholine receptors produced a condition of muscular weakness that closely resembled human myasthenia. This suggested a role for antibody to the acetylcholine receptor in the human disease. Analysis of the lesion in myasthenic muscles indicated that the disease was not due to an inability to synthesize acetylcholine, nor was there any problem in

secreting it in response to a nerve impulse. It appeared that the released acetylcholine was less effective at triggering depolarization of the muscle (Fig. 20.19).

Examination of neuromuscular endplates by immunochemical techniques has demonstrated IgG, and the complement proteins C3 and C9, on the postsynaptic folds of the muscle (Fig. 20.20). The IgG and complement are thought to act in two ways: by increasing the rate of turnover of the acetylcholine receptors and by some blockage of acetylcholine binding. Myasthenic serum injected into experimental animals reduces the size of the miniature endplate potential (MEPP – the amount of depolarization of a muscle fibre caused by acetylcholine from a single vesicle). Cellular infiltration of myasthenic endplates is rarely seen, so it is assumed that damage does not involve effector cells. The transient muscle weakness in babies born to myasthenic mothers is further evidence for a pathogenetic role for IgG antibody in this disease (IgG can cross the placenta).

In a related condition, the Lambert–Eaton syndrome, there is also a muscular weakness, but this is caused by defective release of acetylcholine from the neuron. Serum or IgG from patients, if transfused into mice, will transfer the condition, mediating the presence of autoantibody. The autoantigen is thought to be associated with an ion channel on the neuron itself and not on the endplate.

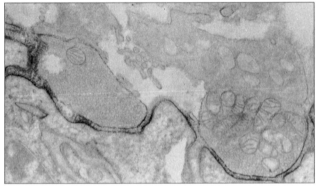

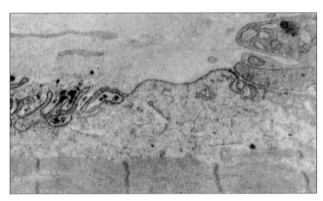

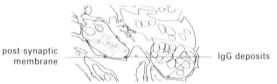

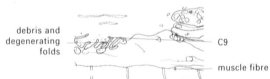

Fig. 20.20 Electronmicrographs showing IgG autoantibody (left) and complement C9 (right) localized at the motor endplate in myasthenia gravis. The upper micrograph shows IgG deposits in discrete patches on the postsynaptic membrane. × 13 000. The micrograph illustrating C9 shows the postsynaptic region denuded of its nerve terminal: it consists of debris and degenerating folds. There is a strong reaction for C9 on this debris. × 9000. (Courtesy of Dr A. G. Engel.)

REACTIONS TO CELLULAR ANTIGENS

Although a great number of autoantibodies react with tissue antigens, their significance in causing tissue damage and pathology *in vivo* is uncertain. It is possible to demonstrate antibody-mediated cytotoxic reactions to thyroid cells using antibody to the thyroid microsomal–microvillous antigen (thyroid peroxidase). Antibody-mediated cytotoxicity to pancreatic islet cells can be detected *in vitro* using sera from some diabetic patients (Fig. 20.21), but it is not certain whether this makes a major contribution to the immunopathological damage, relative to that caused by autoreactive T cells. It is possible that the autoantibodies are formed only after tissue breakdown and release of autoantigens has occurred. Some support for this idea comes from the observation that many of the autoantibodies detected in autoimmune diseases are directed towards intracellular molecules, present in the cytosol or organelles. Nevertheless, traces of these antigens can appear at the surface of the cell to act as potential targets for type II damage mechanisms.

In some cases autoantibodies may actually stimulate receptors on cells, leading to disturbances in physiological regulation but not necessarily to cytotoxic damage (see Chapter 24).

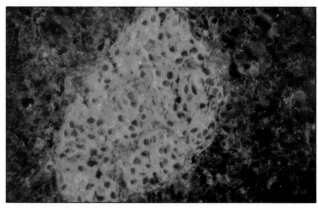

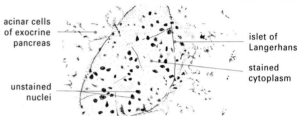

acinar cells of exocrine pancreas

islet of Langerhans

stained cytoplasm

unstained nuclei

Fig. 20.21 Islet cell autoantibodies. Autoantibodies to the pancreas in diabetes mellitus may be demonstrated by immunofluorescence. The antibodies may be cytotoxic for islet cells *in vitro*, indicating a pathological role in disease. (Courtesy of Dr B. Dean.)

FURTHER READING

Anstee DJ. Blood group active substances of the human red blood cell. *Vox Sang* 1990;**58**:1.

Bloy C, Blanchard D, Lambin P, *et al.* Characterization of the D, c, E and G antigens of the Rh blood group system with human monoclonal antibodies. *Mol Immunol* 1988;**25**:926–30.

Burton DR. Immunoglobulin G: Functional sites. *Mol Immunol* 1985;**22**:161–206.

Druet P, Glotz D. Experimental autoimmune nephropathies: induction and regulation. *Adv Nephrol* 1984;**13**:115.

Hughes-Jones NC. Monoclonal antibodies as potential blood-typing reagents. *Immunol Today* 1987;**9**:68.

Lindstrom J. Immunobiology of myasthenia gravis, experimental autoimmune myasthenia gravis and Lambert–Eaton syndrome. *Annu Rev Immunol* 1985;**3**:109–31.

Race R, Sanger R. *Blood Groups in Man.* 6th ed. Oxford: Blackwell Scientific Publications, 1975.

Watkin WM. Biochemical genetics of the blood group antigens: retrospect and propect. *Biochem Soc Trans* 1987;**13**:614–24.

Yamamoto F–I, Clausen H, White T, Marhen J, Hakomori S-I. Molecular genetic basis of the histo-blood group ABO system. *Nature* 1990:**345**:229.

chapter 21

Hypersensitivity – Type III

 TYPES OF IMMUNE COMPLEX DISEASE

Immune complexes are formed every time antibody meets antigen, and generally they are removed effectively by the reticuloendothelial system, but occasionally

Three categories of immune complex disease

cause	antigen	site of complex deposition
persistent infection	microbial antigen	infected organ(s), kidney
autoimmunity	self-antigen	kidney, joint, arteries, skin
inhaled antigen	mould, plant or animal antigen	lung

Fig. 21.1 This table indicates the source of the antigen and the organs most frequently affected.

their formation can lead to a hypersensitivity reaction. Diseases resulting from immune-complex formation can be placed broadly into three groups (Fig. 21.1).

1. The combined effects of a low-grade persistent infection (such as occurs with α-haemolytic *Streptococcus viridans* or staphylococcal infective endocarditis, or with a parasite such as *Plasmodium vivax*, or in viral hepatitis), together with a weak antibody response, leads to chronic immune-complex formation with the eventual deposition of complexes in the tissues (Fig. 21.2).

2. Immune complex disease is a frequent complication of autoimmune disease where the continued production of autoantibody to a self-antigen leads to prolonged immune-complex formation. The mononuclear phagocyte, erythrocyte, and complement systems (which are responsible for the removal of complexes) become overloaded and the complexes are deposited in the tissues, as occurs in systemic lupus erythematosus (SLE) (Fig. 21.3).

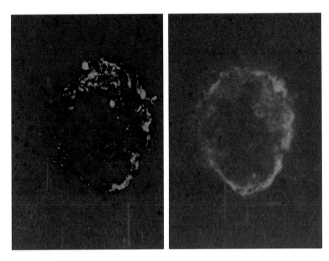

Fig. 21.2 Immunofluorescence study of immune complexes in infectious disease. These serial sections of the renal artery of a patient with chronic hepatitis B infection are stained with fluoresceinated anti-hepatitis B antigen (left) and rhodaminated anti-IgM (right). The presence of both antigen and antibody in the intima and media of the arterial wall indicates the deposition of complexes at this site. IgG and C3 deposits are also detectable with the same distribution. (Courtesy of Dr A. Nowoslawski.)

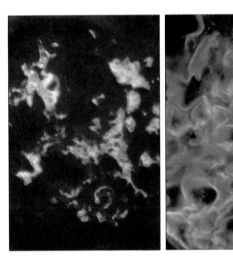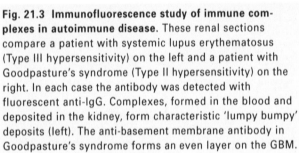

Fig. 21.3 Immunofluorescence study of immune complexes in autoimmune disease. These renal sections compare a patient with systemic lupus erythematosus (Type III hypersensitivity) on the left and a patient with Goodpasture's syndrome (Type II hypersensitivity) on the right. In each case the antibody was detected with fluorescent anti-IgG. Complexes, formed in the blood and deposited in the kidney, form characteristic 'lumpy bumpy' deposits (left). The anti-basement membrane antibody in Goodpasture's syndrome forms an even layer on the GBM.

3. Immune complexes may be formed at body surfaces, notably in the lungs following repeated inhalation of antigenic materials from moulds, plants or animals. This is exemplified in Farmer's lung and Pigeon fancier's

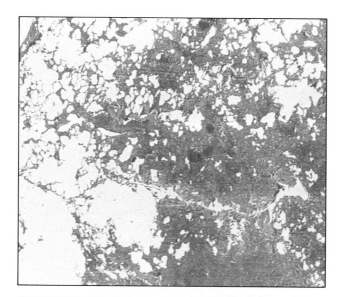

Fig. 21.4 Histological appearance of the lung in extrinsic allergic alveolitis (Pigeon fancier's lung). There is considerable destruction of the alveoli with consolidated areas of darkly stained inflammation and fibrosis due to locally formed immune complexes. H&E stain, × 150. (Courtesy of Dr G. Boyd.)

lung, where there are circulating antibodies to the actinomycete fungi found in mouldy hay, or to pigeon antigens. Both diseases are forms of extrinsic allergic alveolitis, and they only occur after repeated exposure to the antigen. The antibodies induced by these antigens are primarily IgG, rather than IgE, as in immediate (Type I) hypersensitivity reactions. When antigen again enters the body by inhalation, local immune complexes are formed in the alveoli leading to inflammation (Fig. 21.4). Precipitating antibodies to the inhaled actinomycete antigens are found in the sera of 90% of patients with Farmer's lung, but since they are also found in some people with no disease, and are absent from some sufferers, it seems that other factors are also involved, including Type IV hypersensitivity reactions.

The diseases in which immune complexes are important are summarized in Fig. 21.5. The sites of immune-complex deposition are partly determined by the localization of the antigen in the tissues, and partly by how circulating complexes become deposited.

INFLAMMATORY MECHANISMS IN TYPE III HYPERSENSITIVITY

Immune complexes trigger a variety of inflammatory processes. They can interact with the complement system leading to the generation of C3a and C5a (anaphylatoxins), which cause the release of vasoactive amines from mast cells and basophils, thus increasing vascular permeability. These anaphylatoxins are also chemotactic for polymorphs. Cytokines released from macro-

Immune-complex diseases

autoimmune disease	site of deposition					
	circulating complexes	vascular system	kidneys	joints	skin	others
rheumatoid arthritis	+	+		+		
systemic lupus erythematosus	+	+	+	+	+	brain
polyarteritis	+	+	+			muscle, liver
polymyositis/dermatomyositis		+			+	muscle
cutaneous vasculitis	+	+			+	
fibrosing alveolitis	+					lungs
cryoglobulinaemia	+	+	+	+	+	
disease due to microbial antigens						
leprosy	+		+	+	+	eyes
bacterial endocarditis	+	+	+			heart
malaria	+		+			
trypanosomiasis (African)	+	+	+			heart, brain
hepatitis	+	+	+	+		liver
dengue haemorrhagic fever	+		+		+	

Fig. 21.5 Some of the main diseases in which immune-complexes are implicated, indicating sites of deposition. Diseases in the upper part of the table are primarily autoimmune, whereas those in the lower part are due to microbial antigens. There is no distinct site of immune-complex deposition that characterizes a particular disease.

phages, particularly tumour necrosis factor (TNF) and IL-1, are also important in localized immune-complex diseases, such as alveolitis, through a mechanism involving neutrophil recruitment. Platelets can also interact with immune complexes, through their Fc receptors, leading to aggregation and microthrombus formation and hence a further increase in vascular permeability due to the release of vasoactive amines (Fig. 21.6). Platelets are a rich source of growth factors, and release of these may contribute to the cellular proliferation found in immune-complex diseases such as glomerulonephritis and rheumatoid arthritis.

The attracted polymorphs attempt to ingest the complexes, but in the case of tissue-trapped complexes this is difficult and the phagocytes are therefore likely to release their lysosomal enzymes to the exterior, causing tissue damage (Fig. 21.7). If simply released into the blood or tissue fluids these lysosomal enzymes are unlikely to cause much inflammation, because they are rapidly neutralized by serum enzyme inhibitors. But if the phagocyte applies itself closely to the tissue-trapped complexes through Fc binding, then serum inhibitors are excluded and the enzymes may damage the underlying tissue.

EXPERIMENTAL MODELS OF IMMUNE-COMPLEX DISEASE

Experimental models are available for each of the three main types of immune-complex disease described above: serum sickness induced by injections of foreign antigen, to represent the presence of a persistent infection; the NZB/NZW mouse, for autoimmunity; and the Arthus reaction, for local damage by extrinsic antigen. Care must be taken when interpreting animal experiments as the erythrocytes of rodents and rabbits lack the receptor for C3b (known as CR1) which readily binds immune complexes that have fixed complement. This is present on primate erythrocytes.

Deposition of immune-complexes in blood vessel walls – I

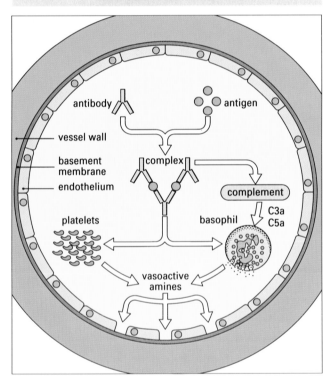

Fig. 21.6 Antibody and antigen combine to form immune-complexes. The complexes act on complement (to release C3a and C5a), which in turn acts on basophils to release vasoactive amines. The complexes also act directly on basophils and platelets (in humans) to produce vasoactive amine release. The amines released include histamine and 5-hydroxytryptamine, which cause endothelial cell retraction and thus increased vascular permeability.

Deposition of immune-complexes in blood vessel walls – II

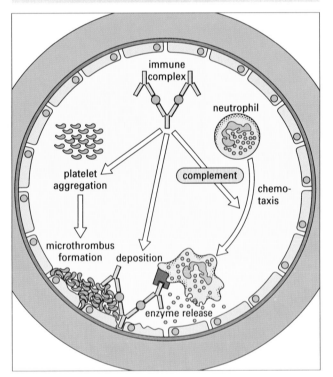

Fig. 21.7 With increased vascular permeability, immune-complexes become deposited in the blood vessel wall. These complexes induce platelet aggregation and complement activation. The platelets aggregate to form microthrombi on the exposed collagen of the basement membrane of the endothelium. Neutrophils (PMNs), which are attracted to the site by complement products, cannot ingest the complexes. They therefore release their lysosomal enzymes, causing further damage to the vessel wall.

INDUCED SERUM SICKNESS

In serum sickness, circulating immune-complexes deposit in the blood vessel walls and tissues leading to increased vascular permeability and thus to inflammatory diseases such as glomerulonephritis and arthritis. In the pre-antibiotic era, serum sickness was a complication of serum therapy with massive doses of antibody for diseases such as diphtheria – horse anti-diphtheria serum was usually used and some people made antibodies against horse proteins.

Serum sickness is now commonly studied in rabbits by giving them an intravenous injection of a foreign soluble protein such as bovine serum albumin (BSA). After about one week antibodies are formed which enter the circulation and complex with antigen in antigen excess (Fig. 21.8). These small complexes (in antigen excess) are only removed slowly by the mononuclear phagocyte system and persist in the circulation. However, with the formation of complexes there is an abrupt fall in total haemolytic complement and the clinical signs of serum sickness develop, due to granular deposits of antigen–antibody and C3 forming along the glomerular basement membrane (GBM) and in small vessels elsewhere. As more antibody is formed, complexes are produced in optimal proportions and are cleared, so the animals recover. Chronic disease is induced by continued daily administration of antigen.

AUTOIMMUNE IMMUNE-COMPLEX DISEASE

Autoimmune immune-complex disease is demonstrated using the F_1 hybrid NZB/NZW mouse which simulates various features of human SLE. These mice make a range of autoantibodies including anti-erythrocyte, anti-nuclear, anti-DNA and anti-SM antibodies. The animals are born clinically normal but within 2–3 months show signs of haemolytic anaemia, and have positive Coombs' tests (for anti-erythrocyte antibody), anti-nuclear antibodies, positive lupus cell tests and circulating immune complexes with deposits in the glomeruli and choroid plexus. The disease is much more marked in the females and these die within a few months of developing symptoms (Fig. 21.9).

THE ARTHUS REACTION

The Arthus reaction takes place at a local site in and around the walls of small blood vessels; it is most frequently demonstrated in the skin. Animals are immunized repeatedly until they have appreciable levels of precipitating, mainly IgG, antibody. On injecting antigen subcutaneously or intradermally a reaction develops which reaches peak intensity in 4–10 hours (Fig. 21.10). Depending on the amount of antigen injected, marked oedema and haemorrhage develop at the site of injection. The reaction then wanes and is usually markedly decreased by 48 hours.

Time course of experimental serum sickness

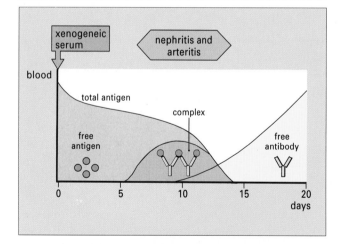

Fig. 21.8 Following an injection of xenogeneic serum there is a lag period of approximately five days in which free antigen is detectable in serum. After this time, antibodies are produced to the foreign proteins and immune-complexes are formed in serum; it is during this period that the symptoms of nephritis and arteritis appear. To begin with, small soluble complexes are found in antigen excess; with increasing antibody titres, larger complexes are formed which are deposited and subsequently cleared. At this stage the symptoms disappear.

Autoimmune disease in NZB/NZW mice

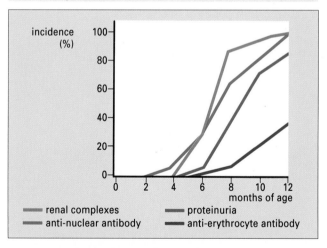

Fig. 21.9 The graph shows the onset of autoimmune disease in female NZB/NZW mice with advancing age. Incidence refers to the percentage of mice with the features identified. Immune-complexes were detected by immunofluorescent staining of a kidney section. Anti-nuclear antibodies were detected in serum by indirect immunofluorescence. Proteinuria reflects kidney damage. Autoantibodies to erythrocytes develop later in the disease and are therefore less likely to relate to kidney pathology. The onset of autoimmune disease is delayed in male mice by approximately three months.

Immunofluorescence studies have shown that initial deposition of antigen, antibody and complement in the vessel wall is followed by neutrophil infiltration and intravascular clumping of platelets (Fig. 21.11). This platelet reaction can lead to vascular occlusion and necrosis in severe cases. After 24–48 hours the neutrophils are replaced by mononuclear cells and eventually some plasma cells appear.

Complement activation via either the classical or alternative pathways is essential for the Arthus reaction to develop. Without complement, neutrophils are not attracted to the site and only a mild oedema will occur in the absence of the neutrophils. Treatment with antibodies to TNF can halve the reaction. The ratio of antibody to antigen is important for producing maximum reactivity. Generally, complexes formed in either antigen or antibody excess are much less toxic than those formed at equivalence.

PERSISTENCE OF COMPLEXES

Normally immune complexes are removed by the mononuclear phagocyte system, particularly in the liver and spleen. Some confusion has arisen owing to the differences between immune-complex removal systems in primates and those in rodents and rabbits. Primate erythrocytes have the CR1 receptor for C3b, whereas erythrocytes in rodents and rabbits do not.

These non-primates rely solely on the receptor for C3b on platelets (a receptor that primates also have). Owing to the large number of erythrocytes, in primates the erythrocyte CR1 constitutes the bulk of CR1 in blood. There are about 700 receptors per erythrocyte, and their effectiveness is enhanced by the grouping of receptors in patches, allowing high-avidity binding to the large complexes. The CR1 receptor readily binds immune complexes which have fixed complement, as shown by experiments with animals lacking complement

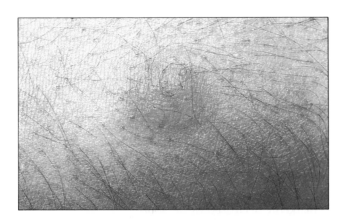

Fig. 21.10 The gross appearance of the Arthus reaction. There is a reddened area of inflammation which is maximal 5–6 hours after injection of antigen.

The Arthus reaction

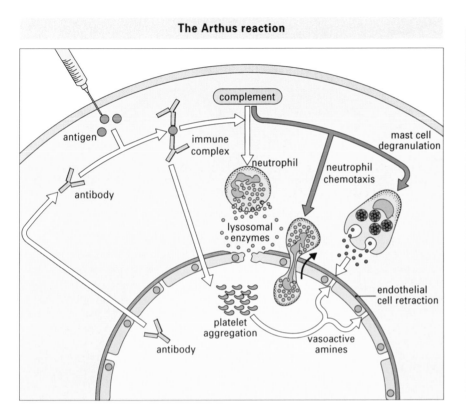

antigen
immune complex
complement
antibody
neutrophil
neutrophil chemotaxis
mast cell degranulation
lysosomal enzymes
platelet aggregation
antibody
vasoactive amines
endothelial cell retraction

Fig. 21.11 Antigen injected intradermally combines with specific antibody from the blood to form immune-complexes. The complexes activate complement and act on platelets, which release vasoactive amines. Immune-complexes also induce macrophages to release TNF and IL-1 (not shown). Complement C3a and C5a fragments cause mast cell degranulation and attract neutrophils into the tissue. Mast cell products, including histamine and leukotrienes, induce increased blood flow and capillary permeability. The inflammatory reaction is potentiated by lysosomal enzymes released from the polymorphs. Furthermore, C3b deposited on the complexes opsonizes them for phagocytes. The Arthus reaction can be seen in patients with precipitating antibodies, such as those with extrinsic allergic alveolitis associated with micropolyspora fungi.

(Fig. 21.12). The complexes are then transported to the liver and spleen, where they are removed by fixed tissue macrophages (Fig. 21.13). Most of the CR1 is removed in the process so, in situations of continuous immune-complex formation, the number of active receptors falls steadily, impairing the efficiency of immune-complex handling. In patients with SLE the number of receptors may well be halved.

Complexes can also be released from erythrocytes in the circulation by the enzymatic action of Factor I, which cleaves C3b, leaving a small fragment, C3dg, attached to the CR1 on the cell membrane. These soluble complexes must then be removed by phagocytic cells bearing receptors for IgG Fc (Fig. 21.14).

In patients with low levels of classical pathway components (either through hereditary deficiency or consumption by complexes) there is poor binding of immune-complexes to erythrocytes. This might be expected to result in persistent immune complexes in the circulation. In fact the reverse occurs, with the complexes disappearing rapidly from the circulation.

Unfortunately these non-erythrocyte-bound complexes are not taken up following passage through the liver and spleen, as might be expected, but are deposited in the tissues such as skin, kidney and muscle, where they can set up inflammatory reactions.

In normal primates the erythrocytes provide a buffer mechanism, binding complexes which have fixed complement and effectively removing them from the plasma. In small blood vessels 'streamline flow' allows the erythrocytes to travel in the centre of the vessel surrounded by the flowing plasma. Thus it is only the plasma that makes contact with the vessel wall (Fig. 21.15). Only in the sinusoids of the liver and spleen, or at sites of turbulence, do the erythrocytes make contact with the lining of the vessels.

The size of an immune complex is very important in regulating its clearance – in general, larger complexes are rapidly removed by the liver within a few minutes, while smaller complexes circulate for longer periods (Fig. 21.16). This is because larger complexes are more effective at fixing complement and thus bind better to erythrocytes. Also, larger complexes are released more slowly from the erythrocytes by the action of Factor I. Anything which affects the size of complexes is therefore likely to influence clearance. It has been suggested

Effects of complement depletion on handling of immune-complexes

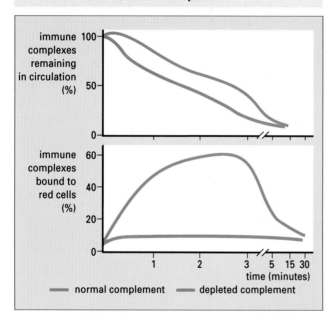

Fig. 21.12 A bolus of immune-complexes was infused into the circulation of a primate. In animals with a normal complement system the complexes were bound quickly by the CR1 receptor on erythrocytes. In animals whose complement had been depleted by treatment with cobra venom factor, the erythrocytes hardly bound immune-complexes at all. Paradoxically, this results in slightly faster removal of complexes in the depleted animals, with the complexes being deposited in the tissues rather than being removed by the spleen and liver. (Based on data from Waxman *et al.*)

Clearance of immune-complexes in the liver

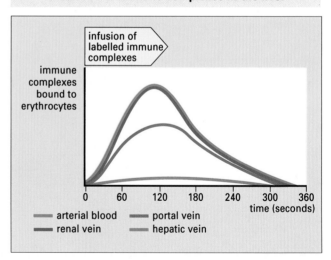

Fig. 21.13 ¹²⁵I-BSA/anti-BSA complexes were infused into a primate over a period of 120 seconds. Blood was sampled from renal, portal and hepatic veins, and the level of immune-complexes bound to the erythrocytes was measured by radioactive counting. The levels of complexes in the renal and portal veins were similar to that in arterial blood. However, complexes were virtually absent from hepatic venous blood throughout, indicating that complexes bound to erythrocytes are removed during a single transit through the liver. (Based on data from Cornacoff *et al.*)

Immune-complex transport and removal

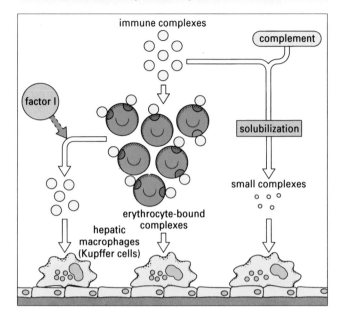

Fig. 21.14 In man and other primates, complexes may be bound by the CR1 receptor on erythrocytes and transported to the liver where they are removed by hepatic macrophages. Complexes released from erythrocytes by Factor I are taken up by cells (including macrophages) bearing receptors for Fc and complement. Complement solubilization of large complexes produces small soluble complexes which may be taken up directly by tissue macrophages.

that a genetic defect which favours production of low-affinity antibody could well lead to formation of smaller complexes, and so to immune-complex disease. Generally, when an individual forms antibodies to self-antigens, only a few epitopes are recognized and this results in small complexes since the formation of a cross-linked lattice is restricted.

Striking differences have been observed in the clearance of complexes with different immunoglobulin classes. IgG complexes are bound by erythrocytes and are gradually removed from the circulation, whereas IgA complexes bind poorly to erythrocytes but disappear rapidly from the circulation, with increased deposition in the kidney, lung and brain. When large amounts of complex are present, the mononuclear phagocyte system may become overloaded. Certainly in experimental animals it is possible to block the mononuclear phagocyte system, which then leads to prolonged circulation of immune complexes with some deposition in the glomerulus. There is evidence for a defective mononuclear phagocyte system in human immune complex disease, but this may well be the result of overload rather than a primary defect.

Recently the carbohydrate groups on immunoglobulin molecules have been shown to be important for removal of immune complexes by phagocytic cells, and there may be abnormalities of these carbohydrates in certain immune complex diseases, particularly rheumatoid arthritis and SLE. It is not certain, however, whether the abnormalities of carbohydrate are primary, or are themselves caused by the disease.

Streamline flow of blood

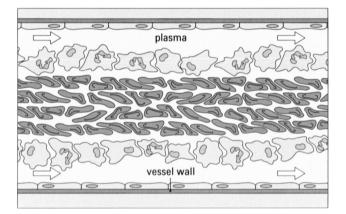

Fig. 21.15 Blood passes through blood vessels in a streamline flow, with erythrocytes in the centre, surrounded by white cells, and then a plasma sheath making contact with vessel walls. Immune-complexes attached to erythrocytes through the CR1 receptor are kept away from vessel walls. Deficiencies in complement prevent attachment to erythrocytes and allow complexes to contact and bind to vessel walls.

Complex clearance by the reticuloendothelial system

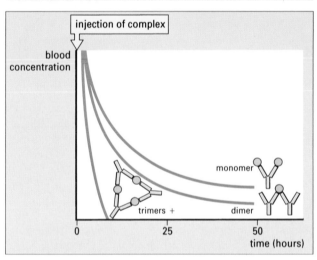

Fig. 21.16 Large immune-complexes are cleared most quickly because they present an IgG–Fc lattice to reticuloendothelial cells with Fc receptors, permitting higher avidity binding to these cells. They also fix complement better than small complexes.

Although immune complexes may persist in the circulation for prolonged periods. simple persistence is not usually harmful in itself. Problems only start to occur when they deposit in the tissues.

DEPOSITION OF COMPLEXES IN TISSUES

Two questions are relevant to tissue deposition:
1. why do complexes deposit?
2. why do complexes show affinity for particular tissues in different diseases?

INCREASE IN VASCULAR PERMEABILITY
The most important trigger for tissue deposition of immune complexes is probably an increase in vascular permeability. Even inert substances, for example colloidal carbon, can be made to deposit in vessel walls if animals are given vasoactive substances such as histamine or serotonin. Similarly, circulating immune complexes may be caused to deposit by the infusion of agents which cause liberation of mast cell vasoactive amines, including histamine. Pretreatment with antihistamines blocks this effect. In studies of experimental immune-complex disease, long-term administration of vasoactive amine antagonists, such as chlorpheniramine or methysergide, considerably reduced complex deposition (Fig. 21.17). More importantly, young NZB/NZW mice treated with methysergide showed less renal pathology than controls (Fig. 21.18).

Increases in vascular permeability can be initiated by a range of mechanisms which may vary in importance in various diseases and in different species. This makes interpretation of some of the animal models difficult. Complement, mast cells, basophils and platelets must all be considered as potential contributors to the release of vasoactive amines.

HAEMODYNAMIC PROCESSES
Immune-complex deposition is most likely where there is high blood pressure and turbulence (Fig. 21.19). Many macromolecules deposit in the glomerular capillaries, where the blood pressure is approximately four times that of most other capillaries. If the glomerular blood pressure is reduced, by partially constricting the renal artery or by ligating the ureter, deposition is reduced. On the other hand, experimentally-induced hypertension enhances the development of acute serum sickness in the rabbit. Similarly at other sites, such as the walls of arteries, the most severe lesions occur at sites of turbulence, such as vessel bifurcations, or in vascular filters such as the choroid plexus or the ciliary body of the eye.

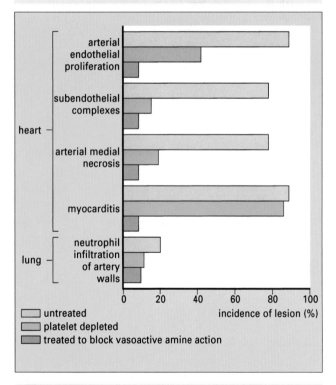

Fig. 21.17 Serum sickness was induced in rabbits with a single injection of bovine serum albumin. The animals were either untreated, platelet depleted or treated with drugs to block vasoactive amine action. The incidence of serum sickness lesions in the heart and lung was scored. Drug treatment considerably reduced the signs of disease by lowering vascular permeability and thus minimizing complex deposition.

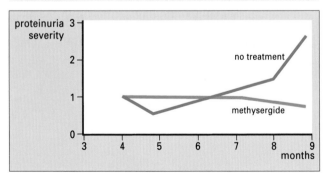

Fig. 21.18 Kidney damage, assessed by proteinuria, was measured in NZB/NZW mice over five months. Untreated animals developed severe proteinuria, while methysergide-treated animals did not. Methysergide blocks formation of the vasoactive amine, 5-HT, and thus blocks a variety of inflammatory events, e.g. deposition of complexes, neutrophil infiltration of capillary walls and endothelial proliferation, all of which produce the glomerular pathology.

TISSUE BINDING OF ANTIGEN

Local high blood pressure explains a general tendency for deposits to form in certain organs, but it does not explain why complexes home in on different organs in different diseases. For example, in SLE the kidney is a particular target, whereas in rheumatoid arthritis, although circulating complexes are present, the kidney is usually spared and the joints are the principal target. It is possible that the antigen in the complex provides the organ specificity. A convincing model has been established where mice are given endotoxin, causing cell damage and release of DNA, which binds to healthy glomerular basement membrane. Anti-DNA is then produced, by polyclonal activation of B cells, and is bound by the fixed DNA leading to local immune complex formation (Fig. 21.20). It is possible that in other diseases antigens will be identified with affinity for particular organs.

The charge of the antigen and antibody may be important in some systems. For example, positively charged (cationic) antigens and antibodies are more likely to deposit in the negatively charged glomerular basement membrane. The degree of glycosylation also affects the fate of complexes containing glycoprotein antigens. In certain diseases the antibodies and antigens are both produced within the target organ. The extreme of this is reached in rheumatoid arthritis where the anti-IgG antibody is produced by plasma cells within the synovium; the antibodies combine with each other (self-associating), so setting up an inflammatory reaction.

Haemodynamic factors affecting complex deposition

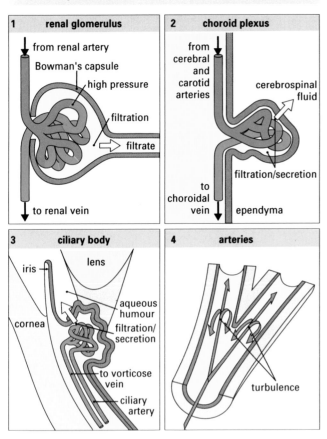

Fig. 21.19 Factors include filtration, which occurs in the formation of the glomerular ultrafiltrate (1), the formation of the cerebrospinal fluid by the choroid plexus (2), and in the formation of the aqueous humour by the epithelium of the ciliary body in the eye (3). High pressure in the renal glomerulus also favours deposition. Turbulence at curves or bifurcations of arteries (4), is another factor favouring deposition.

Tissue binding of antigen with local immune-complex formation

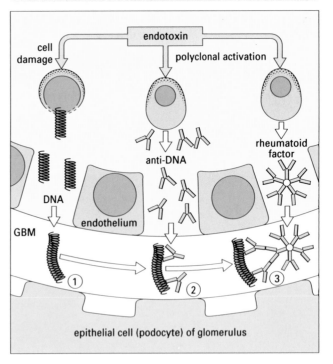

Fig. 21.20 Endotoxin, injected into mice, induces cell damage and consequent release of DNA. The DNA can then become deposited (1) on the collagen of the glomerular basement membrane (GBM). Endotoxin can also induce a polyclonal stimulation of B cells, some of which produce autoantibodies such as anti-DNA and anti-IgM – the latter are known as rheumatoid factors (RFs). Anti-DNA antibody can then bind to the deposited DNA forming a local immune-complex (2). RFs have a low affinity for monomeric IgG, but bind with high avidity to the assembled DNA–anti-DNA complex (3). Thus further immune-complex formation occurs in situ.

SIZE OF IMMUNE COMPLEXES

The exact site of immune-complex deposits depends partly on the size of the complex. This is exemplified in the kidney, where small immune-complexes can pass through the glomerular basement membrane so ending up on the epithelial side of the membrane; large complexes are unable to cross the membrane and generally accumulate between the endothelium and the basement membrane or the mesangium (Fig. 21.21). The size of immune complexes depends on the valency of the antigen, and both the titre and affinity of the antibody.

IMMUNOGLOBULIN CLASS

The class of immunoglobulin in an immune complex can influence its deposition. With anti-DNA antibodies in SLE, there are marked age- and sex-related variations in the class and subclass of antibodies. As NZB/NZW mice grow older there is a class switch, from predominantly IgM to IgG2a. This occurs earlier in females than in males and coincides with the onset of renal disease, indicating the importance of antibody class in the tissue deposition of complexes (Fig. 21.22). Death occurs 2–3 months later.

COMPLEMENT SOLUBILIZATION OF IMMUNE COMPLEXES

It has been known since the work of Heidelberger on the Precipitin Curve, that complement delays precipitation of immune complexes, although this information was forgotten for a long time. This ability to keep complexes soluble is a function of the classical complement pathway. It is thought that, by intercalating into the lattice of the complex, the complement components reduce the number of antigen epitopes the antibodies can bind (i.e. reduce the valency), resulting in smaller complexes which remain soluble. In primates these complement-bearing complexes are readily bound by the receptor for C3b (CR1 receptor) on erythrocytes.

Even if complexes have deposited in the tissues, a mechanism exists for making them soluble once more. Again, this mechanism involves complement.

Complement can rapidly resolubilize precipitated complexes through the alternative pathway (Fig. 21.23). The solubilization appears to occur by the insertion of complement C3b and C3d fragments into the complexes. It may be that complexes are continually being deposited in normal individuals, but are removed by solubil-

Immune-complex deposition in the kidney

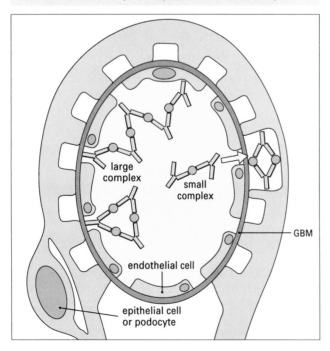

Fig. 21.21 The site of complex deposition in the kidney is dependent on the size of the complexes in the circulation. Large complexes become deposited on the glomerular basement membrane, while small complexes pass through the basement membrane and are seen on the epithelial side of the glomerulus.

Antibody classes in immune-complex disease

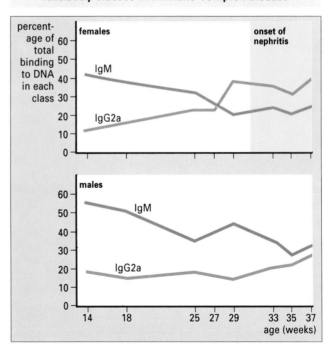

Fig. 21.22 Immune-complex disease is automatic in the NZB/NZW mouse and follows a class switch during early development, from IgM to IgG2a. The graphs show the titres of anti-DNA antibodies (IgM and IgG2a) in females and males. Both the class switch and fatal renal disease occur earlier in the female mice of this strain.

ization. If this is the case, the process would be inadequate in hypocomplementaemic patients and lead to prolonged complex deposition. Solubilization defects have been observed in sera from patients with systemic immune complex disease, but whether the defect is primary or secondary is not known.

DETECTION OF IMMUNE COMPLEXES

There are many techniques for detecting and quantifying immune complexes. The ideal place to look for complexes is in the affected organ. Tissue samples may be examined by immunofluorescence for the presence of immunoglobulin and complement. The composition, pattern and particular area of tissue affected, all provide useful information on the severity and prognosis of the disease. For example, patients with the continuous, granular, sub-epithelial deposits of IgG found in membranous glomerulonephritis have a poor prognosis, in contrast to those whose complexes are localized in the mesangium, where the prognosis is fairly good. Not all tissue-bound complexes give rise to an inflammatory response; for example in SLE, complexes are frequently found in skin biopsies from unaffected areas, as well as from inflamed skin. Complexes may also be found in the circulation, where they may be detected physically as high molecular weight immunoglobulin.

Circulating complexes are found in two separate compartments: bound to erythrocytes and free in plasma. Erythrocyte-bound complexes are less likely to be damaging, so it is of more interest to determine the level of free complexes. Care is required when collecting the sample, as bound complexes can easily be released during clotting by the action of Factor I. To obtain more accurate assays of free complexes, the erythrocytes should be rapidly separated from the plasma to prevent the release of bound complexes.

Precipitation of the immune complex with polyethylene glycol, and estimation of the precipitated IgG, is frequently used to identify high molecular weight IgG; it forms the basis for one of the commercial assays (Fig. 21.24). Circulating complexes are often identified by their affinity for complement, C1q, using either radiolabelled C1q or C1q linked to a solid support (solid phase C1q) (see Fig. 21.25). Other receptors may be used to bind immune complexes for measurement, such as the C3 receptor on RAJI (B0 cell tumour) cells, or the Fc receptor on platelets.

Solubilization of immune-complexes by complement

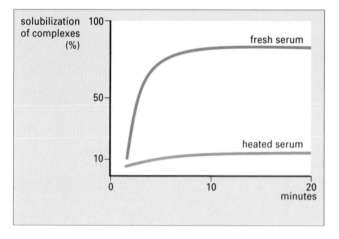

Fig. 21.23 Complement can solubilize precipitable complexes *in vitro*. Addition of fresh serum containing active complement to insoluble complexes induces solubilization over about 15 minutes at 37°C. Some of the complexes resist resolubilization. Heated serum (56°C for 30 minutes) lacks active complement and cannot resolubilize the complexes. It appears that intercalation of complement components C3b and C3d into the complex causes their solubilization.

An assay for immune-complexes based on polyethylene glycol (PEG)

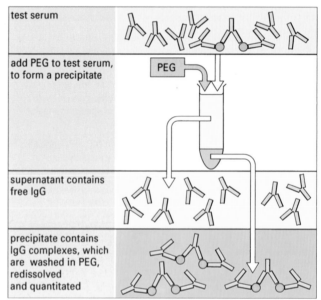

Fig. 21.24 PEG is added to the test serum containing complexes of IgG and IgG monomer, to produce a final concentration of 2% PEG. At 2% PEG, complexes are selectively precipitated and the supernatant contains free antibody. The test tube is then centrifuged and the complexes form a pellet at the bottom. The supernatant containing free antibody is removed and after, washing, the precipitate is redissolved so that complexed IgG can be quantitated (e.g. by single radial immunodiffusion, nephelometry, or radioimmunoassay).

Care must be taken when determining complexes from patients with autoimmune diseases. Frequently these patients will have antibodies to components of the test system. In SLE, patients produce anti-lymphocyte and anti-DNA antibodies which bind to the RAJI cells giving a false positive for immune complexes. C1q has a structure similar to collagen and anti-C1q antibodies have also been found in a number of connective tissue dis-

eases. Furthermore, it is always important to check that what is thought to be an immune complex is actually of higher molecular weight than monomeric IgG. Evaluation of the importance of circulating complexes requires even more care than the interpretation of tissue complexes. Many circulating complexes will not in themselves be harmful. Damage only occurs if they deposit in the tissue.

Radioimmunoassay for immune-complexes

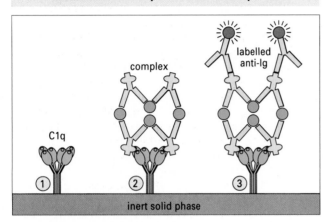

Fig. 21.25 A three layer radioimmunoassay for immune-complexes based on the use of C1q.
1. C1q is linked to an inert solid phase support, usually a polystyrene tube or plate.
2. Serum containing complexes is added and the complexes bind to the solid phase C1q via the array of Fc regions presented to the C1q.
3. The amount of complex bound to the C1q is detected using a radiolabelled antibody to IgG and the radioactivity measured in a gamma counter.

FURTHER READING

Agnello V. Immune complex assays in rheumatic diseases. *Hum Pathol* 1983;**14**:343.

Arthus M. Injections repeté de serum de cheval chez le lapin. *C R Seances Soc Biol Filiale*s 1903;**55**:817.

Birmingham DJ, Herbert LA, Cosio FG, Van Aman ME. Immune complex erythrocyte complement receptor interactions *in vivo* during induction of glomerulonephritis in non-human primates. *J Lab Clin Med* 1990;**116**:242

Cornacoff JB, Hobart LA, Smead WL, Vanaman ME, Birmingham DJ, Waxman FJ. Primate erythrocyte immune complex clearing mechanism. *J Clin Invest* 1983;**71**:236.

Czop J, Nussenweig V. Studies on the mechanism of solubilization of immune precipitates by serum. *J Exp Med* 1976;**143**:615.

Davies KA, Hird V, Stewart S *et al.* A study of *in vivo* immune complex formation and clearing in man. *J Immunol* 1990;**144**:4613.

Dixon FJ, Feldman JD, Vazquez JJ. Experimental glomerulonephritis: the pathogenesis of a laboratory model resembling the spectrum of human glomerulonephritis. *J Exp Med* 1961;**113**:899.

Dixon FJ, Vazquez JJ, Weigle WO, Cochrane CG. Pathogenesis of serum sickness. *Arch Pathol* 1958;**65**:18.

Emlen W, Mannik, M. Clearance of circulating DNA–anti-DNA immune complexes in mice. *J Exp Med* 1982;**155**:1210.

Finbloom DS, Magilvary DB, Harford JB, Rifai A, Plotz PH. Influence of antigen on immune complex behaviour in mice. *J Clin Invest* 1981;**68**:214.

Heidelberger M. Quantitative chemical studies on complement or alexin. *J Exp Med* 1941;**73**:681.

Inman, RD. Immune complexes in SLE. *Clin Res Dis* 1982;**8**:49.

Kjilstra H, Van Es LA, Daha MR. The role of complement in the binding and degradation of immunoglobulin aggregates by macrophages. *J Immunol* 1979;**123**:2488.

Lachman, PJ. Complement deficiency and the pathogenesis of autoimmune complex disease. *Chem Immunol* 1980;**49**:245.

Medof ME, Oger JJ-F. Competition for immune complexes by red cells in human blood. *J Clin Lab Immunol* 1982;**7**:7.

Miller GW, Nussenzweig V. A new complement function: solubilization of antigen–antibody aggregates. *Proc Natl Acad Sci* 1975;**72**:418.

Sedlacek HH, Seiler FR, eds. Immune complexes. *Behring Inst Mitt* 1979;**64**.

Schifferli JA, Ng YC, Peters DK. The role of complement and its receptor in the elimination of immune complexes. *N Engl J Med* 1986;**315**:488.

Takata Y, Tamura N, Fujita T. Interaction of C3 with antigen–antibody complexes in the process of solubilisation of immune precipitates. *J Immunol* 1984;**132**:2531.

Theofilopoulos AN, Dixon FJ. The biology and detection of immune complexes. *Adv Immunol* 1979;**28**:89.

Warren JS, Yabroff KR, Remick DG *et al.* Tumour necrosis factor participates in the pathogenesis of acute immune complex alveolitis in the rat. *J Clin Invest* 1989;**84**:1873.

Waxman FJ, Hebert LE, Cornacoff JB, Van Aman ME, *et al.* Complement depletion accelerates the clearance of immune complexes from the circulation of primates. *J Clin Invest* 1984;**74**:1329.

Whaley K. Complement and immune complex diseases. In: Whaley K, ed. *Complement in Health and Disease.* Lancaster: MTP Press Ltd, 1987.

Williams RC. *Immune Complexes in Clinical and Experimental Medicine.* Massachusetts: Harvard University Press, 1980.

World Health Organization Scientific Group. *Technical Report 606. The Role of Immune Complexes in Disease.* Geneva: WHO, 1977.

chapter 22

Hypersensitivity – Type IV

In the Coombs & Gell classification of hypersensitivity, Type IV (delayed) hypersensitivity is used as a general category to describe all those hypersensitivity reactions which take more than 12 hours to develop, and which involve cell-mediated immune reactions rather than humoral immune reactions. However, it is now recognized that other reactions, such as the late-phase IgE-mediated reaction, may peak between 12 and 24 hours after contact with the allergen. Although an IgE-mediated mechanism is primarily involved, it also involves T-helper cells of the TH2 type, and so the picture becomes more complicated. Other reactions (such as Jones–Mote hypersensitivity, which may be analogous to cutaneous basophil reactions in guinea-pigs) have also been included as delayed hypersensitivity reactions in the past, but the mechanisms involved and the clinical significance remain obscure: these reactions will therefore not be discussed further in this chapter.

Unlike other forms of hypersensitivity, Type IV hypersensitivity cannot be transferred from one animal to another by serum, but can be transferred by T cells (TH1 cells in mice). It is obviously associated with T-cell protective immunity but does not necessarily run parallel with it – there is not always a complete correlation between delayed hypersensitivity and protective immunity. The T cells necessary for producing the delayed response are cells which have become specifically sensitized to the particular antigen by a previous encounter, and they act by recruiting other cell types to the site of the reaction.

Three types of delayed hypersensitivity reaction are recognized (Fig. 22.1). Contact hypersensitivity and tuberculin-type hypersensitivity both occur within 72 hours of antigen challenge, whereas granulomatous reactions develop over a period of weeks. The granulomas are formed by the aggregation and proliferation of

The variants of delayed hypersensitivity

delayed reaction	maximal reaction time
contact	48–72 hours
tuberculin	48–72 hours
granulomatous	21–28 days

Fig. 22.1 Contact and tuberculin-type hypersensitivity have a similar time course and are maximal at 48–72 hours. In certain circumstances (e.g. with insoluble antigen) granulomatous reactions also develop at 21–28 days (e.g. skin testing in leprosy).

macrophages, and may persist for weeks. This reaction is, in terms of its clinical consequences, by far the most serious type of delayed type hypersensitivity response. The position is complicated because these different types of reaction may overlap, or occur sequentially following a single antigenic challenge.

The three types of delayed hypersensitivity were originally distinguished according to the reaction they produced when antigen was applied directly to the skin (epicutaneously) or injected intradermally. The degree of the reaction is assessed in animals by measuring thickening of the skin. This is accompanied by a variety of immune reactions. In addition to the difference in timing and degree of skin swelling, the variants of delayed hypersensitivity are characterized in other ways which will now be described.

CONTACT HYPERSENSITIVITY

Contact hypersensitivity is characterized clinically by an eczematous reaction at the site of contact with the allergen. In Europe the most common agents are haptens, such as nickel, chromate and certain chemicals found in rubber (Fig. 22.2). In the USA, poison ivy and poison oak are also important.

Haptens are molecules that are too small to be antigenic by themselves, having a molecular weight often less than 1 kDa. In contact hypersensitivity they penetrate the epidermis where they conjugate, mostly covalently, to normal body proteins. Metals such as nickel form hapten–carrier complexes with 'carrier' proteins. It is difficult to predict the sensitizing potential of a hapten from its chemical structure, although there may be some correlation with the number of haptens attached to the carrier and the penetrability of the molecule; also, certain contact allergens have unsaturated carbon bonds and are easily oxidized to provide further bonding. Some haptens, for example dinitrochlorobenzene (DNCB), sensitize nearly all individuals. About 85% of epicutaneously applied DNCB binds to epidermal-cell proteins through the -NH₂ group of the amino acid lysine; the conjugates thus formed act as sensitizers. T-cell recognition is specific for the hapten–carrier protein conjugate and does not depend on separate recognition of the hapten and carrier, such as occurs in antibody formation.

THE LANGERHANS' CELL

Contact hypersensitivity is primarily an epidermal phenomenon (as distinct from tuberculin-type hypersensitivity which predominantly takes place in the dermis).

The Langerhans' cell, derived from the family of follicular dendritic cells, is the principal antigen-presenting cell (APC) in contact hypersensitivity (Fig. 22.3). Langerhans' cells are located in the suprabasal epidermis and are derived from the bone marrow. They express the cortical thymocyte antigen CD1, MHC class II antigens and surface receptors for Fc and complement. Electron microscopy shows an organelle, the Birbeck granule (Fig. 22.4), that is specific for the Langerhans' cell. Its function is not known. Langerhans'-like cells (veiled cells) are found in the efferent lymph after antigen is applied to the skin of sensitized animals. *In vitro*, Langerhans' cells can act as APCs and are more potent than blood monocytes. As early as 4 hours after DNCB challenge in mice, Langerhans' cells appear in the paracortical areas of draining lymph nodes. In mice there is a second population of epidermal dendritic cells characterized by the Thy-1 surface antigen and the absence of class II molecules. No equivalent cell has been found in humans.

SENSITIZATION

The process of sensitization takes about 10–14 days in man. Once it has been absorbed, the hapten combines with a protein and is then internalized by epidermal Langerhans' cells which leave the epidermis and migrate, via the efferent lymphatics, to the paracortical areas of regional lymph nodes. Here they present processed hapten–protein conjugate (with class II HLA-DR molecules) to CD4$^+$ lymphocytes, producing a population of 'memory' CD4$^+$ T cells (Fig. 22.5). Studies using DNCB in humans have shown a dose-response effect (higher doses produce both greater reactivity and a higher proportion of subjects sensitized). There is also a concentration effect: doses (DNCB per unit area) below a certain critical level produce no reaction at all; doses increased above a certain level fail to produce further increases in sensitization, i.e. there is a plateau to the response curve. This suggests that antigen dose per unit area, rather than total dose or total area, is the main determinant of sensitization.

ELICITATION

The earliest histological change in contact hypersensitivity is seen after 4–8 hours when mononuclear cells appear around sweat glands, sebaceous glands, follicles or blood vessels and then begin to infiltrate the epidermis. At 48–72 hours, the number of cells infiltrating the epidermis and dermis peaks, and both become oedematous (Fig. 22.6). The majority of infiltrating lymphocytes are CD4$^+$, with lesser numbers of CD8$^+$ cells. Langerhans' cells (CD1$^+$) increase in the epidermis at

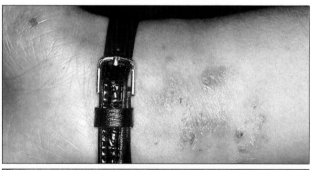

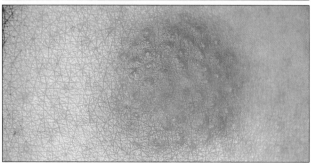

Fig. 22.2 Clinical and patch-test appearances of contact hypersensitivity. Upper: The eczematous area at the wrist is due to sensitivity to nickel in the watch-strap buckle. Lower: The suspected allergy may be confirmed by applying potential allergens, in the relevant concentrations and vehicles, to the patient's upper back (patch testing). A positive reaction causes a localized area of eczema at the site of the offending allergen, 2–4 days after application.

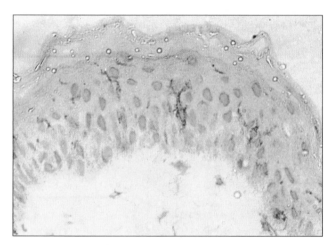

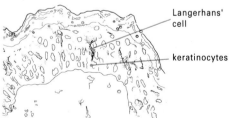

Fig. 22.3 Langerhans' cells seen in a section of normal skin. These dendritic cells constitute 3% of all cells in the epidermis. They express a variety of surface markers which allow them to be visualized. Here they have been revealed using a monoclonal antibody which reacts with the CD1 antigen (counterstained with Mayer's haemalum). × 312.

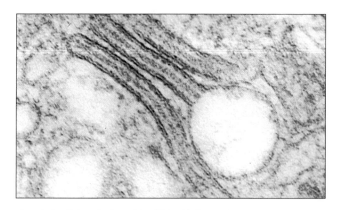

Fig. 22.4 Electron micrograph of a Langerhans' cell, showing the characteristic 'Birbeck granule'. This organelle is a plate-like structure with a distinct central striation and often has a bleb-like extension at one end. × 132 000.

The sensitization phase of contact hypersensitivity

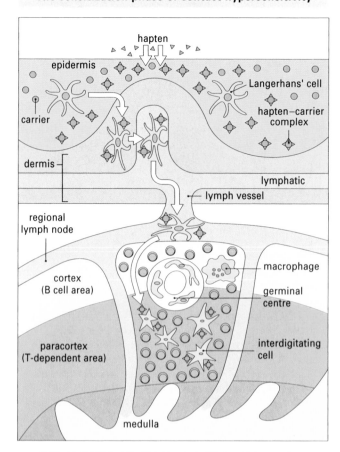

Fig. 22.5 The hapten forms a hapten–carrier complex in the epidermis. Langerhans' cells bearing the antigen migrate via afferent lymphatics to the paracortical area of the regional lymph node where, as interdigitating cells, they present antigen to CD4⁺ T cells.

24 and 48 hours, and CD1⁺ cells are found in the dermal infiltrate. Macrophages invade the dermis and epidermis by 48 hours. Basophils have been observed in some reactions and some mast cells are seen lacking granules, indicating that they have degranulated.

MECHANISM

Details of the pathophysiological mechanisms underlying this reaction have been revealed over the last decade. When Langerhans' cells present the processed hapten–protein conjugate to sensitized 'memory' CD4⁺ T cells, this activates the transduction CD3 receptor of the T cells, and they release cytokines. These include IL-2, IL-3, IFN$_\gamma$ and GM–CSF. The T cells also express IL-2 receptors. Proliferation of T cells is induced by the binding of IL-2 to its receptor on the cells. IFN$_\gamma$ and tumour necrosis factor (TNF) induce the keratinocytes in the epidermis to express intercellular adhesion molecules (e.g. ICAM-1) 24–48 hours after antigenic challenge. At around 48 hours, IFN$_\gamma$ stimulates the keratinocytes to express HLA-DR (Fig. 22.7). ICAM-1 is the natural ligand for the integrin LFA-1, found on many cells of lymphoid and myeloid lineage, so ICAM-1 expression may be important in the localization of lymphocytes and macrophages to the skin. Activated keratinocytes release IL-1, IL-6 and GM–CSF, which may promote activation and proliferation of T cells. GM–CSF also stimulates Langerhans' cells in the same way (Fig. 22.8). Endothelial cells in the dermis may also express adhesion molecules, and they too can be involved in the movement of lymphocytes to the site of inflammation.

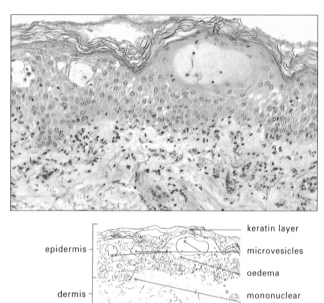

Fig. 22.6 Histological appearance of the lesion in contact hypersensitivity. Mononuclear cells infiltrate both dermis and epidermis. The epidermis is pushed outwards and microvesicles form within it due to oedema. H&E stain, × 130.

The reaction begins to wane after 48–72 hours. This down-regulation is thought to be mediated by a number of mechanisms. Macrophages and keratinocytes produce prostaglandin E (PGE) which inhibits IL-1 and IL-2 production, and T cells bind to activated keratinocytes. There is also degradation (enzymatic and cellular) of the hapten conjugate.

TUBERCULIN-TYPE HYPERSENSITIVITY

This form of hypersensitivity was originally described by Koch. He observed that if patients with tuberculosis were given a subcutaneous injection of tuberculin (a lipoprotein antigen derived from the tubercle bacillus) they reacted with fever and generalized sickness. An area of hardening and swelling developed at the site of injection. Soluble antigens from a number of organisms, including *Mycobacterium tuberculosis*, *M. leprae* and *Leishmania tropica*, induce similar reactions in sensitive people. The skin reaction is frequently used as the basis of a test for sensitivity to the organisms, following previous exposure (Fig. 22.9). This form of hypersensitivity may also be induced by non-microbial antigens, such as beryllium and zirconium.

The elicitation phase of contact hypersensitivity

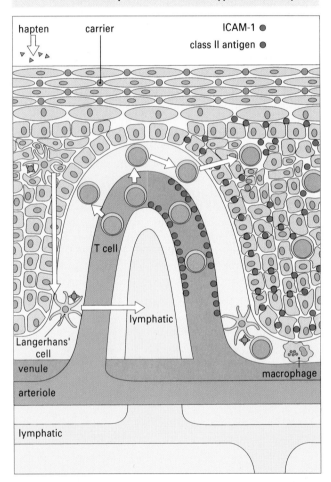

Cytokines, prostaglandins and cellular interactions in contact hypersensitivity

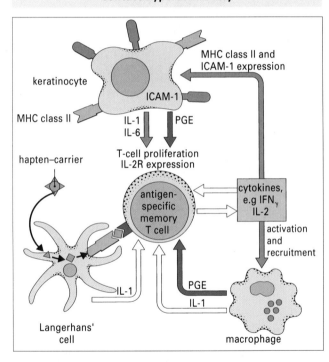

Fig. 22.7 Langerhans' cells carrying the hapten–carrier complex move from the epidermis to the dermis (and thence to regional lymph nodes), where they present the hapten–carrier complex to memory CD4+ T cells. Activated CD4+ T cells release IFN$_\gamma$, which induces expression of ICAM-1 and, later, MHC class II molecules on the surface of keratinocytes and on endothelial cells of dermal capillaries. Activated keratinocytes release proinflammatory cytokines, for example IL-1, IL-6 and GM–CSF, and also possibly eicosanoids, for example PGE, which may inhibit lymphocytes. Non-antigen specific CD4+ T cells are attracted to the site by cytokines and may be bound to keratinocytes by ICAM-1 and class II molecules. Activated macrophages are also attracted to the skin, but this occurs later, when the reaction has started to down-regulate.

Fig. 22.8 Cytokines and prostaglandins are central to the complex interactions between Langerhans' cells, CD4+ T cells, keratinocytes, macrophages and endothelial cells in contact hypersensitivity. The act of antigen presentation causes the release of a cascade of cytokines. This cascade initially results in the activation and proliferation of CD4+ T cells, the induction of expression of ICAM-1 and MHC class II molecules on keratinocytes and endothelial cells, and the attraction of T cells and macrophages to the skin. Subsequent PGE production by keratinocytes and macrophages may have an inhibitory effect on IL-1 and IL-2 production. Production of PGE, binding of activated T cells to keratinocytes and enzymatic and cellular degradation of the hapten–carrier complex all contribute to the down-regulation of the reaction.

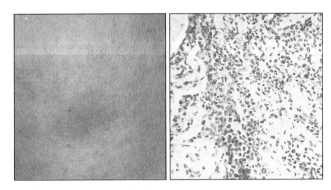

Fig. 22.9 Clinical and histological appearances of tuberculin-type sensitivity. The response of the leprosy bacillus, when injected into a sensitized individual, is known as the Fernandez reaction. The reaction is characterized by an area of firm red swelling of the skin and is maximal at 48–72 hours after challenge (left). Histologically (right), there is a dense dermal infiltrate of leucocytes and macrophages. H&E stain, × 80.

Tuberculin-type hypersensitivity

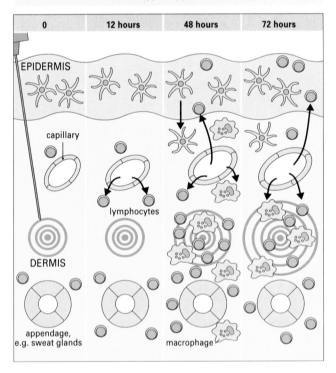

Fig. 22.10 This diagram illustrates cellular movements following intradermal injection of tuberculin. At 12 hours, lymphocytes begin to migrate from local blood vessels and accumulate around appendages. By 48 hours, macrophages are also present and Langerhans' cells start to migrate out of the epidermis. The cellular traffic continues over the next 24 hours, and class II molecules appear on keratinocytes; there is no oedema of the epidermis (cf. contact hypersensitivity).

TUBERCULIN SKIN TEST

Twelve hours after intradermal tuberculin challenge in a sensitive individual, T cells migrate out of the capillaries. This infiltrate, which extends outwards and disrupts the collagen bundles of the dermis, increases to a peak at 48 hours. CD4$^+$ cells outnumber CD8$^+$ cells by about 2:1. CD1$^+$cells (Langerhans'-like cells but lacking Birbeck granules) are also found in the dermal infiltrate at 24 and 48 hours, and a few CD4$^+$ cells infiltrate the epidermis between 24 and 48 hours. Macrophages start to accumulate around dermal vessels at 12 hours, their numbers increasing up to 72 hours. Infiltrating lymphocytes and macrophages express HLA-DR. Overlying keratinocytes express HLA-DR molecules 48–96 hours after the appearance of the lymphocytic infiltrate. These events are summarized in Fig. 22.10.

Macrophages are probably the main APCs in the tuberculin hypersensitivity reaction. However, there are CD1$^+$ cells in the dermal infiltrate, which suggests that Langerhans' cells or indeterminate dendritic cells may also be involved. The circulation of immune cells to and from the regional lymph nodes is thought to be similar to that for contact hypersensitivity.

As the tuberculin lesion develops it may become a granulomatous reaction, probably due to the persistence of antigen in the tissues. Subepidermal infiltration with basophils is not a characteristic of this reaction, but can be seen in some contact hypersensitivity reactions and skin tests with heterologous proteins, as in the Jones–Mote reaction.

GRANULOMATOUS HYPERSENSITIVITY

Granulomatous hypersensitivity is clinically the most important form of delayed hypersensitivity, causing many of the pathological effects in diseases which involve T-cell-mediated immunity. It usually results from the persistence, within macrophages, of microorganisms or other particles, which the cell is unable to destroy. On occasion it may also be caused by persistent immune complexes, for example in allergic alveolitis. This process results in epithelioid cell granuloma formation.

The histological appearance of the granuloma reaction is quite different from that of the tuberculin-type reaction, which is usually a self-limiting response to antigen rather than being due to the persistence of antigen. However, they often result from sensitization to similar microbial antigens, for example the antigens of *Mycobacterium tuberculosis* and *M. leprae* (Fig. 22.11). Immunological granuloma formation also occurs in the sensitivity reactions to zirconium and beryllium, and in sarcoidosis, although in the latter the antigen is unknown. Foreign-body granuloma formation occurs with talc, silica and a variety of other particulate agents. In this case macrophages are unable to digest the inorganic matter. These non-immunological granulomas may be distinguished by the absence of lymphocytes in the lesion.

EPITHELIOID CELLS

This is the characteristic cell of granulomatous hypersensitivity. It is large and flattened with increased endoplasmic reticulum (Fig. 22.12). The nature of epithelioid cells is poorly understood. It has been suggested that they are derived from activated macrophages, but whereas activated macrophages have many phagosomes, epithelioid cells do not.

GIANT CELLS

Also seen in this type of reaction are multinucleate giant cells (Fig. 22.13), sometimes referred to as Langhans' giant cells (not to be confused with the Langerhans' cell discussed earlier). Giant cells have several nuclei, but these are not at the centre of the cell. The giant cell has little endoplasmic reticulum, and its mitochondria and lysosomes appear to be undergoing degeneration. For this reason it is thought that the cell may be a terminal differentiation stage of the monocyte/macrophage line.

THE GRANULOMA

An immunological granuloma typically has a core of epithelioid cells and macrophages, sometimes with giant cells. In some diseases, such as tuberculosis, this central area may have a zone of necrosis (cell death), with complete destruction of all cellular architecture. The macrophage/epithelioid core is surrounded by a cuff of lymphocytes, and there may also be considerable fibrosis (deposition of collagen fibres). This is caused by proliferation of fibroblasts and increased collagen synthesis. An example of a granulomatous reaction can be seen in the Mitsuda reaction to leprosy antigens (see Fig. 22.13) or in the Kveim test, where patients suffering from sarcoidosis (a disease of unknown aetiology) react to unknown splenic antigens derived from other sarcoid patients. The three types of delayed hypersensitivity are summarized in Fig. 22.14.

Antigen stimulation of T cells

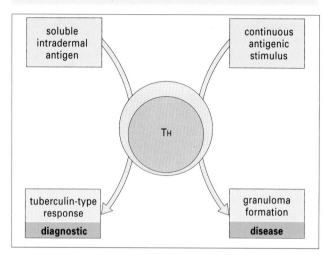

Fig. 22.11 Both tuberculin and granulomatous hypersensitivity reactions depend on CD4+ T cells. Where there is continuous stimulation due to persistent or recurrent infection, or where macrophages cannot destroy an antigen, granuloma formation occurs. The presence of antigen-sensitized TH cells can be detected by the tuberculin-type response to intradermal injection of antigen.

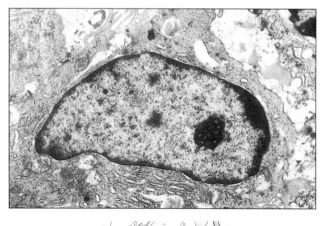

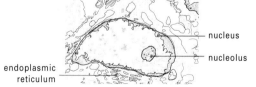

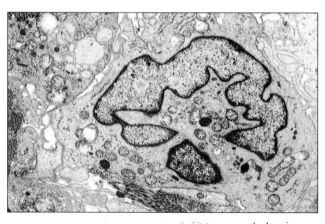

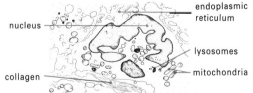

Fig. 22.12 Electron micrograph of an epithelioid cell. This is the characteristic cell of granulomatous hypersensitivity. Compare the extent of the endoplasmic reticulum in the epithelioid cell (left, × 4800) with that of a tissue macrophage (right, × 4800). (Courtesy of M. J. Spencer.)

CELLULAR REACTIONS IN DELAYED HYPERSENSITIVITY

Delayed hypersensitivity reactions are initiated by cells rather than antibody. In 1942 Landsteiner and Chase showed that the reactivity may only be transferred to a non-sensitive individual by cell suspensions containing lymphocytes. Eliminating T lymphocytes in the transfer shows that these cells are the effectors in tuberculin-type hypersensitivity (Fig. 22.15).

T cells are also responsible for initiating the other delayed hypersensitivity reactions. Sensitized T cells, stimulated with the appropriate antigen, undergo lymphoblastoid transformation prior to cell division (Fig. 22.16). This forms the basis of the lymphocyte stimulation test (see Chapter 25). Lymphocyte stimulation is accompanied by DNA synthesis and this can be measured by assaying the uptake of radiolabelled thymidine, a nucleoside which is required for DNA synthesis. Lymphocytes from a patient are cultured with the suspect antigen to determine whether it induces transformation. It is important to stress that this is a test for T-cell memory only, and does not necessarily imply the presence of protective immunity.

Delayed hypersensitivity reactions

DTH type	characteristics			
	reaction time	clinical appearance	histological appearance	antigen
contact	48–72 hours	eczema	infiltration of lymphocytes and, later, macrophages, oedema of epidermis	epidermal: e.g. nickel, rubber, poison ivy usually a hapten
tuberculin	48–72 hours	local hardening and swelling ± fever	infiltration of lymphocytes, monocytes, and macrophages	intradermal injection used diagnostically: tuberculin, mycobacterial and leishmanial antigens
granulo-matous	4 weeks	hardening e.g. in skin or lung	granuloma containing epithelioid cells, giant cells, and macrophages; fibrosis ± necrosis	persistent Ag or Ag–Ab complexes in macrophages; or 'non-immunological', e.g talcum powder

Fig. 22.14 A summary of the most important characteristics of the three types of DTH. They can be differentiated not only by their time of onset, but also by the cell types involved.

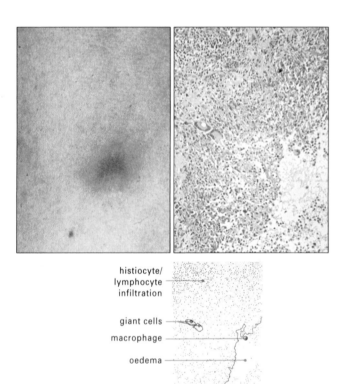

histiocyte/lymphocyte infiltration

giant cells

macrophage

oedema

Fig. 22.13 Clinical and histological appearances of the Mitsuda reaction in leprosy seen at 28 days. Left: The resultant skin swelling (which may be ulcerated) is much harder and better defined than at 48 hours.
Right: Histology shows a typical epithelioid-cell granuloma (H&E stain, × 60). Giant cells are visible in the centre of the lesion, which is surrounded by a cuff of lymphocytes. This response is more akin to the pathological processes in delayed hypersensitivity diseases than the self-resolving tuberculin-type reaction. The reaction is due to the continued presence of mycobacterial antigen.

Demonstration of the role of T cells in the tuberculin response

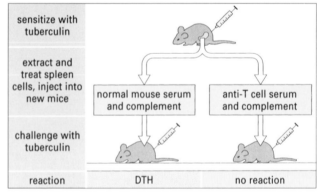

sensitize with tuberculin

extract and treat spleen cells, inject into new mice

normal mouse serum and complement

anti-T cell serum and complement

challenge with tuberculin

reaction   DTH   no reaction

Fig. 22.15 A mouse is sensitized to tuberculin by intradermal injection. Its spleen cells are later removed and treated with either normal serum and complement, or anti-T-cell serum and complement. The treated cells are injected into recipient mice which are then challenged with tuberculin. The mouse with spleen cells treated with normal serum develops a tuberculin-type reaction, whereas the other mouse fails to respond.

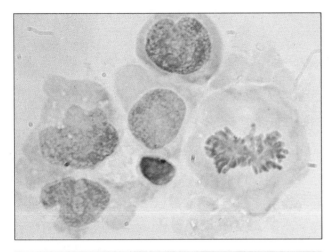

Fig. 22.16 Transformed lymphocytes. Following stimulation with appropriate antigen, T cells undergo lymphoblastoid transformation prior to cell division. Blast cells with expanded nuclei and cytoplasm (as well as one lymphocyte in the metaphase of cell division) are shown.

Following activation by APCs carrying antigen, T cells produce a number of cytokines which attract and activate macrophages. These cytokines include IFN$_\gamma$, TNF, IL-3 and IL-6. In granulomatous reactions the accumulating macrophages become a major source of TNF and the granulomas develop by auto-amplification, with differentiation of macrophages into epithelioid cells (Figs 22.17 and 22.18). These secrete more TNF, with further epithelioid cell formation, and fusion of epithelioid cells to form giant cells (Fig. 22.19).

DISEASES MANIFESTING DELAYED HYPERSENSITIVITY

There are many chronic diseases in man which manifest delayed hypersensitivity, and most are due to infectious agents such as mycobacteria, protozoa and fungi. Important diseases in this respect include the following:
1. Tuberculosis
2. Leprosy
3. Leishmaniasis
4. Listeriosis
5. Deep fungal infections (e.g. blastomycosis)
6. Helminthic infections (e.g. schistosomiasis).

These diseases are caused by pathogens which present a persistent chronic antigenic stimulus. The threat they pose is met by lymphocytes and macrophages. Although these diseases are liable to induce protective immunity, protective immunity and delayed hypersensitivity are not always coincident; some patients, even though they show delayed hypersensitivity, may not be immune.

Macrophage differentiation

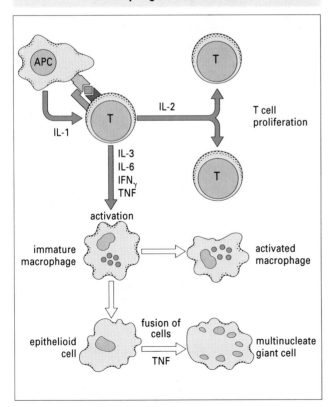

Fig. 22.17 Activated T cells secrete the cytokines IL-3, IL-6, IFN$_\gamma$ and TNF. These cytokines promote differentiation of macrophages into either activated macrophages or epithelioid cells. Epithelioid cells secrete large amounts of TNF; some fuse to form multinucleate giant cells.

The importance of TNF in the formation of granulomas

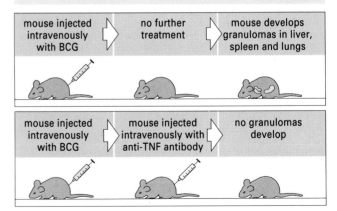

Fig. 22.18 TNF is essential for the development of epithelioid cell granulomas. If BCG-injected mice are injected with anti-TNF antibodies, they do not develop granulomas.

LEPROSY

Established leprosy is divided into three main types, tuberculoid, borderline and lepromatous. In tuberculoid leprosy, the skin shows a few well-defined hypopigmented patches which show an intense lymphocytic and epithelioid infiltrate and no microorganisms. In contrast, the polar reaction of lepromatous leprosy shows multiple confluent skin lesions characterized by numerous bacilli with foamy macrophages and a paucity of lymphocytes. Borderline leprosy has characteristics of both (Fig. 22.20).

A dramatic example of delayed hypersensitivity occurs in the borderline leprosy reaction. Leprosy is a disease where protective immunity depends solely on cell-mediated immunity, with humoral immunity having no protective role. Borderline reactions occur either naturally or following drug treatment. In these reactions, hypopigmented skin lesions, which contain *Mycobacterium leprae*, become swollen and inflamed (Fig. 22.21) due to the patient now being able to mount a delayed-type hypersensitivity reaction. The histological appearance shows more mononuclear cells, i.e. it becomes more tuberculoid. The process may occur in peripheral nerves, where there are mycobacterial antigens, and this is the most important cause of nerve destruction in this disease. The lesion in borderline leprosy is typical of granulomatous hypersensitivity (see Fig. 22.21).

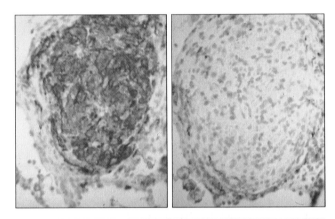

Fig. 22.19 Epithelioid cells in a granuloma from the lung of a patient with sarcoidosis. Left: The epithelioid cells and giant cells in the centre have been stained with the specific antibody RFD 9. Right: Mature tissue macrophages surrounding the granuloma are stained with the specific antibody RFD 7. (Courtesy of C. S. Munro).

Hypersensitivity and the types of leprosy

leprosy type	test			
	delayed type hypersensitivity	lepromin skin test	antibody-antigen complexes	micro-organisms
tuberculoid (TT)	+++	+++	−	−
borderline (BB)	++	++	++	+
lepromatous (LL)	±	−	±	+++

Fig. 22.20 The spectrum of disease in leprosy depends on the competence of the host's delayed hypersensitivity response. Those with good responsiveness to the microorganism have tuberculoid (TT), those with no response have lepromatous (LL) and in between these extremes lies borderline (BB).

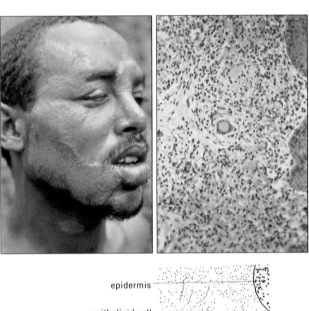

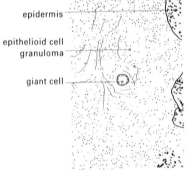

epidermis

epithelioid cell granuloma

giant cell

Fig. 22.21 A borderline leprosy reaction. Left: The previously hypopigmented skin lesions have become swollen and inflamed following sensitization to antigens of *M. Leprae*. Right: The histological appearance is typical of granulomatous hypersensitivity. Note the giant cell and infiltration by monocytes and lymphocytes. H&E stain, × 140.

When a patient develops immunity associated with tuberculoid type hypersensitivity, T-cell sensitization may be assessed *in vitro* by the lymphocyte stimulation test, using either whole or sonicated *M. leprae* as the source of antigen (Fig 22.22).

TUBERCULOSIS

In tuberculosis there is granuloma formation in the lung and other infected organs. Lung damage caused by the granulomatous reaction leads to cavitation and spread of bacteria.

The reactions are frequently accompanied by extensive fibrosis and the lesions may be seen in the chest radiographs of affected patients (Fig. 22.23).

The histological appearance of the lesion is typical of a granulomatous reaction, with central caseous (cheesy) necrosis (Fig. 22.24). This is surrounded by an area of epithelioid cells, with a few giant cells. Mononuclear cell infiltration occurs around the edge.

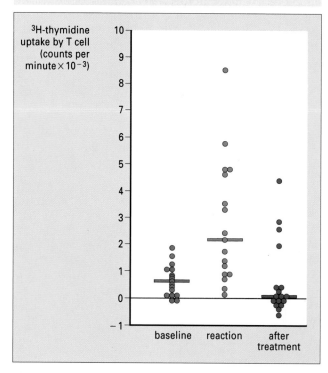

A lymphocyte stimulation test

Fig. 22.22 During a borderline leprosy reaction, the lymphocyte stimulation response to *M. leprae* rises. There is a fall in response when the reaction is treated successfully with corticosteroids. The lymphocyte stimulation responses to sonicated *M. leprae* (measured by uptake of [^{3}H]-thymidine) are shown for 17 patients who developed such reactions: (a) before starting treatment with anti-leprosy drugs (baseline); (b) during the reaction; and (c) following successful treatment with steroids. Medians are indicated by horizontal bars.

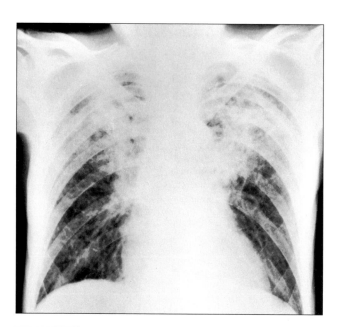

Fig. 22.23 **Chest radiograph of a patient with pulmonary tuberculosis.** There is extensive parenchymal streaking, predominantly in the upper fields of the lungs. These changes are typical of chronic bilateral pulmonary tuberculosis. Some enlargement of the heart is also evident.

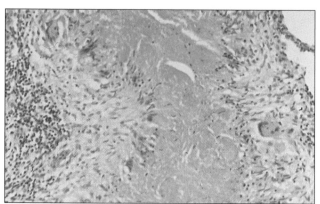

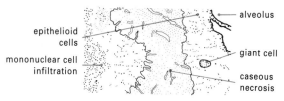

Fig. 22.24 **Histological appearance of a tuberculous section of lung.** This shows an epithelioid cell granuloma with giant cells. There is also marked caseation and necrosis within the granuloma. H&E stain, × 75.

SARCOIDOSIS

Sarcoidosis is a disease of unknown aetiology, although it might be due to an infectious agent such as a mycobacterium, since it involves immunological granuloma formation, frequently accompanied by fibrosis (Fig. 22.25). The disease particularly affects lymphoid tissue, and enlarged lymph nodes may be detected in chest radiographs of affected patients (Fig. 22.26).

One of the paradoxes of clinical immunology is that this disease is usually associated with depression of

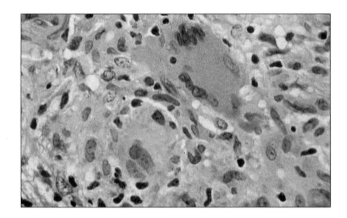

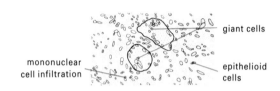

Fig. 22.25 Histological appearance of sarcoidosis in a lymph node biopsy. The granuloma of sarcoidosis is typically composed of epithelial cells and multinucleate giant cells, but without caseation necrosis. There is only a sparse mononuclear cell infiltrate evident at the periphery of the granuloma. H&E stain, × 240.

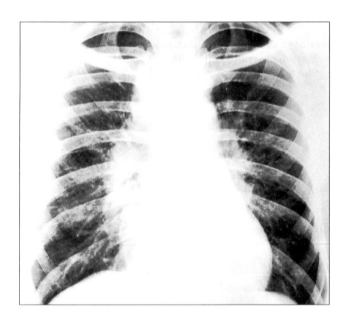

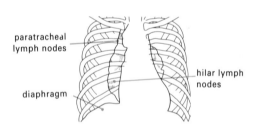

Fig. 22.26 The chest radiograph of a patient with sarcoidosis. There is enlargement of the lymph nodes adjacent to the hilar and paratracheal areas of the lungs, with diffuse pulmonary infiltration characteristic of the disease.

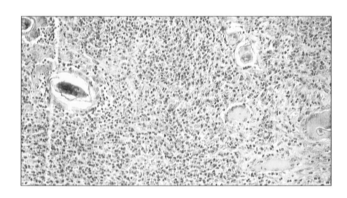

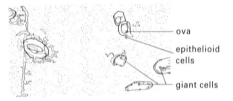

Fig. 22.27 Histological appearance of the liver in schistosomiasis. The epithelioid-cell granuloma surrounds the schistosome ova. Note also the giant cells. H&E stain, × 100.

delayed hypersensitivity both *in vivo* and *in vitro*. These patients are anergic on testing with tuberculin, but when cortisone is injected with tuberculin antigen skin tests become positive, suggesting that cortisone-sensitive T-suppressor cells are responsible for the anergy. Cortisone would normally suppress delayed hypersensitivity.

In sarcoidosis, granulomas develop in a variety of organs, most commonly the lungs, lymph nodes, bone, nervous tissue and skin. Patients may present acutely with fever and malaise, although in the longer term those with pulmonary involvement develop shortness of breath. The diagnosis is often suggested by radiographic changes and confirmed by tissue biopsy or by a Kveim test (see above).

SCHISTOSOMIASIS

Another disease exemplifying granulomatous hypersensitivity is schistosomiasis, caused by parasitic trematode worms (schistosomes). The host becomes sensitized to the ova of the worms, leading to a typical granulomatous reaction in the parasitized tissue (Fig. 22.27; see also Chapter 16).

FURTHER READING

Baadsgaard O, Wang T. Immune regulation in allergic and irritant skin reactions. *Int J Dermatol* 1991;**30**:161–72.

Bjune G, Barnetson RStC, Ridley DS, Kronvall G. Lymphocyte transformation test in leprosy: correlation of the response with inflammation of lesions. *Clin Exp Immunol* 1976;**25**:85–94.

Friedmann PS. The immunology of allergic contact dermatitis: the DNCB story. *Adv Dermatol* 1991;**5**:175–96.

Gawkrodger DJ, McVittie E, Carr MM, Ross JA, Hunter JAA. Phenotypic characterisation of the early cellular responses in allergic and irritant contact dermatitis. *Clin Exp Immunol* 1986;**66**:590–98.

Gawkrodger DJ, Carr MM, McVittie E, Guy K, Hunter JAA. Keratinocyte expression of MHC class II antigens in allergic sensitisation and challenge reactions and in irritant contact dermatitis. *J Invest Dermatol* 1987;**88**:11.

Kindler V, Sappino A-P, Gran GE, Pignet P-F, Vassalli P. The inducing role of tumour necrosis factor in the development of bactericidal granulomas during BCG infection. *Cell* 1989;**56**:731–40.

Munro CS, Campbell DA, Collings LA, Poulter LW. Monoclonal antibodies distinguish macrophages and epithelioid cells in sarcoidosis and leprosy. *Clin Exp Immunol* 1987;**68**,282–87.

Platt JL, Grant BW, Eddy AA, Michael AF. Immune cell populations in cutaneous delayed hypersensitivity. *J Exp Med* 1983;**158**:1227–42.

Poulter LW, Seymour GJ, Duke O, Janossy G, Panayi G. Immunohistochemical analysis of delayed-type hypersensitivity in man. *Cell Immunol* 1982;**74**:358–369.

Sauder DN. Allergic contact dermatitis. In: Thiers BH, Dobson RL, eds. *Pathogenesis of Skin Disease*. New York: Churchill Livingstone, 1986:3–12.

Turk JL. *Research Monographs in Immunology 1. Delayed Hypersensitivity 3e*. Amsterdam: Elsevier, 1980.

Wolff K, Stingl G. The Langerhans cell. *J Invest Dermatol* 1983;**80**(suppl):175–215.

chapter 23

Transplantation and Rejection

The immunobiology of transplantation is important for many reasons. The study of mouse skin-graft rejection led to the discovery of the major histocompatibilty complex (MHC) antigens (see Chapter 4) which function in the presentation of antigens to T lymphocytes (see Chapter 6). T cells are pivotal in transplant rejection and much of our knowledge of T-cell physiology and function, of self tolerance and autoimmunity, and of the role of the thymus in T-cell education, are derived from studies of transplantation. Likewise, transplantation has contributed to our understanding of immune-mediated tissue-damage in hypersensitivity and autoimmunity. Last, but not least, transplantation of tissues is clinically very important. The need to prevent rejection has lead to the development and use of new immunomodulatory drugs and a search for ways to induce tolerance of the grafted tissues, approaches which have a more general application in the treatment of various immune disorders.

Organs are transplanted in clinical practice to make good a functional deficit (Fig. 23.1). Unless the donor and recipient are genetically identical, the graft antigens will elicit an immunological rejection response. Transplantation can stimulate all of the various active mechanisms of humoral and cellular immunity, both specific and non-specific. This is a consequence of the recognition by the recipient's T cells of peptide antigens associated with the foreign MHC antigens on the grafted cells. In this context, the peptide antigens are usually derived from normal cell constituents, but they may also come from viruses within the cells, or from other microbes. (This will be described in more detail later.) By the same token, a transplant can activate all of the regulatory mechanisms that control immune responses (see Chapter 9). Hence, transplantation immunobiology encompasses virtually all aspects of immune function.

BARRIERS TO TRANSPLANTATION

Transplantation barriers can be described in terms of the genetic disparity between the donor and the recipient (Fig. 23.2). Autografts from one part of the body to another are not foreign and do not, therefore, elicit rejection. Similarly, isografts between isogeneic

Clinical transplantation

organ transplanted	examples of disease
kidney	end-stage renal failure
heart	terminal cardiac failure
lung or heart/lung	pulmonary hypertension, cystic fibrosis
liver	cirrhosis, cancer, biliary atresia
cornea	dystrophy, keratitis
pancreas or islets	diabetes
bone marrow	immunodeficiency, leukaemia
small bowel	cancer
skin	burns

Fig 23.1 Organs and tissues are transplanted to treat various conditions. Each type of transplant has its own particular medical and surgical difficulties.

Genetic barriers to transplantation

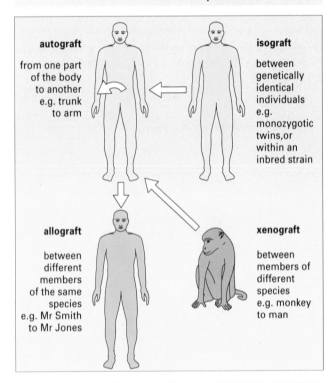

Fig 23.2 The genetic relationship between the donor and recipient determines whether or not rejection will occur. Autografts or isografts are usually accepted while allografts and xenografts are not.

(genetically identical) individuals, such as monozygotic identical twins, or mice of the same inbred strain, do not express antigens foreign to the recipient and do not activate a rejection response. The allograft is the common clinical transplant, where one person donates an organ to a genetically disparate individual. In this case the graft is allogeneic (i.e. between members of the same species having allelic variants of certain genes). The cells of the allograft will express alloantigens which can be recognised as foreign by the recipient.

The maximal genetic disparity is between members of different species, and a xenograft across such a xenogeneic barrier is generally rapidly rejected, either by naturally occurring IgM antibodies in the recipient or by a rapid cell-mediated rejection (see below). Non-viable xenografts such as pig skin, blood vessels or valves, treated to reduce their immunogenicity, can be grafted to human but so far attempts to transplant animal organs to man have been spectacularly unsuccessful, although some success has been achieved in animal models of xenografting. If the immunological problems of xenografting can be overcome, the use of animal donors could alleviate the worldwide shortage of human organs for transplantation. Nevertheless, various non-immunological problems remain, including donor size, animal diseases and the ethics of xenografting.

 GENETICS OF TRANSPLANTATION

The antigens present on genetically disparate tissues are known as histocompatibility (i.e. tissue compatibility) antigens and the genes coding for these antigens are referred to as histocompatibility genes. There are more than 30 histocompatibility gene loci which cause rejection at different rates. Of these, alloantigens encoded by the major histocompatibility complex (MHC) induce particularly strong reactions. These products of the MHC are often called MHC antigens. The products of the other histocompatibility genes individually cause weaker rejection responses and are consequently known as minor histocompatibility antigens. Nonetheless, combinations of minor antigens can elicit strong rejection responses. This is illustrated in Fig. 23.3.

HAPLOTYPE INHERITANCE OF MHC ANTIGENS

The genes of the MHC are subject to simple Mendelian inheritance and are codominantly expressed. In other words, each individual has two 'half-sets' (haplotypes) of genes, one haplotype inherited from each parent (Fig. 23.4). Both of these haplotypes are expressed equally so that each cell in an offspring has both maternal and paternal antigens on its surface (Fig. 23.5). For the Class I MHC antigens, each having only one chain (an α chain) encoded within the MHC, the gene inheritance and antigen expression is straightforward – each Class I gene inherited leads to the cell surface expression of a single antigen. By contrast, MHC Class II antigens are heterodimeric, having an α and a β chain both encoded within the MHC. These α and β genes can be expressed in *cis* (along the DNA strand) or in *trans* (across two DNA strands) configuration. Hence there

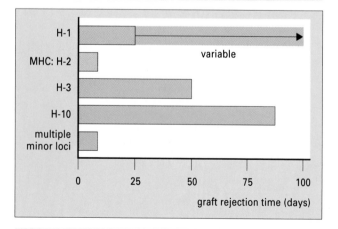

Fig 23.3 This chart gives the rejection time for skin grafts between mice differing at the minor histocompatibility loci (red) or at the MHC locus (H-2) (green) listed. Grafts which differ at multiple minor loci are rejected as quickly as those that differ at H-2. (Data from Graff & Bailey.)

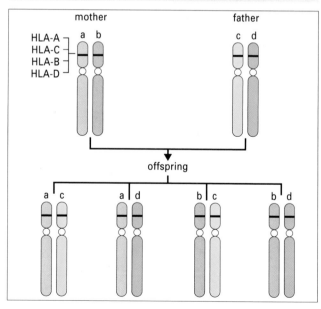

Fig 23.4 The human MHC (HLA) is located on the short arm of chromosome 6. One set (haplotype) of the MHC Class I (HLA-A, B and C) and Class II (HLA-D) antigens are inherited *en bloc* from each parent according to simple Mendelian inheritance.

could be four different combinations of maternal (m) and paternal (p) α and β chains for each Class II molecule.

TISSUE EXPRESSION OF MHC ANTIGENS

MHC antigens are not equally distributed on all cells of the body. Class I molecules are normally expressed on most nucleated cells (and on erythrocytes and platelets in some species), while Class II molecules are restricted to antigen-presenting cells (e.g. dendritic cells, activated macrophages, B cells and, in some species, activated T cells and vascular endothelial cells). MHC expression on cells is controlled by cytokines. Interferon-γ (IFN$_\gamma$) and tumour necrosis factor (TNF) are powerful inducers of MHC antigen expression on many cell types which would otherwise express MHC molecules only weakly. The importance of this and other cytokine effects during graft rejection will be described later.

THE LAWS OF TRANSPLANTATION

The overriding consideration for organ allograft rejection is whether the graft carries any antigens which are not present in the recipient. This principle of host-versus-graft reaction is illustrated in Fig. 23.6. The major exception to this rule is in graft-versus-host (GVH) disease, induced by immunologically competent T cells being transplanted into allogeneic recipients which are unable to reject them. This inability may be due to the genetic relationship of the donor and recipient, or because of a lack of immunocompetence (through immaturity or immunosuppression) of the recipient. In this situation the transplanted immunocompetent T cells can attack the recipient (Fig. 23.7). GVH disease is a major complication of bone marrow transplantation, causing severe damage, particularly to the skin and intestine.

Codominant expression of MHC antigens

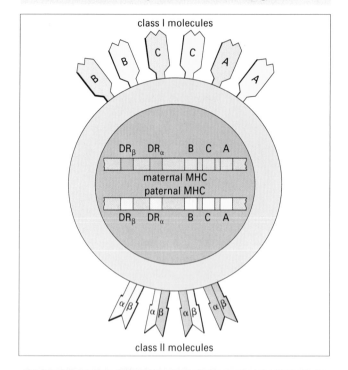

Fig 23.5 Inherited MHC genes are all expressed on the cell surface. For each maternal and paternal Class I gene there are Class I molecules on the membrane. For each Class II α and β gene there are α and β chains on the cell surface but these can associate to form four different molecules. Note that there are other Class II α and β genes coding for DP and DQ antigens as well. B lymphocytes have 23 × 10^5 Class I molecules and the same number of class II molecules per cell.

The laws of transplantation

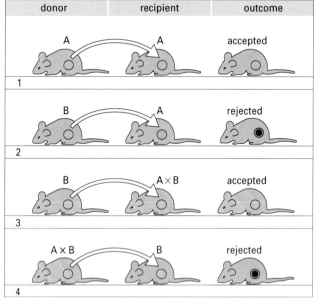

Fig 23.6 Grafts between genetically identical animals are accepted. Grafts between genetically non-identical animals are rejected with a speed which is dependent on where the genetic differences lie. For example, syngeneic animals which are identical at the MHC locus, accept grafts from each other (1). Animals which differ at the MHC locus reject grafts from each other (2). The ability to accept a graft is dependent on the recipient sharing all the donor's histocompatibility genes. This is illustrated by grafting between parental and F$_1$(A×B) animals (3 and 4). Animals which differ at loci other than the MHC reject grafts from each other, but much more slowly.

THE ROLE OF T LYMPHOCYTES IN REJECTION

T cells play a central role in rejection. Rodents born without a thymus (congenitally athymic or 'nude') have no mature T cells and cannot reject transplants. The same is true of normal rats or mice whose thymus is removed in the neonatal period, before mature T cells are released to the periphery. Likewise, thymectomy of adult rats or mice (to stop the production of T cells), followed by irradiation (to remove existing mature T cells) and bone marrow transplantation (to restore haematopoiesis) produces 'ATXBM recipients' which have no T cells and cannot reject grafts.

In any of these animals (nudes, neonatally thymectomized or ATXBM), the ability to reject grafts is restored by the inoculation of T cells from an animal of the same strain. Thus, T cells are necessary for rejec-

Graft versus host disease

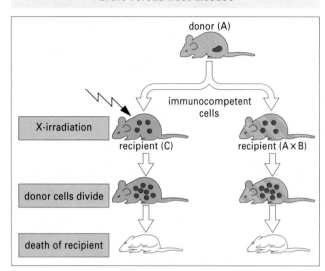

Fig 23.7 Immunocompetent cells from a donor of type 'A' are injected into an immunosuppressed (X-irradiated) host of type 'C', or a normal F$_1$ (A×B) recipient. The immunosuppressed individual is unable to reject the cells and the F$_1$ animal is fully tolerant to parental type 'A' cells. In both cases the donor cells recognize the foreign tissue types 'B' and 'C' of the recipient. They divide and react against the recipient tissue cells and recruit large numbers of host cells to inflammatory sites. Very often the process leads to the death of the recipient.

Intra- and extrathymic induction of tolerance

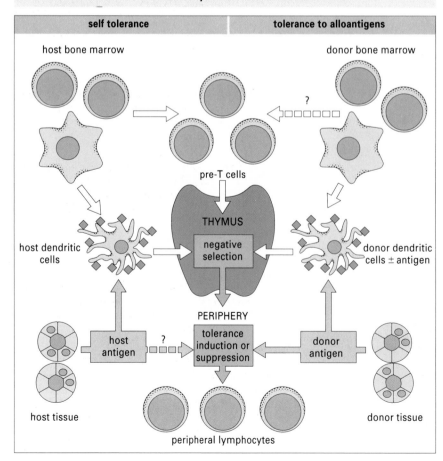

Fig 23.8 Under normal physiological conditions bone marrow-derived pre-T cells enter the thymus and undergo positive selection (rescue from programmed cell death) when they meet epithelial cells in the cortex and negative selection (elimination of self-reactive cells) when they contact dendritic cells at the corticomedullary junction. Newly derived self-reactive T cells can still be inactivated outside the thymus (but not necessarily eliminated) by antigen in the periphery. Alternatively, they can become activated suppressor cells.

In allotolerant animals, foreign antigen may be present in the thymic medulla (as donor-type dendritic cells or as donor antigen presented by recipient dendritic cells) where it can cause tolerance by clonal deletion. Alternatively, foreign antigen in the periphery may cause clonal anergy (unresponsiveness) or stimulate active suppression in allotolerant animals.

tion. This does not imply that antibodies, B cells or other cells play no part. Indeed, antibodies cause graft damage and macrophages may be involved in inflammatory reactions in grafted tissue (see below). However, neither B cells nor macrophages play a necessary or sufficient role in rejection, and they depend on the action of T cells, especially in primary rejection responses.

THE MOLECULAR BASIS OF ALLORECOGNITION

The T cells involved in rejection recognise donor-derived peptides in association with the MHC antigens expressed on the graft. The structure of the T-cell receptor (TCR) (see Chapter 4) is such that T cells can only see peptide antigens associated with MHC molecules; this MHC restriction is reinforced by positive selection in the thymus (see Chapters 10 and 11 and Fig. 23.8).

The structures of different MHC antigens are almost identical. The overall shape of all MHC molecules is of two α helices lying on a β-pleated sheet atop two immunoglobulin-like domains which sit on the cell membrane. Between the α helices is a deep groove into which peptides can be bound. Although antigenic epitopes can be detected serologically on the outside of the molecules, the part of the MHC molecule that is important in T cell recognition, namely the outer surface of the α helices, lacks such epitopes, being highly conserved between different MHC molecules. The only significant amino-acid-sequence differences between two MHC molecules, comparing the HLA-A2 and HLA-Aw68 antigens for example, lie deep in the groove between the α helices, not on the outer surface contacted by the TCR (Fig. 23.9). Hence, as far as T-cell recognition is concerned, the principal difference between MHC molecules is in the shape and charge of the peptide binding groove (Fig. 23.10), and this governs which peptides can be bound and in what orientation they are presented to T-cell receptors (see Chapter 6).

In the normal physiological situation the MHC groove is occupied by polypeptides of normal cellular constituents derived from intracellular degradative pathways. In virus-infected cells, or in specialized antigen-presenting cells, the normal cell-derived peptides are replaced by peptides of foreign origin. T cells then respond to these foreign peptides in association with self-MHC molecules. (Note: T cells that would otherwise have responded to self-peptide–self-MHC complexes are clonally deleted or negatively selected in the thymus – see Chapter 11).

In the case of a genetically distinct transplanted tissue, a different array of the same cellular constituents is presented on the cell surface because of the different shape and charge of the MHC groove. In addition there may be different allelic forms of the normal cellular constituents (determined by minor histocompatibility

Location of amino acid sequence differences between two MHC molecules

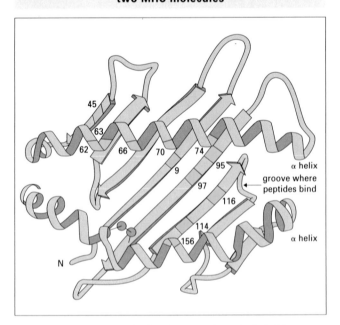

Fig 23.9 Many amino acid sequence differences between MHC molecules are located within the peptide-binding groove either in the walls (α helices) or the floor (β-pleated sheet) of the cleft. In this figure the locations of amino acid differences of HLA-A2 and HLA-Aw68 are shown. (Courtesy of P. Parham, adapted from *Nature*, **342**, 617–8, with permission.

Comparison of the shape of the peptide binding groove of two MHC molecules

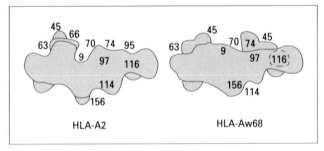

Fig 23.10 The shape of the peptide binding groove of two MHC Class I molecules, HLA-A2 and HLA-Aw68, has been compared by X-ray crystallography and electron density mapping. Within the groove there are 10 amino acid differences, at positions 9, 63, 66, 70, 74, 95, 97, 114, 116 and 156, which alter the shape and charge of the cleft and create different pockets (e.g. at positions 45 and 74) which can accommodate peptide side chains. Consequently, different MHC molecules can bind and present different peptide antigens. (Courtesy of T. P. J. Garrett *et al*, adapted from *Nature*, **342**, 629–6, with permission.)

loci), giving rise to an altogether new selection of peptides. In this way differences between graft donor and recipient in their major histocompatibility antigens (differently shaped and charged grooves) or in their minor histocompatibility antigens (different peptides) leads to the expression on transplanted tissues of a large number of novel antigens which can be recognized by recipient T cells.

THE ROLE OF T HELPER (TH) CELLS IN REJECTION

The relative contribution of T cell subsets to rejection can be tested in athymic animals. Injecting T cells of the CD4+ subpopulation (TH cells) into nude or ATXBM recipients leads to acute skin-graft rejection. Naïve, unsensitized CD8+ T cells are unable to do this, but when CD8+ T cells are mixed with a very low number of CD4+ T cells, or are presensitized to graft antigens (i.e. taken from animals which have already rejected a graft), rapid graft destruction is seen. Further evidence of the importance of CD4+ T cells has been obtained by treating recipients with monoclonal anti-CD4+ antibodies (Fig. 23.11). Hence, CD4+ T cells are both necessary and sufficient to bring about rejection of skin transplants in the absence of CD8+ T cells. By contrast, naïve CD8+ T cells require the presence of CD4+ T cells. However, once sensitized by CD4+ T cells, CD8+ T cells can play a role as well.

THE ROLE OF LYMPHOKINES IN REJECTION

The experiments in athymic animals reconstituted with CD4+ T helper (TH) cells illustrate their central importance in the induction of rejection, but beyond that a multiplicity of immunological mechanisms are involved in rejection. The overall picture is shown in Fig. 23.12.

TH cells are activated by APCs derived from bone marrow and carrying MHC Class II molecules. The APC activating rejection can come from either the donor or

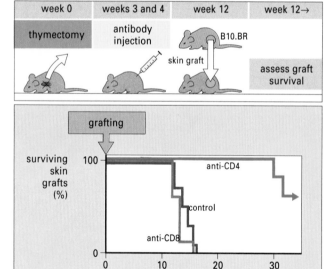

Role of T cells in graft rejection

Fig 23.11 Thymectomized CBA mice were treated with cytotoxic monoclonal antibodies to CD4 or CD8 to selectively deplete those T cell populations. They were then grafted with skin from B10.BR mice which differ at minor histocompatibility loci. The survival of the grafts was assessed. Animals treated with anti-CD4 had greatly extended graft survival by comparison with untreated animals (control) or those treated with anti-CD8. This emphasizes the importance of the CD4+ population in graft rejection. (Based on data of Cobbold & colleagues.)

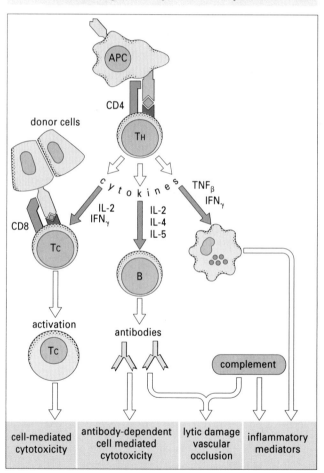

Immunological components of rejection

Fig 23.12 T helper (TH) cells are activated by antigen presenting cells to release lymphokines. IL-2 and IFNγ are required for T cytotoxic (Tc) cell activation; IL-2, IL-4 and IL-5 are involved in B cell activation; a mixture of TNFβ (lymphotoxin) and IFNγ acts as macrophage activating factor (MAF). These cells reject the graft by specific cell-mediated and antibody-mediated immune pathways, or by non-specific inflammatory reactions.

the recipients. Those of donor origin arrive in the graft as 'passenger leucocytes' (interstitial dendritic cells) and they cause 'direct' activation of recipient TH cells. Those of recipient origin are located in draining lymphoid tissues, and acquire antigen which is shed from the transplant and present it to recipient TH cells to cause 'indirect' activation. Direct activation is a more powerful stimulus to rejection than the so-called indirect route since this recipient becomes sensitized to allogenic donor MHC molecules. Hence passenger cells may have a strong influence on graft survival (Fig. 23.13). Regardless of the route of activation, activated TH cells produce the cytokines which are required as growth and differentiation factors for other cells involved in the rejection reaction (Fig. 23.12).

The most important lymphokines in cellular rejection are IL-2 which is required for activation of T cytotoxic cells, and IFN_γ which induces MHC-antigen expression, increases APC activity, activates large granular lymphocytes and, in concert with TNF_β (lymphotoxin), activates macrophages. (Note: the mixture of IFN_γ and TNF_β was formerly known as macrophage activating factor or MAF).

Lymphokines are required, too, for B cell activation leading to the production of anti-graft antibodies. These antibodies fix complement and cause damage to the vascular endothelium, resulting in haemorrhage, platelet aggregation within the vessels, graft thrombosis, lytic damage to cells of the transplant, and the release of the pro-inflammatory complement components C3a and C5a.

Not all parts of the graft need to be attacked for rejection to occur. The critical targets are the vascular endothelium of the microvasculature and the specialized parenchymal cells of the organ such as renal tubules, pancreatic islets of Langerhans or cardiac myocytes.

It is significant that IFN_γ can cause vascular endothelial cells to express high levels of Class II MHC antigens, and can induce the expression of Class I and II antigens on parenchymal cells, which are usually either weakly positive or negative for these antigens. This upregulation of MHC antigen expression can provoke greater stimulation of the rejection response, and provide a greater number of target molecules within the graft for antibodies and activated cells.

TNF_β and IFN_γ also upregulate the expression of adhesion molecules on vascular endothelium. These are required for the adhesion of blood-borne leucocytes to adhere to the walls of blood vessels prior to their migration across the endothelium into the tissues.

THE TEMPO OF REJECTION

The rate of rejection depends in part on the underlying effector mechanisms. Clinicians classify graft damage in patients according to the speed of the rejection observed (Fig. 23.14). Hyperacute rejection occurs very rapidly in patients who already have antibodies against

The role of passenger cells in graft destruction

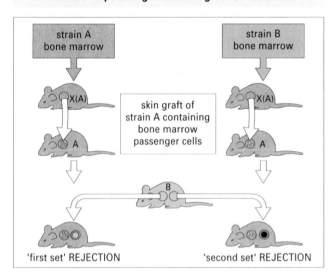

Fig 23.13 Strain A mice were X-irradiated and reconstituted with bone marrow cells of either strain A or strain B. Skin grafts from these mice were accepted by strain A mice. The recipients subsequently received strain B skin grafts. Animals whose first graft came from an animal reconstituted with strain A cells reject the strain B graft more slowly than animals whose first graft came from a mouse reconstituted with strain B cells. This implies that strain B bone marrow cells, carried as passengers in the first graft, primed the recipient to strain B alloantigen.

Tempo of rejection reactions

type of rejection	time taken	cause
hyperacute	minutes–hours	preformed anti-donor antibodies and complement
accelerated	days	reactivation of sensitized T cells
acute	days–weeks	primary activation of T cells
chronic	months–years	causes unclear: antibodies, immune complexes, slow cellular reaction, recurrence of disease

Fig 23.14 Much can be determined about the mechanisms of rejection by observing the speed of graft damage. Preformed antibodies and presensitized lymphocytes cause rapid rejection compared with primary and slowly evolving responses.

the graft. Such antibodies are induced by prior blood transfusions, multiple pregnancies, the rejection of a previous transplant or, in a few cases, by deliberate immunization with foreign cells to induce alloantibodies (e.g. for use in tissue typing). Preformed antibodies fix complement, damaging the endothelial cell lining of the blood vessels which allows the leakage of cells and fluids and causes aggregation of platelets which then block the microvasculature and deprive the graft of a blood supply (Fig. 23.15). Hyperacute rejection can be avoided by performing a crossmatch test in which serum from a prospective recipient is tested for the presence of cytotoxic anti-donor antibodies.

Acute rejection takes days or weeks to become manifest and is due to the primary activation of T lymphocytes and the consequent triggering of various effector mechanisms (Figs 23.16–18). If a transplant is given to someone who has been presensitized to antigens on the graft a secondary reactivation of T cells occurs, leading to an accelerated cell-mediated rejection response. Accelerated or 'second-set' rejection of skin grafts is particularly dramatic, the graft being rejected before it has time to heal in (Fig. 23.19).

Depending on the genetic disparity between donor and recipient and the use of immunosuppressive treatment, graft rejection can be a slow process taking months or years. This is called chronic rejection and may be due to several different causes, such as a low-grade cell-mediated rejection or the deposition of antibodies or antigen-antibody complexes in the grafted tissue. Grafts may also be damaged by any chronic pathological process which necessitated the transplant.

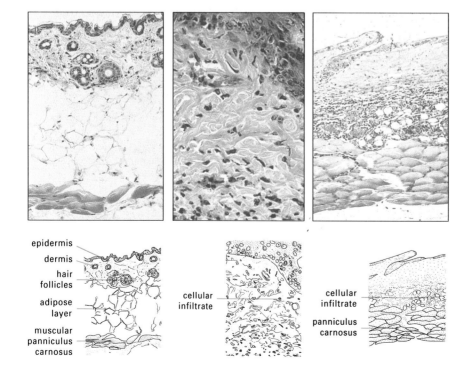

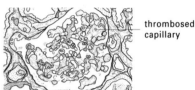

thrombosed capillary

Fig 23.15 Renal histology showing hyperacute graft rejection. There is extensive necrosis of the glomerular capillary associated with massive interstitial haemorrhage. This extensive necrosis is preceded by an intense polymorphonuclear infiltration which occurs within the first hour of the graft's revascularization. The changes shown here occur 24–48 hours after this. H&E stain, × 200.

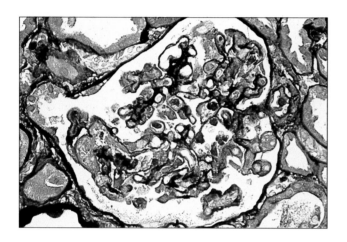

epidermis
dermis
hair follicles
adipose layer
muscular panniculus carnosus

cellular infiltrate
panniculus carnosus

cellular infiltrate
panniculus carnosus

Fig 23.16 Sections of strain A mouse skin showing the normal appearance (left) and the allograft 5 days (middle) and 12 days (right) after transplantation to a CBA host. At 5 days there is a substantial infiltration by host mononuclear cells. At 12 days the epithelium has been totally destroyed and is lifting off the dermis, which is now free of cells; the infiltrating host cells have been destroyed by anoxia but there is still a brisk cellular traffic in the graft bed between the dermis and the panniculus carnosus. (Courtesy of Professor L. Brent.)

PREVENTION OF REJECTION BY TISSUE MATCHING

One way to overcome rejection is by tissue matching for histocompatibility antigens. Obviously, the perfectly matched donor and recipient would be isogeneic, for example monozygotic twins. However, this situation is rare in humans and in all other cases there will be major and/or minor histocompatibility differences between the donor and recipient. Only the MHC (HLA) antigens can be practicably matched. This is usually done by serology, whereby cells from the donor and

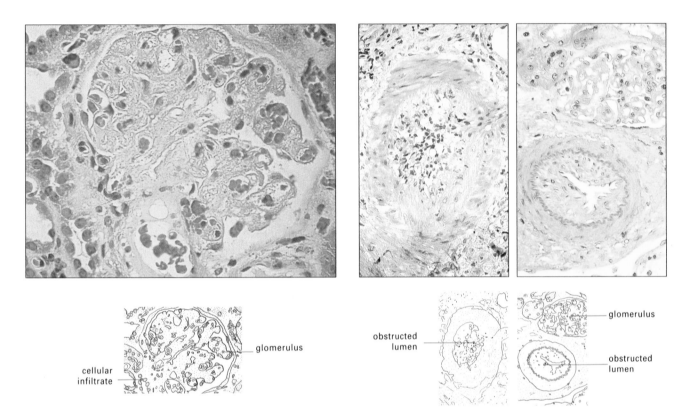

Fig 23.17 Renal histology showing acute graft rejection – I.
Small lymphocytes and other cells are accumulating in the interstitium of the graft. Such infiltration is characteristic of acute rejection and occurs before the appearance of any clinical signs. H&E stain, × 200.

Fig 23.18 Renal histology showing acute graft rejection – II.
The section of acutely rejecting kidney shown on the left (H&E stain) shows vascular obstruction and that on the right (Van Gieson's stain) shows the end stage of this process. × 140.

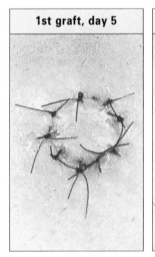
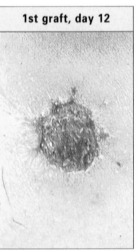
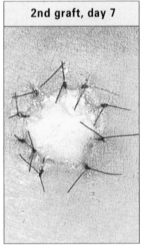

Fig 23.19 Graft rejection displays immunological memory. A human skin allograft at day 5 (left) is fully vascularized and the cells are dividing, but by day 12 (middle) it is totally destroyed. A second graft from the same donor shown here on day 7 (right) does not become vascularized and is destroyed rapidly. This indicates that sensitization to the first graft produces immunological memory.

Serological tissue typing

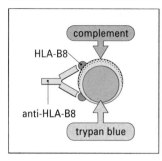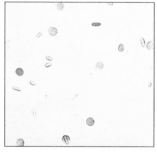

Fig. 23.20 Tissue typing is performed serologically by adding typing antisera of defined specificity (e.g. anti-HLA-B8), complement and trypan blue stain to test cells on a microassay plate. Cell death, as assessed by trypan blue staining, confirms that the test cell carried the antigen in question (HLA–B8). Dead, trypan blue-stained cells (dark staining) are shown on the right.

Serologically detected HLA specificities

locus	class I				class II		
	A	B		C	DR	DQ	DP
antigens	1	5	w50	w1	1	w1	w1
	2	7	51	w2	2	w2	w2
	3	8	w52	w3	3	w3	w3
	9	12	w53	w4	4	w4	w4
	10	13	w54	w5	5	w5	w5
	11	14	w55	w6	w6	w6	w6
	w19	15	w56	w7	7	w7	
	23	16	w57	w8	w8	w8	
	24	17	w58	w9	w9	w9	
	25	18	w59	w10	w10		
	26	21	w60	w11	w11		
	28	w22	w61		w12		
	29	27	w62		w13		
	30	35	w63		w14		
	31	37	w64		w15		
	32	38	w65		w16		
	w33	39	w67		w17		
	w34	40	w70		w18		
	w36	w41	w71		w52		
	w43	w42	w72		w53		
	w66	44	w73				
	w68	45	w75				
	w69	w46	w76				
	w74	w47	w4				
		w48	w6				
		49					

Fig 23.21 There are nearly 80 different Class I HLA-A, B and C) molecules and over 35 different Class II (HLA-DP, DQ and DR) molecules are recognised in humans. The techniques of molecular genetics are leading to the discovery of many more variants which are not serologically distinguishable.

recipient are typed, using a panel of cytotoxic antibodies that react with all the known HLA antigens, to discover which molecules are expressed. Serological typing takes only a few hours and can therefore be performed while the donor organ is preserved on ice (Fig. 23.20). The lists of known Class I (HLA-A, HLA-B and HLA-C) and Class II (HLA-DP, HLA-DQ and HLA-DR) antigens are long (Fig. 23.21) and the chances of a match of two individuals at random are extremely remote. Matching for all known HLA antigens is therefore practically impossible, but good graft survival is obtained when the donor and recipient share only the same MHC Class II (especially HLA-DR) antigens (Fig. 23.22).

Another way to match donors and recipient is by using the mixed lymphocyte reaction (MLR) to test the responsiveness of recipient lymphocytes to antigens expressed on donor cells (Fig. 23.23). Low recipient anti-donor MLR responses are associated with excellent transplant survival. However, the time required for the MLR test precludes its use in most clinical organ transplantation, because organs from dead or brain-dead donors cannot be preserved for more than 24–48 hours. In cases where living donors (e.g. relatives) are to be used, this is possible. The MLR is especially important in bone-marrow transplantation and is often performed to see whether the donor bone marrow cells could respond to recipient antigens and cause graft-versus-host disease (see p.23.3). In such a test, it is the recipient's lymphoid cells that are irradiated, and lymphocytes from the donor that proliferate.

Kidney graft survival and HLA matching

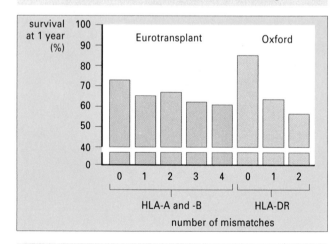

Fig 23.22 The bar chart shows the percentage survival of cadaver kidney grafts at 12 months in humans in two separate studies. In the first study (Eurotransplant), donors were matched for HLA-A and -B (Class I). In the second study (Oxford) donors were matched for HLA-DR (Class II).

TREATMENT OF REJECTION BY NON-SPECIFIC IMMUNOSUPPRESSION

There are two main categories of immunosuppressive treatment, non-specific and specific immunosuppression. Non-specific immunosuppression blunts or abolishes the activity of the immune system regardless of the antigen. For instance, a large dose of X-rays prevents rejection but also has many deleterious effects, as well as abolishing anti-microbial immunity. Most non-specific treatments used today are selective for the immune system, or are used in a way which creates some selectivity. However, the side effects of any non-specific treatment are hard to avoid altogether. The very best treatment would inactivate only those clones of lymphocytes with specificity for donor antigens, leaving other clones intact, so that the patient does not suffer infections or side effects. Such highly specific immunosuppression remains the 'Holy Grail' of transplantation immunobiology and is described later.

The three non-specific agents in current clinical use are steroids, cyclosporine and azathioprine (Fig. 23.24). Steroids have anti-inflammatory properties and suppress activated macrophages, they interfere with APC function and they reduce the expression of MHC antigens. In effect, steroids reverse many of the actions of IFN$_\gamma$ on macrophages and transplanted tissues.

Cyclosporine is a fungal macrolide (see Fig. 23.25) produced by soil organisms isolated in the USA and Norway. Cyclosporine was initially of interest as an antibiotic. Although it is rather poor in this regard it has interesting and potent immunosuppressive properties. Its principal action is to suppress lymphokine production by TH cells and, directly or indirectly, to reduce the expression of the receptors for IL-2 on lymphocytes undergoing activation.

Other macrolides from soil fungi have immunosuppressive properties too, and these are under assessment. One is FK 506, produced by a fungus from Japan. Another is Rapamycin, named after Rapa Pui, the Polynesian name for Easter Island whence the soil sample came. FK 506 suppresses lymphokine production by TH cells although somewhat differently compared with cyclosporine. Rapamycin interferes with the intracellular signalling pathways of the IL-2 receptor and therefore prevents IL-2-dependent lymphocyte activation.

Azathioprine is an anti-proliferative drug. An analogue of 6-mercaptopurine, its incorporation into the DNA of dividing cells prevents further proliferation.

These agents can be effective used alone although high doses are usually required and the likelihood of adverse effects is increased. Used together in various combinations they work in synergy because they interfere with different stages of the same immune pathway.

Tissue typing – mixed lymphocyte reaction

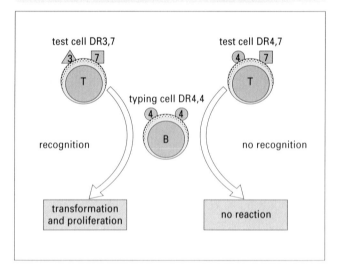

Fig 23.23 The homozygous typing cell here is HLA-DR4,4. (Antigenic specificities are represented by differently numbered shapes.) Two test lymphocytes are shown, DR3,7 and DR4,7. DR4,7 carries the typing cell's specificity (4), and does not recognize the typing cell, while DR3,7 recognizes the typing cell as foreign. This is revealed by the test cell transforming and proliferating. (Typing cells are treated to stop them dividing in response to the test cells.)

Immunosuppression with drugs

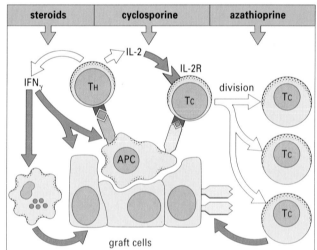

Fig 23.24 The agents in common clinical use, steroids, cyclosporine and azathioprine, suppress the rejection response at different points. Steroids are anti-inflammatory and suppress activated macrophages, decrease antigen-presenting cell function, and reduce MHC antigen expression. Cyclosporine interferes with lymphokine production. Azathioprine prevents the proliferation of activated cells.

The doses of individual agents can thus be reduced and the adverse effects minimized. The clinical results obtained since the introduction of cyclosporine are very good (85–90% graft acceptance at one year for kidneys, hearts and livers), although the problem of chronic rejection remains and long-term use is still associated with adverse effects. Further improvements might be obtained with FK 506 and Rapamycin.

New non-specific but more selective agents are under development (Fig. 23.26). Monoclonal antibodies against lymphocyte surface molecules, especially CD3, CD4, CD8 and the IL-2 receptor (IL-2R) can be used to eliminate cells or to block their function. Cytotoxic drugs can be attached to these antibodies to increase their effectiveness. A related approach is to attach a toxin to IL-2 so that cells undergoing activation in response to graft antigens and expressing receptors for IL-2 are selectively poisoned.

SPECIFIC IMMUNOSUPPRESSION

The immune system is regulated by various 'feedback' mechanisms which control the magnitude, type and specificity of immunological reactions (see Chapter 9). It is possible, in experimental models, to harness these feedback systems to prevent transplant rejection. There are three classical procedures which can be used, neonatally-induced tolerance, active enhancement and passive enhancement.

Neonatal rodents (unlike humans) are born just before mature T cells are first exported from the thymus. (Note: The equivalent stage of human development is 16–20 weeks of gestation.) If a persistent source of antigen, for instance viable cells with potential for growth or repeated injections of antigen, is given to the neonate rodents, the development of mature T cells that react with that antigen is suppressed. Classically, bone marrow cells from an (A×B)F$_1$ mouse are injected into a B neonate. (Note: (A×B)F$_1$ donor cells are used

The structure of immunosuppressive fungal macrolides

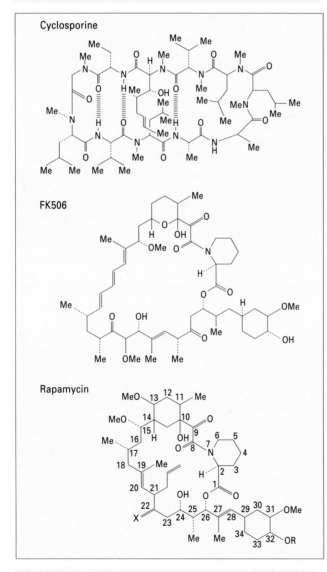

Fig 23.25 The immunosuppressive fungal macrolides, cyclosporine, FK 506 and Rapamycin, have quite different structures. They act on lymphocytes in different ways, cyclosporine and FK 506 affecting lymphokine production and Rapamycin interfering with signalling through the IL-2 receptor.

Selective approaches to immunosuppression

agent	target
heterologous antisera/antibodies	
anti-lymphocyte serum (ALS)	all lymphocytes
anti-thymocyte globulin (ATG)	selective for T cells
monoclonal antibodies	
anti-CD3	mature T cells
anti-CD4	T helper cells
anti-CD25 (IL-2R)	Activated T cells
antibody–toxin conjugates	
anti-CD5 coupled to the	activated (CD5-positive)
A chain of ricin toxin	T cells
lymphokine–toxin conjugates	
IL-2 coupled to diphtheria	activated T cells
toxin	(which express IL-2 receptor)

Fig 23.26 Antibodies and lymphokines can be targeted to cells of the immune system. By contrast, drugs can have adverse effects on non-lymphoid tissue, e.g. nephrotoxicity and hepatotoxicity. The efficacy of biological agents can be increased by coupling drugs or toxins to them.

to obviate the A-strain anti-B GVH reaction which occurs if A donor cells are used.) The bone marrow inoculum produces cells which provide a continuous source of antigen. When the B mouse grows to adulthood it is unresponsive to the A antigens to which it has been exposed and is tolerant of the A antigens on skin grafts and other tissues from A or (A×B)F$_1$ strain donors. Mechanisms to account for neonatal tolerance are outlined in Fig. 23.8 and detailed in chapter 11.

Antigen may selectively activate certain subpopulations of lymphocytes. It is currently proposed that there are two major types of T helper cell, known as TH1 and TH2 cells (see Chapter 7). Neonatally tolerized mice can have a deficit of donor-specific TH1 cells and an increased number of donor-specific TH2 cells. TH1 cells make IFN$_\gamma$ and IL-2 and are the TH cells illustrated in Fig. 23.24, which are involved in rejection. By contrast,

TH2 cells make other lymphokines including IL-10 or cytokine synthesis inhibitory factor (CSIF) which interferes with the synthesis of lymphokines by TH1 cells. For neonatally tolerized mice, fewer donor-specific TH1 cells and more donor-specific TH2 cells means a shift in the balance between rejection and acceptance, leading to tolerance of the graft. This form of tolerance is not strictly unresponsiveness *per se* but is, instead, a deviated response. Interestingly, cyclosporine may have a preferential effect on TH1 cells and spare TH2 cells.

Finally, antigen can activate T suppressor (Ts) cells. The precise identify of these T cells is still shrouded in mystery. What is known is that, when transferred to another animal, T cells from an animal tolerant of a graft from donor A can prevent rejection of a graft carrying A antigens. This is referred to as the adoptive transfer of suppression and the cells responsible are usually CD8$^+$ T cells. Much controversy still exists concerning the Ts cell and its mode of action, but experimental data such as these are a clear indication that functional Ts cells do exist. They are resistant to cyclosporine and may contribute to this agent's mode of action. Ts cells mediate tolerance by active suppression.

A direct equivalent of neonatally-induced tolerance is not possible in humans. However, procedures such as total lymphoid irradiation (TLI), in which mature lymphocytes are severely depleted by radiation while the bone marrow is shielded and therefore remains intact, may create a situation in adults analogous to that in the neonatal rodent. Indeed, TLI followed by antigen exposure induces profound tolerance. However, TLI is rather hazardous for routine clinical use. The use of monoclonal antibodies to mature T cells may achieve their depletion in a much safer but equally effective way.

In some cases prior exposure to donor antigens can cause prolonged or indefinite graft survival (Fig. 23.27). This is, of course, contrary to expectation since one might expect accelerated or hyperacute rejection. The phenomenon is called active enhancement of graft survival. The route of exposure to antigen is important, possibly because it impinges on particular lymphoid tissues. It has been shown in a rat kidney-graft model that a transfusion of donor blood given intravenously to the recipient one week before kidney transplantation leads to long-term organ graft acceptance, while the same dose of blood given subcutaneously causes accelerated rejection. The effect is immunologically specific so that the blood donor and the kidney donor must share at least some antigens.

An active enhancement effect has been employed clinically using donor specific transfusions (DST). For example, if a parent is about to donate a kidney to a child, the recipient can be treated with blood transfusions from the parent before transplantation. Unfortunately, about 20% of patients receiving DST develop anti-donor antibodies and cannot then receive the kidney as planned for fear of hyperacute rejection. However, of the remaining 80% the transplant success rate is 95–100%.

Immunological enhancement of graft survival

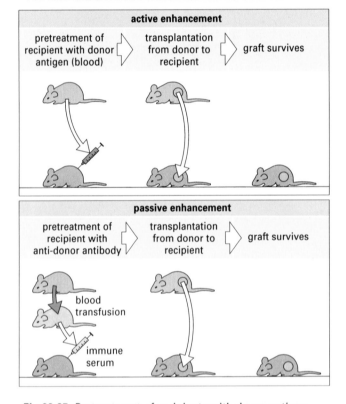

Fig 23.27 Pretreatment of recipients with donor antigen can prolong the survival of a subsequent allograft. This is known as active enhancement of graft survival because the effect requires an active response on the part of the recipient. (Note that the same blood, given by a different route, can result in rapid rejection.) Alternatively, anti-donor antibody given to the recipient at the time of transplantation can cause passive enhancement of graft survival. Both active and passive enhancement are immunologically specific since only the response to the particular donor is suppressed and the survival of third party unrelated grafts is not enhanced.

The beneficial effect of pre-transplant blood transfusion, known as the blood transfusion effect, has also been documented in patients receiving random transfusions, perhaps because of the chance exposure to antigens which happen to be on their transplant (Fig. 23.28). Indeed, the blood transfusion effect increases with the number of random transfusions, and most transplant centres adopted the policy of deliberately transfusing prospective recipients. However, there is always a risk of sensitization of the patient, and improvements in the availability and use of immunosuppressive drugs have largely made this practice redundant.

Active enhancement is so called because it requires an active response by the recipient to the injected donor antigen. The mechanism could be induction of anergy, selective activation of TH2 cells, or activation of Ts cells by the blood transfusion, as described for neonatally-induced tolerance. Alternatively, the mechanism might involve the production of 'enhancing antibodies' specific for donor antigen, thus interfering with the graft rejection process by masking antigens in the graft and preventing their recognition by T cells, or destroying highly immunogenic passenger leucocytes within the graft. Enhancing antibodies may also be formed to antigen receptors, thus eliminating donor-reactive cells or affecting antigen presentation so that, for instance, TH2 and Ts cells are selectively activated after transplantation.

Antibody can play a feedback role in transplanted individuals. Injection of anti-donor antibody into a rat kidney graft recipient at the time of grafting can cause long-term graft acceptance (see Fig. 23.27). (Note: rats have a poor complement system and hyperacute rejection is not usually observed in this species.) The phenomenon of graft protection by injecting anti-donor antibodies is called passive enhancement of graft survival since the product of an immune response (antibody) is transferred rather than the antigen.

The effect of blood transfusion on kidney transplantation

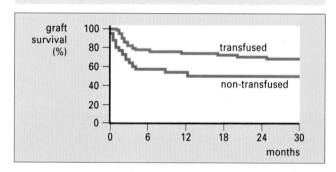

Fig 23.28 This graph plots the survival of kidney grafts in 102 transfused and 71 non-transfused patients.

FURTHER READING

Billingham RE, Silvers ES. *The Immunobiology of Transplantation.* New Jersey: Prentice Hall, 1971.

Cerilli CJ. *Organ Transplantation and Replacement.* Maryland: JB Lippincott, 1988.

Kahan D, ed. *Cyclosporin A – Biological Activity Applications.* New York: Grune & Stratton Inc, 1984.

Klein J. *Natural History of the Major Histocompatibility Complex.* New York: John Wiley & Sons, 1987.

chapter 24

Autoimmunity and Autoimmune Disease

The immune system has tremendous diversity and because the repertoire of specificities expressed by the B and T cell populations is generated randomly, it is bound to include many which are specific for self-components. The complicated mechanisms which the body must establish to distinguish between self and non-self determinants, so as to avoid autoreactivity, have already been discussed (see Chapter 10). However, all mechanisms have a risk of breakdown. The self-recognition mechanisms are no exception, and a number of diseases have been identified in which there is copious production of autoantibodies and autoreactive T cells.

One of the earliest examples in which the production of autoantibodies was associated with disease in a given organ was Hashimoto's thyroiditis. This disease of the thyroid, which is most common in middle-aged women, often leads to formation of a goitre and hypothyroidism. The gland is infiltrated, sometimes to an extraordinary extent, with inflammatory lymphoid cells. These are predominantly mononuclear phagocytes, lymphocytes and plasma cells; secondary lymphoid follicles are common (Fig. 24.1). The gland in Hashimoto's disease often shows regenerating thyroid follicles but this is not a feature of the thyroid in a related condition, primary myxoedema, in which comparable immunological features are seen but the gland undergoes almost complete destruction and shrinks.

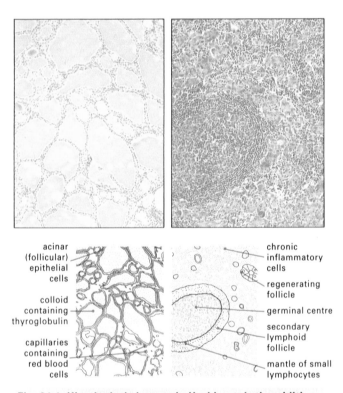

Fig. 24.1 Histological changes in Hashimoto's thyroiditis. A normal thyroid gland (left), showing the follicular cells lining the colloid space into which they secrete thyroglobulin, which is broken down on demand to provide thyroid hormones. A Hashimoto gland (right) in which the normal architecture is virtually destroyed and replaced by invading cells, which consist essentially of lymphocytes, macrophages and plasma cells. A secondary lymphoid follicle with a germinal centre and a small regenerating thyroid follicle are present. H&E stain, × 80.

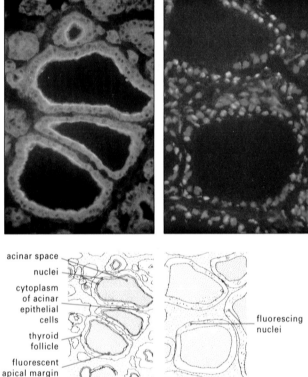

Fig. 24.2 Autoantibodies to thyroid. Healthy, unfixed human thyroid sections were treated with patients' serum, and then with fluoresceinated rabbit anti-human immunoglobulin. Acinar epithelial cells are stained by antibodies from a patient with Hashimoto's disease, which react with the cells' cytoplasm, but not the nuclei (left). Colloid is lost from the unfixed section, so thyroglobulin staining is not seen within the colloid/acinar space. In contrast, serum from a patient with SLE contains antibodies which reacts only with the nucleus of acinar epithelial cells (right).

The serum of patients with Hashimoto's disease usually contains antibodies to thyroglobulin. These antibodies are demonstrable by immunofluorescence (Fig. 24.2) and also, when present in high titre, by precipitin reactions. Many patients also have antibodies directed against a cytoplasmic or microsomal antigen, also present on the apical surface of the microvilli, and now known to be thyroid peroxidase.

THE SPECTRUM OF AUTOIMMUNE DISEASES

The antibodies associated with Hashimoto's disease and primary myxoedema react only with the thyroid, so the resulting lesion is highly localized. In contrast, the serum from patients with diseases such as systemic lupus erythematosus (SLE) reacts with many, if not all, of the tissues in the body. In SLE, one of the dominant antibodies is directed against the cell nucleus (Fig. 24.2). These two diseases represent the extremes of the autoimmune spectrum (Fig. 24.3).

The common target organs in organ-specific disease include the thyroid, adrenals, stomach and pancreas. The non-organ-specific diseases, which include the so-called rheumatological disorders, characteristically involve the skin, kidney, joints and muscle (Fig. 24.4).

Interestingly, there are remarkable overlaps at each end of the spectrum. For example, thyroid antibodies occur with a high frequency in patients with pernicious anaemia who have stomach autoimmunity, and these patients have a higher incidence of thyroid autoimmune disease than the normal population. Similarly, patients with thyroid autoimmunity have a high incidence of stomach autoantibodies and, to a lesser extent, the clinical disease itself, pernicious anaemia.

The cluster of rheumatological disorders at the other end of the spectrum also shows considerable overlap. Features of rheumatoid arthritis, for example, are often associated with the clinical picture of SLE. In these diseases immune complexes are deposited systemically, particularly in the kidney, joints and skin, giving rise to disseminated lesions. In contrast, overlap of diseases at either end of the spectrum is relatively rare (Fig. 24.5).

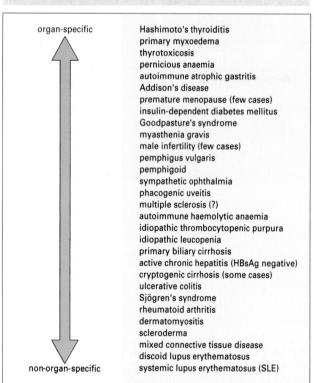

Fig. 24.3. Autoimmune diseases may be classified as organ-specific or non-organ-specific depending on whether the response is primarily against antigens localized to particular organs, or widespread antigens.

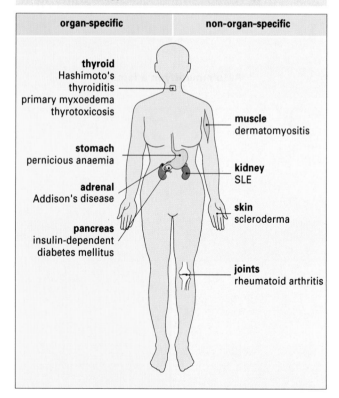

Fig. 24.4 Although the non-organ-specific diseases characteristically produce symptoms in the skin, joints, kidney and muscle, particular organs are more markedly affected by particular diseases, for example the kidney in systemic lupus erythematosus (SLE) and the joint in rheumatoid arthritis.

The mechanisms of immunopathological damage vary depending on where the disease lies in the spectrum. Where the antigen is localized in a particular organ, type II hypersensitivity and cell-mediated reactions are most important (see Chapters 20 and 22). In non-organ-specific autoimmunity, immune complex deposition leads to inflammation through a variety of mechanisms, including complement activation and phagocyte recruitment (see Chapter 21).

GENETICS

There is undoubted familial incidence of autoimmunity, a remarkable example of which is shown in Fig 24.6. This is largely genetic rather than environmental, as may be seen from studies of identical and non-identical twins, and from the association of, for example, thyroid autoantibodies with abnormalities of the X-chromosome.

Autoimmunity within families often shows a bias towards organ-specific reactivity. As well as a general predisposition to develop organ-specific antibodies, it is clear that there are other genetically controlled factors which tend to select the organ that is mainly affected. It is interesting to note that relatives of Hashimoto patients and pernicious anaemia patients both have a higher than normal incidence and titre of thyroid autoantibodies, but the pernicious anaemia patients have a far higher frequency of gastric autoantibodies (Fig. 24.7) indicating that there are genetic factors which differentially select the stomach as the target organ within this group.

Overlap of autoantibodies

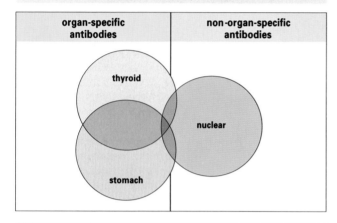

Fig. 24.5 The organ-specific autoantibodies directed against thyroid and stomach often occur together in the same individual, but there is little overlap with non-organ-specific antibodies such as those with reactivity for DNA and nucleoproteins.

Autoimmunity in a family

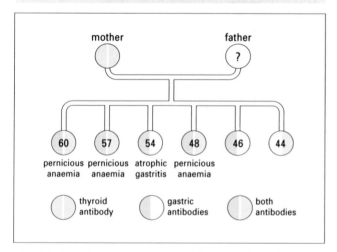

Fig. 24.6 The family chart shows the incidence of organ-specific abnormalities affecting the thyroid and stomach. (At the time of study, the father was dead, and his antibody status unknown.) The siblings all presented with gastric autoimmune disease, unlike the mother who has primary myxoedema. However, there is a striking overlap with thyroid autoimmunity at the serological level, although the siblings lack clinical symptoms of thyroid disease. Autoantibodies are more prevalent with increasing age (ages are given at which autoantibodies were detected).

Autoimmunity in relatives of Hashimoto patients

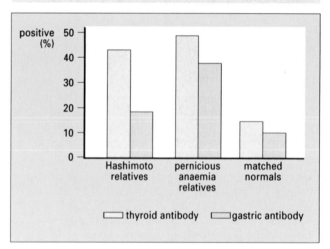

Fig 24.7 A remarkably high proportion of the first degree relatives of patients with Hashimoto's disease have thyroid autoantibodies and to a lesser degree, parietal cell (gastric) autoantibodies. The relatives of patients with pernicious anaemia also have a very high incidence of thyroid autoimmunity, indicating a predisposition to develop organ-specific autoantibodies; the percentage with gastric autoantibodies is also high even when compared with the Hashimoto relatives, suggesting an inherent bias of the immune system for reactivity against particular organs.

Further evidence for the operation of genetic factors in autoimmune disease comes from their tendency to be associated with particular HLA specificities (Fig. 24.8). The haplotype B8, DR3 is particularly common in the organ-specific diseases, though Hashimoto's disease tends to be associated more with DR5. Rheumatoid arthritis showed no HLA associations with the HLA-A and -B loci haplotypes but are associated with HLA-DR4. It is notable that for insulin-dependent (type 1) diabetes mellitus, heterozygotes for DR3 and DR4 have a greatly increased risk of developing the disease. This supports the concept of several genetic factors being involved in the development of autoimmune diseases. These must include genes predisposing individuals to develop autoimmunity, either organ-specific or non-organ-specific, and others which determine the particular antigen or antigens involved.

Confirmation of these views comes from the animal models of autoimmunity discussed in the next section.

PATHOGENESIS

If autoantibodies are found in association with a particular disease there are three possible implications:
1. the autoimmunity is responsible for producing the lesions of the disease
2. there is a disease process which, through the production of tissue damage, leads to the development of autoantibodies
3. there is a factor which produces both the lesions and the autoimmunity.

Autoantibodies secondary to a lesion (proposition 2) have been found in some circumstances. For example, cardiac autoantibodies may develop after myocardial infarction. However, autoantibodies are rarely induced following release of autoantigens by simple trauma. In most diseases associated with autoimmunity, the evidence supports the first proposition, namely that the autoimmune process produces the lesions.

The most direct test of the first proposition is to then deliberately induce autoimmunity in an experimental animal and see if this leads to the production of the lesions. Autoimmunity can be induced in experimental animals by injecting self antigen together with

HLA associations in autoimmune disease

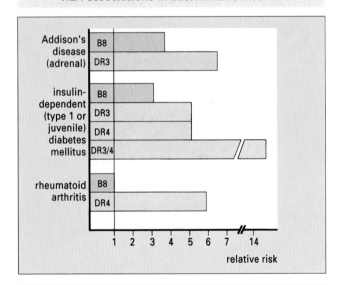

Fig 24.8 The relative risk is a measure of the increased chance of contracting the disease for individuals bearing the HLA antigen, relative to those lacking it. Virtually all autoimmune diseases studied show an association with some HLA specificity. The greater relative risk for Addison's disease associated with DR3 as compared with B8 suggests that DR3 is closely linked to, or even identical with, the 'disease susceptibility gene'. In this case it is not surprising that B8 has a relative risk greater than 1, because it is known to occur with DR3 more often than expected by chance in the general population, a phenomenon termed linkage disequilibrium. Both DR3 and DR4 are associated with type 1 diabetes mellitus, and when a gene for both is present, in the the DR3/4 heterozygote, there is a greatly increased risk, supporting the concept of multiple, additive genetic factors. Rheumatoid arthritis is linked to HLA-DR but not to any HLA-A or HLA-B alleles.

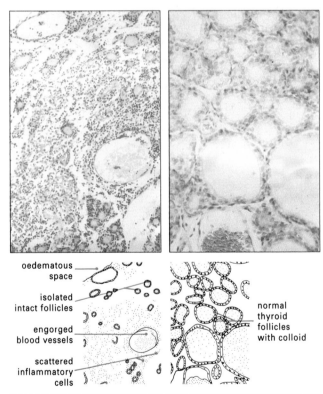

Fig. 24.9 The histological appearance of experimental autoallergic thyroiditis. In the section from a thyroglobulin-injected animal (left) there is gross destruction of the follicular architecture with extensive invasion by mononuclear inflammatory cells, associated with distended blood vessels, oedema and fibrosis. A control section is shown on the right. H&E stain, × 200.

Complete Freund's Adjuvant, and this does indeed produce organ-specific disease in certain organs. For example, thyroglobulin can induce an inflammatory disease of the thyroid while myelin basic protein can cause encephalomyelitis. In the case of thyroglobulin-injected animals, not only are thyroid autoantibodies produced, but the gland becomes infiltrated with mononuclear cells and the acinar architecture crumbles (Fig. 24.9). Although not identical in every respect to Hashimoto's disease, the thyroiditis produced bears a remarkable overall similarity to the human condition.

The ability to induce experimental autoimmune disease depends on the strain of animal used. For example, it is found that the susceptibility of rats and mice to myelin basic protein-induced encephalomyelitis depends on a small number of gene loci, of which the most important are the MHC class II genes. It is also

possible to induce autoallergic encephalomyelitis in susceptible strains by injecting T cells specific for myelin basic protein. These T cells are CD4$^+$ and it has been found that induction of the disease can be blocked by treating the recipients with antibody to CD4, just before the expected time of disease onset. The results indicate the importance of class II restricted autoreactive T_H cells in the development of these conditions, and emphasize the important role of the MHC.

There is much to learn from spontaneous autoimmune disease in animals. One well-established example is the Obese strain chicken (Fig. 24.10) in which thyroid autoantibodies occur spontaneously and the thyroid undergoes the progressive destruction associated with chronic inflammation (Fig. 24.11). The sera of these animals contain thyroglobulin autoantibodies. Furthermore, approximately 15% of the sera react by immunofluorescence with the proventriculus (stomach) of the normal chicken. This is a similar pattern to that obtained when the test is carried out with sera from patients with pernicious anaemia who have parietal cell autoantibodies.

The Obese strain chicken example parallels human autoimmune thyroid disease in terms of the lesion in the gland, the production of antibodies to different components in the thyroid, and the overlap with gastric autoimmunity. So it is of interest that when the immunological status of these animals is altered, quite dramatic effects on the outcome of the disease are seen. For example, if the bursa of Fabricius (in which B cells mature) is removed soon after hatching, the severity of the thyroiditis is greatly diminished, indicating a role for antibody in the pathogenesis of the disease. However, removal of the thymus at birth appears to exacerbate the thyroiditis, suggesting that the thymus exerts a controlling effect on the disease (Fig. 24.12). Paradoxically, destruction of the entire T cell popula-

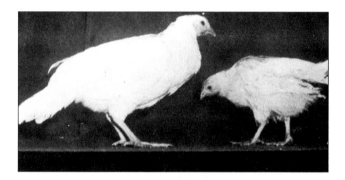

Fig. 24.10 The Obese strain (OS) chicken. This strain of chicken provides an example of spontaneously occurring autoimmune thyroid disease in animals (right). The birds grow poorly and look dishevelled because of the thyroxine deficiency which results from thyroid destruction.

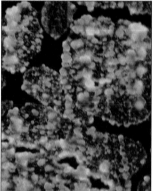 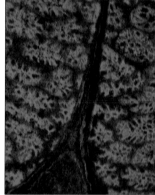

Fig, 24.11 Autoantibodies in OS chickens. Fluorescent staining of a fixed thyroid section showing reaction in the colloid (left). Approximately 15% of the birds have serum antibodies which stain the chicken stomach (proventriculus) giving the characteristic pattern shown (right); this pattern is also seen if human sera containing parietal cell antibodies are tested against this organ.

Modification of thyroiditis in OS chicken by neonatal bursectomy and thymectomy

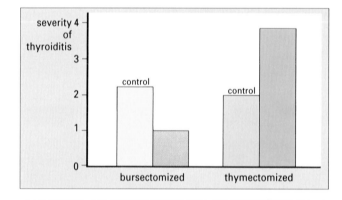

Fig. 24.12 The severity of thyroiditis is assessed by lymphocyte infiltration. Neonatal bursectomy reduces thyroiditis, suggesting an important role for antibody in pathogenesis. Removal of the thymus at birth exacerbates the disease, indicating a controlling effect of Ts cells.

tion in adult animals, by draconian injections of anti-chick T cell serum, completely inhibits both autoantibody production and the attack on the thyroid. T cells clearly play a variety of roles in this disease.

When investigating human autoimmunity directly, rather than animal models, it is of course more difficult to carry out experiments. Nevertheless, there is a great deal of evidence suggesting that autoantibodies are important in the pathogenesis. A number of diseases have been recognized in which autoantibodies to hormone receptors may actually mimic the function of the normal hormone concerned (Fig. 24.13). Thyrotoxicosis was the first disorder in which anti-receptor antibodies were clearly recognized. The phenomenon of neonatal thyrotoxicosis provides us with a natural 'passive transfer' study, because the IgG antibodies from the mother cross the placenta. Many babies born to thyrotoxic mothers and showing thyroid hyperactivity have been reported, but the problem spontaneously resolves as the antibodies derived from the mother are catabolized in the baby over several weeks. A similar phenomenon has been observed with mothers suffering from myasthenia gravis, where antibodies to acetylcholine receptors cross the placenta into the fetus and cause transient muscle weakness in the newborn baby. Somewhat rarely, autoantibodies to insulin receptors and to β-adrenergic receptors can be found, the latter leading to bronchial asthma.

Yet another example of autoimmune disease is seen in rare cases of male infertility where antibodies to spermatozoa lead to clumping of spermatozoa, either by their heads or by their tails, in the semen (Fig. 24.14).

In pernicious anaemia, an autoantibody interferes with the normal uptake of vitamin B_{12}. Vitamin B_{12} is not absorbed directly, but must first associate with a protein called intrinsic factor; the vitamin–protein complex is then transported across the intestinal mucosa. Early studies demonstrated that serum from a patient with pernicious anaemia, if fed to a healthy individual together with intrinsic factor–B_{12} complex, inhibited uptake of the vitamin. Subsequently, the factor in the serum which blocks vitamin uptake was identified as antibody against intrinsic factor. It is now known that plasma cells in the gastric mucosa of patients with pernicious anaemia secrete this antibody into the lumen of the stomach (Fig. 24.15).

Another passive transfer study was carried out in Goodpasture's syndrome, in which antibodies to the glomerular capillary basement membrane are bound to the kidney *in vivo* (see Fig. 21.3). These antibodies were eluted from the kidney of a patient who had died with this disease, and injected into a primate whose kidney antigens were sufficiently similar for the injected antibodies to localize on the glomerular basement membrane. The injected monkeys subsequently died with glomerulonephritis.

In the case of SLE, it can be shown that immune complexes containing autoantigen and antibody, deposited in the kidney of patients, produce the hypersensitivity reactions outlined in Chapter 21. Glomerulonephritis and proteinuria can be induced by repeated injections of high doses of antigen, which lead to chronic immune complex disease and deposition in the kidney. Even a single large dose of antigen can produce acute damage.

Turning to experimental animals, the hybrid of the New Zealand Black and New Zealand White strains of mice spontaneously develops murine SLE in which immune-complex glomerulonephritis and anti-DNA antibodies are major features (see Chapter 9). The fact

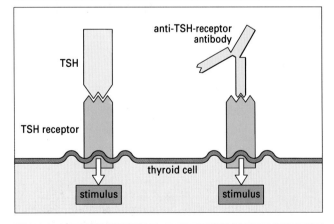

Autoimmunity to cell surface receptors

Fig. 24.13 The thyroid cell is stimulated when thyroid stimulating hormone (TSH) binds to its receptors (left). Antibody to the TSH receptor, present in the serum of a patient with thyrotoxicosis (Graves' or Basedow's disease), combines with the receptor in a similar fashion, thereby delivering a comparable stimulus to the thyroid cell (right).

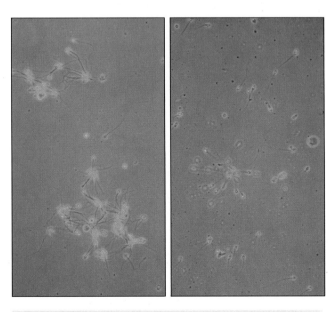

Fig. 24.14 Sperm agglutination. The presence of sperm autoantibodies produces either head-to-head (left) or tail-to-tail (right) agglutination.

that measures which suppress the immune response in these animals (for example the drug cyclophosphamide) also suppress the disease and prolong survival, adds to the evidence for autoimmune reactions causing such disease (Fig. 24.16).

AETIOLOGY

Despite the complex mechanisms operating during lymphocyte development to establish self-tolerance, the body contains large numbers of lymphocytes which are potentially self-reactive.

For example many autoantigens, when injected in adjuvants, make autoantibodies in normal animals and it is possible to identify a small number of autoreactive B cells (e.g. anti-thyroglobulin) in the normal population. Autoreactive T cells are also present in normal individuals since it is possible to produce autoimmune lines of T cells by stimulation of normal circulating T cells with the appropriate autoantigen (e.g. myelin basic protein) and IL-2.

Given that self-reactive B cells exist, the question remains whether they are stimulated to proliferate and produce autoantibodies by interaction with self antigens or by some other means, such as non-specific polyclonal activators or idiotypic interactions. Evidence that B cells are selected by antigen comes from the existence of somatic mutations and high affinity in the autoantibody response, a process which requires both

T cells and autoantigen. Additionally, autoantibodies occur to antigen clusters, consisting of several epitopes on the same autoantigenic molecule. It is really difficult to envisage a mechanism which could account for the co-existence of antibody responses to different epitopes on the same molecule, apart from the presence of autoantigen itself. Similarly, different molecular components of intracellular organelles (e.g. nucleosomes) or antigens linked within the same organ (e.g. thyroglobulin and thyroid peroxidase) can induce autoantibodies in one individual.

The most direct evidence for autoimmunity being antigen-driven comes from studies of the Obese strain chicken which, as described above, spontaneously develops thyroid autoimmunity. If the thyroid gland (the source of antigen) is removed at birth, the chickens grow up without developing thyroid autoantibodies (Fig. 24.17). Furthermore, once thyroid autoimmunity has developed, removal of the thyroid leads to a gross decline of thyroid autoantibodies, usually to undetectable levels.

Suppression of autoimmune disease in NZB/NZW hybrid mice

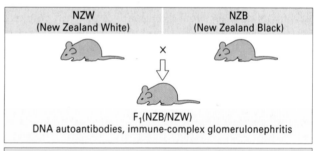

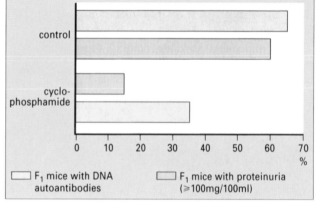

Fig. 24.16 The New Zealand Black mouse spontaneously develops autoimmune haemolytic anaemia. The hybrid between this and the New Zealand White strain develops DNA autoantibodies and immune-complex glomerulonephritis, like patients with SLE. Immunosuppression with cyclophosphamide (an anti-mitotic agent) considerably reduces the severity of the glomerulonephritis and the number of DNA autoantibodies, showing the relevance of the immune processes to the generation of the disease.

Failure of vitamin B_{12} absorption in pernicious anaemia

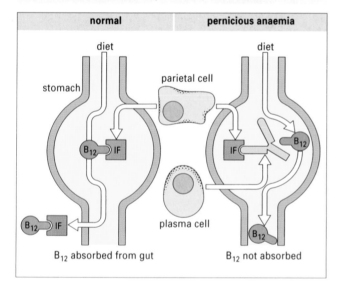

Fig. 24.15 Normally, dietary vitamin B_{12} is absorbed by the small intestine as a complex with intrinsic factor (IF), which is synthesized by parietal cells in gastric mucosa. In pernicious anaemia, locally synthesized autoantibodies, specific for intrinsic factor, combine with intrinsic factor to inhibit its role as a carrier for vitamin B_{12}.

T-cells are utterly pivotal for the development of autoimmune disease. The high affinity and somatic mutations which are characteristic of the IgG autoantibodies are dependent on the cooperative action of T-helper cells. Direct evidence for an involvement of T cells comes from animal models of autoimmune disease (as discussed above in relation to pathogenesis), but is more difficult to obtain in human disorders. However, thyroid-specific T-cell clones have been isolated from the glands of patients with thyrotoxicosis and anti-CD4 therapy is beneficial in rheumatoid arthritis (cf. autoimmune disease in animals). Furthermore, associations between autoimmune diseases and certain MHC types are probably related to the role of MHC molecules in presentation of antigen to T cells.

In organ-specific disorders, there is ample evidence for T cells responding to antigens present in the organs under attack. But in non-organ-specific autoimmunity, we have very little idea which antigens are recognized by the T cells. One possibility is that the T cells do not see conventional peptide antigen at all (clearly true of anti-DNA responses) but instead recognize idiotypes. In this view SLE, for example, would be an 'idiotype disease' (Fig. 24.18). In this scheme, autoantibodies are produced normally at low levels by B cells using germ-line genes. If these then form complexes with the autoantigen, the complexes can be taken up by APCs (including B cells) and components of the complex, including the antibody-idiotype presented to T cells. Idiotype-specific T cells would then help the autoantibody-producing B cells.

CONTROL MECHANISMS

The stimulation of self-reactive lymphocytes that occurs in autoimmune disease must be under control in the normal individual, either by lack of antigen presentation in adequate concentrations, or by some other regulatory mechanisms. Fig. 24.19 outlines possible ways in which such controls might be bypassed. In all these schemes the control on self reactivity is evaded due to stimulation of the autoreactive TH cell or by its being bypassed. A specific way in which autoreactive T cells are bypassed is where the autoantibody-producing B cells are helped by non-self-reactive T cells. This can occur when a self antigen and non-self antigen share an epitope (molecular mimicry – Fig. 24.20).

A disease in which molecular mimicry operates is rheumatic fever, in which autoantibodies to heart valve antigens can be detected. These develop in a small proportion of individuals several weeks after a streptococcal infection of the throat. Carbohydrate antigens on the streptococci cross-react with an antigen on heart valves, so the infection may bypass T cell self-tolerance to heart valve antigens. There may also be cross-reactivity between HLA-B27 and certain strains of *Klebsiella* in connection with ankylosing spondylitis, and cross-reactivity between *Proteus mirabilis* and DR4 in relationship to rheumatoid arthritis. Close similarities between the highly conserved heat-shock proteins of mycobacteria and those of humans might also be a contributory factor in rheumatoid arthritis.

Effect of neonatal thyroidectomy on Obese chickens

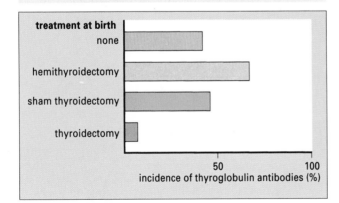

Fig. 24.17 Since removal of the thyroid at birth prevents the development of thyroid autoantibodies, it would appear that the autoimmune process is driven by the autoantigen in the thyroid gland. (Based on data from de Carvalho LCP *et al.* 1982 *J Exp Med*:**155**;1255.)

T-cell help for intermolecular complexes in the induction of autoimmunity

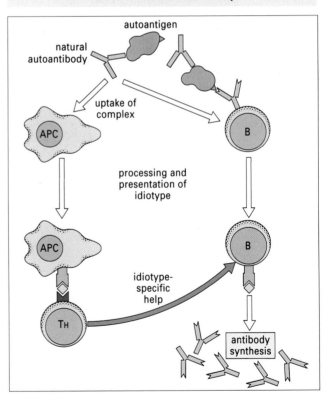

Fig. 24.18 An immune complex consisting of autoantigen and a naturally occurring (germ line) autoantibody is taken up by an APC, and idiotype parts of the antibody (Id) are presented to a TH cell. These T cells can subsequently help cells expressing an autoantibody which captures the complex, and presents processed idiotype to the TH cell.

Cross-reactive antigens may also induce autoimmunity by acting on T cells. For example an exogenous antigen may stimulate a naïve T cell, so that it can now recognize self-antigen, which was previously at too low a concentration, or inadequately presented (Fig. 24.21). Another mechanism to bypass the tolerant self-reactive TH cell is where antigen or another stimulator directly stimulates the autoreactive effector cells. For example, lipopolysaccharide or Epstein–Barr virus causes direct B-cell stimulation and some of the clones of activated cells will produce autoantibodies, although in the absence of T cell help these are normally of low titre and affinity.

Evasion of controls on self-reactivity

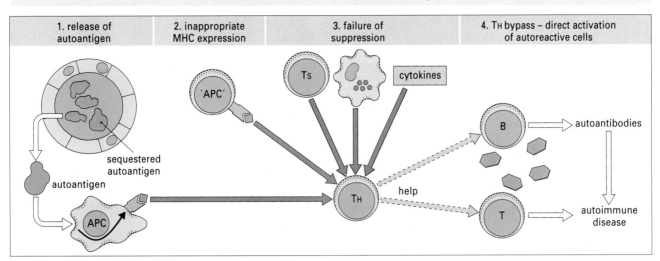

Fig 24.19 Self-reactive TH cells are normally functionally deleted and therefore cannot help self-reactive effector T cells and autoreactive B cells (broken green arrows). Release of a normally sequestered autoantigen (1) may lead to its uptake by APCs and hence stimulation of the TH cells.

Alternatively, a cell may come to express MHC class II inappropriately (2) and thus act as an APC for its own molecules. Failure of suppressive signals on the TH cell (3) may allow it to become active. Some antigens are polyclonal activators (4), so bypassing TH-cell control.

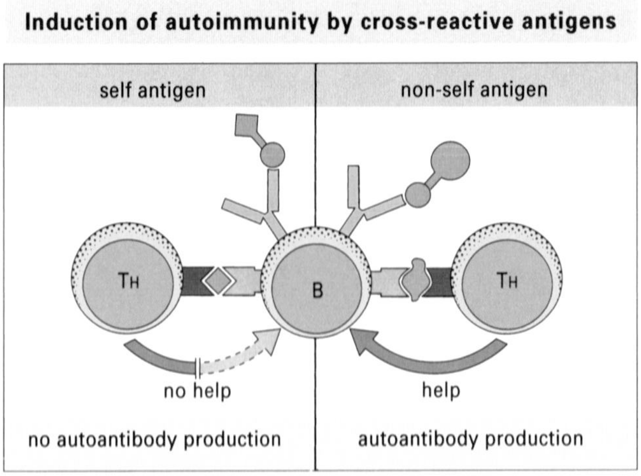

Induction of autoimmunity by cross-reactive antigens

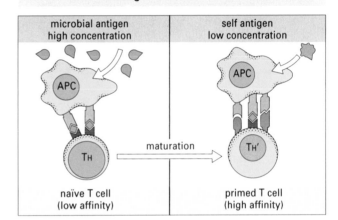

Fig. 24.20 The B cell recognizes an epitope present on self antigen, but coincidentally present also on a non-self antigen. Normally the B cell presents the self antigen but receives no help from self-reactive TH cells, which are functionally deleted. If the cross-reacting non-self antigen is encountered, the B cell can present peptides of this molecule to non-self reactive T cells and thus be driven to proliferate, differentiate and secrete autoantibodies.

Cross-reactive antigens induce autoimmune TH cells

Fig. 24.21 The inability of naïve TH cells to recognize auto-antigen, whether because of low concentration or low affinity, can be circumvented by a cross-reacting microbial antigen at higher concentration or with higher innate affinity, which primes the TH cells (left). Due to increased expression of accessory molecules (e.g. LFA-1 and CD2) the TH cells now have high affinity and can interact with autoantigen to produce autoimmune disease (right).

Controlling factors which restrain the development of autoimmune responses include Ts cells and the suppressive action of hormones (e.g. steroids), cytokines (e.g. TGF$_\beta$) and products of macrophages (Fig. 24.22). This subject is discussed more fully in Chapter 10. It is possible that more than one element of the suppressor network has to fail for an autoimmune response to develop. It is interesting to note that apparently healthy relatives of patients with SLE show a defect in the generation of non-specific Ts cells (as in the patients themselves) suggesting that this defect is just one factor contributing towards SLE. In SLE patients, there may be further abnormalities in either antigen- or idiotype-specific regulatory T cells. Imbalanced cytokine production may also contribute to dysregulation and it is intriguing that TNF (by introduction of a TNF transgene) ameliorates autoimmune disease in NZB × NZW hybrids.

Another important factor in the maintenance of self-tolerance must be the inability of autoreactive T$_H$ cells to recognize potentially autoantigenic molecules on cells which do not normally express MHC class II genes. In these circumstances 'immunological silence' prevails because these T cells can only recognize antigen when it is presented in association with class II molecules. This immunological silence could be broken by inappropriate expression of class II. It was therefore most exciting when cells in thyrotoxic thyroiditis were

found to be actively synthesizing class II MHC molecules (Fig. 24.23) and were thus able to be recognized by CD4$^+$ T cells.

Subsequently it has been shown that many human cell types can be induced to express class II molecules following treatment with IFN$_\gamma$. We are thus presented with an unresolved conundrum – is autoimmunity initiated by some factor causing inappropriate class II expression, or is the class II expression induced by a pre-existing autoimmunity? Even in the latter case, class II expression could contribute to the continuation of the pathogenetic process. It is notable that several strains which are susceptible to autoimmunity are also more readily induced to express MHC class II, on cell types which would not normally do so. These include the Lewis rat (experimental autoimmune encephalomyelitis), the Obese strain chicken (thyroiditis) and the

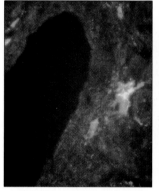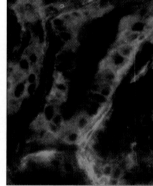

Fig. 24.23 Human thyroid sections stained for MHC class II. Left: Normal thyroid with unstained follicular cells, and an isolated dendritic cell that is strongly positive for MHC class II. Right: Thyrotoxic (Graves' disease) thyroid with abundant MHC class II molecules in the cytoplasm, indicating that rapid synthesis of MHC class II is occurring. (Courtesy of Dr R. Pujol-Borrel and Blackwell Scientific Publications.)

Bypass of regulatory mechanisms

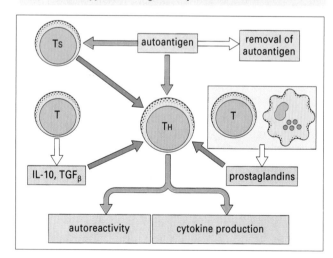

Fig. 24.22 Autoreactive T$_H$ cells are normally held in check by a network of suppressive signals including antigen-specific suppression by T cells, which may be mediated directly or via suppressive cytokines such as IL-10 and TGF$_\beta$. Removal of the autoantigen and non-specific suppression (e.g. mediated by prostaglandins) also limit the capacity of the T$_H$ cell to respond. Should the T$_H$ cell show an enhanced capacity to respond, e.g. increased levels of IL-2 receptor, or the suppressive influences fail, the balance is shifted towards autoimmune disease.

MHC class II expression and diabetes

islet cells	stimulant	expression of class II on:		
		insulin cells	somatostatin cells	glucagon cells
diabetic human (*in vivo*)	none	+ +	–	–
normal human	IFN$_\gamma$	–	–	–
normal human	IFN$_\gamma$ + TNF	+ +	+ +	+ +
BB rat (prone to diabetes)	IFN$_\gamma$	+ +	–	–
rat resistant to diabetes	IFN$_\gamma$	–	–	–

Fig. 24.24 MHC class II expression and diabetes.

BB rat (susceptible to autoimmune diabetes). What is striking about the BB rats is that the results parallel the events occurring in the human disease. It is the insulin-

Thyroid ^{131}I uptake in TSH-suppressed chickens

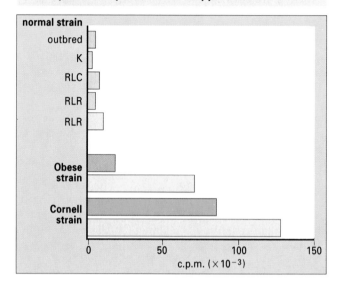

Fig. 24.25 Abnormal thyroid ^{131}I uptake in Obese strain chickens, and the related Cornell strain, compared with normal strains. Endogenous TSH production was suppressed by administration of thyroxine, so that the experiment measured TSH-independent ^{131}I uptake. Values were far higher than normal in Obese strain chickens which spontaneously develop thyroid autoimmunity and even higher in the non-autoimmune Cornell strain from which the Obese strain was bred. This abnormality was not due to immune mechanisms since immunosuppression (blue bars) increased ^{131}I uptake.

Diagnostic value of anti-mitochondrial antibodies

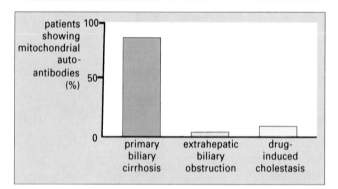

Fig. 24.26 Mitochondrial antibody tests using indirect immunofluorescence, together with percutaneous liver biopsy, can be used to assist in the differential diagnosis of these three diseases. A large proportion of patients with primary biliary cirrhosis have anti-mitochondrial antibodies but this is rare in the other diseases.

producing cells, not the glucagon- and somatostatin-producing cells, which express class II in the diabetic pancreas. Although normal human islets do not express class II when stimulated by IFN_γ, a combination of IFN_γ and TNF does upregulate the class II genes, but here the effect is seen on all cell types in the islets of Langerhans (Fig. 24.24).

Other evidence also suggests that there may be a pre-existing defect in the organ which becomes the target of autoimmune disease. Sundick and colleagues, studying the Obese strain chicken model of spontaneous thyroid autoimmunity (see p. 24.5), showed that the uptake of iodine into the thyroid glands of these animals in which endogenous TSH had been suppressed by thyroxine treatment, was far higher than that seen in a variety of normal strains. Furthermore, this was not due to any stimulating effect of the autoimmunity, since immunosuppressed animals showed even higher uptakes of radio-iodine (^{131}I) (Fig 23.25). Interestingly, the Cornell strain, from which the Obese strain was derived by breeding, showed even higher uptakes of ^{131}I, yet these animals do not develop spontaneous thyroiditis. This could be indicative of abnormal thyroid behaviour which in itself is insufficient to induce autoimmune disease, but contributes to susceptibility in the Obese strain. Confirmation of this idea comes from experiments in which lymphoid cells from older Obese strain chickens with thyroid disease were transferred to other chickens. These cells induced thyroiditis in young Obese strain chickens and the Cornell strain, but not in other histocompatible strains. This re-emphasizes the considerable importance of multiple factors in the establishment of prolonged autoimmunity.

DIAGNOSTIC AND PROGNOSTIC ASPECTS

Whatever the relationship of autoantibodies to the disease process, they frequently provide valuable markers for diagnostic purposes. A particularly good example is the test for mitochondrial antibodies, used in diagnosing primary biliary cirrhosis (Fig. 24.26). Exploratory laparotomy was previously needed to obtain this diagnosis, and was often hazardous because of the age and condition of the patients concerned.

Autoantibodies may also have a predictive value, as shown in Fig. 24.27.

TREATMENT

Often, in organ-specific autoimmune disorders, the symptoms can be corrected by metabolic control. For example, hypothyroidism can be controlled by administration of thyroxine, and thyrotoxicosis by antithyroid drugs. In pernicious anaemia, metabolic correction is achieved by injection of Vitamin $B_{12,}$ and in myasthenia gravis by administration of cholinesterase inhibitors. Where function is lost and cannot be substituted by hormones, as may occur in lupus nephritis or chronic rheumatoid arthritis, mechanical substitutes or tissue grafts may be appropriate. In the case of tissue grafts, protection from the immunological processes which necessitated the transplant may be required.

Conventional immunosuppressive therapy with anti-mitotic drugs can be used to damp down the immune response but, because of the dangers involved, tends to be used only in life-threatening disorders such as SLE and dermatomyositis. The potential of cyclosporin and possible derivatives has yet to be fully realized but quite dramatic results have been reported in the treatment of type I diabetes mellitus. Anti-inflammatory drugs are, of course, prescribed for rheumatoid diseases.

As we understand more about the precise defects in autoimmune diseases, and learn how to manipulate the immunological status of the patient, a number of less well-established approaches may become practical (Fig. 24.28). In particular, some experimental autoimmune diseases have been treated successfully by 'vaccination' with autoantigen-specific T-cell clones. This suggests that stimulating normally suppressive functions, including the idiotype network, could be promising.

The predictive value of autoantibodies

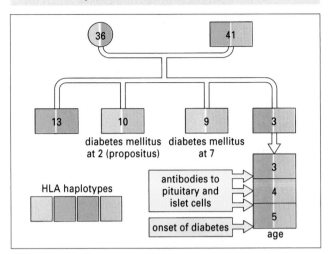

Fig. 24.27 Prospective study of a family with insulin-dependent diabetes mellitus. The sibling sharing a haplotype with the propositus, and having complement-fixing islet-cell antibodies, became diabetic over two years later.

The treatment of autoimmune disease

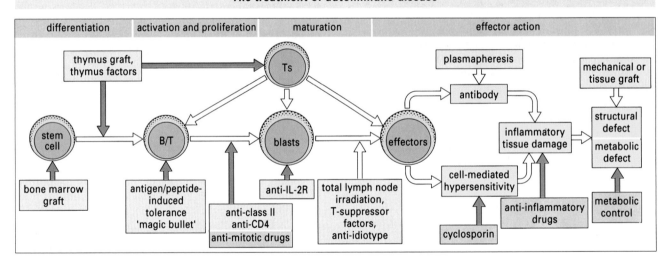

Fig. 24.28 Current treatments (blue boxes) for arresting the pathological developments in autoimmune disease, and those that may become feasible (green boxes). Anti-mitotic drugs are given in severe cases of SLE or chronic active hepatitis, and anti-inflammatory drugs are widely prescribed in rheumatoid arthritis. Organ-specific disorders (e.g. primary myxoedema), can be treated by supplying the defective component (e.g. thyroid hormone). When a live graft is necessary, immunosuppressive therapy can protect the tissue from damage.

FURTHER READING

Chapel HM, Haeney M. *Essentials of Clinical Immunology*. 3rd ed. Oxford: Blackwell Scientific Publications, 1992.

Lachmann PJ, Peters DK, Rosen FS, Walport MJ, eds. *Clinical Aspects of Immunology*. 5th ed. Oxford: Blackwell Scientific Publications, 1992.

McGregor AM, ed. *Immunology of Endocrine Diseases*. Lancaster: MTP Press, 1986.

Morrow J, Isenberg DA, eds. *Autoimmune Rheumatic Disease*. Oxford: Blackwell Scientific Publications, 1987.

Roitt IM, Hutchings PR, Dawe KI, Sumar N, Bodman KB, Cooke AJ. The forces driving autoimmune disease.
J Autoimmun 1992;**5(Suppl A)**:11–26

Schoenfeld Y, Isenberg D. *The Mosaic of Autoimmunity (Factors Associated with Autoimmune Disease)*. Amsterdam: Elsevier, 1989.

Sites DP, Terr AI. *Basic and Clinical Immunology*. 7th ed. California: Lange Medical Publications, 1991

chapter 25

Immunological Techniques

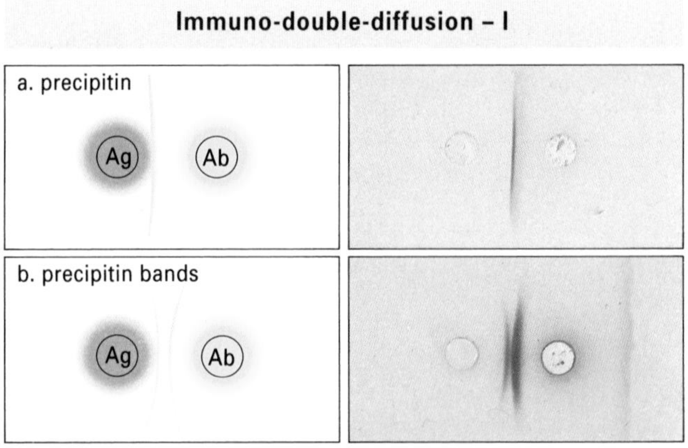

Immuno-double-diffusion – I

a. precipitin

Ag   Ab

b. precipitin bands

Ag   Ab

Fig. 25.1 Agar gels are poured onto slides and allowed to set (1–2% agar in buffer at pH 7–8.5). Wells are then punched in the gel and the test solutions of antigen (Ag) and antibody (Ab) are added. The solutions diffuse out and where Ag and Ab meet they bind to each other, cross-link and precipitate leaving a line of precipitation (a). If two antigens are present in the solution and both can be recognized by the antibody two lines of precipitation form independently (b). The precipitin bands can be better visualized by washing the gel to remove soluble proteins and then staining the precipitin arcs with a protein stain such as Coomassie Blue (right).

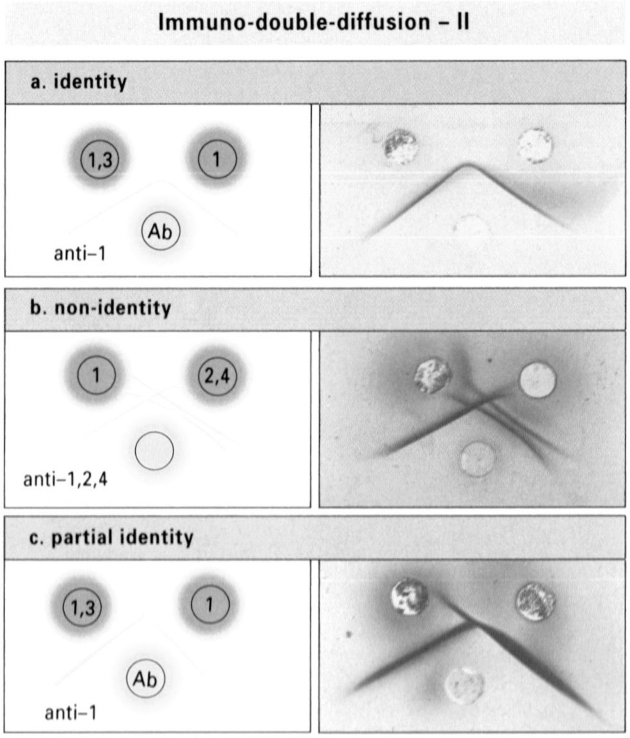

Immuno-double-diffusion – II

a. identity

1,3   1
anti-1   Ab

b. non-identity

1   2,4
anti-1,2,4

c. partial identity

1,3   1
anti-1   Ab

Immunologists employ a number of techniques which are common to other biological sciences. For example, the methods used to isolate antigens and antibodies are those of biochemistry and protein fractionation, while the gene sequences of immunologically important molecules have been elucidated by the standard techniques of molecular genetics. Immunology has, however, developed a number of its own techniques, particularly those based on the specificity of the antigen–antibody interaction. These are finding increasing use in many of the biological sciences. For example, any molecule that acts as antigen can be identified in tissues by immunocytochemical methods. Very low concentrations of such molecules can be quantified by radioimmunoassay (RIA) and enzyme-linked immunosorbent assay (ELISA). There are hundreds of different immunological methods now in use and some of the most common are outlined in this chapter.

ANTIGEN—ANTIBODY INTERACTIONS

PRECIPITATION REACTION IN GELS

One of the first observations of antigen–antibody reactions was their ability to precipitate when combined in proportions at or near equivalence. By performing these reactions in agar gels it is possible to distinguish separate antigen–antibody reactions produced by different populations of antibody present in a serum – the immuno-double-diffusion technique. This technique has been extended to the examination of the relationship between different antigens (Figs 25.1 and 25.2).

Fig. 25.2 The immuno-double-diffusion technique may be used to determine the relationship between antigens (blue) and a particular test antibody (yellow). Three basic patterns appear. The numbers in the blue wells refer to the epitopes present on the test antigen. In reaction (a) the precipitin arcs formed between the antibody and the two test antigens fuse indicating that the antibody is precipitating identical epitopes in each preparation (epitope 1). This does not mean that the antigens are necessarily identical; they are only identical as far as the antibody can distinguish the difference. In reaction (b) the antibody preparation distinguishes the three different antigens which form independent precipitin arcs. In reaction (c) the antigens share epitope 1 but one antigen also has epitope 2. This is the same situation as in (a), but in this case the antibody can distinguish them, by virtue of being able to react against both epitopes. A line of identify forms with anti-epitope 1, with the addition of a 'spur' where the anti-epitope 2 has reacted with the second epitope, thus indicating partial identity between the antigen preparations.

Some antigen mixtures however, are too complex to be resolved by simple diffusion and precipitation and so the technique of immunoelectrophoresis was developed – antigens are separated on the basis of their charge before being visualized by precipitation (Fig. 25.3).

These gel techniques only identify antigens and antibodies qualitatively, but by further modification, using the technique of single radial immunodiffusion, they can be made quantitative (Fig. 25.4).

By applying a voltage across the gels to move the antigens and antibodies together, immuno-double-diffusion becomes countercurrent electrophoresis, and

single radial immunodiffusion becomes rocket electrophoresis (Fig. 25.5). These techniques operate in the range of 20 μg/ml to 2 mg/ml of antigen or antibody.

HAEMAGGLUTINATION AND COMPLEMENT FIXATION

Antibody may be detected and measured by haemagglutination at lower concentrations than those detectable by countercurrent electrophoresis and rocket electrophoresis. This relies on the ability of antibody to cross-link red blood cells by interacting with the antigens on their surface (Fig. 25.6).

Immunoelectrophoresis

1. separation of antigens

2. antiserum in trough

trough

3. diffusion and precipitation

Fig. 25.3 Immunoelectrophoresis. 1. Antigens are separated in an agar gel by placing an electric charge across it. The pH is chosen so that positively charged proteins move to the negative electrode and negatively charged proteins to the positive. 2. A trough is then cut between the wells and filled with the antibody, which is left to diffuse. 3. The antigens and antibody form precipitin arcs. This method allows the comparison of complicated mixtures of antigen such as found in serum.

Single radial immunodiffusion

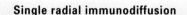
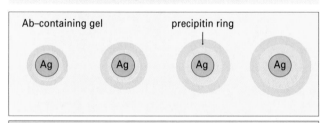

Ab–containing gel   precipitin ring

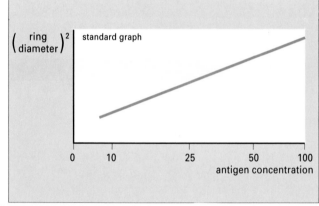

$\left(\dfrac{\text{ring}}{\text{diameter}}\right)^2$ standard graph

antigen concentration

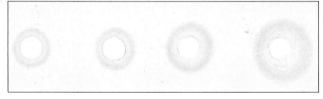

Fig. 25.4 Single radial immunodiffusion. Antibody is added to the agar gel which is then poured onto slides and allowed to set. Wells are punched in the agar and standard volumes of test antigen of different concentration are put in the wells. The plates are left for at least 24 hours, during which time the antigen diffuses out of the wells to form soluble complexes (in antigen excess) with the antibody. These continue to diffuse outwards, binding more antibody until an equivalence point is reached and the complexes precipitate in a ring. The area within the precipitin ring, measured as ring diameter squared, is proportional to the antigen concentration. Unknowns are derived by interpolation from the standard curve (graph). The whole process may be reversed using an antigen-containing gel to determine unknown concentrations of antibody.

Countercurrent electrophoresis and rocket electrophoresis

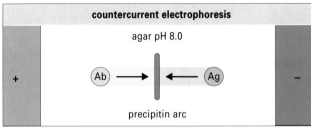

countercurrent electrophoresis

agar pH 8.0

+ (Ab) → | ← (Ag) −

precipitin arc

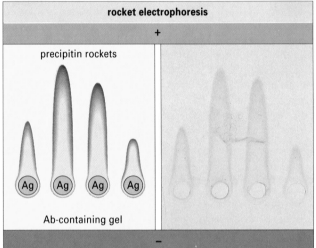

rocket electrophoresis

+

precipitin rockets

(Ag) (Ag) (Ag) (Ag)

Ab-containing gel

−

Fig. 25.5 Countercurrent electrophoresis is performed in agar gels where the pH is chosen so that the antibody is positively charged and the antigen is negatively charged. By applying a voltage across the gel the antigen and antibody move towards each other and precipitate. The principle is the same as immuno-double-diffusion but the sensitivity is increased 10–20-fold. Antigens may be quantitated by electrophoresing them into an antibody-containing gel in the technique termed rocket electrophoresis. The pH of the gel is chosen so that the antibodies are immobile and the antigen is negatively charged. Precipitin rockets form; the height of the rocket is proportional to antigen concentration, and unknowns are determined by interpolation from standards. The appearance of stained rockets is shown on the right. Both techniques rely on the antigen and antibody having different charges at the selected pH; this is true for most antigens since antibodies have a relatively high isoelectric point (i.e. they are neutrally charged at a more alkaline pH than most antigens). If the charges on the antigen and antibody do not differ sufficiently, the antibody or antigen can be chemically modified to alter its isoelectric point. Rocket electrophoresis can be reversed to estimate antibody concentration if a suitable pH gel to immobilize the antigen, without damaging it or preventing the antigen–antibody reaction, can be found.

Haemagglutination

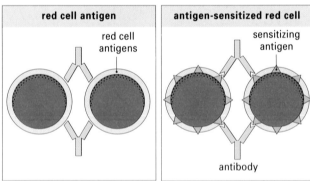

red cell antigen

red cell antigens

antigen-sensitized red cell

sensitizing antigen

antibody

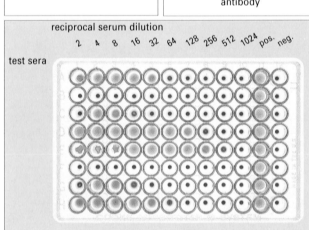

reciprocal serum dilution

2 4 8 16 32 64 128 256 512 1024 pos. neg.

test sera

Fig. 25.6 The active haemagglutination test (upper left panel) detects antibodies to red blood cell antigens. The antibody is serially diluted (usually in doubling dilutions) in physiological saline and placed in the wells (rows 1–10) of the haemagglutination plate. Positive controls (row 11) and negative controls (row 12) are included. A suspension of red cells (containing a protein to prevent the red cells agglutinating non-specifically) is added to each well to given a final concentration of about 1% cells. If sufficient antibody is present to agglutinate (cross-link) the cells they sink as a mat to the bottom of the well (direct Coombs' test). If insufficient antibody is present, the cells roll down the sloping sides of the plate to form a red pellet at the bottom. Some antibodies do not agglutinate red cells very effectively and may be detected in the indirect agglutination test (indirect Coombs' test) by the addition of a second antibody which binds to the antibody on the red cell. By binding different antigens onto the red cell surface, covalently or non-covalently, the test an be extended to detect antibodies to antigens other than those on red cells (upper right panel). Chromic chloride, tannic acid, glutaraldehyde and a number of other chemicals are used to cross-link the antigen to the cells.

Antigen–antibody reactions lead to immune complex formation which produces complement fixation via the classical pathway, and this may be exploited to determine the amount of antigen or antibody present (Fig. 25.7). Haemagglutination and complement fixation can detect antibody at levels of less than 1 μg/ml.

DIRECT AND INDIRECT IMMUNOFLUORESCENCE

Immunofluorescence is used extensively to detect autoantibodies and antibodies to tissue and cellular antigens (Fig. 25.8). Although techniques are more cumbersome than those described above if a quantitative measure of antibody concentration is required, they do have advantages. By using tissue sections (which contain a large number of antigens), antibodies to several different antigens can be identified on a single slide according to their distribution between cells or in different subcellular compartments.

Furthermore, the immunofluorescence tests can be used to identify particular cells in suspension, that is, to identify antigens on live cells. When a live stained cell suspension is put through a fluorescence-activated cell sorter (FACS), the machine measures the fluorescence intensity of each cell and then the cells are separated according to their particular fluorescent brightness. This technique permits the isolation of different cell populations with different surface antigens (stained with antibodies of different specificity carrying different fluorescent dye (Fig. 25.9).

Complement fixation

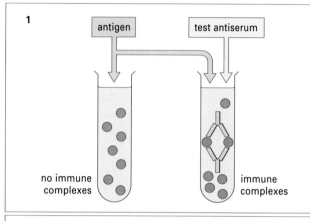

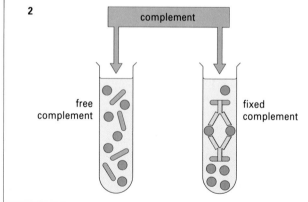

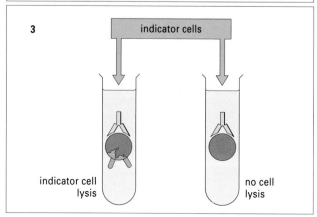

Fig. 25.7 The complement fixation test detects antibody. 1. A test antiserum is titred in doubling dilutions and a fixed amount of antigen is added to each well or tube. If antibody is present in the test serum, immune complexes will form. 2. Complement is then added to the mixture. If complexes are present, they will fix complement and consume it. 3. In the final step, indicator cells (red cells) together with subagglutinating amount of antibody (erythrocyte antibody) are added to the mixture. If there is any complement remaining these cells will be lysed; if it was consumed by immune complexes there will be insufficient to lyse the red cells. A quantity of complement is used which is just enough to lyse the indicator cells if none is consumed by the complexes. The assay is often performed on plastic plates. By using constant amounts of antibody and titrations of antigen, the assay can be applied to testing for antigens. Appropriate controls are most important in this assay because some antibody preparations consume complement without the addition of antigen, for example, if the antibody preparation is serum already containing immune complexes. Some antigens can also have anti-complement activity. The controls should therefore include antibody alone and antigen alone to check that neither fix complement by themselves.

Direct and indirect immunofluorescence

direct	indirect	indirect complement amplified
fluoresceinated antibody	antibody	antibody
tissue section		
wash	wash	wash
	add fluoresceinated anti-Ig	add complement
	wash	wash
		add fluoresceinated anti-C3 antibody
		wash

Fig. 25.8 A section is cut on a cryostat from a deep frozen tissue block. This ensures that labile antigens are not damaged by fixatives.
Direct. The test solution of fluoresceinated antibody is applied to the section in a drop, incubated and washed off. Any bound antibody is then revealed under the microscope; UV light is directed onto the section through the objective, thus the field is dark and areas with bound fluorescent antibody fluoresce green. The pattern of fluorescence is characteristic for each tissue antigen.
Indirect. Antibody applied to the section as a solution is visualized using fluoresceinated anti-immunoglobulin.
Indirect complement amplified. This is an elaboration of the indirect method for the detection of complement fixing antibody. In the second step fresh complement is added which becomes fixed around the site of antibody binding. Due to the amplification steps in the classical complement pathway one antibody molecule can cause many C3b molecules to bind to the section; these are then visualized with fluoresceinated anti-C3.

Fluorescence Activated Cell Sorter (FACS)

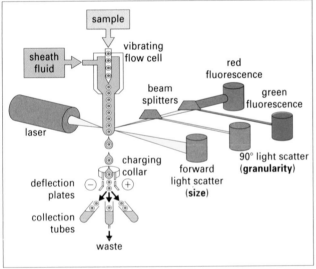

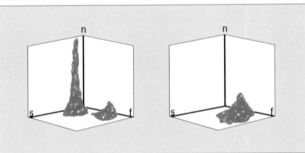

Fig. 25.9 Cells in the sample are stained with specific fluorescent reagents to detect surface molecules and are then introduced into a vibrating flow chamber. The cell stream passing out of the chamber is encased in a sheath of buffer fluid. The stream is illuminated by laser and each cell is measured for size (forward light scatter) and granularity (90° light scatter), as well as for red and green fluorescence, to detect two different surface markers. The vibration in the cell stream causes it to break into droplets which are charged and may then be steered by deflection plates under computer control to collect different cell populations according to the parameters measured. The 3-dimensional graphs plot size (s), number (n) and fluorescence (f) for a whole lymphocyte population (left) and a CD8+ population obtained by cell sorting (right), stained with anti-CD8.

Radioimmunoassay (RIA)

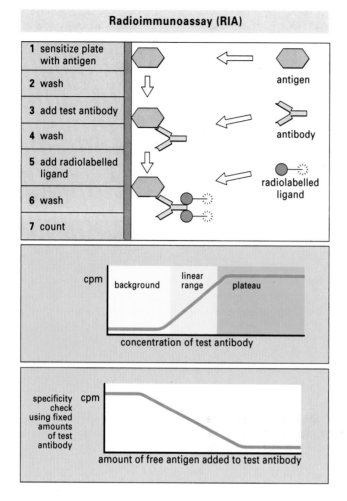

Fig. 25.10 Radioimmunoassay. 1. Antigen in saline is incubated on a plastic plate or tube, and small quantities become absorbed onto the plastic surface. 2. Free antigen is washed away. (The plate may then be blocked with excess of an irrelevant protein to prevent any subsequent non-specific binding of proteins.) 3. Test antibody is added, which binds to the antigen. 4. Unbound proteins are washed away. 5. The antibody is detected by a radiolabelled ligand. The ligand may be a molecule such as staphylococcal protein A which binds to the Fc region of IgG – more often it is another antibody specific for the test antibody. By using a ligand which binds to particular classes or subclasses of test antibody it is possible to distinguish isotypes. 6. Unbound ligand is washed away. 7. The radioactivity of the plate is counted on a gamma counter. A typical titration curve is shown in the upper graph. With increasing amounts of test antibody the counts per minute (cpm) rise from a background level through a linear range to a plateau. Antibody titres can only be detected correctly within the linear range. Typically the plateau binding is 20–100 times the background. The sensitivity of the technique is usually about 1–50 ng/ml of specific antibody. Specificity of the assay may be checked by adding increasing concentrations of free test antigen to the test antibody at step 3; this binds to the antibody and blocks it from binding to the antigen on the plate. Addition of increasing amounts of free antigen reduces the cpm (lower graph).

Enzyme linked immunosorbent assay (ELISA)

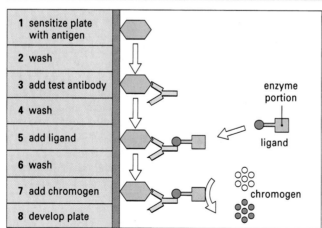

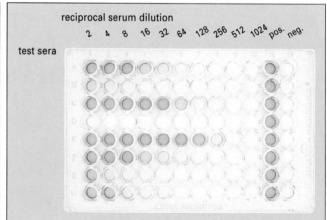

Fig. 25.11 The ELISA plate is prepared in the same way as an RIA plate up to step 4. At this point a different kind of ligand is used. The ligand is a molecule which can detect the antibody and is covalently coupled to an enzyme such as peroxidase. This binds the test antibody and after free ligand is washed away (6) the bound ligand is visualized by the addition of chromogen (7) – a colourless substrate which is acted on by the enzyme portion of the ligand to produce a coloured end product. A developed plate is shown on the right. The amount of test antibody is measured by assessing the amount of coloured end-product by optical density scanning of the plate.

RADIOIMMUNOASSAY AND ENZYME-LINKED IMMUNOSORBENT ASSAY

The techniques of radioimmunosassay (RIA) and enzyme-linked immunosorbent assay (ELISA) are exquisitely sensitive for detecting antigens and antibodies, and are extremely economical in the use of reagents (Figs 25.10 and 25.11).

RIA and ELISA are probably the most widely used of all immunological assays for antibodies since large numbers of tests can be performed in a relatively short time. Modification of the basic system in the radio-allergosorbent test (RAST) allows identification of IgE antibodies which occur at very low levels in serum (Fig. 25.12).

RIA can also be turned into a competition type of assay as illustrated by the radioimmunosorbent test (RIST) which may be used as a very sensitive assay for IgE and for a number of drugs and hormones (Fig. 25.13). (Note that in the RIST, the IgE being measured is acting as an antigen during the test.)

IMMUNOBLOTTING AND IMMUNOPRECIPITATION

The methods described above are particularly useful for measuring levels of certain known antigens or antibodies, but in many case it is necessary to identify and characterize previously unknown antigens from a complex mixture, in which case immunoblotting is very useful.

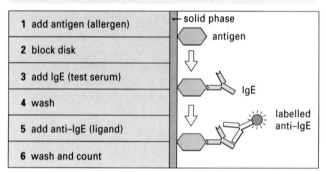

The radioallergosorbent test (RAST)

1 add antigen (allergen)	
2 block disk	
3 add IgE (test serum)	
4 wash	
5 add anti–IgE (ligand)	
6 wash and count	

solid phase
antigen
IgE
labelled anti–IgE

Fig. 25.12 This test measures antigen-specific IgE in a radioimmunoassay where the ligand is a labelled anti-IgE antibody. The steps are identical to the standard radio-immunoassay except that the antigen (allergen) is covalently bound to a cellulose disc rather than non-covalently to a radiolabelled plate. The availability of much more antigen on the disc permits the high sensitivity necessary to bind the small quantities of IgE present in the test serum.

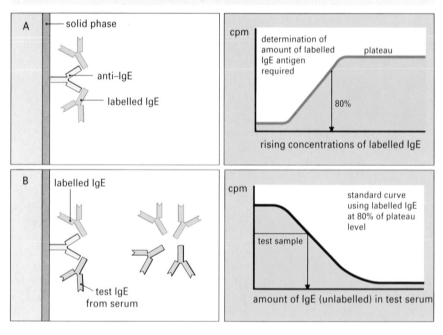

The radioimmunosorbent test (RIST)

A — solid phase
anti–IgE
labelled IgE

cpm
determination of amount of labelled IgE antigen required
plateau
80%
rising concentrations of labelled IgE

B labelled IgE
test IgE from serum

cpm
standard curve using labelled IgE at 80% of plateau level
test sample
amount of IgE (unlabelled) in test serum

Fig. 25.13 This is a competition radioimmunosassay for total serum IgE. The plate is sensitized with anti-IgE and increasing amounts of labelled IgE are added to the plate to determine the maximum amount of IgE that the plate can bind (A). A quantity of labelled IgE equivalent to approximately 80% of the plateau binding is chosen. In the test experiments (B) this amount of labelled IgE is mixed with the serum containing the IgE to be tested. The test IgE competes with the labelled IgE. Thus the more IgE present in the test serum the less the amount of labelled IgE that binds. This produces a standard curve of the type shown where dilutions of a serum containing known IgE concentrations are used. This type of test is widely used to measure hormone concentrations in serum.

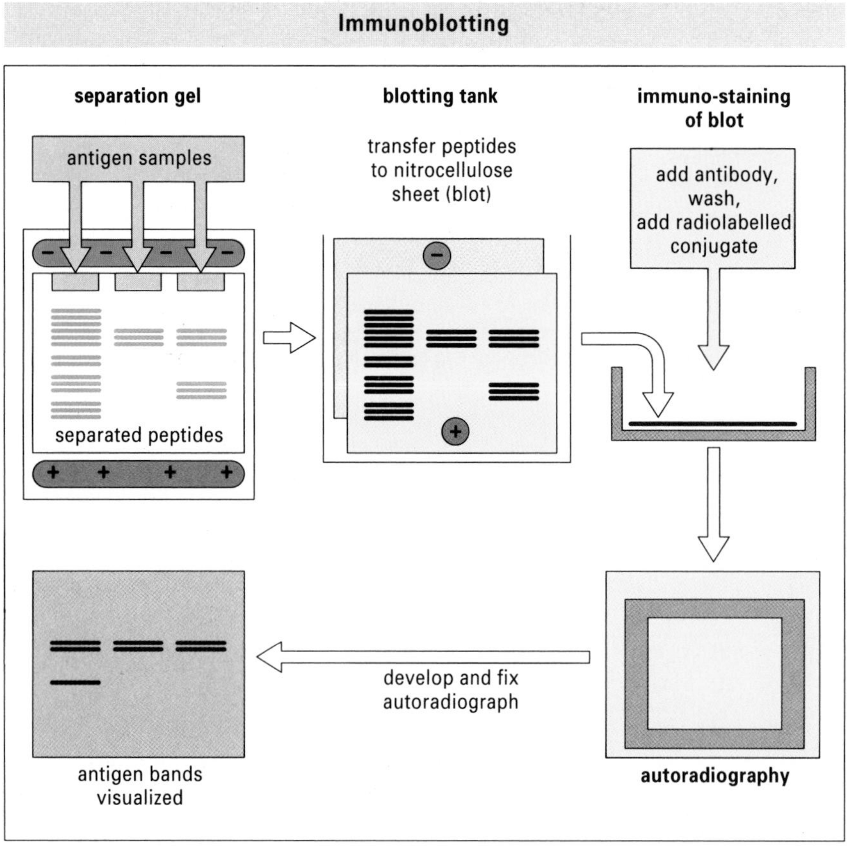

Immunoblotting

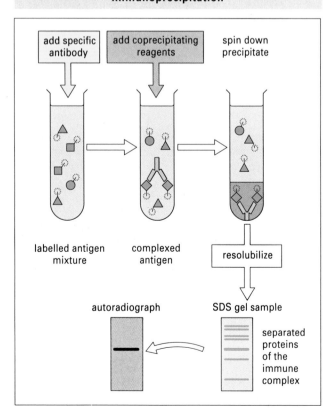

separation gel

antigen samples

separated peptides

antigen bands
visualized

blotting tank

transfer peptides
to nitrocellulose
sheet (blot)

develop and fix
autoradiograph

**immuno-staining
of blot**

add antibody,
wash,
add radiolabelled
conjugate

autoradiography

Fig. 25.14 Antigen samples are separated in an analytical gel, for example an SDS polyacrylamide gel or an isoelectric focusing gel. The resolved molecules are transferred electrophoretically to a nitrocelluose membrane in a blotting tank. The blot is then treated sequentially with antibody to the specific antigen, and washed, and then a radiolabelled conjugate to detect antibodies is bound to the blot. The principle is similar to that of a radioimmunoassay or ELISA. After washing again, the blot is placed in contact with X-ray film in a cassette; the autoradiograph is developed and the antigen bands which have bound the antibody are visible. The technique can be modified for use with an enzyme coupled conjugate, and the bound material can be detected by treatment with a chromogen which deposits an insoluble reagent directly onto the blot.

Immunoprecipitation

add specific
antibody

add coprecipitating
reagents

spin down
precipitate

labelled antigen
mixture

complexed
antigen

resolubilize

autoradiograph

SDS gel sample

separated
proteins
of the
immune
complex

Fig. 25.15 Antigens are labelled with ^{125}I, and antibody is added, which binds just to its specific antigen. The complexes are precipitated by the addition of coprecipitating agents, such as anti-immunoglobulin antibodies or staphylococcal protein A. The insoluble complexes are spun down and washed to remove any unbound, labelled antigens. Then the precipitate is resolubilized, for example in SDS, and the components separated on analytical gels. After running, the fixed gels are autoradiographed, to show the position of the specific labelled antigen. Frequently the antigens are derived from the surface of radiolabelled cells, which are solubilized with detergents before the immunoprecipitation. It is also possible to label the antigens with biotin, and detect them at the end chromatographically using streptavidin (binds biotin) coupled to an enzyme such as peroxidase (cf. ELISA technique).

In immunoblotting, complex mixtures are resolved in analytical separation gels and then the molecules are transferred to membranes (blots) for the identification of individual antigens by specific antisera. By using SDS gels, isoelectric focusing gels or peptide mapping gels in the initial separation, it is possible to obtain data on the size, isoelectric point and molecular relationships of the antigens under investigation (Fig 25.14).

In some cases an antigen becomes so denatured by the gel separations and blotting procedures that some of its epitopes are destroyed and it can no longer bind to particular antibodies. In this case it is necessary to use immunoprecipitation instead to identify which antigen an antibody binds to. The technique can be used either with soluble antigens or with cell surface antigens (Fig. 25.15).

ISOLATION OF PURE ANTIBODIES

Immunologists often need to isolate pure antibodies, which may be either antigen-specific or non-specific immunoglobulin. Isolation of non-specific immunoglobulin from serum is usually carried out by sequential protein fractionation steps which may include:

1. precipitation of the gammaglobulins in 30–50% ammonium sulphate
2. gel filtration to obtain molecules of the correct size
3. ion exchange chromatography to isolate molecules which are positively charged at neutral pH
4. affinity chromatography on natural ligands for immunoglobulin, such as protein A (protein A is a component of staphylococcal cell walls which binds to a region in Cγ2 and Cγ3 of most IgG subclasses i.e. IgG$_1$, IgG$_2$ and IgG$_4$).

Isolation of antigen-specific immunoglobulin is carried out by affinity chromotography using antigen coupled to Sepharose; pure antibody is eluted from the immunoabsorbant with chaotropic agents such as sodium thiocyanate, or glycine–HCl buffer, or diethylamine buffer. Affinity chromatography is the technique used where the isolation of pure antibody or pure antigen is the objective (Fig. 25.16).

Another way of obtaining pure antibody of a defined specificity is to produce monoclonal antibodies from cells in culture. By creating an immortal clone of cells which manufacture a single antibody of defined specificity, production can be maintained indefinitely, obviating the vagaries of antiserum production (Fig. 25.17). Monoclonal antibodies have found widespread use in many biological sciences, where the antibody is used as a highly specific probe.

Affinity chromatography

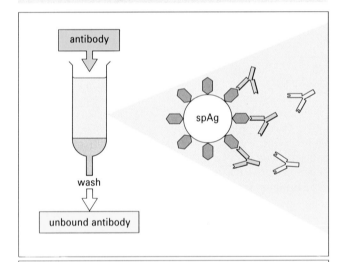

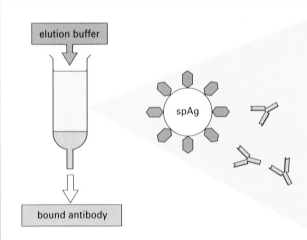

Fig. 25.16 By using affinity chromatography a pure population of antibodies may be isolated. A solid phase immunoabsorbent is prepared (spAg); this is an antigen covalently coupled to an inert support (e.g. cross-linked dextran beads). The immunoabsorbent is placed in a column and the antibody mixture is run in under physiological conditions. Antibody to the antigen is bound to the column while unbound antibody washes through (1). In the second step the column is eluted to obtain the bound antibody using elution buffer (e.g. acetate pH 3.0, diethylamine pH 11.5, 3M guanidine, HCl), which dissociates the antigen–antibody bond (2). By placing antibody on the column the process can be reversed to obtain pure antigen. The technique can also be used to obtain other types of molecule. For example, a lectin column will absorb all molecules with particular sugar residues and these can be eluted in buffer containing the free sugar, which competes with the bound protein for the attachment site on the lectin.

Since any particular B cell is effectively producing a monoclonal antibody, the requirement is to immortalize and propagate individual B cells. Most monoclonal antibodies are generated by the fusion of mouse splenocytes with a B cell myeloma from the same strain which does not secrete its own antibody. It is also possible to produce interstrain or even interspecies hybrids, but these are often unstable. An alternative method is to transform B cells; for example human B cells may be immortalized for monoclonal antibody production by infecting them with Epstein–Barr virus.

Although a monoclonal antibody is a well-defined reagent it does not have a greater specificity than a polyclonal antiserum which recognizes the antigen via a number of different epitopes.

ASSAYS FOR COMPLEMENT

The simplest measurement of complement activity is to determine the concentration of serum which will cause lysis of 50% of a standardized preparation of antibody-sensitized erythrocytes (EA). This is carried out in tubes or microwells. A simpler system, which provides a crude measure of complement activity is single radial haemolysis. The technique is similar to that of single radial immunodiffusion (see Fig. 25.4) except that the wells contain the test serum and the gel contains EA.

A zone of haemolysis develops around wells containing active complement, and the size of the zone is proportional to the amount of complement in the well. This technique measures the total activity of the classical and lytic pathways (C1–C9), but if a serum is deficient in complement activity it cannot identify which complement protein is lacking.

Individual components may be measured separately to determine either their total level or their functional level. This is an important distinction, since a component may be present in normal quantities, but be functionally inactive. Total levels of individual complement proteins are usually measured by RIA or by ELISA using antibody specific for the protein under investigation. Functional levels are measured in assays tailored to detect each individual complement protein by providing a cocktail of sensitized red cells plus all the components required for lysis, except the one under investigation (Fig. 25.18).

ISOLATION OF LYMPHOCYTE POPULATIONS

Many of the experiments performed by immunologists use populations of lymphocytes for either *in vivo* or *in vitro* work. The main sources of lymphocytes from experimental animals are the thymus, the spleen or the peripheral lymph nodes. Specialized studies may

Monoclonal antibody production

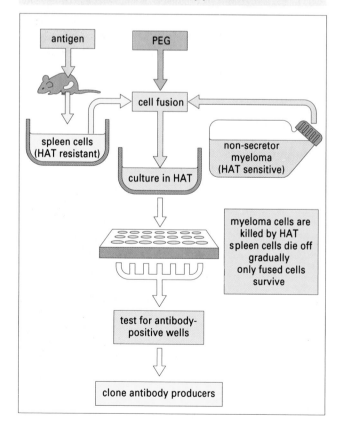

Fig. 25.17 Animals (usually mice or rats) are immunized with antigen. Once the animals are making a good antibody response the spleens are removed and a cell suspension prepared (lymph nodes cells may also be used). These cells are fused with a myeloma cell line by the addition of polyethylene glycol (PEG) which promotes membrane fusion. Only a small proportion of the cells fuse successfully. The fusion mixture is then set up in culture with medium containing 'HAT'. HAT is a mixture of Hypoxanthine, Aminopterin and Thymidine. Aminopterin is a powerful toxin which blocks a metabolic pathway. This pathway can be bypassed if the cell is provided with the intermediate metabolites hypoxanthine and thymidine. Thus spleen cells can grow in HAT medium, but the myeloma cells die in HAT medium because they have a metabolic defect and cannot use the bypass pathway. When the culture is set up in HAT medium it contains spleen cells, myeloma cells and fused cells. The spleen cells die in culture naturally after 1–2 weeks and the myeloma cells are killed by the HAT. Fused cells survive however as they have the immortality of the myeloma and the metabolic bypass of the spleen cells. Some of them will also have the antibody producing capacity of the spleen cells. Any wells containing growing cells are tested for the production of the desired antibody (often by RIA or ELISA) and if positive the cultures are cloned, that is, plated out so that only one cell is in each well. This produces a clone of cells derived from a single progenitor, which is both immortal and produces monoclonal antibody.

require isolation of cells from other areas such as Peyer's patches. Recirculating cells may be obtained by cannulating the thoracic duct and collecting the draining lymphocytes over a number of hours. In studies on humans, peripheral blood lymphocytes are the most readily available source of cells, but spleen, tonsil or lymph nodes may become available following surgical resection. Problems can however arise with surgical material due to the presence of infectious agents or tumour cells, depending on the circumstances that led to surgery. It should be emphasized that the cell populations derived from each of these tissues is quite distinct, with respect to the maturity of the lymphocytes and the proportions of different cell populations. The thymus is a source of fairly pure T cells but these are at varying stages of maturity. When working on lymphocytes from other sources, it is often desirable to separate the different cell populations so as to distinguish their effects.

Assays for complement components

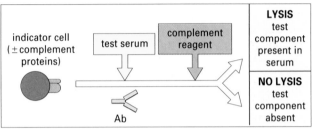

test	indicator	complement reagent
C1	EAC 4 (guinea pig)	C1 reagent
C4	EA	C4–deficient guinea pig serum
C2	EAC 4 (human) (antrypol)	C2 reagent
C3	EAC 142 (guinea pig)	C5-9(NH$_3$ treated guinea pig serum)
C5	EAC 14 oxy 23	C5-deficient mouse serum
C6	EAC 143 (human) (antrypol)	C6-deficient rabbit serum
FB	EA+EGTA+Mg^{2+}	B-deficient serum (50°C treated)
FD	EA+EGTA+Mg^{2+}	D-deficient serum (Sephadex G75 exclusion peak)

Fig. 25.18 These assays detect specific complement components in a test serum. The principle of the assay is to mix sensitized red cells, with a 'complement reagent' so that the sensitized cells plus the reagent contain all the complement components needed to lyse the red cells except for the component being tested. For example to test for C4, erythrocytes sensitized with antibody (EA) are placed with C4-deficient guinea pig serum. The cells will be lysed if there is C4 in the test serum, otherwise they will not. The table lists the combinations of reagents used for each test component. The red cells are prepared by blocking the reactions of EA with complement at a specific point. The complement reagents may be sera deficient in one component or sera treated physicochemically to remove or inactivate one component. In practice the assay would be performed quantitatively, for example, by single radial haemolysis, or in tubes to determine the point at which 50% of the red cells are lysed.

Lymphocyte separation on Ficoll Isopaque

Fig. 25.19 Whole blood is defibrinated by shaking with glass beads and the resulting clot removed. The blood is then diluted in tissue culture medium and layered on top of a tube half full of Ficoll. Ficoll has a density greater than that of lymphocytes but less than that of red cells and granulocytes (e.g. neutrophils). After centrifugation the red cells and PMNs pass down through the Ficoll to form a pellet at the bottom of the tube while lymphocytes settle at the interface of the medium and Ficoll. The lymphocyte preparation can be further depleted of phagocytes by the addition of iron filings; these are taken up by the phagocytes which can

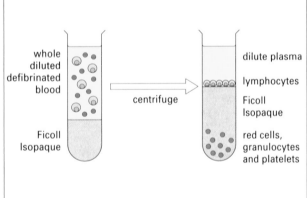

then be drawn away with a strong magnet. Alternatively, macrophages can be removed by leaving the cell suspension to settle on a plastic dish. Macrophages adhere to plastic, whereas the lymphocytes can be washed off.

Isolation of lymphocyte subpopulations – rosetting

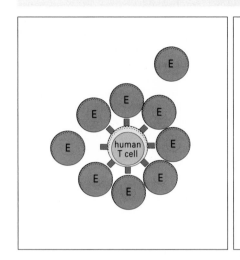 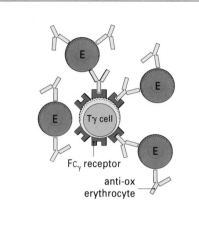 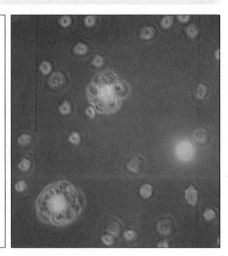

Fig. 25.20 Some lymphocytes have receptors for erythrocytes. Human T cells have receptors for sheep erythrocytes (E); these are CD2 molecules (left). They are not present on mouse T cells in sufficient quantities. When mixed together the T cells form rosettes with the erythrocytes and may be separated from non-rosetting B cells on Ficoll gradients. A modification of this technique to isolate cells with other receptors is also shown (middle). For example, some T cells have a receptor for the Fc of IgG (Fc_γ). These cells may be identified and isolated by rosetting with ox erythrocytes sensitized with a subagglutinating amount of anti-ox erythrocyte. A rosetted lymphocyte is shown on the right.
(Courtesy of Dr P. M. Lydyard.)

Isolation of lymphocyte subpopulations – panning

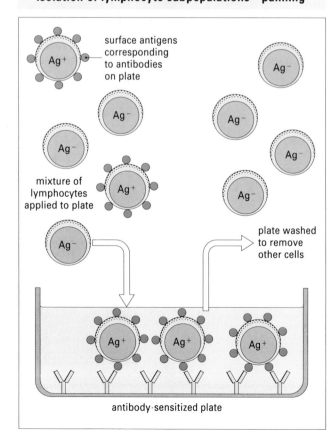

Fig. 25.21 Cell populations can be separated on antibody-sensitized plates. Antibody binds non-covalently to the plastic plate (as for RIA) and the cell mixture is applied to the plate. Antigen-positive cells (Ag^+) bind to the antibody and the antigen-negative cells (Ag^-) can be carefully washed off. By changing the culture conditions or by enzyme-digestion of the cells on the plate it is sometimes possible to recover the cells bound to the plate. Often the cells that have bound to the plate are altered by their binding, for example, binding to the plate cross-links the antigen which can cause cell activation. Thus, the method is most satisfactory for removing a cell population. Examples of the application of this method include separating TH and TC cell populations using antibodies to CD4 or CD8, and separating T cells from B cells using anti-Ig (which binds to the surface antibody of the B cell). By sensitizing the plate with antigen, antigen-binding cells can be separated from non-binding cells.

Reference has already been made to the use of the fluorescence activated cell sorter (FACS) for the isolation of lymphocyte populations, based on their surface markers. The number of cells isolated is, however, limited by the flow-through rate, which is slow since each cell is individually sorted. A number of bulk methods are also available for separating lymphocytes and the specific subpopulations. These include density gradient separation, rosetting, panning and magnetic separations.

Density gradient separation relies on lymphocytes being less dense than erythrocytes and granulocytes, (Fig. 25.19), and is used to isolate the majority of blood lymphocytes. Rosetting and panning (or plating) are used to isolate sub-populations (Figs 25.20 and 25.21).

Lymphocyte panning is a type of affinity chromatography applied to lymphocytes. A related technique uses magnetic beads coated with specific antibodies (e.g. anti-CD4). The beads are mixed with the cell population and bind to those recognized by the antibody. These cells can then be removed or isolated by applying a magnetic field.

Another useful method for removing unwanted cell populations relies on antibody and complement. When a specific antibody (e.g. anti-CD8) is added to a mixture of cells, followed by complement, that subpopulation of cells will be lysed. Naturally this will only work with antibodies that fix complement, and where the target population of cells has sufficient surface antigens to fix a lytic dose of complement.

Another approach to the preparation of lymphocytes is to generate antigen-specific lines of T cells, and propagate them for an extended period (Fig. 25.22). This obviates the need for frequent isolation of primary cultures from animals.

EFFECTOR CELL ASSAYS

Various methods have been developed for assaying lymphocyte effector functions, including antibody production, cytotoxicity, and T-cell-mediated help and suppression.

Antibody-forming cells are measured by plaque-forming cell assay (Fig. 25.23). By modifying the plaque

T cell lines

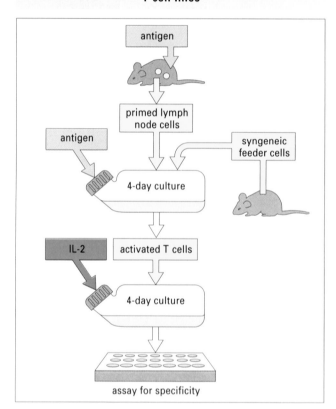

Fig. 25.22 The figure illustrates one protocol for the preparation of T cell lines, although many other protocols are used. Mice are primed with antigen (usually subcutaneously in the rear foot pad), and the draining lymph nodes (in this case the popliteal and inguinal) are removed 1 week later and set up in co-culture with syngeneic feeder cells (e.g. normal thymocytes or splenocytes) and antigen. After 4 days the lymphoblasts are isolated and induced to proliferate with interleukin-2 (IL-2). When the population of cells has expanded sufficiently they are checked for antigen and MHC specificity in a lymphocyte transformation test, and are maintained by alternate cycles of culture on antigen treated feeder cells and culture in IL-2 containing medium.

Plaque forming cell assay – I

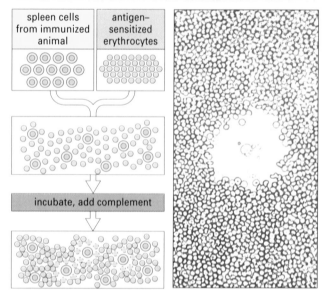

Fig. 25.23 Antibody-forming cells are measured by mixing the test population with antigen-sensitized red cells. Following incubation, the red cells surrounding the cells secreting specific antibody become coated with the antibody and may be lysed by complement.

forming cell assay, it is possible to separately identify IgG-producing and IgM-producing cells specific for an antigen, as well as to identify the total number of antibody-forming cells (Fig. 25.24). An alternative way of detecting antibody-producing cells is by an enzymatic test called the ELISPOT assay. (Fig. 25.25). A development of this assay allows the detection of functional T cells according to the soluble mediators they release, i.e. cytokines. In this assay the plate is sensitized with an antibody to the specific cytokine (e.g. anti-IFN$_\gamma$). This captures the specific cytokine, released in a spot around the active T cell.

Antigen-specific T cells are often detected by the lymphocyte stimulation test, which measures their response to antigen as shown by their entering the cell cycle and incorporating precursors of DNA synthesis (see Figs 25.19 and 25.26). The cytotoxic activity of cell populations is usually detected by their ability to lyse target cells (e.g. virally infected cells, tumour cells, allogeneic tissue cells). Target cell lysis is determined in the chromium release assay (Fig. 25.27).

Experiments for the detection of lymphocyte migration *in vivo* usually involve tracking of labelled lymphocytes to particular tissues after intravenous infusion. The cell may be radiolabelled or be marked with stable fluorescent dyes. Radiolabelled cells are used for quantitative measurements of cell migration. Localization patterns within organs can be seen by autoradiography of labelled cells, or by direct visualization of fluorescent cells by microscopy under ultraviolet illumination.

Analysis of the adhesion molecules involved in lymphocyte migration has mostly been carried out *in vitro*.

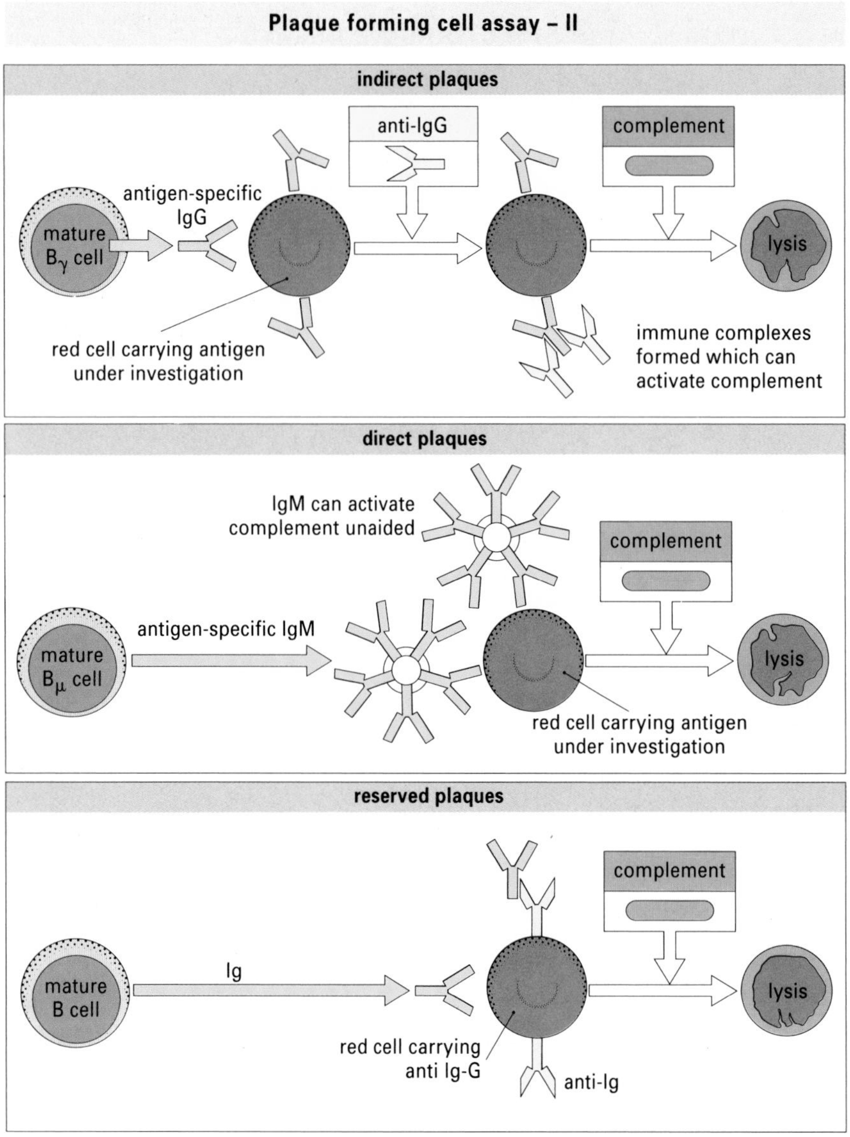

Plaque forming cell assay – II

Fig. 25.24 Plaque forming cell assays are used to detect antibody-forming cells. The assay may be performed in three different ways. **Indirect plaques.** Cells producing antibody to a particular antigen release it, whence it diffuses and binds onto antigen on red cells. This may be red cell surface antigen, or the red cells may be sensitized with another antigen as in the haemagglutination assay. To detect the IgG antibodies bound to the red cells it is necessary to add anti-IgG antibody and then complement. Complexes formed on the cell fix complement and produce a zone of erythrocyte lysis around the B cell. **Direct plaques.** Antigen-specific IgM antibodies are capable of causing complement-mediated lysis without the addition of an extra layer of anti-immunoglobulin. Thus the numbers of antigen-specific IgM and IgG plaque forming cells can be estimated separately. **Reversed plaques.** The reversed plaque method measures total immunoglobulin-producing cells (not just antigen-specific cells). Released Ig binds onto red cells sensitized with anti-Ig. This complex can now fix complement and cause cell lysis. (Protein A, which binds IgG Fc regions, can be substituted for the anti-Ig on the red cells in this assay).

ELISPOT assays

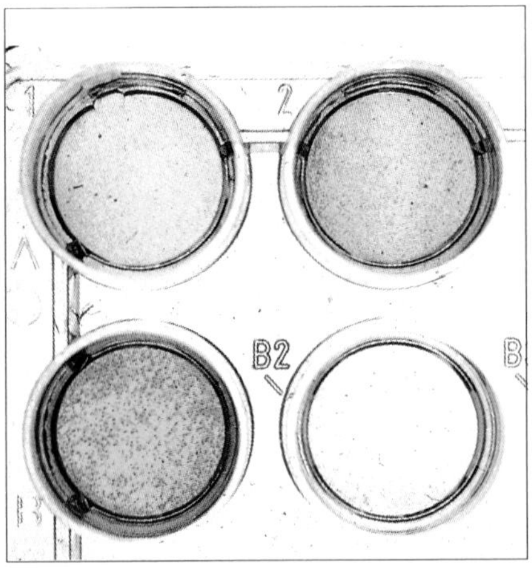

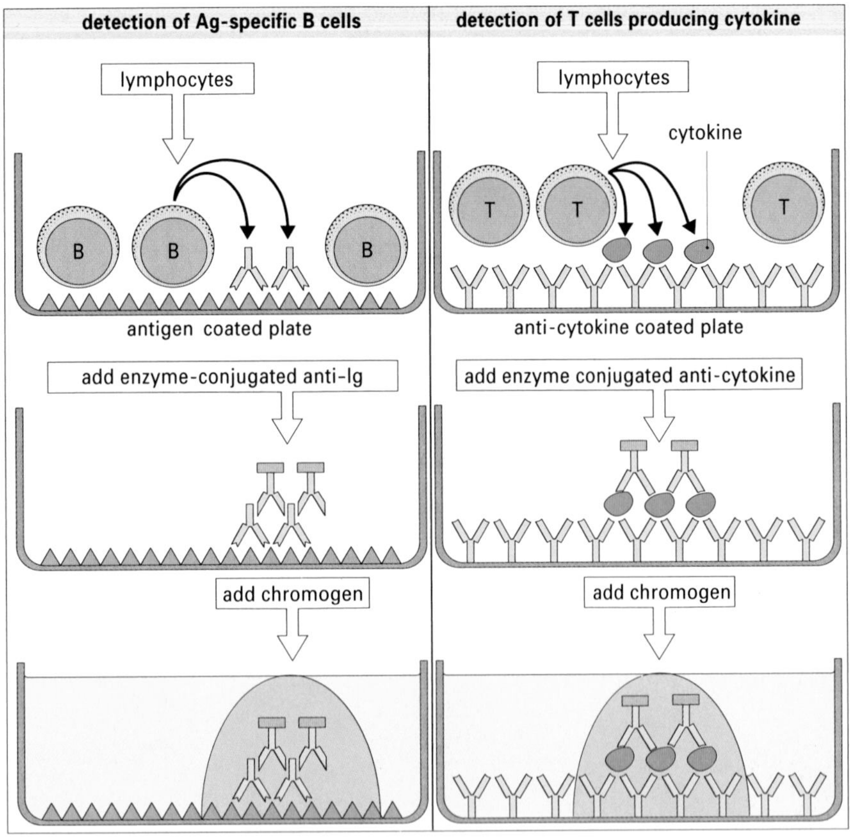

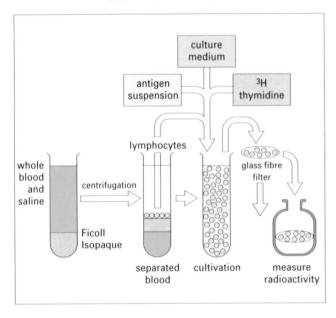

Fig. 25.25 Individual B cells producing specific antibody or individual T cells secreting particular cytokines may be detected by ELISPOT assay. For detection of antibody-producing cells, the lymphocytes are plated onto an antigen-sensitized plate. Antibody binds antigen in the immediate vicinity of cells producing the specific antibody. The spots of bound antibody are then detected chromatographically using enzyme coupled to anti-immunoglobulin and a chromogen. For detection of cytokine-producing cells the plates are coated with anti-cytokine and the captured cytokine is detected with enzyme-coupled antibody to a different epitope on the cytokine. The appearance of a developed plate is shown top left. (Photograph courtesy of P. Hutchings and Blackwell Scientific Press.)

detection of Ag-specific B cells

lymphocytes

antigen coated plate

add enzyme-conjugated anti-Ig

add chromogen

detection of T cells producing cytokine

lymphocytes

cytokine

anti-cytokine coated plate

add enzyme conjugated anti-cytokine

add chromogen

The lymphocyte stimulation test

culture medium

antigen suspension

³H thymidine

lymphocytes

glass fibre filter

whole blood and saline

centrifugation

Ficoll Isopaque

separated blood

cultivation

measure radioactivity

Fig. 25.26 Whole blood in saline solution is layered on Ficoll Isopaque (which has a density between, and therefore separates, white cells and red cells) and centrifuged (400×G). This separates the lymphocytes from the other cell and serum constituents. The cells are washed (to remove contaminants such as antigen) and then put into test tubes with a suspension of antigen and culture medium (cells from lymphoid tissues may also be used). Tritiated thymidine (³H-thymidine) is added 16 hours before the cells are harvested. The cells are harvested on a glass fibre filter disc and their radioactivity is measured by placing the disc in a liquid scintillation counter. A high count indicates that the lymphocytes have undergone transformation and confirms their sensitivity to the antigen.

In the Stamper–Woodroofe assay, the direct binding of lymphocytes to high endothelial venules is measured by allowing the lymphocytes to adhere to tissue sections of lymph node, Peyer's patch or other tissues containing high endothelial venules. Adherent cells are counted under the microscope. Antibodies to intercellular adhesion molecules will reduce the level of binding, provided that the antibodies attach to the adhesion molecules near their active sites. The adhesion of lymphocytes to endothelial cell monolayers can also be blocked *in vitro*. The identity of the adhesion molecules may then be confirmed by labelling the lymphocytes or endothelial cells and using the antibodies which block adhesion, to immunoprecipitate the specific adhesion molecules.

Although this account is by no means exhaustive, the techniques described do form the basis of a great many experiments when used in combination. Furthermore, even complicated techniques found in research papers are frequently modifications of these basic systems.

Cytotoxicity assay by chromium release

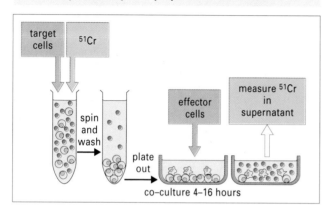

co-culture 4–16 hours

Fig. 25.27 Target cells are incubated with ^{51}Cr, which is taken up into the cells and binds to protein. After incubation the free ^{51}Cr is washed away and the target cells plated out. They are then co-cultured with the effector cells for 4–16 hours and the supernatant is removed and counted to detect chromium released from lysed target cells.

FURTHER READING

Hudson L, Hay FC. *Practical Immunology*. 3rd ed. Oxford: Blackwell Scientific Publications, 1989.

Johnstone A, Thorpe R. *Immunochemistry in Practice*. 2nd ed. Oxford: Blackwell Scientific Publications, 1987.

Nairn RC, ed. *Practical Methods in Clinical Immunology*. Series. Edinburgh: Churchill Livingstone, 1980–1984.

Weir DM. *Handbook of Experimental Immunology*. Vols I & II. 4th ed. Oxford: Blackwell Scientific Publications, 1986.

Appendices

Appendix I: HLA specifications

| | DP | | DQB / DQA | | DR | | B | | C | | A |

DP

Allele	Specificity
DPA1*0101	—
DPA1*0102	—
DPA1*0103	—
DPA1*0201	—
DPB1*0101	DPw1
DPB1*0201	DPw2
DPB1*0202	DPw2
DPB1*0301	DPw3
DPB1*0401	DPw4
DPB1*0402	DPw4
DPB1*0501	DPw5
DPB1*0601	DPw6
DPB1*0801	—
DPB1*0901	DP"Cp63"
DPB1*1001	—
DPB1*1101	—
DPB1*1301	—
DPB1*1401	—
DPB1*1501	—
DPB1*1601	—
DPB1*1701	—
DPB1*1801	—
DPB1*1901	—

DQB / DQA

Allele	Specificity
DQA1*0101	—
DQA1*0102	—
DQA1*0103	—
DQA1*0201	—
DQA1*0301	—
DQA1*0401	—
DQA1*0501	—
DQA1*0601	—
DQB1*0501	DQw5(w1)
DQB1*0502	DQw5(w1)
DQB1*0503	DQw5(w1)
DQB1*0601	DQw6(w1)
DQB1*0602	DQw6(w1)
DQB1*0603	DQw6(w1)
DQB1*0604	DQw6(w1)
DQB1*0201	DQw2
DQB1*0301	DQw7(w3)
DQB1*0302	DQw8(w3)
DQB1*0303	DQw9(w3)
DQB1*0401	DQw4
DQB1*0402	DQw4

DR

Allele	Specificity
DRB1*0101	DR1
DRB1*0102	DR1
DRB1*0103	DR"BR"
DRB1*1501	DRw15(2)
DRB1*0502	DRw15(2)
DRB1*0601	DRw16(2)
DRB1*0602	DRw16(2)
DRB1*0301	DRw17(3)
DRB1*0302	DRw18(3)
DRB1*0401	DR4
DRB1*0402	DR4
DRB1*0403	DR4
DRB1*0404	DR4
DRB1*0405	DR4
DRB1*0406	DR4
DRB1*0407	DR4
DRB1*0407	DR4
DRB1*1101	DRw11(5)
DRB1*1102	DRw11(5)
DRB1*1103	DRw11(5)
DRB1*1104	DRw11(5)
DRB1*1201	DRw12(5)
DRB1*1301	DRw13(w6)
DRB1*1302	DRw13(w6)
DRB1*1303	DRw13(w6)
DRB1*1401	DRw14(w6)
DRB1*1402	DRw14(w6)
DRB1*0701	DR7
DRB1*0702	DR7
DRB1*0801	DRw8
DRB1*0802	DRw8
DRB1*0803	DRw8
DRB1*0901	DR9
DRB1*1001	DR1w10
DRB3*0101	DRw52a
DRB3*0201	DRw52b
DRB3*0202	DRw52b
DRB3*0301	DRw52c
DRB4*0101	DRw53
DRB5*0101	DRw15(2)
DRB5*0102	DRw15(2)
DRB5*0201	DRw16(2)
DRB5*0202	DRw16(2)

B

Allele	Specificity
B*0701	B7
B*0702	B7
B*0801	B8
B*1301	B13
B*1302	B13
B*1401	B14
B*1402	Bw65(14)
B*1501	Bw62(15)
B*1801	B18
B*2701	B27
B*2702	B27
B*2703	B27
B*2704	B27
B*2705	B27
B*2706	B27
B*3501	B35
B*3701	B37
B*3801	B38(16)
B*3901	B39(16)
B*4001	Bw60(40)
B*4002	Bw40
B*4101	Bw41
B*4201	Bw42
B*4401	B44(12)
B*4402	B44(12)
B*4601	Bw46
B*4701	Bw47
B*4901	B49(21)
B*5101	B51(5)
B*5202	Bw52(5)
B*5701	Bw57(17)
B*5801	Bw58(17)

C

Allele	Specificity
Cw*0101	Cw1
Cw*0201	Cw2
Cw*0202	Cw2
Cw*0301	Cw3
Cw*0501	Cw5
Cw*0601	Cw6
Cw*0701	Cw7
Cw*1101	Cw11
Cw*1201	—
Cw*1301	—
Cw*1401	—

A

Allele	Specificity
A*0101	A1
A*0201	A2
A*0202	A2
A*0203	A2
A*0204	A2
A*0205	A2
A*0206	A2
A*0207	A2
A*0208	A2
A*0209	A2
A*0210	A2
A*0301	A3
A*0302	A3
A*1101	A11
A*2401	A24(9)
A*2501	A25(10)
A*2601	A26(10)
A*2901	A29(w19)
A*3001	A30(w19)
A*3101	A31(w19)
A*3201	A32(w19)
A*3301	Aw33(w19)
A*6801	Aw68(28)
A*6802	Aw68(28)
A*6901	Aw69(28)

The right hand column of each subregion lists the distinct antigenic specificities detected serologically. HLA-D specificities are also detected in the MLR. Specificities not yet sufficiently defined are designated by 'w' (workshop).

Allelic variants of MHC genes at each locus are also shown. (Based on data from Bodmer JG, Marsh SGE, Parham P, et al. Nomenclature for factors of the HLA system, 1989. *Hum Immunol* 1990;**28**:327–42.)

CD	identity/function	mol. wt ($\times 10^3$)	T cell	B cell	NK/non-lineage	monocyte	macrophage	granulocyte	platelet	Langerhans cell/ dendritic cell	stem cell
CD1a		49	Thy								
CD1b		45	Thy							LC	
CD1c		43	Thy							DC	
CD2	LFA-3 receptor	50									
CD2R		50	★								
CD3	TCR subunit (γ,δ,ε,ζ,η)	25,20,19,16,22									
CD4	MHC class II receptor	55									
CD5	CD72 receptor	67									
CD6		100									
CD7		40			●				●		
CD8	MHC class I receptor	36/32									
CD9		24		pre-B							
CD10	CALLA, neutral endopeptidase	100		pre-B							Lymph
CD11a	LFA-1 (α chain)	180									
CD11b	CR3 (α chain)	165									
CD11c	CR4 (α chain)	150									
CDw12		90–120							●		
CD13	Aminopeptidase N	150									
CD14	LPS-binding protein	55						●		● (LC)	
CD15	ELAM receptor					●					
CD16	FcγRIII	50–70									
CDw17	Lactosylceramide										
CD18	(β chain of CD11)	95									
CD19		95									
CD20	ion channel?	37/35									
CD21	CR2	140		Mat						FDC	
CD22		135									
CD23	FcεRII	45–50		Mat, ★		★		E			
CD24		41/38									
CD25	IL-2 receptor (β)	55	★	★		★					
CD26	Dipeptidylpeptidase IV	120	★								
CD27		55									
CD28		44		★							
CD29	VLA (β chain)	130									
CD30		120	★	★							
CD31	PECAM-1	140									
CDw32	FcγRII	40									
CD33		67									BM
CD34		105–120									BM
CD35	CR1	160–260									
CD36		90			●						
CD37		40–52	●	Mat			●				
CD38		45	Thy, ★	PC							Lymph
CD39		70–100		Mat			●			FDC	
CD40		50								FDC	
CD41		120/25									
CD42a		23									

Appendix II: CD markers

CD	identity/function	mol. wt (× 10³)	T cell	B cell	NK/non-lineage	monocyte	macrophage	granulocyte	platelet	Langerhans cell/ dendritic cell	stem cell
CD42b		135/25									
CD43	Leukosialin	95									
CD44		80—95									
CD45	Leucocyte common antigen(LCA)	T200									
CD45RA	Restricted LCA	220			●		●				
CD45RB	Restricted LCA	190/205/220									
CD45RO	Restricted LCA	190									
CD46	MCP(membrane cofactor protein)	66/56									
CD47		47—52									
CD48		41									
CDw49b	VLA$_{\alpha2}$	165									
CDw49d	VLA$_{\alpha4}$	150									
CD49f	VLA$_{\alpha6}$	120/30	●								
CDw50		148/108									
CD51	Vitronectin receptor α	120/24									
CDw52	Campath-1	21—28									
CD53		32—40									BM
CD54	ICAM-1										
CD55	DAF(Decay accelerating factor)	70									
CD56	NKH1＝NCAM	220/135		●							
CD57		110			●						
CD58	LFA-3	40—65									
CD59	TAP, protectin	18—20									
CDw60	NeuAc—NeuAc—Gal										
CD61	Vitronectin receptor β	105									
CD62	P-selectin	140									
CD63		53	●	●				●			
CD64	Fc$_\gamma$RI	70									
CDw65	Ceramide dodecasaccharide										
CD66		180—200									
CD67		100									
CD68		110									
CD69		32/28	★	★							
CDw70			★	★							
CD71	Transferrin receptor	95	★	★	★	★					
CD72	CD5 receptor	43/39									
CD73	Ecto-5'-nucleotidase	69									
CD74	MHC class II invariant chain	41/35/33									
CDw75	α 2,6 sialyltransferase	53		Mat							
CD76		85/67		Mat							
CD77	Globotriaosylceramide										
CDw78											

This table shows the recognized CD markers of haemopoietic cells and their distribution. Thy, thymocytes; DC, dendritic cells; LC, Langerhans' cells; N, Neutrophils; E, Eosinophils; GC, germinal centre B cell; FDC, follicular dendritic cell; PC, plasma cell; BM, bone marrow cell.

= present; = subpopulation;
● = subject to further analysis; ★ = activated cells only;
Rest = resting cells only; Lymph = lymphoid cells;
Mat = mature cells only.

Appendix III: The major cytokines

cytokine	immune system source	other cells	principal targets	principal effects
IL-1$_\alpha$ IL-1$_\beta$	macrophages, LGLs, B cells	endothelium, fibroblasts, astrocytes, etc.	T cells, B cells, macrophages, endothelium, tissue cells	lymphocyte activation, macrophage stimulation, ↑ leucocyte/endothelial adhesion, pyrexia, acute phase proteins
IL-2	T cells		T cells	T cell proliferation and differentiation, activation of cytotoxic lymphocytes and macrophages
IL-3	T cells		stem cells	multilineage colony stimulating factor
IL-4	T cells		B cells, T cells	B-cell growth factor, isotype selection, IgE, IgG1
IL-5	T cells		B cells	B-cell growth and differentiation, IgA selection
IL-6	T cells, B cells, macrophages	fibroblasts	B cells, hepatocytes	B cell differentiation, induces acute phase proteins
IL-7		bone marrow stromal cells	pre-B cells, T cells	B cell and T cell proliferation
IL-8	monocytes		neutrophils, basophils	chemotaxis
IL-10	T cells		T$_H$1 cells	inhibition of cytokine synthesis
TNF$_\alpha$	macrophages, lymphocytes, mast cells		macrophages, granulocytes, tissue cells	activation of macrophages, granulocytes and cytotoxic cells, ↑leucocyte/endothelial cell adhesion, cachexia, pyrexia, induction of stimulation of acute phase protein, stimulation of angiogenesis, enhanced MHC class I production
TNF$_\beta$(LT)	T cells			
IFN$_\alpha$ IFN$_\beta$	leucocytes	epithelia, fibroblasts	tissue cells	MHC class I induction, antiviral effect, stimulation of NK cells
IFN$_\gamma$	T cells, NK cells	epithelia, fibroblasts	leucocytes, tissue cells, T$_H$2 cells	MHC class I and II induction, macrophage activation,↑ endothelial cell/lymphocyte adhesion, ↓ cytokine synthesis
M–CSF	monocytes	endothelium, fibroblasts		proliferation of macrophage precursors
G–CSF	macrophages	fibroblasts	stem cells	stimulate division and differentiation
GM–CSF	T cells, macrophages	endothelium, fibroblasts		proliferation of granulocyte and macrophage precursors and activators
MIF	T cells		macrophages	migration inhibition

The cytokines in this list have all been identified as distinct by genomic cloning. Note that only the principal sources, targets and effects have been included in this table. Most cytokines act in concert with others to produce their biological effects *in vivo*.

Glossary

Acute phase proteins. Serum proteins whose levels increase during infection or inflammatory reactions.

ADCC (antibody-dependent cell-mediated cytotoxicity). A cytotoxic reaction in which Fc receptor-bearing killer cells recognize target cells via specific antibodies.

Adjuvant. A substance that non-specifically enhances the immune response to an antigen.

AFCs (antibody-forming cells). Functionally equivalent to plasma cells.

Affinity. A measure of the binding strength between an antigenic determinant (epitope) and an antibody-combining site (paratope).

Affinity maturation. The increase in average antibody affinity frequently seen during a secondary immune response.

Agretope. The portion of an antigen or antigen fragment which interacts with an MHC molecule.

Allele. Intraspecies variance at a particular gene locus.

Allergen. An agent, e.g. pollen, dust, animal dander, that causes IgE-mediated reactions.

Allergy. Originally defined as altered reactivity on second contact with antigen; now usually refers to a Type I hypersensitivity reaction.

Allogeneic. Refers to intraspecies genetic variations.

Allotype. The protein product of an allele which may be detectable as an antigen by another member of the same species.

Altered self. The concept that the combination of antigen and a self MHC molecules interacts with the immune system in the same way as an allogeneic MHC molecule.

Alternative pathway. The activation pathways of the complement system involving C3 and factors B, D, P, H and I, which interact in the vicinity of an activator surface to form an alternative pathway C3 convertase.

Amplification loop. The alternative complement activation pathway, which acts as a positive feedback loop when C3 is split in the presence of an activator surface.

Anaphylatoxins. Complement peptides (C3a and C5a) which cause mast cell degranulation and smooth muscle contraction.

Anaphylaxis. An antigen-specific immune reaction mediated primarily by IgE which results in vasodilation and constriction of smooth muscles, including those of the bronchus, and which may result in death of the animal.

Antibody. A molecule produced by animals in response to antigen which has the particular property of combining specifically with the antigen which induced its formation.

Antigen. A molecule which induces the formation of antibody.

Antigen presentation. The process by which certain cells in the body (antigen-presenting cells) express antigen on their cell surface in a form recognizable by lymphocytes.

Antigen processing. The conversion of an antigen into a form in which it can be recognized by lymphocytes.

APCs (antigen-presenting cells). A variety of cell types which carry antigen in a form that can stimulate lymphocytes.

Atopy. The clinical manifestation of Type I hypersensitivity reactions including eczema, asthma and rhinitis.

Autologous. Part of the same individual.

Autosomes. Chromosomes other than the X or Y sex chromosomes.

Avidity The functional combining strength of an antibody with its antigen which is related to both the affinity of the reaction between the epitopes and paratopes, and the valencies of the antibody and antigen.

β_2-microglobulin. A polypeptide which constitutes part of some membrane proteins including the Class I MHC molecules.

BCG (Bacille Calmette Guérin). An attenuated strain of *Mycobacterium tuberculosis* used as a vaccine an adjuvant or a biological response modifier in different circumstances.

Biozzi mice. Lines of mice selectively bred to produce low or high antibody responses to a variety of antigens (originally sheep erythrocytes).

Bradykinin. A vasoactive nonapeptide which is the most important mediator generated by the kinin system.

Bursa of Fabricius. A lymphoepithelial organ found at the junction of the hind gut and cloaca in birds which is the site of B cell maturation.

Bystander lysis. Complement-mediated lysis of cells in the immediate vicinity of a complement activation site, which are not themselves responsible for the activation.

C domains. The constant domains of antibody and the T-cell receptor. These domains do not contribute to the antigen-binding site and show relatively little variability between receptor molecules.

C genes. The gene segments which encode the constant portion of the immunoglobulin heavy and light chains and the α, β, γ and δ chains of the T-cell antigen receptor.

C1–C9. The components of the complement classical and lytic pathways which are responsible for mediating inflammatory reactions, opsonization of particles and lysis of cell membranes.

Capping. A process by which cell surface molecules are caused to aggregate (usually using antibody) on the cell membrane.

Carrier. An immunogenic molecule, or part of a molecule that is recognized by T cells in an antibody response.

CD markers. Cell surface molecules of leucocytes and platelets that are distinguishable with monoclonal antibodies and may be used to differentiate different cell populations.

CDRs (complementarity-determining regions). The sections of an antibody or T-cell receptor V region responsible for antigen or antigen–MHC binding.

Cell cycle. The process of cell division which is divisible into four phases G1, S, G2 and M. DNA replicates during the S phase and the cell divides in the M (mitotic) phase.

Chemokinesis. Increased random migratory activity of cells.

Chemotaxis. Increased directional migration of cells particularly in response to concentration gradients of certain chemotactic factors.

Chimaerism. The situation in which cells from genetically different individuals coexist in one body.

Class I/II/III MHC molecules. Three major classes of molecule coded within the MHC. class I molecules have one MHC encoded peptide complexed with β_2-microglobulin, class II molecules have two MHC encoded peptides which are non-covalently associated, and class III molecules are other molecules including complement components.

Class I/II restriction. The observation that immunologically active cells will only cooperate effectively when they share MHC haplotypes at either the class I or class II loci.

Classical pathway. The pathway by which antigen–antibody complexes can activate the complement system, involving components C1, C2 and C4, and generating a classical pathway C3 convertase.

Class switching. The process by which an individual B cell can link immunoglobulin heavy chain C genes to its recombined V gene to produce a different class of antibody with the same specificity. This process is also reflected in the overall class switch seen during the maturation of an immune response.

Clonal selection. The fundamental basis of lymphocyte activation in which antigen selectively stimulates only those cells which express receptors for it to divide and differentiate.

Clone. A family of cells or organisms having a genetically identical constitution.

CMI (cell-mediated immunity). A term used to refer to immune reactions that are mediated by cells rather than by antibody or other humoral factors.

Cobra venom factor. A cobra complement component equivalent to mammalian C3b.

Complement. A group of serum proteins involved in the control of inflammation, the activation of phagocytes and the lytic attack on cell membranes. The system can be activated by interaction with the immune system.

ConA (concanavalin A). A mitogen for T cells.

Congenic. Animals which are genetically constructed to differ at one particular locus.

Conjugate. A reagent which is formed by covalently coupling two molecules together, such as fluorescein coupled to an immunoglobulin molecule.

Contrasuppression. The action of a group of T cells which renders T-helper cells resistant to action of T-suppressors.

Constant regions. The relatively invariant parts of immunoglobulin heavy and light chains, and the α, β, γ, and δ chains of the T-cell receptor.

CR1 CR2 CR3. Receptors for activated C3 fragments.

CSFs (colony stimulating factors). A group of cytokines which control the differentiation of haemopoietic stem cells.

Cyclophosphamide. A cytotoxic drug frequently used as an immunosuppressive.

Cyclosporin. An immunosuppressive drug that is particularly useful in suppression of graft rejection

Cytokines. A generic term for soluble molecules which mediate interactions between cells.

Cytophilic. Having a propensity to bind to cells.

Cytostatic. Having the ability to stop cell growth.

Cytotoxic. Having the ability to kill cells.

D genes. Sets of gene segments lying between the V and J genes in the immunoglobulin heavy chain genes, and in the T-cell receptor β and δ chain genes which are recombined with V and J genes during ontogeny.

Degranulation. Exocytosis of granules from cells such as mast cells and basophils.

Dendritic cells. A set of cells present in tissues, which capture antigens and migrate to the lymph nodes and spleen, where they are particularly active in presenting the processed antigen to T cells.

Desetope. The part of an MHC molecule which links to antigen or processed antigen.

DTH (delayed type hypersensitivity). This term includes the delayed skin reactions associated with Type IV hypersensitivity.

DNP (dinitrophenol). A commonly used hapten.

Domain. A region of a peptide having a coherent tertiary structure. Both immunoglobulins and MHC Class I and Class II molecules have domains.

Dominant idiotypes. Individual idiotypes which are present on a large proportion of the antibodies generated to a particular antigen.

dsDNA. Double-stranded DNA.

Epstein–Barr virus (EBV). Causal agent of Burkitt's lymphoma and infectious mononucleosis, which has the ability to transform human B cells into stable cell lines.

Effector cells. A functional concept which in context means those lymphocytes or phagocytes which produce the end effect.

Endogenous. Originating within the organism.

Endothelium. Cells lining blood vessels and lymphatics.

Enhancement. Prolongation of graft survival by treatment with antibodies directed towards the graft alloantigens.

Epitope. A single antigenic determinant. Functionally it is the portion of an antigen which combines with the antibody paratope.

Exon. Gene segment encoding protein.

Fab. The part of an antibody molecule which contains the antigen-combining site, consisting of a light chain and part of the heavy chain; it is produced by enzymatic digestion.

Factors B, P, D, H, and I. Components of the alternative complement pathway.

Fc. The portion of an antibody that is responsible for binding to antibody receptors on cells and the C1q component of complement.

Framework segments. Sections of antibody V regions which lie between the hypervariable regions.

Freund's adjuvant. An emulsion of aqueous antigen in oil. Complete Freund's adjuvant also contains killed *Mycobacterium tuberculosis*, while incomplete Freund's adjuvant does not.

GALT (gut-associated lymphoid tissue). Refers to the accumulations of lymphoid tissue associated with the gastrointestinal tract.

Genetic association. A term used to describe the condition where particular genotypes are associated with other phenomena, such as particular diseases.

Genetic restriction. The term used to be describe the observation that lymphocytes and antigen-presenting cells cooperate most effectively when they share particular MHC haplotypes.

Genome. The total genetic material contained within the cell.

Genotype. The genetic material inherited from parents; not all of it is necessarily expressed in the individual.

Germ line. The genetic material which is passed down through the gametes before it is modified by somatic recombination or maturation.

Giant cells. Large multinucleated cells sometimes seen in granulomatous reactions and thought to result from the fusion of macrophages.

GVH (graft versus host) disease. A condition caused by allogeneic donor lymphocytes reacting against host tissue in an immunologically compromised recipient.

H–2. The mouse major histocompatibility complex.

Haplotype. A set of genetic determinants located on a single chromosome.

Hapten. A small molecule which can act as an epitope but is incapable by itself of eliciting an antibody response.

Helper (TH) cells. A functional subclass of T cells which can help to generate cytotoxic T cells and cooperate with B cells in production of antibody response. Helper cells recognize antigen in association with class II MHC molecules.

Heterologous. Refers to interspecies antigenic differences.

HEV (high endothelial venule). An area of venule from which lymphocytes migrate into lymph nodes.

Hinge. The portion of an immunoglobulin heavy chain between the Fc and Fab regions which permits flexibility within the molecule and allows the two combining sites to operate independently. The hinge region is usually encoded by a separate exon.

Histamine. A major vasoactive amine released from mast cell and basophil granules.

Histocompatibility. The ability to accept grafts between individuals.

HLA. The human major histocompatibility complex.

Homologous. The same species.

hnRNA (heteronuclear RNA). The fraction of nuclear RNA which contains primary transcripts of the DNA prior to processing to form messenger RNA.

Humoral. Pertaining to the extracellular fluids, including the serum and lymph.

Hybridoma. Cell line created *in vitro* by fusing two different cell types, usually lymphocytes, one of which is a tumour cell.

5-hydroxytryptamine. A vasoactive amine present in platelets and a major mediator of inflammation in rodents.

Hypervariable region. The most variable areas (3) of the V domains of immunoglobulin and T-cell receptor chains. These regions are clustered at the distal portion of the V domain and contribute to the antigen-binding site.

ICAM-1 (intercellular adhesion molecule-1). Cell surface molecule found on a variety of leucocytes and non-haematogenous cells which interacts with LFA-1 and is involved in cell traffic.

Idiotype. A single antigenic determinant on an antibody V region.

Idiotype. The antigenic characteristic of the V region of an antibody.

Immune-complex. The product of an antigen–antibody reaction which may also contain components of the complement system.

Immunofluorescence. A technique used to identify particular antigens microscopically in tissues or on cells by the binding of a fluorescent antibody conjugate.

Interferons (IFNs). A group of mediators which increase the resistance of cells to viral infection, and act as cytokine. IFN$_\gamma$ is also an important immunological mediator.

Interleukins (IL-1–IL-10). A group of molecules involved in signalling between cells of the immune system.

Intron. Gene segment between exons not encoding protein.

Ir gene. A group of immune response (Ir) genes determining the level of an immune response to a particularly antigen or foreign stimulus. A number of them are found in the major histocompatibility complex.

Isoelectric focusing. Separation of molecules on the basis of charge. Each molecule will migrate to the point in a pH gradient where it has no net charge.

Isologous. Of identical genetic constitution.

Isotype. Refers to genetic variation within a family of proteins or peptides such that every member of the species will have each isotype of the family represented in its genome (e.g. immunoglobulin classes).

J chain. A monomorphic polypeptide present in polymeric IgA and IgM, and essential to their formation.

J genes. Sets of gene segments in the immunoglobulin heavy and light chain genes, and in the genes for the chains of the T-cell receptor, which are recombined during lymphocyte ontogeny and contribute towards the genes for variable domains.

K cell. A group of lymphocytes which are able to destroy their target by antibody-dependent cell-mediated cytotoxicity. They have Fc receptors.

κ (kappa) chains. One of the immunoglobulin light chain isotypes.

Karyotype. The chromosomal constitution of a cell which may vary between individuals of a single species, depending on the presence or absence of particular sex chromosomes or on the incidence of translocations between sections of different chromosomes.

Kinins. A group of vasoactive mediators produced following tissue injury.

Kupffer cells. Phagocytic cells which line the liver sinusoids.

λ (lambda) chains. One of the immunoglobulin light chain isotypes.

Langerhans' cells. Antigen-presenting cells of the skin which emigrate to local lymph nodes to become dendritic cells; they are very active in presenting antigen to T cells.

Large granular lymphocytes (LGLs). A group of morphologically defined lymphocytes containing the majority of K cell and NK cell activity They have both lymphocyte and monocyte/macrophage markers.

Leukotrienes. A collection of metabolites of arachidonic acid which have powerful pharmacological effects.

LFAs (leucocyte functional antigens). A group of three molecules which mediate intercellular adhesion between leucocytes and other cells in an antigen non-specific fashion.

Ligand. A linking (or binding) molecule.

Line. A collection of cells produced by continuously growing a particular cell culture *in vitro*. Such cell lines will usually contain a number of individual clones.

Linkage. The condition where two genes are both present. In close proximity on a single chromosome and are usually inherited together.

Linkage disequilibrium. A condition where two genes are found together in a population at a greater frequency than that predicted simply by the product of their individual gene frequencies.

Locus. The position on a chromosome at which a particular gene is found.

LPR (lymphoproliferation gene). A gene found in MRL mice which is involved in the generation of autoimmune phenomena.

LPS (lipopolysaccharide). A product of some Gram-negative bacterial cell walls which can act as a B cell mitogen.

Lymphokines. A generic term for molecules other then antibodies which are involved in signalling between cells of the immune system and are produced by lymphocytes (cf. interleukins).

Ly antigens. A group of cell surface markers found on murine T cell which permit the differentiation of T cell subpopulations.

Lytic pathway. The complement pathway effected by components C5–C9 that is responsible for lysis of sensitized call plasma membranes.

MALT (mucosa-associated lymphoid tissue). Generic term of lymphoid tissue associated with the gastrointestinal tract, bronchial tree and other mucosa.

Membrane attack complex (MAC). The assembled terminal complement components C5b–C9 of the lytic pathway which becomes inserted into cell membranes

MHC (major histocompatibility complex). A genetic region found in all mammals whose products are primarily responsible for the rapid rejection of grafts between individuals, and function in signalling between lymphocytes and cells expressing antigen.

MHC restriction. A characteristic of many immune reactions in which cell cooperate most effectively with other cells sharing an MHC haplotype.

β_2-microglobulin. A monomorphic polypeptide encoded outside the MHC that is non-covalently associated with the MHC-encoded polypeptides of class I molecules.

MIF (migration inhibition factor). A group of peptides produced by lymphocytes which are capable of inhibiting macrophage migration.

MLR/MLC (mixed lymphocyte reaction/mixed lymphocyte culture). Assay system for T cell recognition of allogeneic cells in which response is measured by proliferation in the presence of the stimulating cells.

Mitogens. Substances which cause cells, particularly lymphocytes, to undergo cell division.

Monoclonal. Derived from a single clone, for example, monoclonal antibodies, which are produced by a single clone and are homogenous.

Myeloma. A lymphoma produced from cells of the B cell lineage.

Neoplasm. A synonym for cancerous tissue.

Network theory. A proposal first put forward by Jerne (since developed) which states that T cells and B cells mutually inter-regulate by recognizing idiotypes on their antigen receptors.

NIP (4-hydroxy, 5-iodo, 3-nitrophenylacetyl). A commonly used hapten.

NK (natural killer) cells. A group of lymphocytes which have the intrinsic ability to recognize and destroy some virally infected cells and some tumour cells.

NP (4-hydroxy, 3-nitrophenylacetyl). A hapten which partially cross-reacts with NIP.

Nude mouse. A genetically athymic mouse which also carries a closely linked gene producing a defect in hair production.

NZB/W. An F_1 strain of mouse which is a model for systemic lupus erythematosus. The parental NZB strain also suffers from autoimmunity.

OKT. A group of monoconal antibodies used to identify T cell surface markers in humans, now superseded by the CD nomenclature.

Opsonization. A process by which phagocytosis is facilitated by the deposition of opsonins (e g. antibody and C3b) on the antigen.

PAF (platelet activating factor). A factor released by basophils which causes platelets to aggregate.

PALS (periarteriolar lymphatic sheath). The accumulations of lymphoid tissue constituting the white pulp of the spleen.

Paratope The part of an antibody molecule which makes contact with the antigenic determinant (epitope).

Pathogen. An organism which causes disease.

PC (phosphorylcholine). A commonly used hapten which is also found on the surface of a number of microorganisms.

PCA (passive cutaneous anaphylaxis). The technique used to detect antigen-specific IgE, in which the test animal is injected intravenously with the antigen and dye, the skin having previously been sensitized with antibody.

PFC (plaque forming cell). An antibody-producing cell detected *in vitro* by its ability to lyse antigen-sensitized erythrocytes in the presence of complement.

PHA (phytohaemagglutinin). A mitogen for T cells.

Phagocytosis. The process by which cells engulf material and enclose it within a vacuole (phagosome) in the cytoplasm.

Phenotype. The expressed characteristics of an individual (cf. genotype).

Pinocytosis. The process by which liquids or very small particles are taken into the cell.

Plasma cell. An antibody-producing B cell which has reached the end of its differentiation pathway.

Pokeweed mitogen. A mitogen for B and T cells.

Polyclonal. A term which describes the products of a number of different cell types (cf. monoclonal).

Primary lymphoid tissues. Lymphoid organs in which lymphocytes complete their initial maturation steps; they include the fetal liver, adult bone marrow and thymus, and bursa of Fabricius in birds.

Primary response. The immune response (cellular or humoral) following an initial encounter with a particular antigen.

Prime. To give an initial sensitization to antigen.

Prostaglandins. Pharmacologically active derivatives of arachidonic acid. Different prostaglandins are capable of modulating cell mobility and immune responses.

Pseudoalleles. Tandem variants of a gene: they do not occupy a homologous position on the chromosome (e.g C4).

Pseudogenes. Genes which have homologous structures to other genes but which are incapable of being expressed, e.g. *Jκ3* in the mouse.

Radioimmunoassay (RIA). A number of different, sensitive techniques for measuring antigen or antibody titres, using radiolabelled reagents.

Receptor. A cell surface molecule which binds specifically to particular extracellular molecules.

Recombination. A process by which genetic inform rearranged during meiosis. This process also occurs during the somatic rearrangements of DNA which occur in the formation of genes encoding antibody molecules and T-cell antigen receptors.

Recurrent idiotype. An idiotype present in the immune response of different animals or strains to a particular antigen.

Respiratory burst. Increase in oxidative metabolism of phagocytes following uptake of opsonized particles.

Reticuloendothelial system. A diffuse system of phagocytic cells derived from the bone marrow stem cell which are associated with the connective tissue framework of the liver, spleen, lymph nodes and other serous cavities.

Rosetting A technique for identifying or isolating cells by mixing them with particles or cells to which they bind (e.g. sheep erythrocytes to human T cells) The rosettes consist of a central cell surrounded by bound cells.

Secondary response. The immune response which follows a second or subsequent encounter with a particular antigen.

Secretory component. A polypeptide produced by cells of some secretory epithelia which is involved in transporting secreted polymeric IgA across the cell and protecting it from digestion in the gastrointestinal tract.

Skin test. A reaction in the skin following injection or contact with an antigen/allergen.

SLE (systemic lupus erythematosus). An autoimmune disease of humans usually involving anti-nuclear antibodies.

Somatic mutation. A process occurring during B cell maturation and affecting the antibody gene region, which permits refinement of antibody specificity.

Suppressor (Ts) cell. A subpopulation of T cells which act to reduce the immune responses of other T cells or B cell suppression may be antigen-specific, idiotype-specific, or non-specific in different circumstances.

Synergism. Cooperative interaction.

Syngeneic. Strains of animals produced by repeated inbreeding so that each pair of autosomes within an individual is identical.

T15. An idiotype associated with anti-phosphorylcholine antibodies, named after the TEPC15 myeloma prototype sequence.

Tandem duplicates. Adjacent copies of related genes linked together on a chromosome.

T-cell receptor (TCR). The T-cell antigen receptor consisting of either an αβ dimer (TCR-2) or a γδ dimer (TCR-1) associated with the CD3 molecular complex.

T-dependent/T-independent antigens. T-dependent antigens require immune recognition by both T and B cells to produce an immune response. T-independent antigens can directly stimulate B cells to produce specific antibody.

Thy. A cell surface antigen of mouse T cells which has allotypic variants.

TNF (tumour necrosis factor). A cytokine released by activated macrophages that is structurally related to lymphotoxin released by activated T cells.

Tolerance. A state of specific immunological unresponsiveness.

Transformation. Morphological changes in a lymphocyte associated with the onset of division. Also used to denote the change to the autonomously dividing state of a cancer cell.

V domains. The N-terminal domains of antibody heavy and light chains and the α, β, γ and δ chains of the T-cell receptor which vary between different clones and form the antigen-binding site

V genes. Sets of genes which encode the major part of the V domains of antibody heavy and light chains and the α, β, γ and δ chains of the T-cell receptor, and become recombined with appropriate sets of D and J genes during lymphocyte ontogeny.

Vasoactive amines. Products such as histamine and 5-hydroxytryptamine released by basophils, mast cells and platelets which act on the endothelium and smooth muscle of the local vasculature.

White pulp. The lymphoid component of spleen, consisting of periarteriolar sheaths of lymphocytes and antigen-presenting cells.

Xenogeneic. Referring to interspecies antigenic differences (cf. heterologous).

Index

Location references are page numbers. The following abbreviations are used in subheadings: HLA (human leucocyte antigen); Ig (immunoglobulin); IL (interleukin); MHC (major histocompatibility complex).